Common Issues in Breast Cancer Survivors

Gretchen G. Kimmick
Rebecca A. Shelby • Linda M. Sutton
Editors

Common Issues in Breast Cancer Survivors

A Practical Guide to Evaluation and Management

Springer

Editors
Gretchen G. Kimmick
Medical Oncology
Duke University School of Medicine/
Duke Cancer Institute
Durham, NC
USA

Rebecca A. Shelby
Department of Psychiatry and
Behavioral Sciences
Duke University
Durham, NC
USA

Linda M. Sutton
Duke University School of Medicine
Duke Cancer Network
Durham, NC
USA

ISBN 978-3-030-75376-4 ISBN 978-3-030-75377-1 (eBook)
https://doi.org/10.1007/978-3-030-75377-1

This Springer imprint is published by the registered company Springer Nature Switzerland AG
The registered company address is: Gewerbestrasse 11, 6330 Cham, Switzerland

We dedicate this book to our patients, for allowing us the honor of providing them care and for driving us to find ways to make life after breast cancer as best as it can be. Our heartfelt thanks go to our colleagues, collaborators, mentors, and students for stimulating our continuous curiosity and desire to educate and to our families and loved ones for their unwavering support.

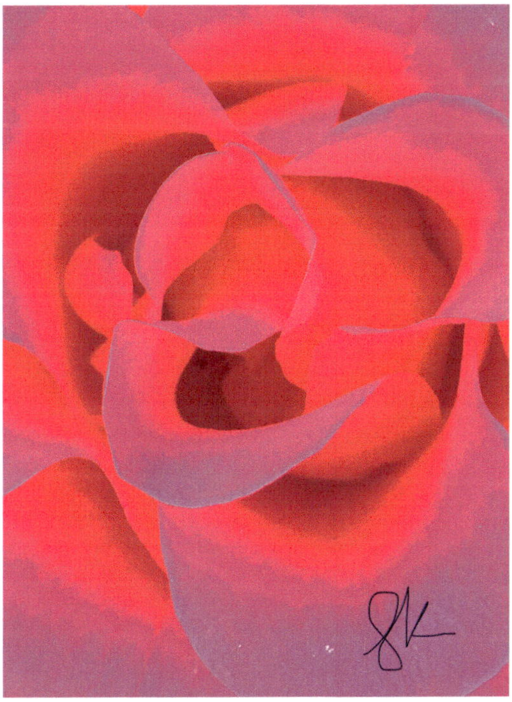

Editors' Note

The contents of this book are primarily based on research that includes patients of female sex who are cisgender (i.e., people whose gender identity matches their sex assigned at birth) but may also include patients who belong to a gender minority group (e.g., patients who identify as gender fluid, non-binary, or transgender) who are not taking hormones. Although patients belonging to this latter group may often have medical needs consistent with that described within this textbook, patients who identify as trans and are opting into medical gender-affirming care may have separate and important needs beyond what is covered herein. For recommendations on providing gender-inclusive care, several resources are available including the ASCO position statement on reducing cancer health disparities among sexual and gender minority populations. (Griggs J, Maingi S, Blinder V, et al: American Society of Clinical Oncology Position Statement: Strategies for reducing cancer health disparities among sexual and gender minority populations. J Clin Oncol 35:2203–2208, 2017.)

Preface

From the Editors:

With improvements in screening and treatment for breast cancer, more patients than ever before are cured after local definitive and systemic therapies. In fact, because of the great number of survivors, those who have specialized in treating breast cancer find themselves under administrative pressure to "discharge" survivors from their practice in order to care for women with new diagnoses. It has become absolutely necessary to share care of survivors among providers, which requires that primary care providers and specialists become familiar with the issues that are faced by breast cancer survivors. Medicine is, however, becoming more and more subspecialized, which subsequently increases care fragmentation. As a result of this progressive entropy of medical care, close collaboration between medical subspecialties becomes essential to providing effective health care. In addition, concise resources are needed to guide providers in approaching issues faced by breast cancer survivors.

The goal for composing this textbook was to provide a clinically useful resource containing knowledge about how to evaluate and manage symptoms and issues that cause burden in those who have been diagnosed and treated for breast cancer. The book has been edited by two oncologists, each with over two decades of experience treating breast cancer and taking care of survivors, and one clinical psychologist, who is specifically trained in both psycho-oncology and sex therapy, with the purpose of integrating the two specialties within each chapter to provide comprehensive evaluation and management recommendations.

As much as possible, each chapter is coauthored by at least one oncologist and one specialist outside the field of oncology, in order to include the perspective of relevant disciplines and make the text comprehensive, user-friendly, and clinically applicable. We also asked that, where appropriate, authors provide: (1) a reasonable approach to evaluating each issue, including a list of baseline evaluations especially to rule out other, non-cancer, causes that are potentially treatable and (2) an algorithmic approach to management. We believe that this is the first textbook to provide a single resource for common issues faced by breast cancer survivors from a truly multidisciplinary standpoint.

We hope that you find this text engaging and informative and that it is useful for improving the overall health and quality of survival in patients who survive after diagnosis and treatment for breast cancer. Perhaps by using this text, non-cancer specialists and practitioners who care for breast cancer survivors will feel empowered to address these common issues that impact patient quality of life.

Durham, NC, USA Gretchen G. Kimmick, MD
Durham, NC, USA Rebecca A. Shelby, PhD
Durham, NC, USA Linda M. Sutton, MD

Acknowledgments

We acknowledge Julie Hughes at the Duke Cancer Institute, whose administrative assistance was invaluable in completing this work, and Susan Kane, RN, an amazing nurse who served our patients and us for many years and was a tremendous help with final editing and proofreading.

We thank the publisher, Springer, for recognizing the importance of the book's topic, and our project coordinator in book production, Sheik K Mohideen, for patience and guidance through the publication process, which was made even more complicated through the COVID-19 pandemic.

Contents

Contributors

Kelly S. Acharya Department of Obstetrics and Gynecology, Duke University, Durham, NC, USA

Ivy Altomare, MD Department of Medicine, Division of Medical Oncology, Duke University Medical Center, Durham, NC, USA

Carey Anders, MD Department of Medicine – Oncology, Duke University Hospital, Durham, NC, USA

Barbara L. Andersen, PhD Department of Psychology, The Ohio State University, Columbus, OH, USA

Comprehensive Cancer Center and Solove Research Institute, The Ohio State University, Columbus, OH, USA

Nicole A. Arrato, MA Department of Psychology, The Ohio State University, Columbus, OH, USA

Sarah S. Arthur, MA Department of Psychology and Neuroscience, Duke University, Durham, NC, USA

Andrew Atia, MD Department of Plastic Surgery, Duke University Hospital, Durham, NC, USA

Elizabeth K. Belcher, PhD The University of Rochester Medical Center, Rochester, NY, USA

Annabelle Brennan, MBBS, LLB Royal Women's Hospital, Melbourne, VIC, Australia

Patrick B. Cacchio, MHS, PA-C, CCD Duke University Department of Medicine, Durham, NC, USA

Devon Check, PhD Department of Population Health Sciences, Duke University School of Medicine, Durham, NC, USA

Daniel S. Childs, MD Department of Oncology, Mayo Clinic, Rochester, MN, USA

Sharon Clancy, MD Department of Plastic and Reconstructive Surgery, Duke University, Durham, NC, USA

Jessica N. Coleman Department of Psychology and Neuroscience, Duke University, Durham, NC, USA

Leonor Corsino, MD, MHS Department of Medicine, Division of Endocrinology, Metabolism, and Nutrition, Duke University School of Medicine, Durham, NC, USA

Ryan D. Davidson, PhD Gastroenterology, Hepatology, and Nutrition, Boston Children's Hospital, Boston, MA, USA

Division of Psychiatry, Harvard Medical School, Boston, MA, USA

Susan F. Dent, MD Duke Cancer Institute, Durham, NC, USA

Caroline S. Dorfman, MD, PhD Department of Psychiatry and Behavioral Sciences, Duke University Medical Center, Durham, NC, USA

Margaret D. Flather Department of Gynecology, Augusta Health, Fishersville, VA, USA

Lauren Pontius Floyd, MD Duke University Medical Center, Durham, NC, USA

Anne Marie Fras, MD Department of Anesthesiology, Duke University Hospital, Durham, NC, USA

Susan C. Gilchrist, MD, MS Clinical Cancer Prevention and Cardiology, the University of Texas MD Anderson Cancer Center, Houston, TX, USA

Nikesha J. Gilmore, PhD The University of Rochester Medical Center, Rochester, NY, USA

Karthik V. Giridhar, MD Department of Oncology, Mayo Clinic, Rochester, MN, USA

Lars Grimm, MD Department of Radiology, Duke University Medical Center, Durham, NC, USA

Arjun Gupta, MBBS Sidney Kimmel Comprehensive Cancer Center, Johns Hopkins University, Baltimore, MD, USA

Sara J. Hardy, MD The University of Rochester Medical Center, Rochester, NY, USA

Amanda A. Heath Department of Physical Therapy and Occupational Therapy, Duke University, Durham, NC, USA

Martha Hickey, BA, MSc, MBChB, FRANZCOG, MD University of Melbourne, Royal Women's Hospital, Melbourne, VIC, Australia

Karen S. Johnson, MD Department of Radiology, Duke University Medical Center, Durham, NC, USA

Physical Therapy and Occupational Therapy Department, Duke University Hospital, Durham, NC, USA

Padma Kamineni, MD Duke University School of Medicine, Durham, NC, USA

Sarah Kelleher, PhD Department of Psychiatry and Behavioral Sciences, Duke University Medical Center, Durham, NC, USA

Robin Kikuchi, BS Duke University, Durham, NC, USA

Gretchen G. Kimmick, MD, MS Medical Oncology, Duke University School of Medicine/Duke Cancer Institute, Durham, NC, USA

Carmen Kloer, BA Department of Plastic Surgery, Duke University Hospital, Durham, NC, USA

Jeffrey Klotz, MD Duke University School of Medicine, Scotland Cancer Treatment Center, Laurinburg, NC, USA

Jordan T. Lee, MA Department of Exercise and Sport Science, University of North Carolina at Chapel Hill, Raleigh, NC, USA

Roberto A. Leon-Ferre, MD Department of Oncology, Mayo Clinic, Rochester, MN, USA

Po-Ju Lin, PhD, MPH The University of Rochester Medical Center, Rochester, NY, USA

Charles L. Loprinzi, MD Department of Oncology, Mayo Clinic, Rochester, MN, USA

Kenneth W. Lyles, MD Duke University School of Medicine, Durham VA Medical Center, Durham, NC, USA

P. Kelly Marcom, MD Department of Medicine, Duke Cancer Institute, Durham, NC, USA

Lisa Massa, PT, CLT Department of Physical and Occupational Therapy, Duke University Hospital, Durham, NC, USA

Jasmine Mcneill, MD, MPH Keck School of Medicine of University of Southern California, Los Angeles, CA, USA

Chiara Melloni, MD, MHSc Duke University, Durham, NC, USA

IQVIA, Durham, NC, USA

Carolyn Menendez, MD, FACS, CGRA Duke University, Duke Cancer Institute, Durham, NC, USA

Heather Moore, PharmD, BCOP Department of Pharmacy – Oncology, Duke University Hospital, Durham, NC, USA

Hyman B. Muss, MD Department of Medicine, University of North Carolina at Chapel Hill School of Medicine and Lineberger Comprehensive Cancer Center, Chapel Hill, NC, USA

Karen M. Mustian, PhD, MPH The University of Rochester Medical Center, Rochester, NY, USA

Kirsten A. Nyrop, PhD Department of Medicine, University of North Carolina at Chapel Hill School of Medicine, Chapel Hill, NC, USA

Erin A. O'Hare, MPH, RD, LDN Lineberger Comprehensive Cancer Center, University of North Carolina at Chapel Hill School of Medicine, Hillsborough, NC, USA

Elise A. Olsen, MD Hair Disorders Research and Treatment Center, Duke University Medical Center, Durham, NC, USA

Chelsea Osterman, MD Department of Medicine, Division of Oncology, University of North Carolina at Chapel Hill, Chapel Hill, NC, USA

Mallika P. Patel, PharmD, CPP Department of Pharmacy – Oncology, Duke University Hospital, Durham, NC, USA

Jennie Petruney, MSN, ANP-BC, AOCNP® Duke University Cancer Center, Durham, NC, USA

Rachel Anne Pienknagura, PA-C, MMS Medical Oncology, Duke University Medical Center/Duke Cancer Institute, Durham, NC, USA

Kathryn J. Ruddy, MD, MPH Department of Oncology, Mayo Clinic, Rochester, MN, USA

Rebecca A. Shelby, PhD Department of Psychiatry and Behavioral Sciences, Duke University, Durham, NC, USA

Kimberly Slawson, MSN, FNP-C Department of Cancer Center Support and Survivorship, Duke University Hospital, Durham, NC, USA

Tamara Somers, PhD Department of Psychiatry and Behavioral Sciences, Duke University School of Medicine, Durham, NC, USA

Mary Scott Soo, MD Department of Radiology, Duke University Medical Center, Durham, NC, USA

Linda M. Sutton, MD Duke University School of Medicine, Duke Cancer Network, Durham, NC, USA

Cindy S. Tofthagen, PhD Department of Nursing, Mayo Clinic, Jacksonville, FL, USA

Sophia C. Weinmann, MD Rheumatology and Immunology, Duke University Medical Center, Durham, NC, USA

Austin Wesevich, MD Departments of Medicine and Pediatrics, Duke University Medical Center, Durham, NC, USA

Kelly E. Westbrook Department of Medicine, Division of Medical Oncology, Duke University, Durham, NC, USA

Huiwen Xu, PhD The University of Rochester Medical Center, Rochester, NY, USA

Siddhartha Yadav, MD Department of Oncology, Mayo Clinic, Rochester, MN, USA

Eric S. Zhou, PhD Perini Family Survivor's Center, Dana-Farber Cancer Institute, Boston, MA, USA

Neurology, Boston Children's Hospital, Boston, MA, USA

Division of Sleep Medicine, Harvard Medical School, Boston, MA, USA

Abbreviations

AASM	American Academy of Sleep Medicine
ABCSG	Austrian Breast & Colorectal Cancer Study Group
AC	Adriamycin-Cytoxan chemotherapy regimen
ACC	American College of Cardiology
ACE	Angiotensin converting enzyme
ACMG	American College of Medical Genetics and Genomics
ACOG	American College of Obstetricians and Gynecologists
ACP	American College of Physicians
ACPA	Anti-citrullinated peptide antibody
ACS	American Cancer Society
ACSM	American College of Sports Medicine
ACT	Acceptance and Commitment Therapy
ACTH	Adrenocorticotropic hormone
ADA	American Diabetes Association
ADHD	Attention deficit hyperactivity disorder
AE	Adverse event
AGREE	Appraisal for Guidelines for Research and Evaluation
AHA	American Heart Association
AHFS	American Hospital Formulary Service
AI	Aromatase inhibitor
AIAA	Aromatase inhibitor-associated arthralgia
AICR	American Institute for Cancer Research
AIMSS	Aromatase inhibitor musculoskeletal symptoms
ALA	Alpha-lipoic acid
ALC	Acetyl-L-carnitine
ALCL	Anaplastic large cell lymphoma
ALL	Acute lymphocytic leukemia
ALND	Axillary lymph node dissection
ALNT	Axillary lymph node transfer
ALTTO	Adjuvant lapatinib and/or trastuzumab treatment optimization study
AMP	Association for Molecular Pathology
AMPK	AMP-activated protein kinase
ANA	Antinuclear antibody
ANCA	Anti-neutrophil cytoplasmic antibodies
ASBS	American Society of Breast Surgeons
ASC	Ambulatory Surgery Center or Active Symptom Control

ASCO	American Society of Clinical Oncology
ASE	American Society of Echocardiography
ASRM	American Society for Reproductive Medicine
ATAC	Arimidex, Tamoxifen Alone or in Combination study
ATM	Ataxia-telangiectasia mutated
ATOLL	Articular tolerance of letrozole study
BC	Breast cancer
BCRL	Breast cancer-related lymphedema
BCS	Breast conserving surgery
BCT	Breast conservation therapy
BETTER	Bring up, Explain, Tell, Timing, Educate, and Record
BFI	Brief Fatigue Inventory
BHGI	Breast Health Global Initiative
BID	Twice daily
BIG	Breast International Group
BIS	Bioimpedance spectroscopy
BLAST	Barcelona lymphedema algorithm for surgical treatment
BLE	Breast lymphedema
BMD	Bone mineral density
BMI	Body mass index
BNP	Brain natriuretic peptides
BP	Blood pressure
BPI	Brief Pain Inventory
BWEL	Breast cancer weight loss study
CABG	Coronary artery bypass graft
CAM	Complementary and alternative medicine
CBC	Complete blood count
CBT	Cognitive-behavioral therapy
CC	Craniocaudal
CCCA	Central centrifugal cicatricial alopecia
CDT	Complex decongestive therapy
CED	Cyclophosphamide equivalent dose or Center for Eating Disorders or Cumulative Energy Demand
CFQ	Chalder Fatigue Scale
CFS	Cancer Fatigue Scale
CI	Confidence interval
CIA	Chemotherapy-induced alopecia
CINV	Chemotherapy-induced nausea and vomiting
CIPN	Chemotherapy-induced peripheral neuropathy
CMF	Cyclophosphamide, methotrexate, and 5-fluorouracil chemotherapy regimen
CMR	Cardiac magnetic resonance
CNS	Central nervous system
CO-OP	Cognitive orientation to daily occupational performance
CORE	Cardio-oncology rehabilitation
COX	Cyclooxygenase-2
CPM	Cancer predisposing mutation
CR	Cognitive rehabilitation

CRCI	Cancer-related cognitive impairment
CRF	Cancer-related fatigue
CRP	C-reactive protein
CSD	Clinically significant distress
CSF	Cerebrospinal fluid
CT	Computed tomography
CTC	Circulating tumor cells or Common Toxicity Criteria
CTCAE	Common terminology criteria for adverse events
CTD	Connective tissue disease
CTE	Chronic telogen effluvium
CTRCD	Cancer treatment-related cardiovascular dysfunction
CV	Cardiovascular
CVD	Cardiovascular disease
CYPTAM	Study involving CYP2D6 genotype related to TAMoxifen metabolism
DASH	Dietary approaches to stop hypertension study
DBT	Digital breast tomosynthesis
DCCT	Diabetes Control and Complications Trial
DCLE	Discoid cutaneous lupus erythematosus
DDP	Dipeptidyl peptidase or Dyadic developmental psychotherapy
DDX	Differential diagnosis
DENSE	Dense Tissue and Early Breast Neoplasm Study
DEXA	Dual energy x-ray absorptiometry
DHEA	Dehydroepiandrosterone
DHT	Dihydrotestosterone
DIEAP	Deep inferior epigastric artery perforator
DM	Diabetes mellitus
DNA	Deoxyribonucleic acid
DSM	Diagnostic and Statistical Manual of Mental Disorders
DXA	Dual-energy X-ray absorptiometry
EACVI	European Association of Cardiovascular Imaging
ECF	Extracellular fluid
EDS	Ehlers-Danlos syndrome
EGFR	Estimated glomerular filtration rate
EIA	Endocrine therapy-induced alopecia
EMG	Electromyography
EORTC	European Organization for Research and Treatment of Cancer
ER	Extended release or Estrogen Receptor
ESC	European Society of Cardiology
ESMO	European Society of Medical Oncology
ESR	Erythrocyte sedimentation rate
ET	Endocrine treatment
EU	European Union
FAC	Fluorouracil, adriamycin, and cyclophosphamide chemotherapy regien

FACIT-F	Functional Assessment of Chronic Illness Therapy-Fatigue Subscale
FACT-G	Functional assessment of cancer therapy (general)
FACT-GOG	Functional assessment of cancer therapy/gynecologic oncology group
FDA	Food and Drug Administration
FEC	Fluorouracil, epirubicin, and cyclophosphamide chemotherapy regimen
FFA	Frontal fibrosing alopecia
FIQ	Fibromyalgia Impact Questionnaire
FPHL	Female-pattern hair loss
FRAX	Fracture risk assessment tool
FSFI	Female Sexual Function Index
FSH	Follicle-stimulating hormone
FSI	Fatigue Symptom Inventory
FU	Fluorouracil
GABA	Gamma-aminobutyric acid
GAD	Generalized anxiety disorder
GAIT	Glucosamine/chondroitin arthritis intervention trial
GBCM	Gadolinium-based contrast media
GDM	Gestational diabetes mellitus
GEP	Gene expression profile
GFR	Glomerular filtration rate
GI	Gastrointestinal
GLP	Glucagon-like peptide
HADS	Hospital Anxiety and Depression Scale
HALT-BC	Hormone Ablation Bone Loss Trial - Breast Cancer
HAQ-DI	Health Assessment Questionnaire-Disability Index
HDD	Hereditary Desmoid Disease
HDL	High-density lipoprotein
HEAL	Health, eating, activity, and lifestyle study
HER	Human epidermal growth factor receptor
HFS	Hand-foot syndrome
HIV	Human immunodeficiency virus
HOPE	Hormones and physical exercise study
HPA	Hypothalamic-pituitary-adrenal
HR	Hormone Receptor, HR gene or heart rate
HRQOL	Health-related quality of life
HRT	Hormone replacement therapy
HSCT	Hematopoietic stem cell transplant
HSDD	Hypoactive sexual desire disorder
IASP	International Association for the Study of Pain
ICBN	Intercostobrachial nerve
ICG	Indocyanine green
ICP	Intermittent pneumatic compression
ICSI	Intracytoplasmic sperm injection
IES	Intergroup Exemestane Study
IFE	Immunofixation

IFG	Impaired fasting glucose
IGF	Insulin-like growth factor
IGT	Impaired glucose tolerance
IL	Interleukin
IM	Intramuscular
IOM	Institute of Medicine
IPC	Intermittent compression pump
IQ	Intelligent quotient
ISCD	International Society for Clinical Densitometry
ISI	Insomnia Severity Index
IU	International unit
IV	Intravenous
IVF	In vitro fertilization
JHS	Joint hypermobility syndrome
LDL	Low-density lipoprotein
LFP	Liver function panel
LH	Luteinizing hormone
LHRH	Luteinizing hormone-releasing hormone
LIQ	Lower inner quadrant
LLLT	Low-level laser treatment
LS	Lymphoscintigraphy
LVA	Lymph-venous anastomosis
LVEF	Left ventricular ejection fraction
MAAT	Memory and Attention Adaptation Training
MAO	Monoamine oxidase inhibitors
MARIBS	Magnetic Resonance Imaging for Breast Screening study
MBI	Molecular breast imaging
MCP	Metacarpophalangeal joint
MCST	Metacognitive strategy training
MDD	Major depressive disorder
MDT	Multidisciplinary team
MET	Metabolic equivalent
MFI	Multidimensional Fatigue Inventory
MFSI-SF	Multidimensional Fatigue Symptom Inventory-Short Form
MGUS	Monoclonal gammopathy of undetermined significance
MI	Myocardial infarction
MIPS	Maximal Intesity Projection
MLD	Manual lymph drainage
MLO	Mediolateral oblique
MOCA	Modifier of cell adhesion
MPA	Medroxyprogesterone acetate
MPHL	Male-pattern hair loss
MR	Magnetic resonance
MRA	Magnetic resonance angiography
MRI	Magnetic resonance imaging
MRV	Magnetic resonance venography
MUGA	Multi-Gated acquisition

MYME	Metformin with chemotherapy vs chemotherapy without metformin study
NAC	N-Acetylcysteine
NASBP	National Surgical Adjuvant Breast and Bowel Project
NCCN	National Comprehensive Cancer Network
NCI	National Cancer Institute
NCS	Nerve conduction study
NECST	Normal, ectasis, contraction and sclerosis type
NEH	Neutrophilic eccrine hidradenitis
NGS	Next-generation sequencing
NGSP	National Glycohemoglobin Standardization Program
NH	Non-Hispanic or Nursing Home or Natiuretic Hormone
NIH	National Institute of Health
NIMH	National Institute of Mental Health
NPH	Natural Protamine Hagedorn (insulin)
NPLD	Non-pegylated liposomal doxorubicin
OA	Osteoarthritis
OAC	Oral anticoagualtion
OGTT	Oral glucose tolerance testing
OR	Odds ratio
OSA	Obstructive sleep apnea
OT	Occupational therapy
OTC	Ovarian tissue cryopreservation or Over-the-counter
PA	Physical activity
PARP	Poly-adenosine diphosphate ribose polymerase
PBP	Persistent breast pain
PCI	Percutaneous coronary intervention
PCS	Pain Catastrophizing Scale
PCT	Porphyria cutanea tarda or Post-coital test
PD	Panic disorder
PDD	Persistent depressive disorder
PDL	Pegylated liposomal doxorubicin
PET	Positron emission tomography
PFS	Piper Fatigue Scale or Progression-free survival
PHL	Pattern hair loss
PHQ	Patient health questionnaire
PLISSIT	Permission, Limited Information, Specific Suggestions, and Intensive Therapy
PLMD	Periodic limb movement disorder
PMPS	Post-mastectomy pain syndrome
POEMS	Prevention of Early Menopause Study
POMS-F	Profile of Mood Sates-Fatigue Subscale
PPMP	Persistent post-mastectomy pain
PR	Progesterone receptor
PREDICOP	Prevention of Breast Cancer Recurrence Through Weight Control, Diet, and Physical Activity Intervention study
PRO	Patient reported outcome

PROMIS	Patient Reported Outcomes Measurement Information System
PRP	Platelet-rich plasma or Pityriasis rubra pilaris
PSEQ	Pain Self-Efficacy Questionnaire
PT	Physical therapy
PTH	Parathyroid hormone
PVC	Polyvinyl chloride or Premature ventricular contraction
QHS	Every night at bedtime
QLQ-CIPN20	Quality of Life Questionnaire-Chemotherapy-Induced Peripheral Neuropathy
QOL	Quality of life
QT	Start of Q-wave to end of T-wave
RA	Rheumatoid arthritis
RANKL	Receptor activator of nuclear factor kappa-beta ligand
RBC	Red blood cell
RCT	Randomized controlled trial
RD	Registered dietitians
REM	Rapid-eye-movement
REMS	Risk evaluation and mitigation strategy
RF	Rheumatoid factor
RFP	Renal function panel
RNA	Ribonucleic acid
ROS	Reactive oxygen species
RR	Risk ratio
RRB	Risk reducing behaviors
RT	Radiotherapy
SCFS	Schwartz Cancer Fatigue Scale
SCISD	Structured Clinical Interview for Sleep Disorders
SCLE	Subacute cutaneous lupus erythematosus
SD	Standard deviation
SEER	Surveillance, Epidemiology, and End Results
SERM	Selective estrogen receptor modulator
SGLT	Sodium-glucose linked transporter
SIADH	Syndrome of inappropriate antidiuretic hormone
SLN	Sentinel lymph node
SLNB	Sentinel lymph node biopsy
SNFSHC	Scientific Network on Female Sexual Health and Cancer
SPEP	Serum protein electrophoresis
SSRI	Selective serotonin reuptake inhibitor
STEP	Sleep Training Education Program
STOP-BANG	Snoring, Tiredness, Observed apnea, high blood Pressure - Body Mass Index, Age, Neck circumference, and gender
STS	Stewart-Treves syndrome
SWAN	Study of Women Across the Nation
SWOG	Southwest Oncology Group
TAT	Total adipose tissue
TBI	Total body irradiation
TBS	Trabecular bone scores

TCA	Tricyclic antidepressants
TENS	Transcutaneous electrical nerve stimulation
TID	Three times daily
TMT	Trail Making Test
TNBC	Triple-negative breast cancer
TNF	Tumor necrosis factor
TNS	Total neuropathy score
TRAM	Transverse rectus abdominal muscle
TSH	Thyroid-stimulating hormore
TTG	Tissue transglutaminase
UCV	Uncertain variant
UI	International unit
UPBEAT	Understanding and Predicting Breast Cancer Events After Treatment study
UPEP	Urine protein electrophoresis
USDA	US Department of Agriculture
UV	Uncertain variant
VAS	Visual analog score
VBM	Voxel-based morphometry or Vascular basement membrane or Value-based medicine
VDR	Vitamin D receptor
VFA	Vertebral fracture assessment
VLNT	Vascularized lymph node transplant
VTE	Venous thromboembolism
VUS	Variant of uncertain significance
WCRF	World Cancer Research Fund
WHI	Women's Health Initiative study
WHO	World Health Organization
WOMAC	Western Ontario and McMaster Universities Osteoarthritis Index
WVE	Women's Voices for the Earth study
XRT	Radiation therapy
YOCAS	Yoga for Cancer Survivors study

Overview of the National and International Guidelines for Care of Breast Cancer Survivors

1

Jeffrey Klotz, Padma Kamineni, and Linda M. Sutton

Cancer Survivorship

Cancer survivorship, as a concept developed in response to the unique needs and challenges of the growing number of patients surviving for years following their initial cancer diagnosis, is particularly important for breast cancer. Breast cancer is the most commonly diagnosed cancer in women in the United States [1] and the world [2] with a projection that there will be nearly five million breast cancer survivors in the United States alone by 2030 [3]. The concept of care specifically focused on cancer survivors has been evolving steadily for 35 years since Dr. Fitzhugh Mullan, a physician coping with cancer, first described the survivorship experience as "not one condition but many." [4] The National Cancer Institute (NCI) [5] defines survivorship as the experience living with, through, and beyond the diagnosis of cancer. The NCI emphasizes that survivorship focuses not only on the health but also the holistic well-being of individuals with cancer – as well as their family, caregivers, and friends, from diagnosis until the end of life. Through survivorship, a broad range of issues related to follow-up care, late effects of treatment, cancer recurrence, second cancers, and quality of life are addressed. Driven especially by the Institute of Medicine's (IOM) report "From Cancer Patient to Cancer Survivor: Lost in Transition" in 2006 [6], survivorship care has taken on a particular urgency in the face of the rapidly rising number of cancer survivors [7]. The focus of clinical care during survivorship has expanded from attention to surveillance for cancer recurrence to wide-ranging clinical issues including fatigue, anxiety, depression, cognitive impairment, cardiac toxicity, lymphedema, hormone-related symptoms, bone health, genetic risk assessment, sexual dysfunction, infertility, and healthy lifestyle choices with regard to diet and exercise. While the "common sense" appeal of providing survivorship care remains strong, some elements of the IOM report, particularly the recommendation for Survivorship Care Plans (SCPs), have been controversial due to lack of consistent evidence for their benefit [8–10]. It is therefore vital to get the best answers to the key questions that accompany improved long-term survival including what are the best evidence-based guidelines for breast cancer survivorship care [11].

J. Klotz
Duke University School of Medicine, Scotland Cancer Treatment Center, Laurinburg, NC, USA

P. Kamineni
Duke University School of Medicine, Durham, NC, USA

L. M. Sutton (✉)
Duke University School of Medicine, Duke Cancer Network, Durham, NC, USA
e-mail: linda.sutton@duke.edu

G. G. Kimmick et al. (eds.), *Common Issues in Breast Cancer Survivors*,
https://doi.org/10.1007/978-3-030-75377-1_1

Clinical Practice Guidelines

Clinical practice guidelines are statements that formulate specific recommendations intended to optimize patient care. Formal guidelines are informed by a systematic review of relevant evidence supporting an assessment of the benefits and harms of alternative options for clinical care [12]. It is generally agreed, in the United States [12] and internationally [13–15], that the development of high-quality, trustworthy clinical practice guidelines do all of the following:

1. Utilize a systematic review of existing evidence
2. Establish transparency and disclose the methods used for all development steps
3. Involve a multidisciplinary development group, including patients
4. Disclose and manage both financial and nonfinancial conflicts of interest
5. Have clear and direct guideline recommendations
6. Utilize a specific grading system to rate the strength of evidence and recommendations
7. Be subject to external review
8. Be updated on a regular basis [16]

While it is usually accepted in the dynamic world of oncology that clinical guidelines support optimal health care or patients [17], there are many barriers to implementing clinical guidelines into practice. These barriers include simple lack of awareness that a guideline exists, or knowledge regarding the specific recommendations within the guideline; absence of consensus between health-care providers on the specific recommendations, particularly when produced by one specialty society, government agency, or insurance company; organizational and resource constraints; clinician inertia; patient factors; and the format, language, and usability of the guideline itself [18, 19]. Overcoming the challenges associated with promoting systematic uptake of research findings and high-quality clinical practice guidelines requires well-coordinated efforts in clinical epidemiology, implementation science [20], and systems engineering [21]. Resource constraints are a particular barrier to guideline implementation for breast cancer in low- and middle-income countries (LMICs) and regions. Internet-based document repositories such as the United States' former Guidelines Clearinghouse [22] and international efforts such as the Guidelines International Network [23] help motivate guideline developers to adhere to quality standards, but it is difficult to measure the impact these archives have on delivering better health care across the globe, especially for as heterogeneous an area as breast cancer survivorship care.

Topics of Note in Breast Cancer Survivorship Guidelines

Table 1.1 provides an overview of breast cancer survivorship guidelines [24–34]. Guidelines commonly cover the following topics: (1) surveillance for recurrence, (2) after effects of treatment, and (3) health promotion.

Recommendations for Survivorship Visits

- Family history/genetic evaluation
- Adjuvant/risk-reducing strategies
- Clinical evaluations with history and physical examinations
- Breast health awareness
- Laboratory testing driven by signs/symptoms
- Breast and bone health imaging

Several of the chapters in this book will provide additional detail and guidance on the genetic evaluation (Chap. 20) and breast imaging surveillance of patients following breast cancer (Chap. 2). It is important to note that routine imaging for recurrent regional or metastatic disease, in the absence of suspicious signs or symptoms, is not indicated in breast cancer survivors. Several studies and subsequent meta-analysis have failed to demonstrate any survival benefit for routine surveillance imaging beyond mammography in

Table 1.1 Overview of breast cancer survivorship guidelines

Guideline name	Country	Publication year	Topics of note			Comments	References
			Surveillance for recurrence[a]	After effects of treatment[b]	Health promotion[c]		
ASCO	USA	2016	All – except breast self-exam	All	All	Few prospective randomized control studies were performed. At the time of development they were not evaluated by Appraisal for Guidelines for Research and Evaluation (AGREE II) instrument (Runowicz et al. 2016)	Runowicz et al. 2016
National Comprehensive Cancer Network	USA	2020	All – except breast self-exam	All	All	Surveillance for immune-mediated toxicities and immunizations were also covered	Gradishar WJ et al. 2020 NCCN Guidelines Survivorship Version 1.2020 NCCN Guidelines Breast Cancer Version 3.2020
ESMO	EU	2019	All	All – except lymphedema, fertility, cognitive impairment	All – except smoking cessation and alcohol use	Most European countries developed their own guidelines. Recommended to perform mammography ± ultrasound. Ultrasound can also be considered in the follow-up of lobular invasive carcinomas. (Cardoso et al. 2019)	Cardoso et al. 2019 Spronk et al. 2017
Alberta Health Services[d]	Canada	2015	All	All	All	Other Canadian guidelines – Health Canada, and Ministry of Health have not covered all key areas and their references are included for review	Alberta Health Services 2015 Grunfeld et al. 2005 Ministry of Health, British Columbia 2013
National Health Commission of the People's Republic of China	China	2018	All – except breast self-exam	None	None	Breast ultrasound, chest imaging, abdominal ultrasound, and blood test are recommended. Evidence-based guidelines exist for diagnosis and treatment, but no specific guidelines exist for survivorship	National Health Commission of the People's Republic of China 2018 Li Q 2019

(continued)

Table 1.1 (continued)

Guideline name	Country	Publication year	Topics of note: Surveillance for recurrence[a]	After effects of treatment[b]	Health promotion[c]	Comments	References
National Cancer Center, Japan	Japan	2019	All – except family history/ genetic evaluation	All – except body image, cardiotoxicity, cognitive impairment, fatigue, sexual health, psychosocial issues	None	There is no single comprehensive breast cancer survivorship guideline	Okubo R et al. 2019

[a]Surveillance for breast cancer recurrence includes family history/genetic evaluation, adjuvant/risk-reducing strategies, surveillance visits, breast self-exam, laboratory testing, and imaging

[b]After effects of breast cancer treatment include assessment and treatment of complications – lymphedema, cardiotoxicity, body image, fertility, sexual health, cognitive impairment, fatigue, bone health, psychosocial: distress, depression, anxiety, fear, financial/employment, and interpersonal

[c]Health promotion includes physical activity, nutrition, weight management, smoking cessation, lifestyle behaviors – alcohol use

[d]Evolutions to Canadian Approach to guidelines

breast cancer survivors [35]. Estimates suggest that 96% of locoregional recurrences are detected by the patient (42%), the clinician on examination (30%), or mammographically (25%) [36]. In contrast to regional or distance surveillance imaging, many guidelines endorse the use evaluations of the remaining breast tissue for cancer development. Based on robust data, ASCO, NCCN, and ESMO guidelines support the routine use of clinical examinations (history and physical examinations) and mammography for women surviving Stage 0-III Breast Cancer. A subset of women at significantly increased risk of developing breast cancer, such as those survivors with genetic predispositions or other factors that provide >20% risk of developing breast cancer, may also benefit from annual breast MRI as an adjunct to mammography [37, 38].

After Effects of Breast Cancer Treatment

- Lymphedema
- Cardiotoxicity
- Body image
- Fertility
- Sexual health
- Cognitive impairment
- Fatigue
- Bone health
- Psychosocial issues
  - Distress
  - Depression
  - Anxiety
  - Fear
- Financial/employment issues
- Interpersonal/relationship issues

Monitoring for complications and long-term side effects after the initial diagnosis and treatment of breast cancer is part of routine follow-up care. Assessment and management of issues unique to breast cancer survivors are covered in other chapters in this book, as are recommendations regarding health promotion.

Health Promotion

- Physical activity
- Nutrition
- Weight management
- Smoking cessation
- Lifestyle behaviors
- Alcohol use

United States Breast Cancer Survivorship Guidelines

Although the United States did not have a dedicated Breast Cancer Survivorship guideline until the publishing of the American Cancer Society/American Society of Clinical Oncology (ACS/ASCO) Guideline in December 2015 [39], prior guidelines related to breast cancer care focused on important aspects of the modern concept of survivorship [40–42]. Additionally, several ASCO guidelines and endorsements have focused on important aspects of breast cancer care that impact survivorship including the role of bisphosphonates [43], integrative therapies [44], and extended adjuvant endocrine therapy [45]. As survivorship recommendations have broadened from surveillance for breast cancer recurrence to more diverse topics including body image concerns, cardiotoxicity, cognitive impairment, distress, depression, and anxiety, the evidence basis for these recommendations remains limited with only 16% of the guideline citations coming from randomized trials and only 2% supported by level I evidence (meta-analysis of RCTs) [46] (See Fig. 1.1).

The National Comprehensive Cancer Network (NCCN) has a comprehensive Breast Cancer guideline [47] that contains recommendations related to breast cancer surveillance and follow-up after initial diagnosis and treatment, but survivorship care is addressed more explicitly in its Survivorship guideline [48]. The NCCN Survivorship guideline focuses on several highly

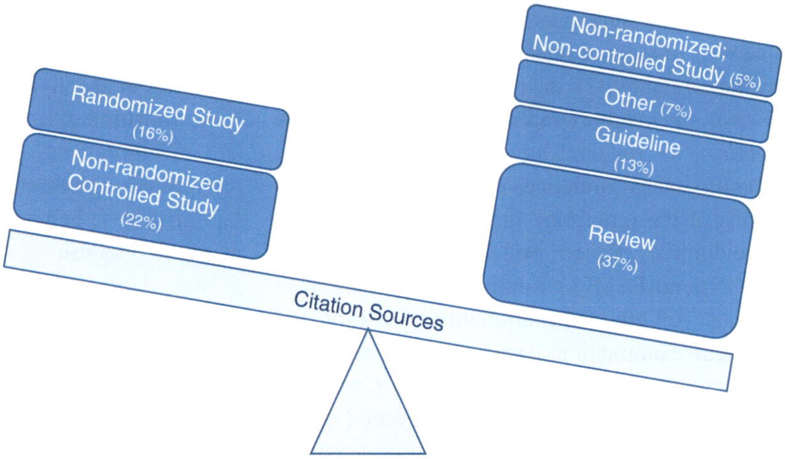

Fig. 1.1 Weight of citation. (Sources: ACS/ASCO Breast Cancer Survivorship Care Guideline 2016; adapted from Pan et al. 2018)

relevant clinical areas for breast cancer survivors including physical activity, nutrition, anthracyclines-induced cardiac toxicity, lymphedema, hormone-related symptoms, and sexual function concerns. Both the ASCO/ACS and NCCN guidelines emphasize the need for coordinated care between oncologists and primary care physicians along with thresholds for subspecialty referrals. As initially conceived, SCPs were intended to provide a tool to clarify the details of a patient's treatment and its aftermath, thereby improving communication between oncologists, other members of the health-care team, and patients themselves. Despite their uncertain benefits [49–51], SCPs continue to be recommended for all patients as part of the ASCO/ACS and NCCN guidelines. However, the mandate for SCPs driven by accreditation bodies may be waning. The 2020 Commission on Cancer (CoC) Standards [52] removed the requirement for SCPs for the majority of patients.

Inequities in access to care translates into widely variable breast cancer survivorship experience across the United States. At many comprehensive cancer centers in the United States, efforts are extended to prioritize, fund, and research innovations in survivorship care. Some organizations network with surrounding community cancer centers [53] to disseminate best practices. Nonetheless, the survivorship care experience in rural areas is more likely to be fragmented due to limited oncology provider access, fewer ancillary survivorship providers (e.g., physical therapists with specialized training in lymphedema treatment, behavioral health specialists, or cardiologists with interest in cardio-oncology), and financial barriers [54]. Additionally, the US survivorship experience is influenced by individual patient perceptions and the culturally specific context of the survivor [55, 56].

International Breast Cancer Survivorship Guidelines

Despite significant differences in 5-year relative survival rates for breast cancer between high-income countries (80–90%) and low-income countries (40% or less), usually attributed to limited early detection, lack of access to treatment, and social and cultural barriers [57], the number of breast cancer survivors is increasing throughout the world [58]. This improved survival has led to an increased global recognition for the need to provide breast cancer survivorship care and an increase in the development of international guidelines [59–61]. The European Society of Medical Oncology (ESMO) and other high-income countries' guidelines include survivorship recommendations with the guidelines for breast cancer treatment and are less explicit about breast cancer survivorship itself. Whereas the long-term physical and psychological consequences of breast cancer diagnosis and treatment are acknowledged in the ASCO/ACS and NCCN guidelines for cancer survivorship [59], the ESMO guidelines are less specific about these issues. Some high-income countries, such as Japan, have taken the approach of largely adopting Western countries' survivorship care guidelines, while acknowledging "cultural and health system differences" that purportedly precluded use of specific recommendations regarding cognitive function, fatigue, sexual function, and menopause [62].

In LMICs and regions, where the primary focus is primary treatment of breast cancer care, available resources, societal values and priorities, and health-care infrastructure limit the focus on survivorship. Some progress in developing breast cancer care guidelines for resource-constrained regions has been made through international cooperative efforts, such as the Breast Health Global Initiative (BHGI) [63] and Initiative 2.5 [64, 65]. The BHGI stratifies its guideline-based recommendations according to a resource allocation scale. *Basic services* are those "fundamental services absolutely necessary for any breast health care system to function"; *limited services* are those "intended to produce major improvements in outcome, and are attainable with limited financial means"; *enhanced services* are "optional but important"; and *maximal resources* "may be used in some high-income countries, and/or may be recommended by breast care guidelines that do not adapt to resource constraints" with heavy emphasis on education for health-care providers, survivors, and family members [66]. As the awareness of need for survivorship care becomes apparent in LMICs and regions, the need for culturally and regionally specific implementation of guideline-based recommendations, rather than adoption of United States or European recommendations, is also evident [67–69].

The Future of Survivorship Guidelines

The future of survivorship guidelines is intimately linked with the direction of survivorship itself, both nationally and internationally. This future is largely dependent on expanding the quality and depth of the survivorship research base. While there has been a steady rise in survivorship research, with more focus on breast cancer survivors than any other cancer survivor group [70], much of this research has focused on limited time point patient reported outcomes and quality of care. A research agenda that is driven by impact on survival, utilization of social support, nutritional, and rehabilitation services, costs, and impact on health equity [71] may be more effective at demonstrating the value of survivorship care in the United States and other high-income countries. While the primary focus of cancer research in LMICs remains epidemiology, prevention, screening, and acute cancer treatment, there must be an increased focus on higher quality research into survivorship care that meets the needs of individual international communities.

This same recognition that survivorship care needs to be specific to varied global circumstances also extends to individuals within those systems. Personalized survivorship care models which stratify patients to self-management, limited primary care and oncology-based survivorship care, and multidisciplinary management for high needs patients have been piloted with success in non-US high-income countries [72]. Given the challenges of adhering to the complex recommendations for breast cancer survivorship care, such a personalized approach might also be extended to the guidelines themselves, triaged by survivor acuity and ethnoculturally specific circumstances. Finally, as with all guidelines, high-quality evidence and well-written recommendations by themselves are insufficient to improve breast cancer survivorship if the information and recommendations are not understood and acted upon by the intended audience. Therefore, the success of improving the standard for breast cancer survivorship care through guidelines will be dependent on its effective dissemination and implementation both in the United States and the world.

References

1. American Cancer Society. Breast cancer facts & figures 2019-2020. Atlanta: American Cancer Society, Inc; 2019.
2. Worldwide Cancer Research Fund International. 2020. https://www.wcrf.org/dietandcancer/cancer-trends/worldwide-cancer-data. Accessed 24 Feb 2020.
3. Miller K, Nogueira L, Mariotto A, et al. Cancer treatment and survivorship statistics, 2019. CA Cancer J Clin. 2019;69:363–85.
4. Mullan F. Seasons of survival: reflections of a physician with cancer. N Engl J Med. 1985;313:270–3.
5. National Cancer Institute. 2020. https://www.cancer.gov/publications/dictionaries/cancer-terms/def/survivorship. Accessed 23 Feb 2020.
6. National Research Council. From cancer patient to cancer survivor: lost in transition. Washington, DC: The National Academies Press; 2006. https://doi.org/10.17226/11468.
7. Miller KD, Noguiera L, Mariotto AB, et al. Cancer treatment and survivorship statistics, 2019. CA Cancer J Clin. 2019;69:363–85.
8. Grunfeld E, Julian J, Pond G, et al. Evaluating survivorship care plans: results of a randomized, clinical trial of patients with breast cancer. J Clin Oncol. 2011;29:4755–62.
9. Stricker C, Jacobs L, Palmer S. Survivorship care plans: an argument for evidence over common sense. J Clin Oncol. 2012. https://doi.org/10.1200/JCO.2011.40.7940.
10. Tevaarwerk AJ, Sesto ME. Continued challenges to the adoption and implementation of survivorship care plans. J Oncol Pract. 2018;14:573–6.
11. Shapiro C, Jacobsen P, Henderson T, et al. ASCO core curriculum for cancer survivorship education. J Oncol Pract. 2016. https://doi.org/10.1200/JOP.2015.009449.
12. Institute of Medicine. Clinical practice guidelines we can trust. Washington, DC: The National Academies Press; 2011. https://doi.org/10.17226/13058.
13. Qaseem A, Forland F, Macbeth F, et al. Guidelines international network: toward international standards for clinical practice guidelines. Ann Intern Med. 2012;156:525–31.
14. Van der Wees P, Qaseem A, Kaila M, et al. Prospective systematic review registration: perspective from the Guidelines International Network (G-I-N). Syst Rev. 2012;1:3.
15. Schunemann H, Al-Ansary L, Forland F, et al. Guidelines international network: principles for disclosures of interests and management of conflicts in guidelines. Ann Intern Med. 2015;163:548–53.
16. Shekelle P. Overview of clinical practice guidelines. In: Givens J, editor. UpToDate. 2020. Retrieved 25 Feb 2020 from https://www.uptodate.com/contents/overview-of-clinical-practice-guidelines/.
17. Ettinger D, Kuettel M, Malin J, et al. NCCN roundtable: what are the characteristics of an optimal clinical practice guideline? J Natl Compr Cancer Netw. 2015;13:640–2.
18. Cabana M, Rand C, Powe N, et al. Why don't physicians follow clinical practice guidelines? A framework for improvement. JAMA. 1999;282:1458–65.
19. Gupta S, Rai N, Bhattacharrya O et al. Optimizing the language and format of guidelines to improve guideline uptake. CMAJ. 2016. https://doi.org/10.1503/cmaj.151102.
20. Eccles M, Mittman B. Welcome to implementation science communication. Implement Sci Commun. 2006;1:1.
21. Pronovost P. Enchancing physicians' use of clinical guidelines. JAMA. 2013;310:2501–2.
22. Munn Z, Qaseem A. Disappearance of the National Guideline Clearinghouse: a huge loss for evidence-based health care. Ann Intern Med. 2018;169:648–9.
23. Guidelines International Network. 2020. https://g-i-n.net/about-g-i-n/introduction. Accessed 23 Feb 2020.
24. Alberta Health Services. Follow-up care for early-stage breast cancer. 2nd ed. Alberta: Alberta Health Services; 2015.
25. Cardoso F, Kyriakides S, Ohno S, Penault-Llorca F, Poortmans P, Rubio IT, Zackrisson S, Senkus E. Early breast cancer: ESMO Clinical Practice Guidelines for diagnosis, treatment and follow-up. Ann Oncol. 2019;30:1194–220.
26. Gradishar WJ, Anderson BO, Abraham J, Aft R, Agnese D, Allison KH, et al. NCCN clinical practice guidelines in oncology. J Natl Compr Cancer Netw. 2020;18(4):452–78. https://doi.org/10.6004/jnccn.2020.0016.
27. Grunfeld E, Dhesy-Thind S, Levine M. Clinical practice guidelines for the care and treatment of breast cancer: follow-up after treatment for breast cancer (summary of the 2005 update). CMAJ. 2005;172(10):1319–20.
28. Luctkar-Fludea M, Aiken A, McColl MA, Tranmer J. A comprehensive framework and key guideline recommendations for the provision of evidence based breast cancer survivorship care within the primary care setting. Fam Pract. 2015;32(2):129–40. https://doi.org/10.1093/fampra/cmu082.
29. Ministry of Health, British Columbia 2013. https://www2.gov.bc.ca/gov/content/health/practitioner-professional-resources/bc-guidelines/breast-cancer-management#followup-care.
30. National Comprehensive Cancer Network NCCN Clinical Practice Guidelines in Oncology Survivorship Version 1.2020 March 17, 2020.
31. Spronk I, Korevaar JC, Schellevis FG, Albreht T, Burgers JS. Evidence-based recommendations on care for breast cancer survivors for primary care providers: a review of evidence-based breast cancer guidelines. BMJ Open. 2017;7:e015118. https://doi.org/10.1136/bmjopen-2016-015118.
32. National Health Commission of the People's Republic of China. Chinese guidelines for diagnosis and treatment of breast cancer 2018 (English version). Chin J Cancer Res. 2019;31(2):259–77. https://doi.org/10.21147/j.issn.1000-9604.2019.02.02.

33. Li Q, Lin Y, Xu Y, Molassiotis A. Cancer survivorship care after curative treatment: Chinese oncology practitioners' practices. Support Care Cancer. 2019;27:1287–98.
34. Okubo R, Wada S, Shimizu Y, Tsuji K, Hanai A, Imai K, et al. Expectations of and recommendations for a cancer survivorship guideline in Japan: a literature review of guidelines for cancer survivorship. Jpn J Clin Oncol. 2019;49(9):812–22. https://doi.org/10.1093/jjco/hyz070.
35. Rojas MP, Telaro E, Russo A, et al. Followup strategies for women treated for early breast cancer. Cochrane Database Syst Rev. 2005;(1):CD001768.
36. Bychkovsky GL, Lin NU. Imaging in the evaluation and follow-up of early and advanced breast cancer; when, why and how often? Breast. 2017;31:318–24.
37. NCCN. Genetic/familial high-risk assessment: breast, ovarian and pancreatic. Version 1.2021. 8 Sept 2020. Nccn.org
38. Saslow D, Boetes C, Burke W, et al. American Cancer Society guidelines for breast screening with MRI as an adjunct to mammography. CA Cancer J Clin. 2007;57:75–89.
39. Runowicz C, Leach C, Henry L, et al. American Cancer Society/American Society of Clinical Oncology breast cancer survivorship care guideline. J Clin Oncol. 2016;34:611–35.
40. Schapira D, Davidson N, Bluming M, et al. Recommended breast cancer surveillance guidelines. J Clin Oncol. 1997;15:2149–56.
41. Khatcheressian J, Wolff A, Smith T, et al. American Society of Clinical Oncology 2006 update of the breast Cancer follow-up and management guidelines in the adjuvant setting. J Clin Oncol. 2006;31:5091–7.
42. Khatcheressian J, Hurley P, Bantug E, et al. Breast cancer follow-up and management after primary treatment: American Society of Clinical Oncology clinical practice guideline update. J Clin Oncol. 2013;31:961–5.
43. Dhesy-Thind S, Fletcher G, Blanchette P, et al. Use of adjuvant bisphosphonates and other bone-modifying agents in breast cancer: a Cancer Care Ontario and American Society of Clinical Oncology clinical practice guideline. J Clin Oncol. 2017;35:2062–81.
44. Lyman G, Greenlee H, Bohlke K, et al. Integrative therapies during and after breast cancer treatment: ASCO endorsement of the SIO clinical practice guideline. J Clin Oncol. 2018;36:2647–55.
45. Burstein H, Lacchetti C, Anderson H, et al. Adjuvant endocrine therapy for women with hormone receptor-positive breast cancer: ASCO clinical practice guideline focused update. J Clin Oncol. 2018;37:423–38.
46. Pan K, Hurria A, Chlebowski R. Breast cancer survivorship: state of the science. Breast Cancer Res Treat. 2018;168:593–600.
47. National Comprehensive Cancer Network. Breast cancer (Version 3.2020). https://www.nccn.org/professionals/physician_gls/pdf/breast.pdf. Accessed 3 Apr 2020.
48. National Comprehensive Cancer Network. Survivorship (Version 1.2020). https://www.nccn.org/professionals/physician_gls/pdf/survivorship.pdf. Access 3 Apr 2020.
49. Smith T, Snyder C. Is it time for (survivorship care) plan B? J Clin Oncol. 2012;29:4740–1.
50. Maly R, Liang L, Liu Y, et al. Randomized controlled trial of survivorship care plans among low-income, predominantly Latina breast cancer survivors. J Clin Oncol. 2017;35:1814–21.
51. Boekhout AH, Maunsell E, Pond G, et al. A survivorship care plan for breast cancer survivors: extended results of a randomized clinical trial. J Cancer Surviv. 2015;9:683–91.
52. American College of Surgeons. 2020. https://www.facs.org/-/media/files/quality-programs/cancer/coc/optimal_resources_for_cancer_care_2020_standards.ashx. Accessed 3 Apr 2020.
53. Shapiro C, McCabe M, Syrjala K, et al. The Livestrong survivorship center of excellence network. J Cancer Surviv. 2009;3:4–11.
54. Anbari A, Wanchai A, Graves R. Breast cancer survivorship in rural settings: a systematic review. Support Care Cancer. 2020. https://doi.org/10.1007/s00520-020-05308-0.
55. Gonzales F, Sangaramoorthy M, Dwyer L, et al. Patient-clinician interactions and disparities in breast cancer care: the equality in breast cancer study. J Cancer Surviv. 2019;13:968–80.
56. Polek C, Hardie T, Deatrick J. Breast cancer survivorship experiences of urban hispanic women. J Cancer Educ. 2019. https://doi.org/10.1007/s13187-019-01543-0.
57. Coleman M, Quaresma M, Berrino F, et al. Cancer survival in five continents: a worldwide population-based study (CONCORD). Lancet Oncol. 2008;9:730–56.
58. Breast Cancer Initiative 2.5. 2020. http://globam.fredhutch.org. Accessed 14 Mar 2020.
59. Cardoso F, Kyriakides S, Ohno S, et al. Early breast cancer: ESMO clinical practice guidelines for diagnosis, treatment, and follow up. Ann Oncol. 2019;30:1194–220.
60. Spronk I, Korevar J, Schellevis F, et al. Evidence-based recommendations on care for breast cancer survivors for primary care providers: a review of evidence-based breast cancer guidelines. BMJ Open. 2017;7:e015118. https://doi.org/10.1136/bmjopen-2016-015118.
61. Sussman J, Souther LH, Grunfeld E, Howell D, Cage C, Keller-Olaman S, et al. Models of care for cancer survivorship. Sussman J, Fletcher G, reviewers. Toronto: Cancer Care Ontario; 2012 Oct 26 [ENDORSED 2017 March 28]. Program in Evidence-based Care Evidence-Based Series No.: 26-1 Version 2 ENDORSED.
62. Matsuoka Y, Okubo R, Shimizu Y, et al. Developing the structure of Japan's cancer survivorship guidelines using an expert panel and modified Delphi method. J Cancer Surviv. 2019. https://doi.org/10.1007/s11764-109-00840-3.

63. Breast Health Global Initiative. 2020. https://www.fredhutch.org/en/research/divisions/public-health-sciences-division/research/epidemiology/breast-health-global-initiative.html. Accessed 14 Mar 2020.
64. Breast Cancer Initiative 2.5. 2020. https://www.fredhutch.org/en/research/divisions/public-health-sciences-division/research/epidemiology/breast-cancer-initiative-2-5.html. Accessed 14 Mar 2020.
65. Koczwara B, Birken S, Perry C, et al. How context matters: a dissemination and implementation primer for global oncologists. JCO Glob Oncol. 2016. https://doi.org/10.1200/JGO.001438.
66. Ganz P, Yip C, Gralow J, et al. Supportive care after curative treatment for breast cancer (survivorship care): resource allocations in low- and middle-income countries. A Breast Health Global Initiative 2013 consensus statement. Breast. 2013;22:606–15.
67. Chan A, Zheng K, Ng T, et al. Perceptions and barriers of survivorship care in Asia: perceptions from Asian Breast Cancer Survivors. JCO Glob Oncol. 2017;3:98–104.
68. Abdel-Raqeq H, Mansour A, Jaddan D. Breast cancer care in Jordan. JCO Glob Oncol. 2020;6:260–8.
69. Ristevski E, Thompson S, Kingaby S, et al. Understanding aboriginal peoples' cultural and family connections can help inform the development of culturally appropriate cancer survivorship models of care. JCO Glob Oncol. 2020;6:124–32.
70. Harrop J, Dean J, Paskett E. Cancer survivorship research: a review of the literature and summary of current NCI-designated cancer center projects. Cancer Epidemiol Biomark Prev. 2011;20:2042–7.
71. Halpern M, Argenbright K. Evaluation of effectiveness of survivorship programmes: how to measure success? Lancet Oncol. 2017;18:e51–9.
72. Alfano C, Jefford M, Maher J, et al. Building personalized cancer follow-up care pathways in the United States: lessons learned from implementation in England, Northern Ireland, and Australia. Am Soc Clin Oncol Educ Book. 2019;39:625–39.

2 Breast Imaging: Screening for New Breast Cancers and for Cancer Recurrence

Mary Scott Soo, Karen S. Johnson, and Lars Grimm

Long-term survival of breast cancer patients is common, with a 5-year survival rate of 90% [1]. With more than 3.5 million breast cancer survivors in the United States as of January 2020, a frequent and key component of daily clinical encounters is screening for new or recurrent cancers; the screening and diagnostic imaging guidelines are somewhat complex.

Patient age, risk factors, and surgical and other treatment history need to be considered when selecting appropriate imaging studies for surveillance. Because breast cancer is a heterogeneous disease, management is tailored to the individual, differing for in situ versus invasive lesions and numerous other factors. Therapies may involve surgery, radiation therapy, and hormonal and/or chemotherapy, based on tumor size, axillary nodal involvement, distant metastases, tumor biology, genetic history, and social factors among others. Screening is therefore tailored to the patient's specific medical history and situation.

Likewise, appropriate workup of physical symptoms is essential in these patients. Imaging recommendations vary depending on the type of surgical treatment, use of radiation therapy, and timing after surgery; these and other factors impact the imaging workup of clinical symptoms that occur after treatment. This chapter reviews imaging recommendations for both screening and diagnostic evaluations in women who have undergone breast cancer treatment.

M. S. Soo (✉) · K. S. Johnson · L. Grimm
Department of Radiology, Duke University Medical Center, Durham, NC, USA
e-mail: mary.soo@duke.edu

Breast Imaging Modalities for Screening Breast Cancer Survivors

An array of breast imaging modalities are available for screening residual native breast tissue in women with a personal history of breast cancer, including mammography, digital breast tomosynthesis (DBT), magnetic resonance imaging (MRI), and ultrasound. Choosing the most appropriate modality or modalities depends on the patient's cancer history, surgical therapy, age, and overall risk status.

Breast Imaging Modalities

- Digital mammography (two-dimensional mammography)
- Digital breast tomosynthesis (three-dimensional mammography)
- Magnetic resonance imaging
- Ultrasound

G. G. Kimmick et al. (eds.), *Common Issues in Breast Cancer Survivors*,
https://doi.org/10.1007/978-3-030-75377-1_2

Digital Mammography and Digital Breast Tomosynthesis (DBT)

In conjunction with history and physical exam, annual digital mammography (i.e., traditional two-dimensional mammography) and digital breast tomosynthesis (DBT) (i.e., three-dimensional mammography) are the indicated imaging modalities for screening the bilateral breasts in patients who have undergone breast conserving surgery (BCS), or for screening the contralateral breast after mastectomy. DBT is a newer, advanced mammography technology that uses low-dose radiation to acquire multiple initial projection images; data from these images are then used to reconstruct numerous image "slices" which provide a simulated three-dimensional view of the entire breast. Compared to standard two-dimensional (2D) digital mammography, DBT also requires breast compression, and uses only a minimally higher radiation dose overall. The ability of DBT to evaluate breast tissue at thin slices (usually 1 mm each) allows for identification of small cancers that are often obscured by superimposed tissue on standard 2D digital mammograms (Fig. 2.1). This results in improved cancer detection rates and reduced false positives, and is particularly beneficial in women with dense breast tissue, including younger women, who tend to have dense tissue.

Although the sensitivity of digital mammography can decrease by as much as 11% in breast cancer survivors compared to women without a personal history of breast cancer [2, 3], studies have shown that surveillance mammography still significantly reduces the risk of dying from breast cancer in survivors of all ages [2–4]. In addition, mammography detects lesions earlier, resulting in more favorable prognoses, than lesions detected by physical exam [5]. Further, overall survival is improved when recurrent breast cancer is detected by mammography compared to recurrence detected by physical exam [5]. Regardless of age, the American College of Radiology and the Society of Breast Imaging recommend annual digital mammography or DBT starting 6–12 months after cancer surgery, to establish a new baseline imaging appearance [6].

In all patients, the guiding principle of screening and surveillance should be to consider the individual patient's risk of recurrence in the context of her functional status. There is no fixed upper age limit to stop screening, but consideration to stopping should be given for women whose life expectancy is less than 5–7 years based on age or comorbidities, as well as women who would choose not to act on any abnormal results from screening mammography.

Magnetic Resonance Imaging (MRI)

Contrast-enhanced breast MRI is recommended for surveillance in high-risk women with a greater than 20% lifetime risk of breast cancer. Compared to both 2D mammography and DBT, MRI offers superior sensitivity and an improved cancer detection rate, with only a small decrease in specificity [6–10]. A recently published study of 1249 high-risk women demonstrated a sensitivity of 96% for MRI, but only 31% for mammography, with a cancer detection rate of 21.8 cancers per 1000 MRI examinations but only 7.2 cancers per 1000 mammography examinations [8]. Another recent study of 1355 women with increased familial risk found that more breast cancers were detected and that the breast cancers were smaller and more often node negative in the MRI group compared to the mammography group [11]. During breast MRI examinations, women lie prone with their breasts positioned dependently within a dedicated breast coil that provides high resolution imaging. Gadolinium-based dye is injected through an IV during scan acquisition and concentrates within breast cancers soon after the injection. Typically, breast cancer will vigorously enhance due to the collection of gadolinium within breast cancer. This vigorous enhancement of breast cancer can typically be detected even in a background of dense breast tissue which reduces mammographic sensitivity. This explains why breast MRI has a higher sensitivity than mammography and, in fact, has the highest sensitivity of all current imaging modalities for the detection of breast cancer. In addition, while mammography is not used routinely for

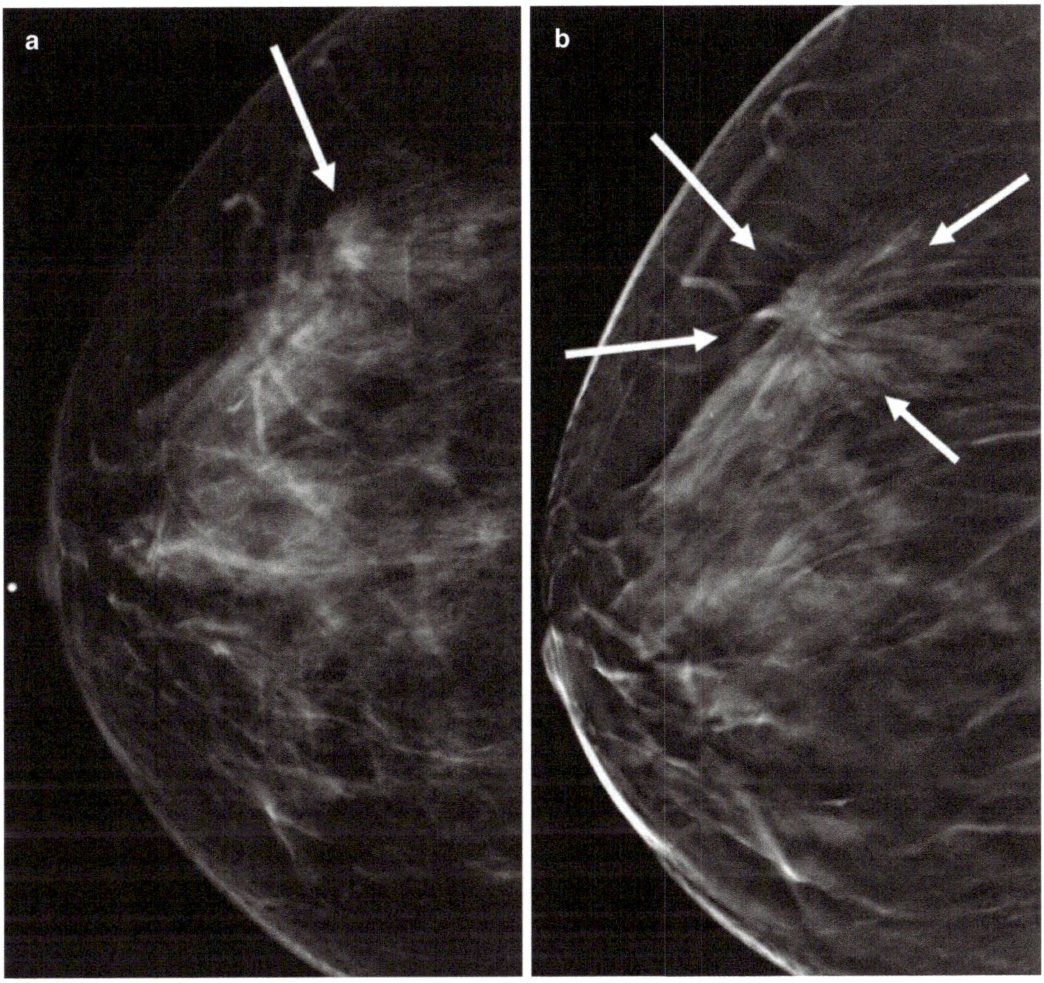

Fig. 2.1 Digital mammography and DBT of invasive ductal carcinoma in the patient's right breast. (**a**) Craniocaudal view from a traditional 2D digital mammogram shows an asymmetry laterally in the right breast (arrow), in the region of the carcinoma. The features of the carcinoma are partly obscured due to surrounding fibroglandular tissue, making it somewhat inconspicuous. (**b**) One of 50 reconstructed craniocaudal images (slices) throughout the right breast, created to produce the 3D tomosynthesis mammogram. Compared to figure **a**, this 1 mm thick slice at the level of the invasive cancer makes the tumor more conspicuous and better defined, seen now as a highly suspicious spiculated mass (arrows)

annual surveillance of a reconstructed breast, chest wall, or ipsilateral axilla following mastectomy, breast MRI can effectively assess these areas with routinely acquired axial images if there is clinical concern for recurrent breast cancer.

Based on the life-time risk assessments, the American Cancer Society (ACS) in 2007 concluded that there was insufficient evidence to recommend for or against routine breast MRI screening in the general breast cancer survivor population [12]. However, women with a personal history of breast cancer who meet high-risk criteria according to the ACS guidelines should undergo yearly screening MRI as part of their survivorship care plan. As stated earlier, high risk is defined as a greater than 20% lifetime risk of developing a second primary cancer and would include women who are BRCA1/BRCA2 mutation carriers or women with a very strong family history of breast cancer. More recently, utilization of screening MRI for women with a personal history of breast cancer has been shown to increase detection of early stage biologically aggressive breast cancers and decrease interval cancers [13]. In addition, MRI also appears to perform better in women with a personal history of breast cancer compared to MRI in women with genetic risk or family history, due to fewer false positive exams (12.3% vs. 21.6%) and higher specificity (94.0% vs. 86.0%), without statistically different sensitivity and cancer detection rates [10].

Increased breast density confers a small additional risk of breast cancer, with a relative risk of 1.45 for women with dense breasts compared to those with scattered fibroglandular density [14]. Increased breast density alone does not confer a high-risk status, but in conjunction with a personal history of breast cancer an individual patient's lifetime risk may cross the >20% lifetime threshold to qualify for high-risk screening MRI. However, many risk-assessment models do not incorporate breast density into their calculations. There is a small, but growing, body of evidence that suggests that screening MRI may be beneficial for non-high-risk women with dense breasts [15–17]. The Dutch DENSE trial randomized women with extremely dense breasts to biennial MRI plus mammography versus mammography alone and found a significant decrease in interval cancers in the MRI group (4.9/1000 vs. 0.8/1000) [16]. Unfortunately, many insurance providers will not cover screening MRI if the patient does not meet high-risk criteria, and so decisions about MRI utilization must be individualized to the patient's risk status, financial circumstances, and insurance coverage.

The steadily growing number of women with greater-than-normal risk for breast cancer who are eligible for MRI screening has raised concerns about access and availability for breast MRI. Breast MRI imaging protocols were designed for comprehensive preoperative staging to define the extent of disease. Newer abbreviated breast MRI protocols have been developed specifically for screening purposes [18–21]. These abbreviated protocols reduce the number of image sequences acquired; therefore, they result in marked reductions in acquisition time (patient time in the MRI scanner) and radiologist interpretation time [21]. This allows more breast MRIs to be scheduled per hour, improving availability, and potentially decreasing patient costs. Multiple retrospective and prospective observational studies have demonstrated comparable sensitivity and positive predictive values for abbreviated versus full breast MRI protocols [18–21]. At least one randomized controlled trial is in progress to evaluate abbreviated MRI protocols more comprehensively [22]. Breast MRI utilization for breast cancer survivors will likely increase over time, based on the high sensitivity and improved access, due to these evolving abbreviated protocols and resultant cost reductions.

There are several drawbacks to MRI compared to other imaging modalities. Breast MRI requires IV access and contrast administration. The adverse event rate for gadolinium-based contrast media (GBCM) ranges from 0.07% to 2.4%, and most reactions are mild and physiologic, including coldness, warmth or pain at the injection site, nausea, headaches, paresthesia, or dizziness [23]. Allergic-like reactions are rare and range from 0.004% to 0.7%, with anaphylactic reactions exceedingly rare [23]. Concerns about nephrogenic sclerosing fibrosis have been raised; however, these are essentially eliminated by appropriately screening patients for risk factors, most notably acute renal disease [24]. Health concerns about gadolinium deposition in the brain are currently theoretical but an area of investigation [25]. The most common reasons that some patients refuse to participate in high-risk screening MRI programs include claustrophobia, financial concerns, referring physician refusal to provide referral, lack of interest, and medical intolerance of MRI [26]. Finally, there may be increased anxiety associated with more frequent screening (MRI plus mammography compared to mammography alone).

Ultrasound

The role for screening ultrasound in women with a personal history of breast cancer is limited.

Regardless of risk status, ultrasound is primarily indicated for supplemental screening of women with mammographically dense breasts, resulting in an incremental increase in the cancer detection rate, but at the cost of increased false-positive findings and a lower positive predictive value [27, 28]. For women with dense breasts who undergo screening ultrasound, the risk of false positives becomes more pronounced and the benefits diminish if DBT is used instead of digital mammography [29]. Ultrasound does have a valuable role in the diagnostic setting and is indicated for women with palpable abnormalities, pain, or other breast symptoms. During ultrasound evaluations, the patient lies supine or in decubitus positions while the radiologist or sonographer pass a handheld or automated device over the skin surface of the breast, acquiring images through use of sound waves to identify abnormalities.

Other Imaging Modalities

Other imaging modalities such as molecular breast imaging [MBI], computed tomography [CT], and positron emission tomography [PET] can also image the breast. However, they do not have an established role in screening women with a personal history of breast cancer, and are most often used in specific clinical settings, such as staging of newly diagnosed breast cancer.

Screening After Breast Conserving Surgery

After BCS for early-stage cancer, ipsilateral recurrent breast tumors occur in approximately 4% of women [30]. The first post-treatment surveillance mammogram can be performed 6–12 months after radiation treatment ends [31]. Breast conserving surgery combined with radiation treatment induces changes in the breast that typically evolve and stabilize over 3 years. Diagnostic mammography provides extra scrutiny of the surgical site and helps to establish a new baseline appearance. Since most local recurrences present within 5 years after treatment, annual diagnostic mammography, which is better able to detect small areas of residual or recurrent disease, is performed for the first 5 years after diagnosis [32]. After 5 years, routine screening mammography is continued.

Diagnostic mammograms in BCS patients typically include routine craniocaudal (CC) and mediolateral oblique (MLO) views plus extra spot magnification or spot compression tomosynthesis views of the lumpectomy site. The addition of a spot compression tomosynthesis view of the lumpectomy site helps to evaluate for abnormal findings such as biopsy scar enlargement, developing masses, and asymmetries. Ultrasound is commonly used in these settings to evaluate for underlying masses or fluid collections and may facilitate biopsy planning when necessary. Spot magnification views of the lumpectomy site are useful for identifying and characterizing indeterminate or suspicious calcifications at or around the scar site that would prompt stereotactic core biopsy. This is particularly important for patients whose initial cancer presentation involved calcifications.

Imaging features of recurrent carcinomas in areas of native breast remote from the lumpectomy scar site are similar to features of cancer detected in patients without a personal history of breast cancer. Radiologists focus their search on new suspicious masses, calcifications, developing asymmetries, areas of architectural distortion, or suspicious axillary adenopathy. Search is also made for any increase in trabecular thickening, skin thickening, skin dimpling/retraction, or nipple inversion that would also warrant further diagnostic evaluation.

Another added benefit of diagnostic mammography after BCS is that a radiologist oversees and interprets the images at the time the images are obtained. Therefore, if a new abnormality is suspected and additional views and/or ultrasound are warranted to ensure a more accurate diagnosis, those can be performed at that same visit, potentially saving the patient from needing to return. Finally, because a diagnostic mammogram is overseen by a radiologist, patients can receive their results immediately which often reduces their anxiety because they do not need to wait for results. After the initial 5-year period of diagnostic mammography surveillance, patients are often recommended for annual bilateral screening protocols which do not include focused views of the lumpectomy site.

Screening After Mastectomy

Annual mammography screening of the contralateral, unaffected breast should continue after mastectomy. Screening mammography of the unaffected breast typically begins 6–12 months after completion of local therapy, followed thereafter by annual screening mammography for healthy women. Imaging features of screen-detected carcinomas in these cases are similar to features of cancers detected in patients without a personal history of breast cancer.

Routine mammograms are no longer required for screening of the residual tissue on the treated side in patients receiving simple, modified radical, or radical mastectomies. Typically, there is not enough breast tissue left to perform a mammogram, and surveillance is performed with physical exam. Breast cancer can still recur immediately below the skin in the subcutaneous tissue or just overlying the pectoralis muscle, and these recurrences should be readily detected if a physical exam is part of the routine surveillance care. For patients who undergo a *skin-sparing* mastectomy, sometimes referred to as a subcutaneous mastectomy, there is still a role for mammography because the nipple and tissue beneath the skin are not removed. This leaves behind enough tissue to necessitate annual routine mammographic screening [33]. Obtaining an accurate surgical history is necessary to ensure correct imaging evaluation.

Patients who undergo mastectomy may also undergo breast reconstruction. Breast reconstruction generally falls into two categories: implant (prosthetic) or flap (autologous) reconstruction. In either case, if the patient has undergone a simple, modified radical, or radical (and not a skin-sparing or subcutaneous) mastectomy, routine mammographic screening *of the reconstructed breast* is usually not necessary. In patients with implant reconstruction, mammographic screening is technically limited because the implant limits compression, and implant density obscures underlying tissues, making physical exam the primary mode of surveillance.

After flap reconstructions, however, the bulk of the reconstructed breast is commonly made up of fatty tissue from other parts of the body (e.g., abdominal, posterior chest, medial thigh, or buttock) so mammography is more technically feasible. While the risk of developing breast cancer in these flap reconstruction tissues is low, small amounts of normal breast tissue can be left behind, below the skin in the subcutaneous soft tissues and immediately overlying the pectoralis muscle, as in mastectomy patients without reconstruction. Recurrences at these sites validate some institutions' use of routine mammographic imaging of autologously reconstructed breast. The data on screening women following autologous reconstruction are sparse, and there is no consensus on this issue. Overall, physical exam is the primary method for surveillance for recurrent cancer in reconstructed breasts, and patients should be encouraged to perform self-exams.

Imaging Management of Breast Symptoms in Breast Cancer Survivors

After breast cancer treatment, patients are often relieved to be finished with their therapy, but many worry about the possibility of breast cancer recurrence. Clinical providers should evaluate for signs and symptoms of disease recurrence. The affected breast undergoes a number of changes at the conclusion of treatment; most are considered a normal evolution in the healing process and are benign. The degree of change varies among patients, with different reactions depending on body habitus, surgical, radiation and medical oncology therapies, and timing after the treatments.

Symptoms After Breast Conserving Surgery and Radiation

Early imaging changes in the months following BCT and radiation therapy often reveal skin erythema and edema on physical examination. While normal skin thickness in an untreated breast is 2 mm, up to 90% of patients with BCT and radiation will commonly develop skin thickness greater than 2 mm as an expected sequela of therapy (Fig. 2.2). After 2–3 years, thickening should stabilize or decrease [34]. Mammography during this time identifies the corresponding skin and trabecular thickening, in addition to prominent asymmetry and vague architectural distortion at the surgical site. These changes often decrease gradually over time, and the surgical site changes become more defined, evolving to a smaller spiculated mass or area of architectural distortion (Fig. 2.3). Areas of fat necrosis with dystrophic calcifications often occur within the lumpectomy site as well. While fat necrosis that may present as round, lucent oil cysts may develop within 6–12 months of surgery, dystrophic calcifications typically appear on mammogram 2–3 years after the completion of treatment. In addition, postoperative seromas can be seen within the surgical cavity in up to 50% of patients 1 month following BCT. While most postoperative seromas spontaneously resolve, a quarter will persist beyond 6 months and a small minority may persist for years.

Although these changes are expected, some progress to complications that present challenges to clinical management, based on associated symptoms and findings on physical examination. For example, evolving scars and fat necrosis seen as oil cysts can present as a new firm palpable lump that feels much like recurrent breast cancer. Fat necrosis and resultant oil cysts often have characteristic benign features on mammography and ultrasound allowing conclusive diagnosis; however, if atypical in appearance, then biopsy may be required to confirm the diagnosis. Likewise, large seromas may be palpable, and cause swelling and pain, or can even become

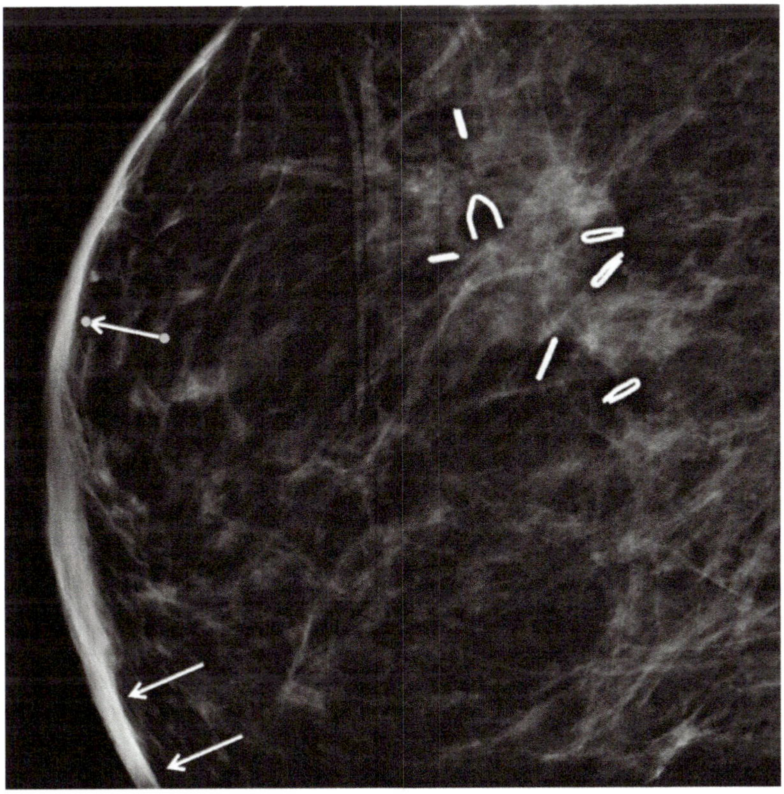

Fig. 2.2 MLO mammogram after lumpectomy and radiation therapy shows skin thickening (arrows) due to treatment changes. Also seen are surgical clips, asymmetry, and architectural distortion at the lumpectomy site

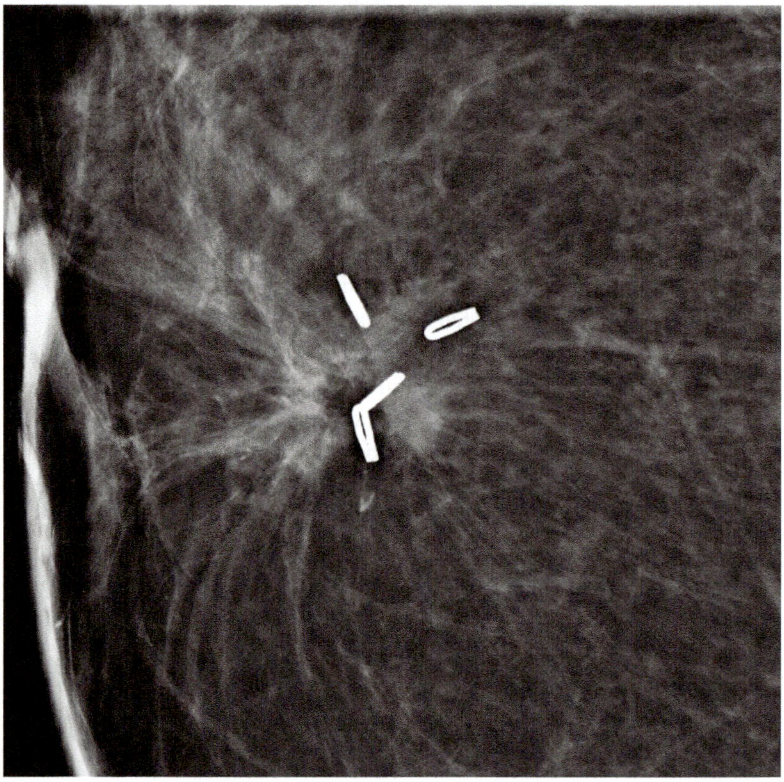

Fig. 2.3 Craniocaudal mammogram demonstrates typical postoperative architectural distortion and surgical clips at a lumpectomy site

infected, requiring drainage and antibiotic therapy. Enlarging seromas over time can also result in suspicious changes at mammography. Diagnostic ultrasound is essential in these cases to identify the seromas and guide drainage procedures and culture when necessary.

On physical examination, any concerning change or increase in size of these common post-treatment sequela (e.g., palpable lumps at the mastectomy or lumpectomy scars; new areas of thickening; focal pain or swelling; nipple discharge, flattening or retraction; skin dimpling and other changes; palpable axillary adenopathy) should raise concern for recurrent breast cancer and require diagnostic imaging evaluation. In most cases, both diagnostic mammography (with DBT when available) and ultrasound are needed for a complete evaluation, although the workup is tailored by the radiologist for each individual situation. The majority (65%) of early recurrences occur at or within a few centimeters of the surgical scar site and within the first 7 years of treatment [35]. Diagnostic mammography with magnification views of the lumpectomy site helps to exclude the presence of suspicious recurring calcifications or an underlying suspicious mass at the surgical site. In patients with concerning physical symptoms, targeted mammographic images plus a diagnostic ultrasound evaluation targeting the area also help detect cancer recurrence. In rare cases when these tests are inconclusive, a problem-solving breast MRI may be helpful, and consultation with the radiologist can help guide management.

Symptoms After Mastectomy

Understanding typical post-treatment changes after mastectomy in patients with or without reconstruction is important for accurate physical exam surveillance. Seromas frequently develop in the surgical cavity immediately following mastectomy; therefore, drains are typically placed at the time of surgery to avoid chronic seromas. Persistent seromas may cause clinical concern or interfere with subsequent treatments, requiring percutaneous drainage. Diagnostic ultrasound alone is commonly used in the immediate postoperative period to identify the seroma and guide drainage procedures when necessary, facilitating culture of fluid if infection is suspected.

Other palpable lumps may develop at the mastectomy site over time. In the absence of reconstruction, patients who have undergone mastectomy can be evaluated for most symptomatic complaints and worrisome physical exam findings with ultrasound alone. Ultrasonography can readily detect and potentially diagnose fat necrosis, lymphadenopathy, and cancer recurrence. However, a diagnostic mammogram, imaging the focal area of concern ("lumpogram") may also be necessary to differentiate fat necrosis from recurrent tumor as the cause of the patient's symptoms, because some forms of fat necrosis and recurrent cancer are indistinguishable at ultrasound. Breast MRI can also be useful in selected cases, as MRI has been shown in one study to have a 100% sensitivity and specificity for the detection of breast cancer in this patient population [36].

For patients who have undergone mastectomy with breast reconstruction, a diagnostic mammogram and ultrasound should be ordered if an area of concern is found on physical exam by the patient or her clinician. Diagnostic mammography is superior to ultrasound for diagnosing findings such as calcified fat necrosis and oil cysts, and is effective for evaluating both implant-reconstructed and the predominantly fat containing autologous flap reconstructions. Ultrasound is superior to mammography in characterizing discrete masses as solid or cystic and detecting intracapsular implant rupture. Breast MRI could also be considered as an adjunct to clarify any concerning physical exam findings if mammography and ultrasound are inconclusive.

Mastectomy with Implant Reconstruction

Women who undergo mastectomy followed by implant reconstruction may develop breast symptoms due to peri-implant fluid collections (seroma, hematoma, abscess), changes in the implant over time (capsular contracture or possible rupture), changes in the tissue due to surgery (scar and fat necrosis), and of course, remain at risk for recurrent cancer. Following implant placement for breast reconstruction or augmentation, a small amount of fluid may normally collect around the implant; however, persistent, large, or rapidly growing seromas can be clinically symptomatic and increase the risk of infection. Diagnostic ultrasound is commonly used in the postoperative period to identify the fluid collection and guide drainage procedures when necessary. Later development of peri-prosthetic fluid collections raises concerns for abscess, chronic seromas, or very rarely implant-associated anaplastic large cell lymphoma (ALCL). Implant-associated ALCL has been reported to present anywhere between 1 and 23 years after implant placement, with a median time of 8 years [37]. The most common presentation of ALCL is a chronic peri-implant seroma, which requires cytological testing of the fluid, usually collected through ultrasound-guided aspiration [38].

Changes in the implant shape or contour over time raise the suspicion of implant rupture. For breast reconstruction, the two most common types of implants are saline and silicone-gel, both of which can leak or rupture. A ruptured saline implant will simply "deflate" and the body absorbs the saline. No imaging is necessary to confirm saline implant rupture since marked changes on physical exam are typically sufficient to make the diagnosis. Silicone gel implants, however, can rupture and be asymptomatic, or cause a range of symptoms. Patients might notice a change in the implant shape, associated pain, hardened areas due to silicone granulomas within the breast, or silicone-associated adenopathy as the silicone gel migrates through the breast tissue and collects in axillary lymph nodes. While mammography and ultrasound can at times demonstrate conclusive evidence of extracapsular silicone implant rupture, non-contrast breast MRI is the most sensitive method. The FDA recommends that women with silicone gel implants undergo screening non-contrasted breast MRI to look for asymptomatic implant rupture at 3 years after implantation and then every 2 years thereafter [39].

Capsular contracture is also a relatively common complication of implant reconstruction occurring in approximately 13% of patients [40]. This is usually identified on physical exam as hardening and rounding of the implant, and imaging is not warranted to make the diagnosis.

The presence of a prosthetic implant, whether saline or silicone gel, does not increase the risk for breast cancer, but it limits the sensitivity of mammography for detecting breast cancer [41]. However, if ultrasound is combined with mammography, the sensitivity for detecting recurrent malignancy increases. Therefore, if a patient has undergone mastectomy with implant reconstruction and presents with concerning physical exam findings, the appropriate first imaging tests include a diagnostic mammogram with ultrasound. If imaging is inconclusive and concern persists, breast MRI can be helpful and has been reported in some series to have 100% sensitivity [42].

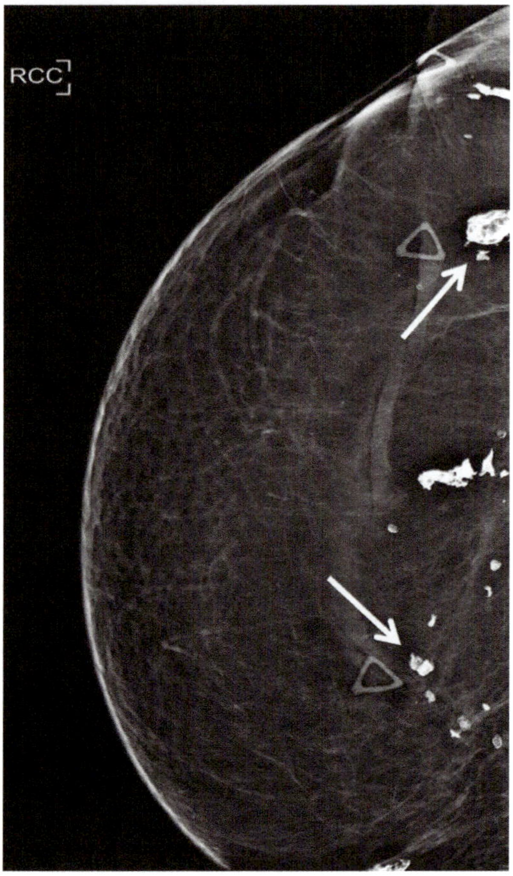

Fig. 2.4 Fat necrosis in the TRAM flap reconstructed breast. The craniocaudal mammogram confirms the diagnosis, showing densely calcified areas of fat necrosis (arrows) underlying triangular-shaped skin markers, correlating with the palpable lumps

Mastectomy with Autologous Flap Reconstruction

Many women undergo breast reconstruction with either autologous flaps or implant prostheses. Overall, women with autologous flap reconstructions have more complications than those with implant reconstruction [43, 44]. Women who receive mastectomy followed by autologous flap reconstruction (e.g., TRAM [transverse rectus abdominal muscle; DIEAP [deep inferior epigastric artery perforator], latissimus dorsi) also experience a range of postoperative complications that require imaging evaluation. Fat necrosis occurs in over 50% of patients with a TRAM flap reconstruction at an average of 2 months following surgery (Fig. 2.4) [45]. Seromas, hematomas, and skin thickening are also common postoperative sequelae of flap reconstruction surgery, all of which can lead to palpable lumps that can mimic malignancy on physical exam [46]. In most cases, diagnostic mammography with ultrasound can distinguish a benign palpable lump such as a seroma, hematoma, oil cyst, or fat necrosis from recurrent breast cancer. If assessment of a clinical abnormality is indeterminate or suspicious with imaging, a diagnostic mammogram and/or ultrasound can often safely facilitate imaging-guided biopsy of the area of concern.

Locally recurrent breast cancers after skin-sparing mastectomy with autologous flap reconstruction are uncommon (2–4%), and most occur in areas of residual breast tissue within 5 years of reconstruction [47]. The majority of these recurrences (50–72%) occur superficially in the contact zone between the skin envelope and the autologous flap tissue (Fig. 2.5) and are easily detected by physical exam [46, 48]. Chest wall recurrences are less common than subcutaneous

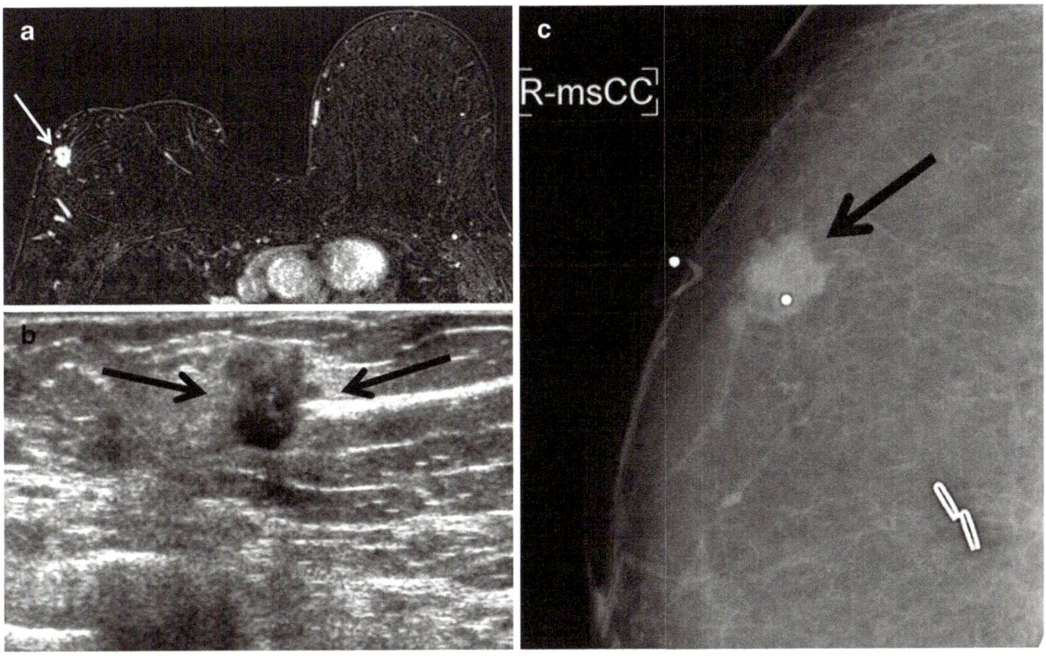

Fig. 2.5 Recurrent invasive cancer in the smaller, right reconstructed breast, seen as (**a**) a high signal irregular enhancing mass (arrow) in the contact zone between residual skin and autologous flap on MRI, (**b**) a superficial irregular hypoechoic mass (arrows) at ultrasound, and (**c**) an irregular superficial mass (arrow) at mammography

cancers because the pectoralis fascia is commonly removed with the mastectomy specimen at surgery. If patients present with focal pain or discomfort rather than a superficial lump, cancer recurrence within the posterior margin of the mastectomy bed along the pectoralis muscle should be considered. Patients with chest wall recurrences have a higher likelihood of metastatic disease, with an associated poorer prognosis [47]. Because the chest wall region can be more difficult to evaluate with physical exam, mammography, or even ultrasound and/or breast MRI imaging should be considered in some cases as a reasonable and reliable tool to exclude the presence of malignancy.

Autologous Fat Grafting

Autologous fat grafting is commonly being used for reconstruction refinements after mastectomy reconstructions and can also be used after BCS [49]. Imaging findings in these patients often show definitively benign changes such as multiple fat-containing oil cysts, dystrophic calcifications, and areas of scarring at mammography, or round benign-appearing oil cysts at ultrasound [50]. However, in approximately 5% of patients, suspicious clinically palpable lesions and imaging detected abnormalities require biopsy [50]. For palpable abnormalities that occur in patients with autologous fat grafting, a detailed history of the reconstructive procedure is helpful in making an accurate diagnosis, along with diagnostic mammography and ultrasound evaluation.

Conclusion

As women with a history of breast cancer are living longer and longer, knowing the appropriate and available options to detect recurrent disease is crucial to the ongoing medical care of breast cancer survivors. Imaging plays a key role in the surveillance of these patients, and tailoring its use to the specific individual based on a variety factors will contribute to ongoing increased longevity of breast cancer survivors.

References

1. Howlander N, Noone AM, Krapcho M, Miller D, Brest A, Yu M, et al. SEER Cancer Statistics Review, 1975-2016. Bethesda: National Cancer Institute; 2019. Available from: https://seer.cancer.gov/csr/1975_2016/.
2. Lash TL, Fox MP, Buist DS, Wei F, Field TS, Frost FJ, et al. Mammography surveillance and mortality in older breast cancer survivors. J Clin Oncol. 2007;25(21):3001–6.
3. Lash TL, Fox MP, Silliman RA. Reduced mortality rate associated with annual mammograms after breast cancer therapy. Breast J. 2006;12(1):2–6.
4. Schootman M, Jeffe DB, Lian M, Aft R, Gillanders WE. Surveillance mammography and the risk of death among elderly breast cancer patients. Breast Cancer Res Treat. 2008;111(3):489–96.
5. Orel SG, Fowble BL, Solin LJ, Schultz DJ, Conant EF, Troupin RH. Breast cancer recurrence after lumpectomy and radiation therapy for early-stage disease: prognostic significance of detection method. Radiology. 1993;188(1):189–94.
6. Houssami N, Abraham LA, Miglioretti DL, Sickles EA, Kerlikowske K, Buist DS, et al. Accuracy and outcomes of screening mammography in women with a personal history of early-stage breast cancer. JAMA. 2011;305(8):790–9.
7. Weinstein SP, Localio AR, Conant EF, Rosen M, Thomas KM, Schnall MD. Multimodality screening of high-risk women: a prospective cohort study. J Clin Oncol. 2009;27(36):6124–8.
8. Lo G, Scaranelo AM, Aboras H, Ghai S, Kulkarni S, Fleming R, et al. Evaluation of the utility of screening mammography for high-risk women undergoing screening breast MR imaging. Radiology. 2017;285(1):36–43.
9. Weinstock C, Campassi C, Goloubeva O, Wooten K, Kesmodel S, Bellevance E, et al. Breast magnetic resonance imaging (MRI) surveillance in breast cancer survivors. Springerplus. 2015;4:459.
10. Lehman CD, Lee JM, DeMartini WB, Hippe DS, Rendi MH, Kalish G, et al. Screening MRI in women with a personal history of breast cancer. J Natl Cancer Inst. 2016;108(3):djv349.
11. Saadatmand S, Geuzinge HA, Rutgers EJT, Mann RM, de Roy van Zuidewijn DBW, Zonderland HM, et al. MRI versus mammography for breast cancer screening in women with familial risk (FaMRIsc): a multicentre, randomised, controlled trial. Lancet Oncol. 2019;20(8):1136–47.
12. Saslow D, Boetes C, Burke W, Harms S, Leach MO, Lehman CD, et al. American Cancer Society guidelines for breast screening with MRI as an adjunct to mammography. CA Cancer J Clin. 2007;57(2):75–89.
13. Cho N, Han W, Han BK, Bae MS, Ko ES, Nam SJ, et al. Breast cancer screening with mammography plus ultrasonography or magnetic resonance imaging in women 50 years or younger at diagnosis and treated with breast conservation therapy. JAMA Oncol. 2017;3(11):1495–502.
14. Cummings SR, Tice JA, Bauer S, Browner WS, Cuzick J, Ziv E, et al. Prevention of breast cancer in postmenopausal women: approaches to estimating and reducing risk. J Natl Cancer Inst. 2009;101(6):384–98.
15. Berg WA, Rafferty EA, Friedewald SM, Hruska CB, Rahbar H. Screening algorithms in dense breasts: AJR expert panel narrative review. AJR Am J Roentgenol. 2021;216(2):275–94.
16. Bakker MF, de Lange SV, Pijnappel RM, Mann RM, Peeters PHM, Monninkhof EM, et al. Supplemental MRI screening for women with extremely dense breast tissue. N Engl J Med. 2019;381(22):2091–102.
17. Kuhl CK, Strobel K, Bieling H, Leutner C, Schild HH, Schrading S. Supplemental breast MR imaging screening of women with average risk of breast cancer. Radiology. 2017;283(2):361–70.
18. Kuhl CK, Schrading S, Strobel K, Schild HH, Hilgers RD, Bieling HB. Abbreviated breast magnetic resonance imaging (MRI): first postcontrast subtracted images and maximum-intensity projection-a novel approach to breast cancer screening with MRI. J Clin Oncol. 2014;32(22):2304–10.
19. Mango VL, Morris EA, David Dershaw D, Abramson A, Fry C, Moskowitz CS, et al. Abbreviated protocol for breast MRI: are multiple sequences needed for cancer detection? Eur J Radiol. 2015;84(1):65–70.
20. Grimm LJ, Soo MS, Yoon S, Kim C, Ghate SV, Johnson KS. Abbreviated screening protocol for breast MRI: a feasibility study. Acad Radiol. 2015;22(9):1157–62.
21. Harvey SC, Di Carlo PA, Lee B, Obadina E, Sippo D, Mullen L. An abbreviated protocol for high-risk screening breast MRI saves time and resources. J Am Coll Radiol. 2016;13(4):374–80.
22. Kuhl CK. Abbreviated breast MRI for screening women with dense breast: the EA1141 trial. Br J Radiol. 2018;91(1090):20170441.
23. Media ACoDaC. ACR manual on contrast media: American College of Radiology; 2020. Available from: https://www.acr.org/Clinical-Resources/Contrast-Manual.
24. Altun E, Martin DR, Wertman R, Lugo-Somolinos A, Fuller ER 3rd, Semelka RC. Nephrogenic systemic fibrosis: change in incidence following a switch in gadolinium agents and adoption of a gadolinium policy--report from two U.S. universities. Radiology. 2009;253(3):689–96.
25. RSNA statement on gadolinium-based MR contrast agents: Radiological Society of North America; 2018.
26. Berg WA, Blume JD, Adams AM, Jong RA, Barr RG, Lehrer DE, et al. Reasons women at elevated risk of breast cancer refuse breast MR imaging screening: ACRIN 6666. Radiology. 2010;254(1):79–87.
27. Nothacker M, Duda V, Hahn M, Warm M, Degenhardt F, Madjar H, et al. Early detection of breast cancer: benefits and risks of supplemental breast ultrasound in asymptomatic women with mammographically dense breast tissue. A systematic review. BMC Cancer. 2009;9:335.

28. Weigert JM. The Connecticut experiment; the third installment: 4 years of screening women with dense breasts with bilateral ultrasound. Breast J. 2017;23(1):34–9.
29. Tagliafico AS, Calabrese M, Mariscotti G, Durando M, Tosto S, Monetti F, et al. Adjunct screening with tomosynthesis or ultrasound in women with mammography-negative dense breasts: interim report of a prospective comparative trial. J Clin Oncol. 2016;34(16):1882–8.
30. Yang SH, Yang KH, Li YP, Zhang YC, He XD, Song AL, et al. Breast conservation therapy for stage I or stage II breast cancer: a meta-analysis of randomized controlled trials. Ann Oncol. 2008;19(6):1039–44.
31. Runowicz CD, Leach CR, Henry NL, Henry KS, Mackey HT, Cowens-Alvarado RL, et al. American Cancer Society/American Society of Clinical Oncology breast cancer survivorship care guideline. J Clin Oncol. 2016;34(6):611–35.
32. Carlson RW. Surveillance of patients following primary therapy. In: Harris JR, Lippman ME, Morrow M, Osborne CK, editors. Disease of the breast. 4th ed. Philadelphia: Lippincott Williams & Wilkins; 2010.
33. Noroozian M, Carlson LW, Savage JL, Jeffries DO, Joe AI, Neal CH, et al. Use of screening mammography to detect occult malignancy in autologous breast reconstructions: a 15-year experience. Radiology. 2018;289(1):39–48.
34. Krishnamurthy R, Whitman GJ, Stelling CB, Kushwaha AC. Mammographic findings after breast conservation therapy. Radiographics. 1999;19 Spec No:S53–62; quiz S262–3.
35. Mendelson EB. Evaluation of the postoperative breast. Radiol Clin N Am. 1992;30(1):107–38.
36. Yilmaz MH, Esen G, Ayarcan Y, et al. The role of US and MR imaging in detecting local chest wall tumor recurrence after mastectomy. Diagn Interv Radiol. 2007;13(1):13–8.
37. Administration USFaD. Anaplastic large cell lymphoma (ALCL) in women with breast implants: preliminary FDA findings and analyses. Available from: http://www.fda.gov/medicaldevices/productsandmedicalprocedures/implantsandprosthetics/breastimplants/ucm239996.htm.
38. Roller R, Chetlen A, Kasales C. Imaging of breast implants and their associated complications. J Am Osteopath Coll Radiol. 2014;3(1):2–9.
39. Administration USFaD. Update on the safety of silicone gel-filled breast implants (2011) - executive summary. Available from: https://www.fda.gov/medical-devices/breast-implants/update-safety-silicone-gel-filled-breast-implants-2011-executive-summary.
40. Coroneos CJ, Selber JC, Offodile AC 2nd, Butler CE, Clemens MW. US FDA breast implant postapproval studies: long-term outcomes in 99,993 patients. Ann Surg. 2019;269(1):30–6.
41. Miglioretti DL, Rutter CM, Geller BM, Cutter G, Barlow WE, Rosenberg R, et al. Effect of breast augmentation on the accuracy of mammography and cancer characteristics. JAMA. 2004;291(4):442–50.
42. McIntosh SA, Horgan K. Augmentation mammoplasty: effect on diagnosis of breast cancer. J Plast Reconstr Aesthet Surg. 2008;61(2):124–9.
43. Xu F, Sun H, Zhang C, Jiang H, Guan S, Wang X, et al. Comparison of surgical complication between immediate implant and autologous breast reconstruction after mastectomy: a multicenter study of 426 cases. J Surg Oncol. 2018;118(6):953–8.
44. Bennett KG, Qi J, Kim HM, Hamill JB, Pusic AL, Wilkins EG. Comparison of 2-year complication rates among common techniques for postmastectomy breast reconstruction. JAMA Surg. 2018;153(10):901–8.
45. Garvey PB, Buchel EW, Pockaj BA, Casey WJ 3rd, Gray RJ, Hernandez JL, et al. DIEP and pedicled TRAM flaps: a comparison of outcomes. Plast Reconstr Surg. 2006;117(6):1711–9; discussion 20–1.
46. Pinel-Giroux FM, El Khoury MM, Trop I, Bernier C, David J, Lalonde L. Breast reconstruction: review of surgical methods and spectrum of imaging findings. Radiographics. 2013;33(2):435–53.
47. Peng C, Chang CB, Tso HH, Flowers CI, Hylton NM, Joe BN. MRI appearance of tumor recurrence in myocutaneous flap reconstruction after mastectomy. AJR Am J Roentgenol. 2011;196(4):W471–5.
48. Howard MA, Polo K, Pusic AL, Cordeiro PG, Hidalgo DA, Mehrara B, et al. Breast cancer local recurrence after mastectomy and TRAM flap reconstruction: incidence and treatment options. Plast Reconstr Surg. 2006;117(5):1381–6.
49. Kaoutzanis C, Ganesh Kumar N, O'Neill D, Wormer B, Winocour J, Layliev J, et al. Enhanced recovery pathway in microvascular autologous tissue-based breast reconstruction: should it become the standard of care? Plast Reconstr Surg. 2018;141(4):841–51.
50. Juhl AA, Redsted S, Engberg DT. Autologous fat grafting after breast conserving surgery: breast imaging changes and patient-reported outcome. J Plast Reconstr Aesthet Surg. 2018;71(11):1570–6.

3 Hot Flashes

Daniel S. Childs, Arjun Gupta, Cindy S. Tofthagen, and Charles L. Loprinzi

Introduction

A majority of women will experience vasomotor symptoms, including hot flashes and night sweats, during menopause; the quality, quantity, and severity of these can vary markedly among individuals [1]. Using symptom logs and other qualitative data, efforts have been made to describe and categorize the range of hot flash severity in breast cancer survivors [2–4]. The milder variety of hot flashes may last only a few minutes and result in warmth or facial reddening but lead to no emotional or behavioral consequences. The spectrum, however, extends all the way to very severe events that have been described as "boiling eruptions," producing profuse diaphoresis and other physical symptoms. When this severe, hot flashes interrupt usual daily activities and may impair sleep. Additionally, they may have significant emotional implications, leading to anxiety, embarrassment, and even panic. For this reason, hot flashes have been ranked by women as the second most bothersome symptom of menopause, behind only weight gain [5]. Hot flashes can be particularly disruptive and bothersome for those with cancer as well.

Vasomotor symptoms are highly prevalent in survivors of breast cancer. Most women who are treated for breast cancer, irrespective of their menopausal status, will experience hot flashes [6]. For example, in one study over half a breast cancer survivors report having experienced a hot flash in the last week, emphasizing the frequency with which this untoward symptom occurs [4]. Vasomotor symptoms, or hot flashes, occur more often in breast cancer patients because of the widespread use of antiestrogen therapies and chemotherapies that can induce ovarian failure. Groups recognize the importance of better managing this symptom and have labeled hot flashes as 1 of 5 key endocrine therapy-associated symptoms warranting close monitoring during breast cancer treatment [7].

The goal of the current chapter is to outline options for treating hot flashes. Estrogen-based pharmacotherapies work well, but there are concerns with these medications, especially regarding breast cancer risk [8]. This chapter will outline multiple non-estrogen approaches for controlling hot flashes, including information on dosing, efficacy, and toxicity. It is designed as an aid to busy clinicians and nurses; the information

D. S. Childs (✉) · C. L. Loprinzi
Department of Oncology, Mayo Clinic, Rochester, MN, USA
e-mail: childs.daniel@mayo.edu; cloprinzi@mayo.edu

A. Gupta
Sidney Kimmel Comprehensive Cancer Center, Johns Hopkins University, Baltimore, MD, USA

C. S. Tofthagen
Department of Nursing, Mayo Clinic, Jacksonville, FL, USA
e-mail: tofthagen.cindy@mayo.edu

G. G. Kimmick et al. (eds.), *Common Issues in Breast Cancer Survivors*,
https://doi.org/10.1007/978-3-030-75377-1_3

provided may also be helpful for informing educated patients, to better help them participate in shared decision-making.

Quick Overview of Treatment Options for Hot Flashes in Breast Cancer Survivors

With regard to the alleviation of hot flashes in breast cancer survivors, a large number of studies have been conducted in the past 30 years. Many have been positive, some negative, and a few others have shown mixed results. Fortunately, there are now a number of accepted therapeutic options to choose from when treating hot flashes, which allows clinicians to make individualized recommendations in the context of a patient's preferences, and risks and benefits with regard to other comorbidities (Fig. 3.1).

As a general approach, for most patients it makes sense to begin with non-prescription options, such as physical measures and lifestyle changes. Some will find lifestyle changes alone to be sufficient in controlling their symptoms. Patients with bothersome enough hot flashes, for which they wish to try drug therapy, can be offered a trial of pharmacotherapy, understanding that some women would rather deal with their hot flashes as opposed to taking a medication for them. There are four main classes of non-estrogenic drugs that have been shown to be helpful for treating hot flashes, those being antidepressant medications, gabapentinoids, anticholinergic medications, and progesterone analogs. The efficacy and potential toxicities of these agents are discussed below.

Tincture of Time and Physical Measures

For most women, hot flashes subside over time even without treatment, but it can take many years as is described in the Study of Women across the Nation (SWAN) [9]. In SWAN, the median duration of menopausal vasomotor symptoms was 7.4 years. There are less data describing the natural history of hot flashes for those receiving modern treatments for breast cancer. Readers may note that in most short-term, placebo-controlled trials, hot flash frequency decreases on average by 20–30% within 4 weeks of starting a placebo [10]. However, the observed reduction actually appears to be from a placebo effect as opposed to the natural history of hot

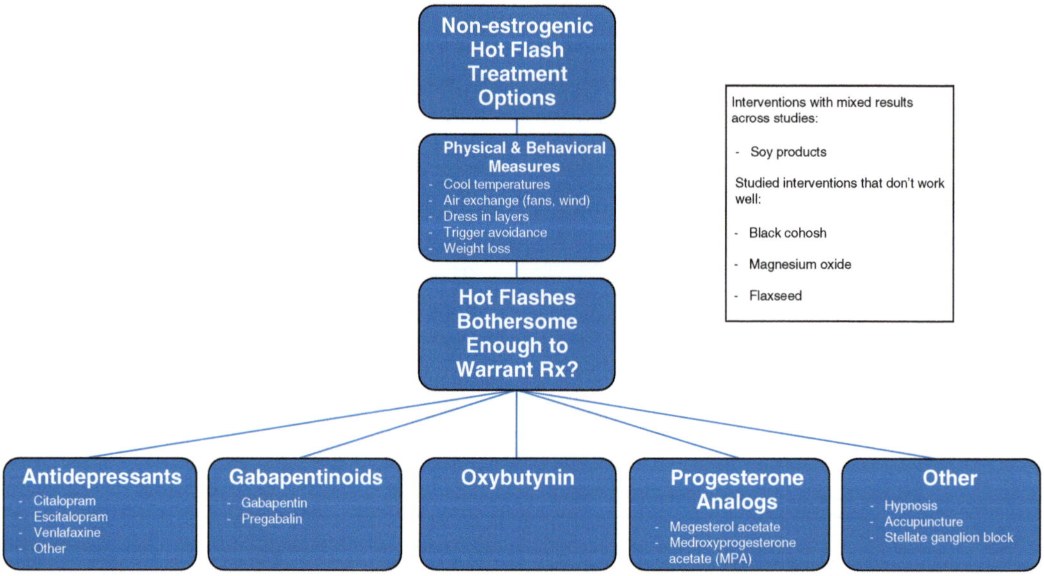

Fig. 3.1 Approach to the treatment of hot flashes in breast cancer patients

flash improvement. This is illustrated in a trial that had a 2-week baseline period, whereby there was no substantial change in mean hot flash scores during the first and second weeks of screening prior to beginning any intervention [11]. With no intervention, hot flashes do improve over time, but it takes much longer than weeks for women to notice a substantial reduction in hot flash frequency and severity.

In additional to watchful waiting, physical measures are sometimes sufficient for patients with mild vasomotor symptoms. Proposed interventions include dressing in layers the can be removed easily, using fans or other means to promote air circulation, and avoiding triggers such as hot baths or spicy foods [12]. A patient once shared a practical tip with us as it relates to this topic. When driving in the winter, she would put her coat on backwards before fastening her seatbelt so that the coat could easily be removed without unfastening the seatbelt if hot flashes occurred while she was driving. Weight loss, too, can be helpful as hot flashes are more prevalent in women who are obese [13], and even modest weight loss leads to fewer bothersome flushing episodes [14].

Antidepressant Medications

Serotonin Norepinephrine Reuptake Inhibitors (SNRIs)

In the 1990s, several providers independently recognized that women taking four different antidepressants (venlafaxine, paroxetine, fluoxetine, and sertraline) seemed to have reductions in their hot flashes. Following such anecdotal evidence, a pilot study was developed to evaluate the efficacy of low-dose *venlafaxine* (12.5 mg twice daily) for alleviating hot flashes in women with a history of breast cancer and in men receiving androgen deprivation therapy [15]. The study enrolled 28 patients who provided hot flash data via daily questionnaires. By the fourth week of treatment, overall hot flash scores had decreased to 45% of their baseline value. Over half of the patients experienced greater than a 50% reduction in hot flash scores following initiation of venlafaxine, and, importantly, the medication was relatively well-tolerated. The positive results of this trial led to a subsequent randomized, placebo-controlled trial evaluating three different doses of venlafaxine [16]. All three doses of venlafaxine outperformed the placebo; the best dose was 75 mg daily as it was more effective than 37.5 mg daily and had fewer side effects, including mouth dryness, decreased appetite, nausea, and constipation than 150 mg daily; additionally, there was no suggestion that the higher dose decreased hot flashes any more than 75 mg daily. When using this drug for management of vasomotor symptoms, it is recommended to start with 37.5 mg daily and, if ineffective, up-titrate to 75 mg per day. The lower dose of venlafaxine may be enough to control hot flashes for some patients, in which case the dose does not need to be increased.

Subsequent, randomized, double-blinded, placebo-controlled trials began evaluating other antidepressants, including another serotonin-norepinephrine reuptake inhibitor, *desvenlafaxine*, which has demonstrated similar efficacy, to venlafaxine, in multiple large placebo-controlled trials [17, 18]. The target dose for desvenlafaxine is 100 mg daily with a starting dose of 50 mg daily.

Selective Serotonin Reuptake Inhibitors (SSRIs)

Another class of antidepressants, selective serotonin reuptake inhibitors (SSRIs), includes the only non-hormonal drug with US Food and Drug Administration (FDA) approval for the treatment of hot flashes. Initial trials with paroxetine showed results similar to what had been seen with venlafaxine [19]. In 2013, the FDA-approved *paroxetine* for treatment of moderate-to-severe vasomotor symptoms of menopause. Approval was largely based on the results of two trials, which involved over 1100 postmenopausal women. The first trial observed a median reduction of 5.9 hot flashes per day in the paroxetine arm as compared to 5.0 in the placebo arm [20].

The second trial demonstrated median reductions of 5.6 and 3.9 hot flashes per day in each group, respectively [20]. Though one might view the absolute reduction in hot flash frequency as not overly impressive, patients did find it to be clinically meaningful. It is possible that some of the benefit was derived from improved sleep quality, as later studies have shown that sleep disturbances caused by hot flashes are significantly reduced by low-dose paroxetine [21].

The SSRIs do not seem to have an entirely uniform class effect in improving vasomotor symptoms. Despite sertraline being one of the drugs that was initially noted to decrease hot flashes in women who were taking it for other indications, such as mood symptoms, multiple studies support that *sertraline* less consistently outperforms placebo in reducing hot flashes [22–25]. Though another SSRI, *fluoxetine*, appears better than a placebo, mixed treatment comparison analysis shows that it has the lowest probability of providing clinically meaningful improvements among all the SSRIs [26]. For these reasons, the authors are less inclined to use sertraline and fluoxetine for the treatment of hot flashes.

Caution should be exercised when using certain SSRIs in patients who have breast cancer. It is worth noting that paroxetine and fluoxetine are both potent inhibitors of the cytochrome P-450 CYP2D6 enzyme, which converts tamoxifen to its more potent metabolite, endoxifen. Paroxetine decreases plasma concentrations of endoxifen by 64%, which may diminish the efficacy of tamoxifen [27]. Indeed, a long-term, population-based cohort study of overlapping treatment with tamoxifen and SSRIs suggested an increased risk of breast cancer-related death for women taking paroxetine (but not other SSRIs) [28]. However, other work, such as the prospective CYPTAM study, did not show a correlation between endoxifen levels and relapse free survival for women with early-stage breast cancer receiving tamoxifen [29]. The topic remains highly debated, and there are not yet definitive answers about the impact of co-prescription of antidepressants and tamoxifen. Lesser degrees of CYP2D6 inhibition are seen with citalopram and venlafaxine, and pragmatically, other options exist such that antidepressants known to show higher inhibition of CYP2D6 (like paroxetine) can be avoided [30].

Among the antidepressant options for cancer patients, the authors feel that *citalopram* may have the best benefit/toxicity/cost ratio (Table 3.1). A phase III, placebo-controlled trial demonstrated a magnitude of benefit that is similar to what has been reported for venlafaxine and paroxetine – a mean reduction in hot flash scores of approximately 50% – but, unlike paroxetine, citalopram is only a moderate inhibitor of the CYP2D6 enzyme [31]. It causes less nausea and vomiting than venlafaxine, which is a particularly important in cancer patients who may already have gastrointestinal symptoms related to cancer-directed therapies [32]. Daily doses of 10 mg, 20 mg, and 30 mg appear to be equivalent in controlling symptoms, but a target dose of 20 mg daily may be more effective for controlling mood symptoms.

The SSRI *escitalopram* is another option that leads to fewer and less severe hot flashes. An

Table 3.1 Recommended dosing and common side effects for antidepressants used for hot flashes

Medication	Starting dose	Target dose	Common or major side effects
Citalopram	20 mg daily	20 mg daily	No more than placebo in some trials; others report drowsiness, insomnia
Escitalopram	10 mg daily	20 mg daily	No more than placebo in some trials; others report headache, insomnia, drowsiness, GI symptoms
Venlafaxine ER	37.5 mg daily	75 mg daily	Xerostomia, nausea, decreased appetite, constipation
Paroxetine[a]	10 mg daily	10 mg daily	Nausea, headache, insomnia
Desvenlafaxine	50 mg daily	100 mg daily	Nausea, insomnia, xerostomia

Abbreviations: *ER* extended release
[a]Potent CYP2D6 inhibition

early study evaluated this antidepressant in healthy menopausal women without concomitant mood disorders [33]. This study lacked a control group but noted a reduction in hot flash frequency and severity after starting escitalopram. Another small study evaluated escitalopram against estrogen-based therapy and reported a greater reduction in climacteric symptoms for those receiving escitalopram [34]. The use of this medication is further supported by a multisite, randomized, placebo-controlled, double-blind clinical trial published in 2011 [35]. By the end of the first week, patients receiving 10–20 mg per day of escitalopram reported significant reduction in hot flash severity that was paralleled by reductions in hot flash frequency. Similar to other studies of SSRIs and SNRIs, approximately 50% of patients experienced at least a 50% reduction in hot flash frequency.

A few additional points about antidepressant use for hot flash symptoms merit discussion. First, some of the trials discussed above included women with natural or surgical menopause, while others included patients with breast cancer, some of whom had cancer treatment-related menopausal symptoms. These non-hormonal therapies seem to be similarly useful regardless of whether a patient has a history of breast cancer, or not, and regardless of whether they were taking tamoxifen, or not [36]. Second, antidepressants improve hot flash symptoms much more quickly than they do mood symptoms with some studies demonstrating significant improvement within a week [35]. Unpublished data from the initial placebo-controlled venlafaxine study reveals significant reductions in hot flashes, compared to the placebo arm, very quickly [16]. Third, per cross-study comparisons, all agents mentioned within this section (except for sertraline and fluoxetine) appear to have a relatively similar efficacy for reducing hot flashes. Finally, if one antidepressant does not work, will another be effective? While there are no good clinical trial data to address this question; anecdotally it appears that changing to another may be helpful for some patients.

Gabapentinoid Medications

In 2000, Dr. Thomas Guttuso, a neurologist, described a series of six cases where *gabapentin* was prescribed for pain indications; he noted that it, incidentally, ameliorated patients' hot flashes [37]. His hypothesis was subsequently tested in a randomized, double-blind, placebo-controlled trial, which reported that gabapentin 900 mg daily resulted in a 54% reduction in a composite score of hot flash severity and frequency, as compared to only a 31% reduction for patients receiving placebo [38]. Since that time, numerous RCTs, comparing gabapentin to placebo, have been completed; these have included diverse patient populations from different practice settings and countries [39–43]. A recent meta-analysis demonstrated that patients benefited from gabapentin but at the expense of more dizziness and somnolence (RR 4.45, 95% CI 2.50–7.94) [44]. Gait instability or ataxia may also occur with gabapentinoids, and lower doses are recommended for individuals with renal impairment [45]. Thus, gabapentin is another reasonable option for controlling hot flashes. It may be particularly useful for those who have another neurologic indication for using gabapentin or those intolerant of antidepressants. Most studies start gabapentin at a dose of 300 mg daily and up-titrate to goal dose of 300 mg three times daily. If a patient primarily has nighttime hot flashes (night sweats), this can be titrated up to a single bedtime dose of 900 mg day.

Pregabalin is a GABA analog that works in a manner similar to gabapentin. It is widely used for neuropathic pain and also is prescribed off-label for several other neurologic indications. The activity of pregabalin for vasomotor symptoms is supported by a phase III, placebo-controlled trial including 163 patients with bothersome hot flash symptoms [46]. After week 6, pregabalin 150 mg twice daily decreased hot flash scores by 71%, pregabalin 75 mg twice daily decreased hot flash scores by 65%, and a placebo decreased hot flash scores by 50%. The side effect profile of pregabalin is similar to what is described above for gabapentin, but the twice daily dosing of pregabalin is

Table 3.2 Recommended dosing and common side effects for gabapentinoid medications used for hot flashes

Medication	Starting dose	Target dose	Common or major side effects
Gabapentin	300 mg daily	300 mg TID	Somnolence, dizziness
Pregabalin	50 mg QHS	75 mg BID	Somnolence, dizziness, weight gain

Abbreviations: *QHS* every night at bedtime, *TID* three times daily, *BID* twice daily

more convenient. For improved tolerability without significant detriment to efficacy, consider a target dose of 75 mg twice daily.

In summary, multiple placebo-controlled, randomized, double-blind clinical trials demonstrate that both gabapentin and pregabalin decrease hot flashes to a similar magnitude as seen with the above-noted antidepressant medications (Table 3.2).

Venlafaxine Versus Gabapentin: Which Do Women Prefer?

As discussed above, both antidepressants and gabapentinoid medications are viable options for treating hot flashes. In one crossover study, breast cancer survivors with hot flashes received 4 weeks of treatment with venlafaxine and 4 weeks of treatment with gabapentin [11]. Each treatment period was separated by a washout interval. Most patients (68%) preferred venlafaxine to gabapentin, though both agents reduced overall hot flash scores to a similar degree. The results of the study support first trying an antidepressant, and, if ineffective, consider a transition to a gabapentinoid. Interestingly, gabapentin and an antidepressant together seems no better than gabapentin alone for hot flash reduction, so the antidepressant can be tapered off if ineffective for control of hot flashes [47].

Oxybutynin

Support for studying oxybutynin in the treatment of hot flashes came from the observation that patients taking the medication for overactive bladder also noticed that it provided relief from sweating [48]. Indeed, a multitude of studies have shown that oxybutynin is efficacious in controlling generalized hyperhidrosis [49]. A Canadian group retrospectively examined the charts of 52 patients who received oxybutynin and reported that 70% had a partial or excellent response to treatment [50].

Extended release oxybutynin at a dose of 15 mg daily was compared to placebo in a multicenter, double-blind, phase II trial [51]. Seventy-three percent of women receiving oxybutynin, compared to 26% receiving placebo, reported that their vasomotor symptoms were "much improved" at the end of treatment; however, about 7% of patients in this study discontinued oxybutynin secondary to side effects, primarily dry mouth. Another phase III trial randomized 150 women with hot flashes to lower doses of oxybutynin, at 2.5 mg twice daily, 5 mg twice daily, versus a placebo [52]. At the end of the study, mean hot flash scores (a composite measure of hot flash frequency and severity) were reduced by 10.6, 16.9, and 5.7 units in each group, respectively. Hot flash frequency was also significantly reduced in the oxybutynin groups as compared to placebo. While the study was not designed to compare the two different doses of the medication, patients receiving the higher doses of oxybutynin seemed to have better improvement in the quality-of-life metrics. In this study, using lower daily doses of oxybutynin than were used in the prior study, side effects were milder than seen in the previous manuscript, and there were no differences in drug discontinuation because of adverse effects between the three study arms.

The anticholinergic effects of oxybutynin lead to dry mouth, constipation, and urinary retention, particularly in the elderly and when the daily dose exceeds 15 mg [53]. This medication should not be used in patients who have urinary retention, narrow angle glaucoma, or gastrointestinal motility disorders [54, 55]. It should be used with caution in older patients with comorbidities and polypharmacy. When using this medication, it may be best to start at low doses and gradually ramp up the dose until symptom control is achieved or toxicity encountered (Table 3.3).

Table 3.3 Recommended dosing and common side effects for oxybutynin used for hot flashes

Medication	Starting dose	Target dose	Common or major side effects
Oxybutynin	2.5 mg BID	5 mg BID	Xerostomia, difficulty urinating, and abdominal pain

Abbreviations: *BID* twice daily

Progesterone Analogs

Oral *megestrol acetate* is a progesterone-type hormonal agent that, by cross study comparison, appears to control hot flashes about as well as estrogen [56]. In a study of 97 women with history of breast cancer and 66 men with prostate cancer receiving androgen deprivation therapy, megestrol acetate (20 mg twice daily) reduced hot flashes by 85%, as compared to 21% in the placebo group [57]. The medication's long-term efficacy and tolerability was described in another study, which contacted patients years after they had been enrolled in a short-term trial of megestrol acetate for hot flashes [58]. Almost half of the patients were still taking megestrol acetate 3 years beyond conclusion of the study, and the treatment still appeared to be well tolerated.

Medroxyprogesterone Acetate (MPA) Medroxyprogesterone acetate has a more convenient dosing scheduled than does megestrol acetate, as MPA is a single-dose intramuscular injection that provides long lasting progestin coverage. The two medications, megestrol acetate and MPA, were compared head-to-head and provided equal relief from hot flashes at 6 weeks [59]. MPA has also been directly compared to venlafaxine; MPA was superior in controlling hot flashes and was well tolerated [60].

In considering the use of MPA or megestrol acetate, one should discuss long-term safety concerns of using a progesterone analog in patients with potentially hormonally sensitive cancers. Some breast cancer oncologists are opposed to using these hormones in patients, despite both of them having been used, in the past, for treating metastatic breast cancer (albeit at higher doses than are used to treat hot flashes). Although large randomized, controlled trials have not addressed the safety of progestin use, a case-control study that matched 75 breast cancer survivors receiving MPA for hot flashes with controls, on the basis of age, stage of disease, HER2 status, and year of diagnosis, did not identify a detrimental effect of MPA on overall survival or oncologic outcomes, though the study may have been underpowered to assess these endpoints [61]. More recently, data were presented suggesting post-menopausal women who receive combined estrogen and progesterone have higher rates of breast cancer, while those who receive estrogen alone experience a lower incidence of breast cancer [62]. In the absence of consensus about safety, before starting a patient on a progestin-type hormonal agent, they should be made aware of potential cancer-related risk along with other side effects, including blood clots and/or increased appetite with or without weight gain (Table 3.4).

Clonidine

Randomized, placebo-controlled, double-blinded clinical trials support that clonidine decreases hot flashes, but not as much as has been seen with multiple other agents such as antidepressants and gabapentinoids. One study with a crossover design compared transdermal clonidine to placebo [63]. Hot flash frequency was reduced only 20% from baseline in the clonidine group. Taking into account adverse effects, patients were asked which drug they preferred at the conclusion of the study. The splits were fairly even with 31% choosing clonidine, 24% choosing placebo, and 45% unable to tell a difference. A later trial evaluated oral clonidine 0.1 mg per day, which resulted in a 37% reduction in hot flash frequency versus 24% for placebo [64]. Patients taking clonidine more commonly experience dry mouth, constipation, sleep, and sedation-related concerns. Given the availability of other suitable pharmacotherapies with less troublesome side effect profiles, clonidine is no longer widely prescribed for hot flashes.

Table 3.4 Recommended dosing and common side effects for progesterone analogs used for hot flashes

Medication	Starting dose	Target dose	Common or major side effects
Megestrol acetate	20 mg daily	20–40 mg daily	Theoretical concerns about breast cancer risk, withdrawal menstrual bleeding, increased appetite, thromboembolic phenomena
Medroxyprogesterone acetate (MPA)	400 mg IM once	400 mg IM once (understanding that repeat doses can be used months later if hot flashes return)	Theoretical concerns about breast cancer risk, irritation at site of injection, withdrawal menstrual bleeding, increased appetite, thromboembolic phenomena

Abbreviations: *IM* intramuscular

Non-pharmacologic Treatment Options

Hypnosis

Hypnosis is non-pharmacologic option used by some in the treatment of hot flashes. It is a form of behavioral mind-body therapy that achieves a state of consciousness where suggestions may lead to a change in perception. For instance, hot flashes may be combated by cooler imagery, such as drinking a cold glass of water, a cool breeze, or a winter day in Minnesota. One study randomized women to receive 5 weekly sessions of hypnosis versus no intervention. Hypnosis appeared better than no treatment and resulted in a 68% reduction in hot flash scores [65]. Similar results were reported in a comparison of hypnosis to a sham intervention that matched therapist exposure between the two groups [66]. In this study, clinical hypnosis resulted in a 74% reduction in hot flash frequency as compared to 17% with the sham procedure.

Another study sought to evaluate the efficacy of hypnosis alone or in combination with antidepressant therapy, versus antidepressant therapy alone [67]. The trial had four arms: venlafaxine + hypnosis, venlafaxine + sham hypnosis, placebo + hypnosis, and placebo + sham hypnosis. Interestingly, patients in each active therapy arm experienced a reduction in hot flashes of approximately 50%, as compared to only 25% for patients receiving placebo + sham hypnosis group. The combination of venlafaxine and hypnosis did not appear to be better than either treatment alone.

Hypnosis is not a widely used approach at this time. It is important to recognize that few providers have experience or expertise as a hypnotherapist. Further, this methodology requires frequent office visits for therapy sessions making it a less convenient treatment option. There is ongoing work evaluating a self-hypnosis approach which, if it works, should be able to become more broadly available [68].

Stellate Ganglion Blocks

A series of small trials, including a randomized, sham-controlled trial, supports that stellate ganglion blocks work; however, they are rarely used for treating hot flashes at this time. The procedure involves injecting a local anesthetic adjacent to a nerve group in the neck. The first randomized, sham-controlled trial compared stellate ganglion block to a sham procedure that involved injecting saline into the subcutaneous tissue of the neck. In total, 40 women with vasomotor symptoms were recruited and followed with regular symptom assessment for 6 months after the injection. While there was no between group difference with regard to hot flash frequency, those receiving the stellate ganglion block experienced fewer moderate to very severe episodes (RR 0.5) [69].

Stellate ganglion block has also been compared to other standards of care. For example, a small trial compared stellate ganglion block to paroxetine, and the two interventions resulted in a similar improvement in hot flash score at 2 weeks, 4 weeks, and 6 weeks [70]. Another small study compared stellate ganglion block to pregabalin 75 mg twice daily [71]. Both interventions resulted in reduced hot flush scores compared to each group's baseline, but at the conclusion of the third month, stellate ganglion block significantly outperformed pregabalin with a percent reduction in hot flash score of 88% versus 74% for pregabalin. Importantly, very few adverse events have been reported in the stellate ganglion block trials.

Acupuncture

Trials have yielded mixed results in the evaluation of acupuncture for hot flashes. For example, one trial with 103 participants compared medical to sham acupuncture [72]. In the medical acupuncture group, needles were placed at appropriate, validated acupuncture points, while the sham procedure involved needling non-acupuncture, non-meridian areas. The verum procedure did not control hot flashes any better than the sham procedure; however, it is recognized that sham acupuncture techniques are not entirely inert [73]. Another study compared 12 weeks of acupuncture to venlafaxine [74]. Both groups experienced approximately a 50% of reduction in vasomotor symptoms. Menopause-specific quality of life measures, including depression, were also similarly improved, but patients receiving acupuncture had fewer adverse events than those taking antidepressant, and the effects of acupuncture on hot flashes appeared to be sustained for a longer period.

In summary, there is some support for this modality, but data are still limited. The state of evidence is well summarized in a meta-analysis of randomized controlled trials, cumulatively including over 1000 women, which notes that acupuncture is more effective than no intervention, but no better than sham procedures and less effective than menopausal hormonal replacement therapy [75].

Dietary Supplements That May Provide Limited Benefit

Vitamin E

Vitamin E is a fat soluble vitamin known for its antioxidant activity [76]. It is widely available and is also affordable. There was anecdotal support and commentary advocating for its use; however, evidence was fairly limited until 1998 when a placebo-controlled trial randomized women to receive vitamin E 800 IU daily or placebo for 4 weeks followed by crossover treatment [77]. Vitamin E resulted in a small benefit over placebo with a magnitude of one fewer hot flashes per day. A second placebo-controlled sequential trial reproduced the results with vitamin E leading to a modest improvement in hot flash frequency and severity [78]. No significant toxicities were observed in either trial. In summary, vitamin E may provide a benefit similar to placebo plus a bit more. Some physicians have recommended that a trial of vitamin E may be reasonable for a women with hot flashes as it is a relatively safe over-the-counter medication which may allow a patient to get the above-described placebo-effect and maybe slightly more benefit. A reasonable dose to recommend is 400 IU twice daily.

Soy Products

Soy products have been touted to have "natural" benefits as they contain phytoestrogens, plant-based compounds with mixed weak estrogenic and antiestrogenic action. Given these properties, it has been proposed that increasing the intake of phytoestrogens may decrease bothersome symptoms, like hot flashes, that occur in low estrogen states. Supplemental soy phytoestrogens have been evaluated as an alternative or complementary approach in several phase III trials, and the results have been mixed. As a representative sampling of studies, some trials show modestly reduced hot flashes with soy product supplementation over placebo [79], while others show no improvement [80–82]. In one trial, women receiving soy isoflavone tablets even experienced more hot flashes [83]. There is a fair amount of heterogeneity among trials, with different doses and formulations of soy-derived phytoestrogens being used. In aggregate, a meta-analysis found no conclusive evidence that phytoestrogen supplements decrease hot flashes [84].

Dietary Supplements That Do Not Appear to Work

Many other supplements available at grocery stores or pharmacies claim to relieve menopause-related symptoms but less consistently demonstrate efficacy. For example, one of the most widely used herbal remedies for hot flashes is *black cohosh*, a phytochemical containing estrogen-like isoflavones. However, in pooled analysis of multiple moderate sized, randomized, placebo controlled trials, black cohosh was found to be no better than placebo at reducing hot flash frequency [85]. At this time, there is insufficient evidence to support the use of black cohosh for vasomotor symptoms.

Similar to the soy products discussed above, *flaxseed* contains phytoestrogens, in particular, a class called lignin. Pilot data suggested a mean reduction in hot flash frequency of 50% with flaxseed [86], but when the phase III trial was conducted, no statistical difference in hot flash outcomes emerged [87]. Approximately a third of patients in both arms achieved a 50% reduction in their hot flash score. These results underscore the importance of placebo-controlled trials in evaluating potential hot flash treatments.

In recent years, *magnesium oxide* also gained attention with publication of a case report describing two women whose hot flashes markedly improved after starting magnesium supplementation for other indications [88]. Subsequently, two open-label pilot studies, each with 20–30 patients, also reported significant reductions in hot flash symptoms [89, 90]. Unfortunately, despite the promise of the pilot studies, a larger, well-designed placebo controlled trial evaluating two doses of magnesium oxide (800 mg and 1200 mg daily) demonstrated no difference in hot flash score or hot flash frequency [91]. As expected, patients receiving magnesium had more diarrhea, owing to the well-known laxative effect of the drug. Thus, magnesium oxide is not recommended for treating vasomotor symptoms.

What About Men with Hot Flashes?

The focus of this book is managing symptoms in breast cancer survivors, the majority of whom are women. However, men with breast cancer may experience hot flashes as well, though they have not been well represented in hot flash trials. Hot flashes in men are most prominent in patients with prostate cancer who have received antiandrogen therapy.

Pilot studies for the antidepressants venlafaxine and paroxetine suggest that they may be useful for men having hot flashes in androgen-deprived states, but they have not been well evaluated in larger placebo-controlled trials [92, 93]. One placebo-controlled trial that compared venlafaxine to a soy protein showed more substantial decreases in hot flashes in the first 4 weeks with venlafaxine, but this effect was not maintained out to 12 weeks [94]. Additionally, this trial started with a 75 mg per day dose of venlafaxine, as opposed to starting at 37.5 mg per day and titrating upward. Thus, patients were more likely to stop venlafaxine than placebo. Gabapentin dosed at 900 mg per day has been shown to outperform placebo and works to a similar degree in men and women [95]. Multiple trials show that progesterone analogs also work well for male hot flashes [57, 96]. The opposite is true for clonidine; though it can work for women, it did not significantly decrease hot flash frequency or severity in men who have undergone surgical or medical orchiectomy [97]. Finally, oxybutynin has not been extensively studied in men, but case reports and anecdotal experience support that it does decrease male hot flashes [98].

Conclusions

There are a variety of non-estrogenic options for treatment of hot flashes associated with cancer. Following a trial of physical and behavioral measures, individuals who continue to experience bothersome symptoms have pharmacologic and non-pharmacologic treatment options. Pharmacologic options include antidepressants, gabapentinoids, oxybutynin, or progesterone analogs. Hypnosis, acupuncture, and stellate ganglion blocks are non-pharmacologic options that can be considered for patients who prefer not to take medications.

References

1. Feldman BM, Voda A, Gronseth E. The prevalence of hot flash and associated variables among perimenopausal women. Res Nurs Health. 1985;8(3):261–8.
2. Finck G, et al. Definitions of hot flashes in breast cancer survivors. J Pain Symptom Manag. 1998;16(5):327–33.
3. Freeman EW, Sherif K. Prevalence of hot flushes and night sweats around the world: a systematic review. Climacteric. 2007;10(3):197–214.
4. Chang HY, et al. Hot flashes in breast cancer survivors: frequency, severity and impact. Breast. 2016;27:116–21.
5. Bernhard LA, Sheppard L. Health, symptoms, self-care, and dyadic adjustment in menopausal women. J Obstet Gynecol Neonatal Nurs. 1993;22(5):456–61.
6. Gupta P, et al. Menopausal symptoms in women treated for breast cancer: the prevalence and severity of symptoms and their perceived effects on quality of life. Climacteric. 2006;9(1):49–58.
7. Zhu YH, et al. Symptom map of endocrine therapy for breast cancer: a scoping review. Cancer Nurs. 2019;42(5):E19–30.
8. Rossouw JE, et al. Risks and benefits of estrogen plus progestin in healthy postmenopausal women: principal results from the Women's Health Initiative randomized controlled trial. JAMA. 2002;288(3):321–33.
9. Avis NE, et al. Duration of menopausal vasomotor symptoms over the menopause transition. JAMA Intern Med. 2015;175(4):531–9.
10. Sloan JA, et al. Methodologic lessons learned from hot flash studies. J Clin Oncol. 2001;19(23):4280–90.
11. Bordeleau L, et al. Multicenter, randomized, crossover clinical trial of venlafaxine versus gabapentin for the management of hot flashes in breast cancer survivors. J Clin Oncol. 2010;28(35):5147–52.
12. Gupta A. Hormone therapy-related hot flashes and their management. JAMA Oncol. 2018;4(4):595.
13. Saccomani S, et al. Does obesity increase the risk of hot flashes among midlife women?: a population-based study. Menopause. 2017;24(9):1065–70.
14. Huang AJ, et al. An intensive behavioral weight loss intervention and hot flushes in women. Arch Intern Med. 2010;170(13):1161–7.
15. Loprinzi CL, et al. Pilot evaluation of venlafaxine hydrochloride for the therapy of hot flashes in cancer survivors. J Clin Oncol. 1998;16(7):2377.
16. Loprinzi CL, et al. Venlafaxine in management of hot flashes in survivors of breast cancer: a randomised controlled trial. Lancet. 2000;356(9247):2059–63.
17. Archer DF, et al. A double-blind, randomly assigned, placebo-controlled study of desvenlafaxine efficacy and safety for the treatment of vasomotor symptoms associated with menopause. Am J Obstet Gynecol. 2009;200(2):172 e1–10.
18. Speroff L, et al. Efficacy and tolerability of desvenlafaxine succinate treatment for menopausal vasomotor symptoms: a randomized controlled trial. Obstet Gynecol. 2008;111(1):77–87.
19. Stearns V, et al. Paroxetine controlled release in the treatment of menopausal hot flashes: a randomized controlled trial. JAMA. 2003;289(21):2827–34.
20. Simon JA, et al. Low-dose paroxetine 7.5 mg for menopausal vasomotor symptoms: two randomized controlled trials. Menopause. 2013;20(10):1027–35.
21. Pinkerton JV, et al. Low-dose paroxetine (7.5 mg) improves sleep in women with vasomotor symptoms associated with menopause. Menopause. 2015;22(1):50–8.
22. Grady D, et al. Ineffectiveness of sertraline for treatment of menopausal hot flushes: a randomized controlled trial. Obstet Gynecol. 2007;109(4):823–30.
23. Kerwin JP, Gordon PR, Senf JH. The variable response of women with menopausal hot flashes when treated with sertraline. Menopause. 2007;14(5):841–5.
24. Wu MF, et al. The efficacy of sertraline for controlling hot flashes in women with or at high risk of developing breast cancer. Breast Cancer Res Treat. 2009;118(2):369–75.
25. Kimmick GG, et al. Randomized, double-blind, placebo-controlled, crossover study of sertraline (Zoloft) for the treatment of hot flashes in women with early stage breast cancer taking tamoxifen. Breast J. 2006;12(2):114–22.
26. Shams T, et al. SSRIs for hot flashes: a systematic review and meta-analysis of randomized trials. J Gen Intern Med. 2014;29(1):204–13.
27. Stearns V, et al. Active tamoxifen metabolite plasma concentrations after coadministration of tamoxifen and the selective serotonin reuptake inhibitor paroxetine. J Natl Cancer Inst. 2003;95(23):1758–64.
28. Kelly CM, et al. Selective serotonin reuptake inhibitors and breast cancer mortality in women receiving tamoxifen: a population based cohort study. BMJ. 2010;340:c693.
29. Sanchez-Spitman A, et al. Tamoxifen pharmacogenetics and metabolism: results from the prospective CYPTAM study. Am J Clin Oncol. 2019;37(8):636–+.

30. Jin Y, et al. CYP2D6 genotype, antidepressant use, and tamoxifen metabolism during adjuvant breast cancer treatment. J Natl Cancer Inst. 2005;97(1):30–9.
31. Barton DL, et al. Phase III, placebo-controlled trial of three doses of citalopram for the treatment of hot flashes: NCCTG trial N05C9. J Clin Oncol. 2010;28(20):3278–83.
32. Carvalho AF, et al. The safety, tolerability and risks associated with the use of newer generation antidepressant drugs: a critical review of the literature. Psychother Psychosom. 2016;85(5):270–88.
33. Defronzo Dobkin R, et al. Escitalopram reduces hot flashes in nondepressed menopausal women: a pilot study. Ann Clin Psychiatry. 2009;21(2):70–6.
34. Soares CN, et al. Escitalopram versus ethinyl estradiol and norethindrone acetate for symptomatic peri- and postmenopausal women: impact on depression, vasomotor symptoms, sleep, and quality of life. Menopause. 2006;13(5):780–6.
35. Freeman EW, et al. Efficacy of escitalopram for hot flashes in healthy menopausal women: a randomized controlled trial. JAMA. 2011;305(3):267–74.
36. Bardia A, et al. Efficacy of nonestrogenic hot flash therapies among women stratified by breast cancer history and tamoxifen use: a pooled analysis. Menopause. 2009;16(3):477–83.
37. Guttuso TJ Jr. Gabapentin's effects on hot flashes and hypothermia. Neurology. 2000;54(11):2161–3.
38. Guttuso T Jr, et al. Gabapentin's effects on hot flashes in postmenopausal women: a randomized controlled trial. Obstet Gynecol. 2003;101(2):337–45.
39. Agarwal N, et al. Evaluation of gabapentin in management of hot flushes in postmenopausal women. Post Reprod Health. 2014;20(1):36–8.
40. Butt DA, et al. Gabapentin for the treatment of menopausal hot flashes: a randomized controlled trial. Menopause. 2008;15(2):310–8.
41. Pandya KJ, et al. Gabapentin for hot flashes in 420 women with breast cancer: a randomised double-blind placebo-controlled trial. Lancet. 2005;366(9488):818–24.
42. Pinkerton JV, et al. Phase 3 randomized controlled study of gastroretentive gabapentin for the treatment of moderate-to-severe hot flashes in menopause. Menopause. 2014;21(6):567–73.
43. Sathyanarayana RM, et al. Effect of gabapentin extended-release (G-Er) on hot flashes in postmenopausal women. Menopause-the Journal of the North American Menopause Society. 2010;17(6):1220.
44. Shan D, et al. Efficacy and safety of gabapentin and pregabalin in patients with vasomotor symptoms: a systematic review and meta-analysis. Am J Obstet Gynecol. 2020;222(6):564–579.e12.
45. Goodman CW, Brett AS. Gabapentinoids for pain: potential unintended consequences. Am Fam Physician. 2019;100(11):672–5.
46. Loprinzi CL, et al. Phase III, randomized, double-blind, placebo-controlled evaluation of pregabalin for alleviating hot flashes, N07C1. J Clin Oncol. 2010;28(4):641–7.
47. Loprinzi CL, et al. Phase III trial of gabapentin alone or in conjunction with an antidepressant in the management of hot flashes in women who have inadequate control with an antidepressant alone: NCCTG N03C5. J Clin Oncol. 2007;25(3):308–12.
48. LeWitt P. Hyperhidrosis and hypothermia responsive to oxybutynin. Neurology. 1988;38(3):506–7.
49. Tupker RA, Harmsze AM, Deneer VH. Oxybutynin therapy for generalized hyperhidrosis. Arch Dermatol. 2006;142(8):1065–6.
50. Sexton T, et al. Oxybutynin for refractory hot flashes in cancer patients. Menopause. 2007;14(3 Pt 1):505–9.
51. Simon JA, et al. Extended-release oxybutynin therapy for vasomotor symptoms in women: a randomized clinical trial. Menopause. 2016;23(11):1214–21.
52. Leon-Ferre RA, et al. A randomized, doubleblind, placebo-controlled trial of oxybutynin (Oxy) for hot flashes (HF): ACCRU study SC-1603. Cancer Res. 2019;79(4). https://pubmed.ncbi.nlm.nih.gov/32337497/
53. Wolosker N, et al. Long-term results of the use of oxybutynin for the treatment of axillary hyperhidrosis. Ann Vasc Surg. 2014;28(5):1106–12.
54. Ouslander JG, et al. Pharmacokinetics and clinical effects of oxybutynin in geriatric patients. J Urol. 1988;140(1):47–50.
55. Yarker YE, Goa KL, Fitton A. Oxybutynin. A review of its pharmacodynamic and pharmacokinetic properties, and its therapeutic use in detrusor instability. Drugs Aging. 1995;6(3):243–62.
56. Maclennan AH, et al. Oral oestrogen and combined oestrogen/progestogen therapy versus placebo for hot flushes. Cochrane Database Syst Rev. 2004;4:CD002978.
57. Loprinzi CL, et al. Megestrol acetate for the prevention of hot flashes. N Engl J Med. 1994;331(6):347–52.
58. Quella SK, et al. Long term use of megestrol acetate by cancer survivors for the treatment of hot flashes. Cancer. 1998;82(9):1784.
59. Bertelli G, et al. Intramuscular depot medroxyprogesterone versus oral megestrol for the control of postmenopausal hot flashes in breast cancer patients: a randomized study. Ann Oncol. 2002;13(6):883–8.
60. Loprinzi CL, et al. Phase III comparison of depomedroxyprogesterone acetate to venlafaxine for managing hot flashes: North Central Cancer Treatment Group Trial N99C7. J Clin Oncol. 2006;24(9):1409–14.
61. Ertz-Archambault NM, et al. Depomedroxyprogesterone acetate therapy for hot flashes in survivors of breast cancer: no unfavorable impact on recurrence and survival. Support Care Cancer. 2020;28(5):2139–43.
62. Chlebowski RT, et al. Association of menopausal hormone therapy with breast cancer incidence and mortality during long-term follow-up of the women's health initiative randomized clinical trials. JAMA. 2020;324(4):369–80. https://doi.

org/10.1001/jama.2020.9482. PMID: 32721007; PMCID: PMC7388026.
63. Goldberg RM, et al. Transdermal clonidine for ameliorating tamoxifen-induced hot flashes. J Clin Oncol. 1994;12(1):155–8.
64. Pandya KJ, et al. Oral clonidine in postmenopausal patients with breast cancer experiencing tamoxifen-induced hot flashes: a University of Rochester Cancer Center Community Clinical Oncology Program study. Ann Intern Med. 2000;132(10):788–93.
65. Elkins G, et al. Randomized trial of a hypnosis intervention for treatment of hot flashes among breast cancer survivors. J Clin Oncol. 2008;26(31):5022–6.
66. Elkins GR, et al. Clinical hypnosis in the treatment of postmenopausal hot flashes: a randomized controlled trial. Menopause. 2013;20(3):291–8.
67. Barton DL, et al. Efficacy of a biobehavioral intervention for hot flashes: a randomized controlled pilot study. Menopause. 2017;24(7):774–82.
68. Alba E, et al. Weekly first-line chemotherapy of metastatic breast cancer with cyclophosphamide and epirubicin. Tumori. 1992;78:338.
69. Walega DR, et al. Effects of stellate ganglion block on vasomotor symptoms: findings from a randomized controlled clinical trial in postmenopausal women. Menopause. 2014;21(8):807–14.
70. Rahimzadeh P, et al. Comparison of the effects of stellate ganglion block and paroxetine on hot flashes and sleep disturbance in breast cancer survivors. Cancer Manag Res. 2018;10:4831–7.
71. Othman AH, Zaky AH. Management of hot flushes in breast cancer survivors: comparison between stellate ganglion block and pregabalin. Pain Med. 2014;15(3):410–7.
72. Vincent A, et al. Acupuncture for hot flashes: a randomized, sham-controlled clinical study. Menopause. 2007;14(1):45–52.
73. Zhang CS, et al. Placebo devices as effective control methods in acupuncture clinical trials: a systematic review. PLoS One, 2015;10(11).
74. Walker EM, et al. Acupuncture versus venlafaxine for the management of vasomotor symptoms in patients with hormone receptor-positive breast cancer: a randomized controlled trial. J Clin Oncol. 2010;28(4):634–40.
75. Dodin S, et al. Acupuncture for menopausal hot flushes. Cochrane Database Syst Rev. 2013;(7):CD007410.
76. Shils ME, Shike M. Modern nutrition in health and disease. 10th ed. Philadelphia: Lippincott Williams & Wilkins; 2006. p. xxv, 2069 p.
77. Barton DL, et al. Prospective evaluation of vitamin E for hot flashes in breast cancer survivors. J Clin Oncol. 1998;16(2):495–500.
78. Ziaei S, Kazemnejad A, Zareai M. The effect of vitamin E on hot flashes in menopausal women. Gynecol Obstet Investig. 2007;64(4):204–7.
79. Upmalis DH, et al. Vasomotor symptom relief by soy isoflavone extract tablets in postmenopausal women: a multicenter, double-blind, randomized, placebo-controlled study. Menopause. 2000;7(4):236–42.
80. MacGregor CA, et al. A randomised double-blind controlled trial of oral soy supplements versus placebo for treatment of menopausal symptoms in patients with early breast cancer. Eur J Cancer. 2005;41(5):708–14.
81. Quella SK, et al. Evaluation of soy phytoestrogens for the treatment of hot flashes in breast cancer survivors: a North Central Cancer Treatment Group Trial. J Clin Oncol. 2000;18(5):1068–74.
82. Van Patten CL, et al. Effect of soy phytoestrogens on hot flashes in postmenopausal women with breast cancer: a randomized, controlled clinical trial. J Clin Oncol. 2002;20(6):1449–55.
83. Levis S, et al. Soy isoflavones in the prevention of menopausal bone loss and menopausal symptoms: a randomized, double-blind trial. Arch Intern Med. 2011;171(15):1363–9.
84. Lethaby A, et al. Phytoestrogens for menopausal vasomotor symptoms. Cochrane Database Syst Rev. 2013;(12):CD001395.
85. Leach MJ, Moore V. Black cohosh (Cimicifuga spp.) for menopausal symptoms. Cochrane Database Syst Rev. 2012;(9):CD007244.
86. Pruthi S, et al. Pilot evaluation of flaxseed for the management of hot flashes. J Soc Integr Oncol. 2007;5(3):106–12.
87. Pruthi S, et al. A phase III, randomized, placebo-controlled, double-blind trial of flaxseed for the treatment of hot flashes: North Central Cancer Treatment Group N08C7. Menopause. 2012;19(1):48–53.
88. Smith TJ. Magnesium supplements for menopausal hot flashes. J Clin Oncol. 2009;27(7):1151–2.
89. Herrada J, et al. Oral magnesium oxide for treatment of hot flashes in women undergoing treatment for breast cancer: a pilot study. J Clin Oncol. 2010;28(15). https://ascopubs.org/doi/abs/10.1200/jco.2010.28.15_suppl.e19530.
90. Park H, et al. A pilot phase II trial of magnesium supplements to reduce menopausal hot flashes in breast cancer patients. Support Care Cancer. 2011;19(6):859–63.
91. Park H, et al. North Central Cancer Treatment Group N10C2 (Alliance): a double-blind placebo-controlled study of magnesium supplements to reduce menopausal hot flashes. Menopause. 2015;22(6):627–32.
92. Loprinzi CL, et al. Pilot evaluation of paroxetine for treating hot flashes in men. Mayo Clin Proc. 2004;79(10):1247–51.
93. Quella SK, et al. Pilot evaluation of venlafaxine for the treatment of hot flashes in men undergoing androgen ablation therapy for prostate cancer. J Urol. 1999;162(1):98–102.
94. Vitolins MZ, et al. Randomized trial to assess the impact of venlafaxine and soy protein on hot flashes and quality of life in men with prostate cancer. J Clin Oncol. 2013;31(32):4092–8.

95. Loprinzi CL, et al. A phase III randomized, double-blind, placebo-controlled trial of gabapentin in the management of hot flashes in men (N00CB). Ann Oncol. 2009;20(3):542–9.
96. Irani J, et al. Efficacy of venlafaxine, medroxyprogesterone acetate, and cyproterone acetate for the treatment of vasomotor hot flushes in men taking gonadotropin-releasing hormone analogues for prostate cancer: a double-blind, randomised trial. Lancet Oncol. 2010;11(2):147–54.
97. Loprinzi CL, et al. Transdermal clonidine for ameliorating post-orchiectomy hot flashes. J Urol. 1994;151(3):634–6.
98. Smith TJ, Loprinzi CL, Deville C. Oxybutynin for hot flashes due to androgen deprivation in men. N Engl J Med. 2018;378(18):1745–6.

Management of Genital Symptoms

4

Annabelle Brennan, Charles L. Loprinzi,
and Martha Hickey

Introduction

Breast cancer continues to affect growing numbers of women globally, with over two million women affected each year [1]. As treatments have become more effective, survival rates have increased, making survivorship issues affecting quality of life increasingly important. Menopausal symptoms are a significant survivorship issue for many breast cancer patients, in particular, vasomotor symptoms (hot flashes and night sweats) and genitourinary symptoms such as vaginal dryness, genital discomfort and pain during sexual activity. While menopausal symptoms are not always bothersome, these may significantly affect physical, mental, and sexual wellbeing. Breast cancer survivors pose a unique dilemma for menopause symptom management as systemic estrogen-based therapies are avoided after breast cancer, even in estrogen receptor-negative disease. This chapter will outline the nature of genitourinary symptoms in breast cancer survivors and the importance of recognizing these symptoms and discuss the options for safe and effective therapies. The topic of vasomotor symptoms will be covered in other chapters of this book.

A. Brennan (✉)
Royal Women's Hospital, Melbourne, VIC, Australia

C. L. Loprinzi
Department of Oncology, Mayo Clinic,
Rochester, MN, USA

M. Hickey
University of Melbourne, Royal Women's Hospital,
Melbourne, VIC, Australia

Genitourinary Symptoms Associated with Menopause and Their Significance

Physiology

Genitourinary symptoms associated with menopause include vulvovaginal discomfort associated with dryness or pain, dyspareunia and urinary symptoms such as dysuria [2]. The physiological decrease in circulating estrogen in postmenopausal women results in a reduction in both vaginal epithelial blood flow and collagen synthesis. Impaired vaginal vascularity results in epithelial atrophy, causing both reduced vaginal secretions and an increased vaginal pH, from a lack of glycogen availability for the dominant vaginal lactobacillus. Ultimately, these changes result in a shorter, more inelastic vagina with a thinner and potentially more fragile epithelium [3].

Prevalence and Significance

Following breast cancer, women may report genitourinary symptoms after premenopausal bilateral oophorectomy, chemotherapy-induced ovarian failure and cessation of menopausal hormone therapy or endocrine therapy [4–6]. While not all menopausal symptoms require treatment,

G. G. Kimmick et al. (eds.), *Common Issues in Breast Cancer Survivors*,
https://doi.org/10.1007/978-3-030-75377-1_4

breast cancer survivors report a higher symptom prevalence compared to non-cancer patients and greater levels of distress [7]. The burgeoning number of breast cancer survivors means that safe and effective treatments for these symptoms are of growing importance.

Genitourinary symptoms associated with menopause may also involve sexual dysfunction, related to both the physical and psychological implications of a cancer diagnosis. In addition to the physical impact of changing estrogen exposure on the genitals, breast cancer treatment may also affect sexual wellbeing through changes to libido associated with medications, physical changes associated with treatment including mastectomy, concurrent psychological illness such as anxiety or depression and/or relationship changes.

Identification of Symptoms

Given the prevalence of genitourinary symptoms among breast cancer patients and the potential impact on quality of life, recognition of these symptoms is the first important step in providing comprehensive care. However, there are multiple patient and clinician factors impacting the provision of targeted care of genitourinary symptoms in breast cancer patients. Patients may be reluctant to raise these issues and associated sexual dysfunction with their care providers. This discomfort may be related to the intimate nature of the symptoms as well as potential feelings of guilt from prioritizing sexual wellbeing during cancer treatment [8].

Clinicians report feeling time pressured in short consultations where significant issues and urgent treatment need to be discussed [9, 10]. Furthermore, there is uncertainty about who is responsible for managing menopausal symptoms, highlighting the need for multidisciplinary, holistic care with open communication between all team members [5].

Comprehensive, patient-centered care should involve a thorough history and examination, pre-treatment counseling and post-treatment symptom review [5]. Appropriate gynecological history and examination should include a menstrual and sexual history, particularly the presence of any pre-treatment genitourinary symptoms and pre-existing vulval dermatoses. Conditions likely to flare during periods of immunosuppression should also be noted, including cervical dysplasia, condyloma and herpes simplex [11]. The gynecological impact of breast cancer treatment should be discussed including the likelihood and nature of genitourinary symptoms, as well as fertility implications for younger premenopausal patients.

All clinicians involved in cancer care should be encouraged to facilitate ongoing discussions about genitourinary symptoms and sexual wellbeing with patients, using supportive communication and open-ended questions. These discussions may be facilitated through the use of validated tools to assess symptom impact on quality of life. A range of tools have been validated across various cancer streams, with some of the most commonly used among women including the Day-to-Day Impact of Vaginal Aging Questionnaire [12], the Sexual Symptom Checklist for Women After Cancer [13], the Fallowfield Sexual Activity Questionnaire [14] and the PROMIS Sexual Function and Satisfaction [15], briefly outlined in Table 4.1. These tools allow the identification of significant symptoms, evaluation of their impact on quality of life, and assessment of treatment efficacy. Clinician-led discussions encourage patients to address these issues, facilitating open and honest communication and optimizing patient care.

Management

While vaginal estrogen has been shown to be the most effective treatment for vaginal dryness in the general menopausal population [16, 17], the safety of vaginal estrogen after breast cancer is not established [18]. Consequently, the management of genitourinary symptoms will often

Table 4.1 Various tools for the assessment of genitourinary symptoms

Tool	Validated in cancer patients	Symptoms	Review period	Strength
Day-to-day impact of vaginal aging questionnaire	No	Impact of vaginal symptoms on daily life	30-day recall	Broad impact examined including emotional wellbeing and body image
PROMIS sexual function and satisfaction	Yes	Sexual activity and function	30-day recall	Customizable to include domains of greatest relevance and available in other languages
Fallowfield sexual activity questionnaire	Yes	Sexual activity and function	30-day recall	Thorough symptom review and widely used
Sexual symptom checklist for women after Cancer	Yes	Sexual activity and function	30-day recall	Easy to administer and quickly identifies most bothersome symptoms

require a multidisciplinary and patient-centered approach involving appropriate counseling and patient education, to enable shared decision making. In addition to conservative management, pharmacological treatments include both non-hormonal and hormonal options, outlined below.

Non-hormonal

Lubricants and Moisturizers

There is a range of vaginal moisturizers and lubricants that have been marketed to reduce genitourinary symptoms. However, there is a lack of high-level evidence supporting the use of any particular product. Vaginal moisturizers should be applied regularly if utilized, and while they may offer a small improvement in symptoms, recent evidence has failed to demonstrate an advantage over placebo in the treatment of genitourinary symptoms of menopause [17]. It is important to note that this recent trial found that neither vaginal moisturizer nor prescribed vaginal estradiol tablet significantly reduced vulvovaginal symptoms compared to placebo. Some women may prefer to trial vaginal moisturizers initially prior to considering use of hormonal treatment.

Lubricants may be silicone-, water- or oil-based and aim to reduce pain and discomfort associated with penetrative intercourse. While high-level comparative data are lacking, one small randomized controlled trial demonstrated some superiority of silicone-based lubricants in reducing discomfort and patient preference for these products [19]. Lubricant may also be used in conjunction with topical lidocaine applied to the vaginal vestibule prior to intercourse, which has been shown to reduce dyspareunia and improve sexual function in breast cancer survivors [20].

There is growing interest in hyaluronic acid vaginal cream, which several small studies have shown to be as effective as vaginal estrogen in reducing vaginal dryness, itching and dyspareunia [21–23]. However, while it may be a useful non-hormonal option, more high-level research is needed regarding its safety, including long-term outcomes as well as its use in the cancer population.

Vaginal Dilators and Pelvic Floor Therapy

Graduated vaginal dilators can be used to gently stretch the vagina over time and assist with the return of comfortable penetrative intercourse, if desired [24]. Their use may also be supported by a pelvic floor physiotherapist to aid in pelvic muscle relaxation associated with painful intercourse [25]. Recent preliminary data demonstrated an intensive program of pelvic floor therapy, including both supervised and independent practice for 12 weeks, was effective in reducing genitourinary symptoms and had positive impact on quality of life and sexual function [26]. There is evidence to suggest that these conservative measures work in a complementary manner to improve symptoms, but they do require continued participation [27].

Vaginal Laser

The two laser types that have been studied in the gynecological context are the microablative carbon dioxide laser and the nonablative erbium laser. Laser treatment aims to stimulate vascularity and promote collagen synthesis, thereby supporting vaginal epithelial tissue. One recent small trial suggested short-term efficacy similar to vaginal estrogen but excluded women with a history of hormone-sensitive malignancies [28]. Retrospective studies evaluating the use of monthly laser treatment in breast cancer patients with genitourinary symptoms have reported a significant reduction in symptoms, particularly dyspareunia and dryness, by up to 80% after three treatments [29, 30]. Further trials are underway with high level evidence on the safety and quality of vaginal laser awaited.

However, potential adverse events such as vaginal burns, scarring, or pain are noted by the FDA, and long-term safety data is lacking. Large randomized controlled trials should be undertaken to confirm both treatment efficacy and long-term safety, particularly in the cancer population, before routine recommendation can be made.

Selective Estrogen Receptor Modulators (SERM)

Ospemifene is a SERM approved for use in the treatment of dyspareunia associated with menopause. While it appears to exert estrogenic effects on the vagina [31], its safety in women with a history of breast cancer has not been established, and it is therefore not currently approved for use in this population.

Hormonal

Systemic Hormone Replacement Therapy (HRT)

The general approach to breast cancer management has been to minimize circulating estrogen levels to prevent the proliferation of breast cancer cells, reducing cancer progression and the risk of recurrence. Consequently, international guidance recommends against the use of systemic HRT in breast cancer survivors [2, 32, 33]. This is especially true of HRT regimens that contain both estrogen and progesterone [34, 35].

Vaginal Estrogen

Vaginal estrogen targets the local (vaginal) area, but there is also a small amount of systemic absorption. The degree of systemic absorption of local therapy depends on a range of factors including the potency and amount of active ingredient used, tissue integrity and mode of application. Circulating concentrations of estrogens with local therapy are substantially lower than systemic hormone therapy and appear to decrease over time. One prospective study of vaginal estrogen in breast cancer survivors taking aromatase inhibitors showed no increase after 12 weeks of vaginal estrogen use compared to baseline levels [36]. The clinical implications of these small increases in circulating estrogens are unclear [37].

Moreover, while randomized data is lacking, observational data from several large studies have not shown an increase in breast cancer with use of vaginal estrogen therapy [38–40]. Crandall et al. used data from over 45,000 women in the Women's Health Initiative Observational Study, although excluded women with a personal history of breast cancer [39]. Le Ray et al. included over 13,000 women specifically evaluating the risk of breast cancer recurrence [40]. Average follow-up in these studies was between 3 and 6 years, so more longer-term follow-up data would be useful.

Consequently, consensus suggests the consideration of vaginal estrogen for women after breast cancer with troublesome genitourinary symptoms not responding to non-hormonal treatment [2, 18, 41]. These treatment decisions should involve multidisciplinary discussions with members of the treating team and adequate patient education regarding current evidence base and risk profile to allow informed and shared decision-making. Relevant considerations may include the grade and stage of cancer, time since diagnosis, hormone receptor status and current treatment including ovarian suppression, aromatase inhibitors or a SERM such as tamoxifen.

This approach may be particularly reasonable in patients with hormone receptor-negative cancers and in patients on tamoxifen, where there is competition for the estrogen receptor [2]. Vaginal estrogen use is harder to support in women on aromatase inhibitors, which are designed to decrease estrogen levels. However, these women often have the most severe genital symptoms. As with any pharmacological intervention, treatment should aim for use of the lowest dose and shortest duration needed to manage symptoms, which requires ongoing monitoring.

There are a range of estrogenic products available including vaginal creams, pessaries and rings, depending on the country of treatment. It is important to review clinical guidance for up-to-date dosages, but international guidelines offer the following clinical practice guidance [2, 18]: There is no strong evidence that one vaginal estrogen product is safer or more effective than another.

- 17ß-estradiol cream: 2 g daily for 1–2 weeks followed by 0.5–1 g twice weekly
- Conjugated equine estrogen cream: continuous use of 0.5 g twice weekly, or cyclical treatment 21 days 0.5 g daily followed by 7 days off
- 17ß-estradiol ring: 2 mg ring for 90 days, releases 7.5μg per day
- Estradiol hemihydrate vaginal tablet: 10μg tablet daily for 2 weeks followed by 10μg tablet twice weekly

Vaginal DHEA and Testosterone

Dehydroepiandrosterone (DHEA) is a steroid in the pathway of testosterone and estradiol production. Vaginal administration has been shown to improve genitourinary symptoms and sexual function via local conversion into testosterone and estradiol and has been approved by the FDA [42, 43]. However, long-term safety is unknown after breast cancer. There have been no head-to-head trials comparing vaginal DHEA and estrogen use in breast cancer survivors. Use of vaginal testosterone is not currently recommended [44]. The peripheral conversion of testosterone into estradiol via aromatase activity has been demonstrated even in patients taking aromatase inhibitors, and there are no approved formulations for use in women.

Conclusions

Genitourinary symptoms including vaginal dryness, itch and dyspareunia arising in the menopausal period are more common in breast cancer survivors. These symptoms may result from surgical menopause, chemoradiation or ongoing medical treatment with aromatase inhibitors or SERMs. With increasing survival rates, survivorship issues such as the management of genitourinary symptoms are becoming increasingly important to improve quality of life after cancer.

A major barrier in the treatment of these symptoms is the recognition of their presence. Comprehensive, patient-centered care demands open discussions between patients and their clinicians to identify and effectively treat genitourinary symptoms after cancer. There are a range of validated tools to assist clinicians with these discussions and monitor response to treatment.

The management of these symptoms requires a multidisciplinary and patient-centered approach involving appropriate counseling and patient education to enable shared decision making. All members of the treating team should be involved in these decisions including oncologists, gynecologists, general practitioners and cancer nurses.

Practice Points

- Use open-ended questions and supportive language to enquire about genitourinary symptoms in breast cancer survivors.
- First-line treatment should involve non-hormonal conservative management including vaginal moisturizers, lubricants, vaginal dilators, and physical therapy with pelvic floor muscle relaxation techniques.
- Vaginal estrogen may be considered as a second-line treatment for women with significant symptoms not responding to first-line treatments. This should be done in consulta-

tion with the treating oncologist and ensuring appropriate patient education to allow shared decision making.

- Long-term safety data in the breast cancer-specific population should be undertaken for other available treatments including vaginal laser therapy and vaginal DHEA.

References

1. The World Health Organization: breast cancer. 2020. https://www.who.int/cancer/prevention/diagnosis-screening/breast-cancer/en/. Accessed 14 Apr 2020.
2. North American Menopause Society. Management of genitourinary syndrome of menopause in women with or at high risk for breast cancer: consensus recommendations from The North American Menopause Society and The International Society for the Study of Women's Sexual Health. Menopause. 2018;25(6):1–13.
3. Melmed S, Auchus RJ, Goldfine AB, Koenig RJ, Rosen CJ. Williams textbook of endocrinology. 14th ed. Philadelphia: Elsevier; 2020. p. 634.
4. Marino JL, Saunders CM, Emery LI, et al. Nature and severity of menopausal symptoms and their impact on quality of life and sexual function in cancer survivors compared with women without a cancer history. Menopause. 2014;21(3):267–74.
5. Szabo R, Marino JL, Hickey M. Managing menopausal symptoms after cancer. Climacteric. 2019;22(6):572–8.
6. Sousa MS, Peate M, Jarvis S, et al. A clinical guide to the management of genitourinary symptoms in breast cancer survivors on endocrine therapy. Ther Adv Med Oncol. 2017;9(4):269–85.
7. Schover LR, Baum GP, Fuson LA, Brewster A, Melhem-Bertrandt A. Sexual problems during the first 2 years of adjuvant treatment with aromatase inhibitors. J Sex Med. 2014;11:3102–11.
8. Brennan A, Hickey M. A GP'S guide to talking about cancer. *AusDoc.Plus*. 2019. April.
9. Park ER, Bober SL, Campbell EG, et al. General internist communication about sexual function with cancer survivors. J Gen Intern Med. 2009;24:S407–11.
10. Wiggins DL, Wood R, Granai CO, et al. Sex, intimacy, and the gynecologic oncologists: survey results of the New England Association of Gynecologic Oncologists (NEAGO). J Psychosoc Oncol. 2007;25:61–70.
11. Brennan A, Hickey M. Gynaecological care after stem cell transplant: an overview. Maturitas. 2017;105:30–2.
12. Huang AJ, Gregorich SE, Kuppermann M, et al. Day-to-day impact of vaginal aging questionnaire: a multidimensional measure of the impact of vaginal symptoms on functioning and well-being in postmenopausal women. Menopause. 2015;22:144–54.
13. Bober SL, Reese JB, Barbera L, et al. How to ask and what to do: a guide for clinical inquiry and intervention regarding female sexual health after cancer. Curr Opin Support Palliat Care. 2016;10:44–54.
14. Atkins L, Fallowfield LJ. Fallowfield's sexual activity questionnaire in women with without and at risk of cancer. Menopause Int. 2007;13(3):103–9.
15. Flynn KE, Lin L, Cyranowski JM, et al. Development of the NIH PROMIS sexual function and satisfaction measures in patient's with cancer. J Sex Med. 2013;10(0 1):43–52.
16. Lethaby A, Ayeleke R, Roberts H. Local oestrogen for vaginal atrophy in postmenopausal women. Cochrane Database Syst Rev. 2016;(8):CD001500.
17. Mitchell CM, Reed SD, Larson JC, et al. Efficacy of vaginal estradiol or vaginal moisturizer vs placebo for treating postmenopausal vulvovaginal symptoms: a randomized clinical trial. JAMA Intern Med. 2018;178(5):681–90.
18. ACOG, Committee Opinion: The use of vaginal estrogen in women with a history of estrogen-dependent breast cancer. Obstet Gynecol. 2016;127(3):e93–e96.
19. Hickey M, Marino JL, Braat S, et al. A randomized, double-blind, crossover trial comparing a silicone- versus water-based lubricant for sexual discomfort after breast cancer. Breast Cancer Res Treat. 2016;158(1):79–90.
20. Goetsch MF, Lim JY, Caughey AB. A practical solution for dyspareunia in breast cancer survivors: a randomized controlled trial. J Clin Oncol. 2015;33(30):3394–400.
21. Jokar A, et al. Comparison of the hyaluronic acid vaginal cream and conjugated estrogen used in treatment of vaginal atrophy of menopause women: a randomized controlled clinical trial. Int J Community Based Nurs Midwifery. 2016;4(1):69–78.
22. Chen J, et al. Evaluation of the efficacy and safety of hyaluronic acid vaginal gel to ease vaginal dryness: a multicenter, randomized, controlled, open-label, parallel-group, clinical trial. J Sex Med. 2013;10(6):1575–84.
23. Stute P. Is vaginal hyaluronic acid as effective as vaginal estriol for vaginal dryness relief? Arch Gynecol Obstet. 2013;288(6):1199–201.
24. Management of symptomatic vulvovaginal atrophy: 2013 position statement of The North American Menopause Society. Menopause. 2013;20:888–902.
25. Faubion SS, Shuster LT, Bharucha AE. Recognition and management of nonrelaxing pelvic floor dysfunction. Mayo Clin Proc. 2012;87:187–93.
26. Mercier J, Morin M, Zaki D, et al. Pelvic floor muscle training as a treatment for genitourinary syndrome of menopause: a single-arm feasibility study. Maturitas. 2015;125:57–62.
27. Carter J, Stabile C, Seidel B, et al. Vaginal and sexual health treatment strategies within a female sexual medicine program for cancer patients and survivors. J Cancer Surviv. 2017;11(2):274–83.
28. Paraiso MFR, Ferrando CA, Sokol ER, et al. A randomized clinical trial comparing vaginal laser therapy

to vaginal estrogen therapy in women with genitourinary syndrome of menopause: the VeLVET trial. Menopause. 2020;27(1):50–6.
29. Pagano T, De Rosa P, Vallone R, et al. Fractional microablative CO_2 laser for vulvovaginal atrophy in women treated with chemotherapy and/or hormonal therapy for breast cancer: a retrospective study. Menopause. 2016;23(10):1108–13.
30. Gambacciani M, Levancini M. Vaginal erbium laser as second-generation thermotherapy for the genitourinary syndrome of menopause: a pilot study in breast cancer survivors. Menopause. 2016;24(3):316–9.
31. Shin JJ, Kim SK, Lee JR, Suh CS. Ospemifene: a novel option for the treatment of vulvovaginal atrophy. J Menopausal Med. 2017;23(2):79–84.
32. SOGC. Use of hormonal replacement therapy after treatment of breast cancer. Int J Gynaecol Obstet. 2005;88:216–21.
33. Management of Menopause After Cancer. Royal Australian and New Zealand College of Obstetricians and Gynaecologists. 2020. https://ranzcog.edu.au/RANZCOG_SITE/media/RANZCOG-MEDIA/Women%27s%20Health/Statement%20and%20guidelines/Clinical%20-%20Gynaecology/Management-of-the-Menopause-after-Breast-Cancer-(C-Gyn-15)-Review-November-2014_1.pdf?ext=.pdf. Accessed 15 Apr 2020.
34. Chlebowski RT, Rohan TE, Manson JE, et al. Breast cancer after use of estrogen plus progestin and estrogen alone: analyses of data from 2 Women's Health Initiative randomized clinical trials. JAMA Oncol. 2015;1:296.
35. Manson JE, Chlebowski RT, Stefanick ML, et al. Menopausal hormone therapy and health outcomes during the intervention and extended poststopping phases of the Women's Health Initiative randomized trials. JAMA. 2013;310:1353.
36. Melisko ME, Goldman ME, Hwang J, et al. Vaginal testosterone cream vs estradiol vaginal ring for vaginal dryness or decreased libido in women receiving aromatase inhibitors for early-stage breast cancer: a randomized clinical trial. JAMA Oncol. 2017;3(3):313–9.
37. Wills S, Ravipati A, Venuturumilli P, et al. Effects of vaginal estrogens on serum estradiol levels in postmenopausal breast cancer survivors and women at risk of breast cancer taking an aromatase inhibitor or a selective estrogen receptor modulator. J Oncol Pract. 2012;8:144–8.
38. Lyytinen H, Pukkala E, Ylikorkala O. Breast cancer risk in postmenopausal women using estrogen-only therapy. Obstet Gynecol. 2006;108:1354–60.
39. Crandall CJ, Hovey KM, Andrews CA, et al. Breast cancer, endometrial cancer, and cardiovascular events in participants who used vaginal estrogen in the Women's Health Initiative Observational Study. Menopause. 2018;25:11–20.
40. Le Ray I, Dell'Aniello S, Bonnetain F, et al. Local estrogen therapy and risk of breast cancer recurrence among hormone- treated patients: a nested case-control study. Breast Cancer Res Treat. 2012;135:603–9.
41. Management of Menopause After Cancer. Royal Australian and New Zealand College of Obstetricians and Gynaecologists. 2020. https://ranzcog.edu.au/RANZCOG_SITE/media/RANZCOG-MEDIA/Women%27s%20Health/Statement%20and%20guidelines/Clinical%20-%20Gynaecology/Management-of-the-Menopause-after-Breast-Cancer-(C-Gyn-15)-Review-November-2014_1.pdf?ext=.pdf. Accessed 15 April 2020.
42. Barton DL, Sloan JA, Shuster LT, et al. Evaluating the efficacy of vaginal dehydroepiandosterone for vaginal symptoms in postmenopausal cancer survivors. Support Care Cancer. 2018;26:643–50.
43. Bouchard C, Labrie F, Derogatis L, et al.; VVA Prasterone Group. Effect of intravaginal dehydroepiandrosterone (dhea) on the female sexual function in postmenopausal women: ERC-230 open-label study. Horm Mol Biol Clin Invest. 2016;25:181–90.
44. Davis SR, Baber R, Panay N, et al. Global consensus position statement on the use of testosterone therapy for women. J Clin Endocrinol Metab. 2019;104(10):4660–6.

5 Sexual and Reproductive Health Concerns

Rebecca A. Shelby, Jessica N. Coleman, Sarah S. Arthur, Kelly S. Acharya, Amanda A. Heath, Margaret D. Flather, Kelly E. Westbrook, and Caroline S. Dorfman

According to the World Health Organization, sexual health is "a state of physical, emotional, mental and social well-being in relation to sexuality; it is not merely the absence of disease, dysfunction or infirmity." [1] Sexual and reproductive health can be profoundly impacted by breast cancer diagnosis and treatments [2, 3]. Rates of sexual dysfunction are significantly higher among breast cancer survivors compared to rates among similarly aged women without a cancer history [3–7]. Among breast cancer survivors, 32–93% of women report sexual problems [6, 8, 9] and 27% to 88% report body image concerns [10]. For women of reproductive age, treatments for breast cancer may also negatively impact fertility [11]. Breast cancer treatment-related changes in sexual and reproductive health are associated with significant distress and often negatively impact women's emotional well-being, relationships, sense of self, and overall quality of life [10, 12–15]. The biopsychosocial approach (see Fig. 5.1) to understanding and treating sexual problems highlights the complex interplay among the biological (e.g., body changes, hormonal alterations, pain), psychological (e.g., emotional distress, perceptions of body and self), interpersonal (e.g., relationship dynamics and quality, communication difficulties), and socio-cultural (e.g., cultural norms, religious influences, background or upbringing) factors that contribute to sexual function and well-being [16]. Because sexuality and the implications of sexual problems are complex, a multidisciplinary approach is often required to address the multiple facets that can affect and are affected by sexual and reproductive health changes. This chapter provides information regarding female sexual response, the impacts of breast cancer treatments on sexual function, approaches for assessment and evaluation of sexual problems, strategies for managing sexual problems, and the management of fertility concerns among breast cancer survivors. Routinely asking about sexual problems and facilitating appropriate referral and treatment for sexual difficulties demonstrates that sexuality is

R. A. Shelby (✉)
Department of Psychiatry and Behavioral Sciences, Duke University, Durham, NC, USA
e-mail: Rebecca.shelby@duke.edu

J. N. Coleman · S. S. Arthur
Department of Psychology and Neuroscience, Duke University, Durham, NC, USA

K. S. Acharya
Department of Obstetrics and Gynecology, Duke University, Durham, NC, USA

A. A. Heath
Department of Physical Therapy and Occupational Therapy, Duke University, Durham, NC, USA

M. D. Flather
Department of Gynecology, Augusta Health, Fishersville, VA, USA

K. E. Westbrook
Department of Medicine, Division of Medical Oncology, Duke University, Durham, NC, USA

C. S. Dorfman
Department of Psychiatry and Behavioral Sciences, Duke University Medical Center, Durham, NC, USA

G. G. Kimmick et al. (eds.), *Common Issues in Breast Cancer Survivors*,
https://doi.org/10.1007/978-3-030-75377-1_5

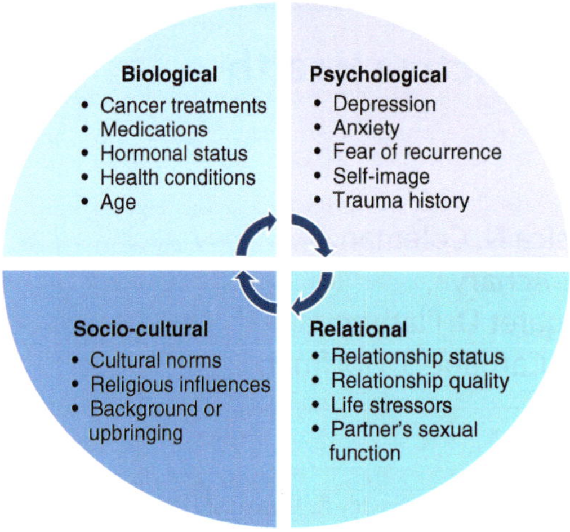

Fig. 5.1 Biopsychosocial factors impacting sexual function

recognized as an important and valued aspect of a woman's health and well-being.

Female Sexual Function

Beginning with the work of Masters and Johnson in the 1960s, researchers have been working to understand the interrelated physiological stages of female sexual response [17–19]. Although research is ongoing and a full consensus on these stages is yet to be reached, the following are the most consistently agreed upon components of typical human sexual response:

- Desire or interest
- Physiologic arousal
- Orgasm
- Resolution

Breast cancer survivors can experience disruptions in all aspects of sexual response [10]. Many breast cancer survivors (39–71%) report experiencing a significant decline in sexual desire after cancer treatment [7, 10, 20, 21], with approximately 35% reporting no interest in sex [5, 22]. Difficulty experiencing subjective arousal and problems with lubrication are extremely common (up to 74% of women) [7, 20, 21], especially among breast cancer survivors treated with chemotherapies or endocrine therapies [13]. Problems experiencing sexual pleasure are frequently reported (64% to 77% of breast cancer survivors) [20, 23], with a significant proportion of breast cancer survivors experiencing difficulty with orgasm (e.g., 42% of women met criteria for orgasmic dysfunction in a study of early-stage breast cancer survivors) [7]. Many breast cancer survivors report decreased sexual satisfaction [20, 23, 24]. Disruptions in the sexual response cycle may contribute to significant declines in sexual activity reported by women following breast cancer (e.g., 75%) [20, 23], with almost 30% of breast cancer survivors reporting no engagement in sexual activity [6, 8, 9, 21, 22].

Box 5.1 Description of terms

Sexual health	State of physical, emotional, mental, and social well-being in relation to sexuality; it is not merely the absence of disease or dysfunction
Sexual dysfunction	Persistent, recurrent difficulty with sexual response, desire, orgasm, or pain that has been present for at least 6 months is associated with patient-reported distress
Sexual problems	Difficulty with sexual response, desire, orgasm, or pain that may interfere with sexual activity and/or cause distress, but does not meet criteria for a sexual dysfunction
Sexual response	Refers to the physical and psychological changes that occur with sexually stimulating activities. The phases of sexual response are typically described as including desire, arousal, orgasm, and resolution

While Masters and Johnson's model conceptualized the stages of sexual response as occurring linearly, more recent models describe a complex circular sexual response cycle. For example, Basson [17] recognized that desire is not always present prior to the initiation of sexual activity, especially in women, and thus differentiated between spontaneous sexual desire and receptive or "responsive" desire. Inclusion of the concept of receptive desire within the conceptualization of sexual response acknowledges that the motivation to engage in sex is complex and can be related to other factors such as emotional intimacy rather than a simplistic biologically driven or pleasure-driven motivation for sex. Basson's model also recognized that a person may be sexually satisfied with or without experiencing orgasm if other factors are driving desire or satisfaction (e.g., feeling cared for by their partner). Basson's conceptualization of the sexual response cycle can be particularly helpful in guiding discussions about sexual health problems with breast cancer survivors who are experiencing changes in desire, arousal, and/or orgasm. For example, a woman whose sexual interest and experiences of arousal were largely driven by spontaneous desire prior to treatment may benefit from education about the different types of desire (i.e., spontaneous and receptive) and how they operate differently. Providing this education, in addition to normalizing the sexual changes often experienced after treatment, can help women to understand that desire is likely, still present but may have shifted from spontaneous desire to predominantly receptive desire.

Box 5.2 Sexual desire

Spontaneous desire	Seemingly sudden wanting or urge for sexual activity, sexual fantasy, or sexual thoughts. Individuals may also experience associated body or genital sensations.
Receptive or responsive desire	Experience of sexual interest or desire that occurs when a person interacts with sexual stimuli (e.g., thoughts, visual stimuli, touch) or participates in sexually stimulating activity.

Moving beyond describing stages of sexual response, Bancroft and colleagues proposed the Dual Control Model for understanding how women build sexual desire and arousal [25]. This model proposes that this building process relies on an interaction between excitatory and inhibitory processes. When describing this to patients, the language of having a gas pedal (i.e., excitatory) and brake pedal (i.e., inhibitory) is often useful [26]. Factors that may increase excitatory processes for an individual could include feeling safe or feeling supported by their partner, interacting with sexual content (e.g., television, movies), or touch. Factors that may contribute to inhibitory processes could include anxious thoughts, trauma, relationship conflict, or changes in body image related to treatment experiences such as body-altering surgeries and treatments impacting vaginal dryness. In order to build desire and arousal, excitatory processes must be prominent and outweigh inhibitory processes [25]. Evidence suggests that inhibitory processes play a more prominent role in female sexual desire and arousal. Thus, the factors that are activating the "brake pedal" often play a larger role in desire and arousal difficulties than factors that activate the "gas pedal" [26].

Impacts of Breast Cancer Treatments on Sexual Function

Breast Surgery

It is widely accepted that the breast can be a sensual organ, and breast sensation frequently changes after breast cancer surgery (including mastectomy and breast-conserving procedures). Altered breast sensation can result in decreases in arousal from breast stimulation and less sexual satisfaction [27, 28]. Scarring, nerve damage, and lymphedema are also potential side effects of breast cancer surgery, which may lead to sexual difficulties. Surgical breast procedures can be accompanied by persistent post-surgical pain, and dissatisfaction with cosmetic outcomes can negatively impact body image [29–31]. Some research suggests that women who undergo mastectomy report lower sexual satisfaction compared to women who undergo breast conserving surgery or reconstruction, but findings are inconsistent [32, 33]. For example, one study found that women reported significantly reduced sexual desire, arousal, and orgasm after mastectomy, while women who had breast-conserving surgeries did not experience significant changes in sexual function [34]. Yet other studies have found that rates of sexual dysfunction are comparable in women who had mastectomy and women who had breast-conserving surgery [7]. These inconsistent findings may suggest that additional factors beyond type of surgery confer risk for sexual dysfunction (e.g., body image, pain, psychological adjustment, response of partner, or partner status) [10]. Several studies have accounted for adjuvant therapies such as chemotherapy, radiation, and endocrine therapies when examining surgical side effects and suggest cumulative sexual side effects when receiving multiple types of treatment [7].

Radiation Therapy

Little empirical work has investigated the impact of breast radiation on sexual function. Research to date suggests that breast radiation can result in fatigue, pain, and long-term tissue and skin changes that subsequently impact aspects of sexual function including desire and arousal [15]. Side effects of radiation therapy that can negatively impact body image and women's sexuality include lymphedema, scarring, and burns [14, 35]. The chest region can become inflamed, tender, swollen, dry, or sensitive during treatment [10], with some changes persisting post-treatment. These effects impact women's body image and sexual desire for years after treatment completion [35].

Chemotherapy

The acute and long-term side effects of chemotherapy negatively impact breast cancer survivors' sexual function. During the course of chemotherapy, low white cell blood counts are a common, transient side effect, which confers risk for infection, and patients may be advised to use barrier methods of protection (i.e., condoms) or to refrain from intercourse in the setting of neutropenia. Side effects from chemotherapy that can impact body image and self-esteem include weight gain or loss, alopecia (hair loss), and generalized edema [35–38]. The changes women experience during chemotherapy can have negative impacts on sexual self-image, sexual function, and sexual relationships (e.g., response of sexual partner to physical changes during treatment could impact the relationship) [2]. Women also may experience suppression of ovarian function, which can result in decreased sexual desire, arousal, and lubrication as well as vaginal pain [39–41]. Chemotherapy can result in premature ovarian failure for 30–96% of premenopausal women [42], with the highest risk found among women who received alkylating agents (e.g., cyclophosphamide) and those older than 40 years [42, 43]. Early menopause and reductions in estrogen place women at increased risk for sexual problems [37, 44]. Research suggests chemotherapy-induced menopause significantly predicts sexual dysfunction and sexual inactivity among breast cancer survivors [6]. Chemotherapy-related depletion of reproductive hormones can have profound negative impacts on vulvar and vaginal health [13]. Resulting vulvovaginal changes and atrophy are characterized by decreased blood flow, thinning of the epithelium, decreased vaginal secretions, pH increases, loss of vaginal rugae, and loss of collagen and elastin that lead to vaginal shortening or narrowing and tissue that can become pale, smooth, and fragile [45]. Chemotherapy-induced menopause can also cause symptoms such as extreme fatigue, gastrointestinal or genitourinary concerns, sexual pain, and hot flashes, which can negatively impact sexual function [10, 35, 37, 46–48].

Endocrine Therapy

Endocrine therapy refers to medications and interventions that augment or block actions of hormones. For breast cancer, this includes medications (e.g., tamoxifen or aromatase inhibitors) which block the action or production of estrogen. As therapy for hormone receptor positive, early-stage breast cancer, endocrine therapy is recommended because it decreases risk of breast cancer recurrence and death [49]. The therapy type varies by whether women are pre- or post-menopausal. Endocrine therapy, for 5–10 years, is standard of care for women with hormone receptor positive breast cancer, which comprises about 80% of breast cancers [49]. Endocrine therapy increases the risk for sexual dysfunction and is associated with profound changes in all aspects of sexual function including desire, arousal, orgasm, and sexual self-image [13, 50, 51]. Women taking endocrine therapy are likely to experience significant vulvovaginal changes (i.e., decreased blood flow; epithelial thinning; decreased vaginal secretions and vaginal dryness; pH increases; loss of rugae, collagen and elastin) resulting in vulvovaginal atrophy and vaginal shortening or narrowing. Additional common sexual side effects of adjuvant endocrine therapies for breast cancer include vaginal and vulvar pain and discomfort, hot flashes, and decreased sexual desire and responsiveness [15, 52, 53]. These side effects significantly contribute to lack of sexual interest and poor sexual satisfaction [5].

Research suggests that both tamoxifen and aromatase inhibitors contribute to reduced sexual desire [50], and rates of distress and sexual problems related to endocrine therapy are highest among younger women [54]. While both tamoxifen and aromatase inhibitors contribute to the vulvovaginal changes described above, women taking aromatase inhibitors experience vulvar and vaginal atrophy and dyspareunia (i.e., painful intercourse) at higher rates than women who are prescribed tamoxifen [55, 56]. Women who take aromatase inhibitors are also more vulnerable to lichen sclerosis [13], which is a perineal skin condition that results in itching and burning as well as thin, crinkled tissue prone to injury and scarring [57, 58]. For premenopausal breast cancer survivors on endocrine therapy who are receiving medications to suppress ovarian function (i.e., leuprolide, goserelin), evidence indicates that treatment-related sexual dysfunction can be severe; all aspects of sexual function (i.e., desire, arousal, orgasm, resolution) are impacted, loss of sexual satisfaction is common, and treatment-related sexual problems do not improve over time [59]. Some premenopausal breast cancer survivors with hormone-receptor-positive breast cancer may undergo oophorectomy, which can also negatively impact all aspects of sexual function and result in severe genitourinary difficulties [46, 47], including vulvovaginal dryness and atrophy, dyspareunia, and urinary symptoms [60]. Oophorectomy can also impact women's sense of self and femininity [5, 10].

Assessment of Sexual Problems

Because treatments for breast cancer often result in sexual health changes, routine assessment of sexual health is an essential part of high-quality survivorship care [14]. Current National Comprehensive Cancer Network (NCCN) guidelines highlight the importance of assessing sexual health in every woman, not only at the time of diagnosis and during treatment but also after treatment completion and in longer-term survivorship [61]. A woman can experience sexual problems, regardless of age, partner status, or current sexual activity. Routinely asking about sexual problems can help to facilitate early identification, referral, and treatment for sexual difficulties. It also demonstrates that sexuality is recognized as an important and valued aspect of a woman's health and well-being. It is important for providers to indicate that they are open to discussing and addressing sexual health problems as part of routine care.

When caring for breast cancer survivors, it is essential to have a clear strategy for initiating discussions about sexual problems, providing appropriate resources, and providing recommendations for treatment and follow-up care. A number of models have been developed to help guide both the assessment and management of sexual health problems including the Permission, Limited Information, Specific Suggestions, and Intensive Therapy (PLISSIT) model; [62] the Bring up, Explain, Tell, Timing, Educate and Record (BETTER) model; [63] and the 5As Model (see below) for sexual health in cancer [14]. An expert group from the Scientific Network on Female Sexual Health and Cancer (SNFSHC) recently endorsed the 5 As communication model specifically for addressing the sexual problems of cancer survivors in medical settings. The 5 As model extends beyond the PLISSIT and BETTER models to provide clear steps for both assessment and delivery of appropriate resources or recommendations. The five elements of this model include Ask, Advise, Assess, Assist, and Arrange Follow-up [14]. Table 5.1 gives an overview of this model as applied to sexual health problems.

Ask highlights the importance of bringing up the topic of sexual problems and validating the patient's experience. *Advise* refers to providing patients with information about their concerns, educating patients about possible treatment options, and normalizing their concerns. Although providers may not be able to answer all questions or know of all available treatment options, providers can convey that they are open to talking about sexual problems and helping patients find appropriate resources (e.g., educational information, referral). Providers can also reassure patients that sexual health problems can be discussed presently or in the future, and the timing of addressing sexual health problems can be based on the patient's preference. *Assess* focuses on the importance of fully evaluating the patient's sexual health problems, which may include clinical conversation, taking a history, conducting a symptom assessment, physical exam, and/or other clinical evaluation. Including symptom checklists or validated screening measures (described below) can facilitate assessment, help to decrease stigma associated with sexual problems, and help to identify specific concerns the patient might have. *Assist* refers to providing patients with education, informational resources, treatment recommendations, and referral to additional resources as needed. For breast cancer survivors, evidence suggests that without intervention, sexual problems will not improve and their impact will likely worsen over time [64, 65]. While many patients will benefit from education or simple interventions (e.g., specific strategies for managing vaginal dryness) [66], it is also important to have multidisciplinary referral resources available (e.g., gynecology, urology, pelvic floor physical therapy, and psychotherapy or counseling) [14]. Finally, *arrange follow-up* underscores the importance of routine follow-up when addressing sexual problems. Follow-up is needed to assess for changes in symptoms,

Table 5.1 The 5 As model for sexual health after cancer developed by a working group of the Scientific Network on Female Sexual Health and Cancer (SNFSHC)

5 As	Description
Ask	Provide validation to the patient by letting them know that changes in sexual health are common. Ask the patient about changes they may have experienced (e.g., *After breast cancer treatment, many women experience changes or have concerns about sexual health. What have you experienced? What concerns do you have?*)
Advise	Reassure patients by normalizing their concerns, letting them know that treatment options exist, and that sexual concerns can be discussed at this time or any time in the future.
Assess	Provide routine assessment of sexual concerns as part of survivorship care. • Using a symptom checklist with items related to sexual health can help to decrease stigma associated with sexual dysfunction and identify specific concerns. • For survivors with sexual concerns or who express interest, a complete evaluation should be conducted including taking a history, assessment of current medical status, review of medications, and physical examination. • If aspects of the evaluation cannot be conducted by the oncology provider team, breast cancer survivors should be referred to appropriate specialty providers to complete these components.
Assist	Provide patients with education, informational resources, treatment recommendations, and referral to additional resources as needed (e.g., gynecology, pelvic physical therapy; psychotherapy).
Arrange follow-up	Schedule follow-up visits, and establish practice routines that ensure patient's sexual health concerns, access to care, and engagement in care are routinely monitored. It is important to initiate follow-up discussions about sexual health concerns at subsequent visits.

Note: A complete description of the model and associated resources can be found in the following publication: Bober et al. [14]

the development of new sexual problems, the patient's use of referral resources or recommended treatments, and additional education as needed.

Screening Measures

In addition to clinical recognition of the issue, obtaining a brief assessment using validated measures can help to identify sexual health problems and assess changes in sexual health over time (see Table 5.2) [51]. It is important to note that the use of screening measures can help to facilitate the clinical conversation and assessment, but such measures do not replace a clinical evaluation.

When screening for sexual problems, a screening measure specifically designed to assess sexual problems is needed, as general distress screening tools often miss the majority of patients with sexual problems [67]. A brief checklist for identifying the presence of sexual problems or concerns in the clinical setting was developed by an international collaboration of sexual medicine experts in 2004 [68] and was further adapted for women with cancer by the expert group from SNFSHC who modified the 5As model above [14]. This brief checklist (completion time < 5 minutes) can be used as a self-report measure, or used by providers as part of clinical conversation about sexual difficulties. The checklist asks about sexual satisfaction, vaginal health concerns, sexual interest, sensation, lubrication, orgasm, pain and discomfort, anxiety about sex, and interest in discussing these concerns with a provider. A copy of the checklist and related resources are provided in the SNFSHC group's 2016 publication [14] and in the recent NCCN survivorship guidelines regarding female sexual function [61].

For breast cancer survivors with sexual difficulties, assessment using multidimensional measures of sexual function and well-being should be considered. Table 5.2 provides a summary of several patient-reported sexual function measures. The Female Sexual Function Index (FSFI) [69] is a widely used measure of sexual function that has been validated in female cancer survivors [70, 71]. The FSFI includes 19 items that assess function over the past 4 weeks in the domains of desire, arousal, lubrication, orgasm, satisfaction, and pain. The FSFI is a measure with cut-off scores that indicate clinically significant sexual problems [69]. The FSFI, instructions for its use, and scoring are available at https://www.FSFIquestionnaire.com. It is important to note that the FSFI has several limitations when used to

Table 5.2 Screening measures of sexual function and foncerns

Measure	Number of items	Time Frame	Domains	Cut-off scores	Completion time
Brief Sexual Symptom Checklist for Women [68]	4	Past 3 months	Satisfaction; concerns about vaginal health; sexual problems checklist (i.e., interest, sensation, lubrication, orgasm, pain, anxiety); need for information or referral	None available	< 5 minutes
Female Sexual Function Index (FSFI) [69]	19	Past 4 weeks	Desire; arousal; lubrication; orgasm; satisfaction; pain	Score ≤ 26 indicate risk of sexual problem	10–15 minutes
PROMIS Sexual Function and Satisfaction Full Profile [72]	25	Past 30 days	Interest; lubrication; vaginal discomfort; labial discomfort; clitoral discomfort; orgasm ability; orgasm pleasure; satisfaction; oral discomfort; oral dryness; anal discomfort	None available (T-score conversion available)	15 minutes
PROMIS Sexual Function and Satisfaction Brief Profile [74]	13	Past 30 days	Interest; lubrication; vaginal discomfort; labial discomfort; clitoral discomfort; orgasm ability; orgasm pleasure; satisfaction	None available (T-score conversion available)	10 minutes

assess sexual problems in breast cancer survivors. The FSFI is unable to differentiate between women with sexual difficulties versus those who are sexually inactive for other reasons. The FSFI does not assess sexual difficulties related to the specific impacts of cancer treatments, and it does not provide information about the use of sexual interventions or aids that can help manage sexual difficulties.

A newer measure is the PROMIS Sexual Function and Satisfaction (PROMIS SexFS) scale [72–74]. Developed for patients with cancer and validated in women with breast cancer, the PROMIS SexFS offers full and brief profile versions that assess function and satisfaction over the past 30 days. The PROMIS SexFS measures can be used for survivors who are sexually active with a partner and for those without a partner, and these measures have been validated among individuals who are identified as heterosexual or straight, lesbian, gay, or bisexual. The PROMIS SexFS Full Profile includes 25 items and assesses eleven domains: sexual interest, lubrication, vaginal discomfort, labial discomfort, clitoral discomfort, orgasm ability, orgasm pleasure, orgasm satisfaction, oral discomfort, oral dryness, and anal discomfort. The PROMIS SexFS Brief Profile includes 13 items and assesses the domains covered in the Full Profile with the exception of oral discomfort, oral dryness, and anal discomfort. The PROMIS SexFS item bank also includes additional scales that can be used to assess the use of sexual aids or interventions. Custom short forms can be made by selecting any items from the PROMIS SexFS item bank and can be scored using the PROMIS Scoring Service which can be accessed online. While the PROMIS SexFS assesses sexual difficulties related to the impacts of cancer treatments, it does not have established cut-off scores to indicate clinically significant sexual problems. PROMIS Full and Brief Profile scores can be converted into T scores, which rescale the raw score into a standardized score with a mean of 50 and a standard deviation (SD) of 10. Therefore, a person with a T-score of 40 is one SD below the mean indicating lower than average sexual function and well-being. The PROMIS measures and additional scales/items, instructions for use, and scoring are available at https://www.healthmeasures.net/index.php.

Clinical Evaluation

NCCN guidelines recommend comprehensive evaluation for women who report sexual problems or those who express interest in further evaluation of sexual health [61]. A comprehensive clinical evaluation is needed to identify and address the range of sexual problems breast cancer survivors might experience. Along with the direct and indirect impacts of breast cancer treatments on sexual function, the causes of sexual problems are often multifactorial including biological, psychological, relational, and sociocultural factors [75, 76]. A comprehensive clinical evaluation should consider the range of biopsychosocial factors (see Fig. 5.1) that might contribute to sexual problems so that appropriate recommendations and referrals can be made. In addition to the assessment of symptoms and sexual problems, a comprehensive clinical evaluation should involve taking a history, assessment of current medical status, review of medications, and physical examination [61, 66, 77]. If aspects of a comprehensive clinical evaluation for sexual health, as described below, cannot be conducted by the oncology provider team, breast cancer survivors should be referred to appropriate specialty providers to complete these components of the evaluation (e.g., gynecology, pelvic floor physical therapy, counseling or psychotherapy, sex therapy, psychiatry, urogynecology, or reproductive endocrinology). For example, if contributing factors related to depression and relationship distress are identified, the survivor could be referred to a sex therapist or other mental health professional for further evaluation.

Evaluation of Sexual Problems Review of the survivor's current sexual problems should be conducted in detail, including the difficulties she is experiencing related to sexual desire, arousal, orgasm, and sexual pleasure, as well as experiences of pain or discomfort during sex [14, 66,

76, 78]. When enquiring about sexual desire, it is important to ask about experiences of both spontaneous and receptive desire, and to clarify whether the survivor is experiencing a normal variation in sexual response versus sexual dysfunction. For example, a survivor who reports experiencing spontaneous or receptive desire but reports a desire discrepancy between herself and her partner is most likely describing a normal variation in sexual response rather than a sexual dysfunction. When asking about arousal difficulties, it is important to assess both subjective feelings of arousal (e.g., feeling "turned on") and physical responses associated with arousal (e.g., lubrication, warmth). For orgasm, both the presence (i.e., is orgasm possible when desired) and quality of orgasm (e.g., is it pleasurable, very delayed, weak/non-intense, or painful) should be evaluated. Review whether desired sexual activities are possible (e.g., is intercourse possible). For women reporting pain, further clarification is needed about when pain is experienced (e.g., with and/or without touch, during penetrative activity), location and depth (e.g., insertional or deeper pain), quality of pain (e.g., burning, stabbing, etc.), constancy, timing (during and/or after sexual activity), and factors that exacerbate pain (e.g., partner's ejaculation fluid, deep thrusting). For all sexual problems, it is important to ask about the duration of difficulties (e.g., lifelong, onset after cancer treatments) and ascertain whether difficulties occur in general or only in specific situations (e.g., during self-stimulation or only during partnered activity). Enquire about other factors that might be negatively impacting sexual function or reasons for avoiding sex, considering aspects of the biopsychosocial model (see Fig. 5.1). Factors to consider include sexual self-image and body image, experiences of distracting thoughts or negative emotions during sex, relationship status and quality, sexual dysfunction of the partner, and other significant life stressors.

Historical Assessment When taking a history, the breast cancer survivor's oncologic, medical, psychosocial, and sexual and reproductive health history should be included. Review of oncologic history would include breast cancer diagnosis (e.g., stage, hormone-receptor status), surgeries, local radiation therapy, systemic therapy (endocrine and chemotherapy), and history of diagnosis and treatment for other malignancies. It is also important to assess the presence of any preexisting gynecologic conditions, dermatological conditions of the genitals, genitourinary symptoms, sexually transmitted illnesses, and conditions likely to be impacted by periods of immunosuppression such as with chemotherapy (e.g., cervical dysplasia, condyloma, and herpes simplex) [78].

Current Medical Status When assessing the survivor's current medical status, special attention should be given to health conditions that can impact sexual function. Table 5.3 provides an overview of the sexual function impacts of common chronic health conditions. Consideration should also be given to the assessment of the cardiorespiratory function, mobility, and continence requirements for sexual activity (including intercourse, self-stimulation, and orgasm) [78].

Review of Medications In addition to the impacts of endocrine therapy on sexual function, many commonly used medications may negatively impact sexual function. For example, difficulties with sexual desire, arousal, and orgasm are frequently experienced with selective serotonin reuptake inhibitor use, with 30–70% of women reporting these side effects [79]. Table 5.4 provides an overview of the sexual side effects associated with common medications.

Physical Examination A full physical examination, including a genital/pelvic examination, should be completed. If the oncology provider team is unable to complete a genital/pelvic examination, the breast cancer survivor should be referred for a gynecologic exam. For survivors reporting pelvic or vulvovaginal pain (with or without sexual activity), a physical exam is particularly important. Physical exams are also important for women taking aromatase inhibitors, as they are at increased risk for lichen

Table 5.3 Medical conditions that may impact sexual function

Condition	Impact on sexual function
Cardiovascular disease	
Coronary artery disease	Decreased arousal [76, 79, 187]
Hypertension	Decreased desire [76, 79, 187], decreased lubrication, difficulty with orgasm [78, 188]
Hyperlipidemia	Decreased arousal, decreased lubrication, difficulty with orgasm, less satisfaction [189]; increase in vascular resistance in clitoris has been found [190]
Heart failure	Decreased desire, decreased lubrication, difficulty with orgasm; increased frequency of unsuccessful intercourse; fear regarding safety of having sex; lack of energy and decreased exercise capacity reduce the ability to be sexually active [191]
Myocardial infarction	Decreased desire, decreased arousal; fear regarding safety of having sex; lack of knowledge about sexual activity after myocardial infarction [78, 192]
Stroke	Decreased desire, decreased lubrication, difficulty with orgasm; greater sexual dysfunction in hemiplegic vs. hemiparetic patients; stroke-related impacts that can affect sexual function (physical limitations, urinary incontinence, excess salivation, facial changes, and body image concerns) [193]
Endocrine disease	
Diabetes mellitus	Decreased desire, decreased lubrication, difficulties with orgasm [76, 194, 195]; increased levels of dyspareunia [194]; comorbid depressive symptoms may impact sexual function [78, 195]
Metabolic syndrome	Decreased desire, difficulty with orgasm; higher prevalence of sexual inactivity; less satisfaction [196]
Hypothyroidism	Decreased arousal, decreased lubrication, difficulties with orgasm; increased pain; less satisfaction [195, 197]
Hyperthyroidism	Decreased arousal, decreased lubrication, difficulties with orgasm; increased pain; less satisfaction [195]
Adrenal insufficiency	Decreased or loss of desire; less satisfaction [195]
Cushing's syndrome	Decreased desire, decreased arousal, decreased lubrication, difficulty with orgasm; less satisfaction; body image concerns [195]
Musculoskeletal conditions and chronic pain	
Osteoarthritis	Body/joint pain, joint stiffness, decreased mobility, and fatigue may interfere with sexual activity [198]
Fibromyalgia	Decreased desire, decreased arousal; body pain, impaired mobility, and fatigue may interfere with sexual activity [199]
Low back pain	Decreased desire; body pain and impaired mobility may interfere with sexual activity [199]
Osteoporosis	Frailty; fear of injury during sexual activity; musculoskeletal pain, decreased trunk and extremity strength, decreased endurance, and fatigue may interfere with sexual activity [199, 200]
Rheumatic Disease	
Rheumatoid arthritis	Decreased desire; genital pain and tissue changes; body/joint pain, reduced mobility, and debility (e.g., cannot use hands) may interfere with sexual activity; self-image concerns [78, 199]
Systemic sclerosis	Vaginal dryness, loss of elasticity, ulcerations, dyspareunia [78]
Gynecologic conditions	
Dermatologic conditions of the genitals	Genital pain associated with vulvar lichen sclerosus, vulvar eczema, psoriasis, or other condition [76]
Sexually transmitted Illnesses	Fear of transmission; fear of disclosure; feelings of stigma; relationship avoidance; reduced sense of intimacy; for HIV, lack of desire, less satisfaction, and less frequent activity; for genital herpes, lesions that prevent activity [201]
Chronic pelvic pain	Pain [76]
Pelvic organ prolapse	Decreased desire, decreased arousal, difficulty with orgasm; increased sexual pain; associated urinary and bowel symptoms that interfere with sexual function [202]

Table 5.3 (continued)

Condition	Impact on sexual function
Endometriosis	Decreased desire, decreased arousal, difficulty with orgasm; increased sexual pain; fear of sexual pain; less satisfaction [203]
Urinary problems	
Urinary incontinence	Decreased desire, decreased arousal, poor lubrication; painful sexual intercourse; less satisfaction; body image concerns; avoidance of intimacy; embarrassment due to incontinence [202]
Urinary tract infections	Avoidance of intimacy due to fear of infection; impacts of associated emotional distress and low self-esteem [202]
Lower urinary tract symptoms	Sexual pain; poor lubrication; genital inflammation [202]
Overactive bladder	Decreased desire, decreased arousal; poor lubrication; difficulty with orgasm; sexual pain [204]
End-stage renal disease or renal failure	Decreased desire or loss of desire; poor lubrication; sexual pain; comorbid conditions that impact sexual function (e.g., depression, cardiac disease, diabetes); impact of associated symptoms (fatigue, nausea, bodily pain) [76, 78]
Inflammatory bowel disease	Decreased desire, difficulty building arousal, difficulty with orgasm; sexual pain; body image concerns; interference of associated depressive symptoms; medication side effects [205]
Neurological disease	
Spinal cord and cauda equina injury	Desire often retained; impairment in sexual function will depend lesions/injury location; orgasm often lost with upper motor neuron damage; loss of reflex lubrication and physical sensations from genital stimulation with lower lesions (S2, 3, 4 nerve roots); complete loss of genital sensation (as well as bladder and bowel control) with cauda equine injury [78]
Multiple sclerosis	Brain and spinal cord damage can impede desire, decrease vaginal/genital sensation and lubrication, impair orgasm, and cause pain with sex; interference of associated symptoms (bladder/bowel dysfunction, fatigue, weakness, and spasticity, cognitive dysfunction, depression) [206, 207]
Parkinson disease	Desire altered by either decrease or increase (hypersexuality); difficulty with arousal and orgasm; poor lubrication; loss of genital sensation [78, 208, 209]
Dementia	Desire altered by either decrease or increase (hypersexuality) [78]
Traumatic brain injury	Desire altered by either decrease or increase (hypersexuality); impairment in sexual function depends on injury location; injury-related impacts affect sexual function (impaired insight and cognition, interpersonal difficulties, depression, body image concerns, disinhibition, eating disturbances) [210]
Seizure	Decreased desire, decreased arousal; enzyme-inducing and multiple anti-seizure drugs associated with sexual dysfunction [211]
Pituitary tumor, hyperprolactinemia	Decreased desire [78]
Psychiatric disorders	
Depression and mood disorders	Decreased desire, decreased arousal, reduced lubrication, difficulty with orgasm; SSRIs, SNRIs and mirtazapine associated with new onset sexual dysfunction [78, 212–214]
Anxiety disorders	Decreased arousal, difficulty with orgasm [78]
Psychotic illness	Antipsychotic medication associated with decreased desire; those with psychotic illness are less likely to have sexual relationships [78]

sclerosus [57, 58]. The physical exam should include visual external and internal (speculum) inspection and bimanual pelvic examination [80]. Physical vaginal characteristics (agglutination, scarring/adhesions, pH, moisture, rugosity, elasticity, length, thickness, epithelial integrity, vascularity, and irritation) and physical vulvar characteristics (vulvar atrophy, irritation, and vestibular irritation) should be assessed [66].

Given that approximately one in three women are estimated to experience gender-based violence (e.g., sexual violence, intimate partner violence) in their lifetime [81, 82] and rates of disclosure to medical providers are low, it is important that, in addition to obtaining a sexual history, providers take universal precautions during the examination to prevent re-traumatization. Survivors of violence

Table 5.4 Medications with sexual side effects

	Sexual side effect				
Medication	Desire	Arousal	Orgasm	Vaginal dryness	Reduced sensation
Amphetamines and related anorexic drugs			X		
Anticholinergics		X			
Anticonvulsant (phenytoin sodium)	X				
Antifungal (ketoconazole)	X				
Antihistamines (e.g., diphenhydramine)	X	X			X
Cardiovascular and antihypertensive medications					
Antilipid medications	X				
Beta blockers	X				
Clonidine	X	X			
Digoxin	X		X		
Methyldopa	X				
Spironolactone	X				
Histamine H2-receptor blockers, pro-motility agents	X				
Hormonal preparations					
Antiandrogens	X	X	X		
Danazol	X				
GnRh agonists	X	X			
Oral hormonal contraceptives	X				
Ultra-low-potency contraceptives	X	X			
Muscle relaxers (e.g., baclofen (Lioresal))			X		
Narcotics			X		
NSAIDs					
Ibuprofen				X	
Indomethacin	X			X	
Naproxen				X	
Psychoactive medications					
Antipsychotics	X		X		
Barbiturates	X	X	X		
Benzodiazepines	X	X	X	X	
Lithium	X	X	X		
MAO inhibitors	X				
SSRIs	X	X	X		X
SSNRIs (Venlafaxine)	X	X	X		X
Tricyclic antidepressants	X	X	X		

Note: Information compiled from a report by the Association of Reproductive Health Professionals [215] and the American Hospital Formulary Service (AHFS) Patient Medication Information database [216]

report that examinations include cues that can remind them of abuse (e.g., being told where to move their body and to "relax", pain from penetration, the position they are in) [83–85]. Before beginning the examination, providers should speak with the patient first while they are fully clothed to describe each part of the examination and ask if they have questions, concerns, or requests (e.g., having another provider present, self-inserting the speculum, using a smaller speculum, conducting the exam in a different position). Providers should convey that patients can tell the provider to pause or stop at any point. During the examination, the provider should seek affirmative consent from the patient before each step and check in with the patient about how they are doing. Ades (2020) provides comprehensive guidance for trauma-sensitive gynecologic examinations [86].

Laboratory Investigations Laboratory testing is usually not needed to identify the causes of sexual dysfunction [87]. For example, while androgens are positively associated with female sexual function (e.g., improved sexual interest, arousal, and orgasm), there is no lower level of testosterone that predicts female sexual dysfunction [79]. While low estradiol levels are associated with genitourinary symptoms (e.g., vaginal dryness) which can be identified by physical exam, studies have not consistently demonstrated an association between sexual desire and level of estradiol [79].

Managing Sexual Problems

All breast cancer survivors should be provided with information about the potential sexual impacts of their breast cancer treatments, including the sexual changes that might occur with treatment-related hormonal changes [61]. There are a number of high-quality patient resources available regarding sexual health and cancer, which are accessible online or in print. The American Cancer Society has published "Sex and the Adult Female with Cancer" (http://www.cancer.org), and this online resource covers a wide range of sexual health topics including female sexual function, the sexual impacts of cancer treatments, and managing sexual problems related to cancer (e.g., moisturizers and lubricants for vaginal dryness, sexual positions for reducing pain or discomfort). The Scientific Network on Female Sexual Health and Cancer provides links to a range of patient and provider educational resources on its website (http://cancersexnetwork.org/). A 2016 publication [14] in the journal *Current Opinion in Supportive and Palliative Care* by an expert group from this organization includes teaching/tip sheets about vaginal dryness and low desire, which can be given to patients. The MacMillan Cancer Support Community in the United Kingdom (http://www.macmillan.org.uk) has several online information resources focused on sex in cancer survivorship in their resource "Impacts of Cancer A to Z." Additional educational resources about sex for cancer survivors can be found through the Cancer Council of Australia (www.cancercouncil.com.au).

While providing sexual health information should be a routine part of quality cancer survivorship care [66], it is also important to recognize when more specialized care is needed and to have multidisciplinary referral resources available [14]. Addressing the sexual difficulties experienced by breast cancer survivors often requires a multidisciplinary approach [14]. A robust referral network for sexual health care would ideally include gynecologists who have experience caring for breast cancer survivors, pelvic floor physical therapists, sex therapists, counselors or psychotherapists, psychiatrists, urogynecologists, and reproductive endocrinologists (see Fig. 5.2). In addition to building referral networks within the health system and community, there are several professional organizations that have resources to help identify health-care professionals by location and areas of expertise. Table 5.5 provides a listing of these organizations.

Below we provide an overview of strategies for managing common sexual problems experienced by breast cancer survivors, including non-pharmacologic and pharmacologic

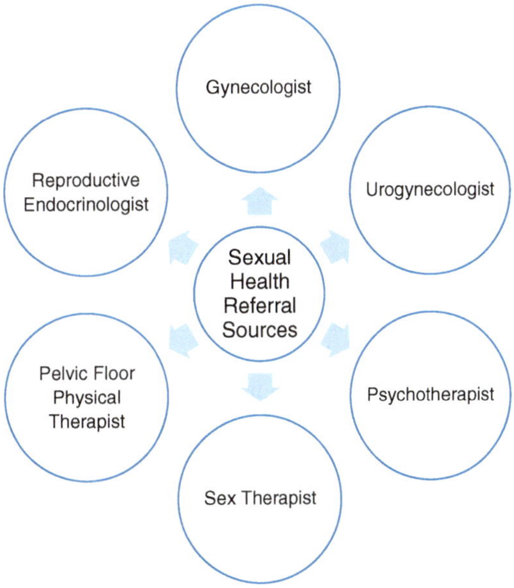

Fig. 5.2 Referral resources for sexual health care

Table 5.5 Resources for sexual health information and referral resources

Professional organization	Internet address
Scientific Network on Female Sexual Health and Cancer	http://www.cancersexnetwork.org
International Society for the Study of Women's Sexual Health	http://www.isswsh.org
The North American Menopause Society	http://www.menopause.org
Society for Sex Therapy and Research	http://www.sstarnet.org
American Association of Sexuality Educators, Counselors, and Therapists	http://www.aasect.org
American Association for Marriage and Family Therapy	http://www.aamft.org
American Physical Therapy Association	https://ptl.womenshealthapta.org/
International Pelvic Pain Society	http://www.pelvicpain.org

approaches. Table 5.6 provides a summary of non-pharmacologic approaches, and Table 5.7 provides a summary of pharmacologic approaches.

Non-pharmacological Approaches

Moisturizers and Lubricants

Vaginal dryness is a common problem for breast cancer survivors, and its associated symptoms are often painful or uncomfortable (e.g., sensations of burning, chafing, and itching), have negative impacts on sexual function, result in pain during sexual activity, and are emotionally distressing [2, 88]. While there is limited data to support the use of over-the-counter vaginal moisturizers and lubricants, these products are considered to be the initial and most widely used approaches for managing vaginal dryness in breast cancer survivors [80, 89]. Providing women with education about vaginal moisturizers and sexual lubricants is vital to properly manage vaginal dryness and dyspareunia as many women are unfamiliar with the difference between these products and how to use them properly.

Vaginal moisturizers are long-acting and should be used on a regular basis, independent of sexual activity, to maintain tissue integrity, elasticity, and pliability [80, 90, 91]. For breast cancer survivors, frequent use is recommended, with expert opinion suggesting that moisturizers should be used several times per week to daily to help maintain vaginal moisture and pH balance [80]. A large number of vaginal moisturizer products are available. These products are poorly characterized for consumers, difficult to differentiate between, and there is no evidence to support the use of any particular moisturizer product or ingredient(s). For example, in a recent 12-week multicenter randomized trial comparing a 10-mcg vaginal estradiol tablet plus placebo gel, placebo tablet plus vaginal moisturizer, and placebo tablet plus placebo gel, all three groups demonstrated similar reductions in bothersome vulvovaginal symptoms and pain during sexual intercourse [92, 93]. Interestingly, vaginal moisturizer with placebo tablet and dual placebo gel and tablet performed equally well, and both of these interventions performed as well as the 10-mcg vaginal estradiol tablet and placebo gel. While there is no evidence to support the use of particular moisturizer products or ingredients, there are products that women should avoid. Below we provide a discussion of product characteristics or ingredients that should be avoided.

Lubricants are short-acting and used to reduce friction and discomfort during sexual activity. Lubricants come in a variety of options including water-based, oil-based, silicone-based, and hybrids of these. Some products can be used as both a moisturizer and lubricant. Women should be instructed to apply lubricant to the genital area shortly before sexual activity (i.e., the inner labia, clitoral area, vaginal entrance, and any other areas that feel dry during sexual activity). Lubricant should also be applied to body parts or items involved in sexual activity (e.g., fingers, penis, or sexual aids or toys), and lubricants should be re-applied as needed during sexual activity. Patient selection of type of lubricant often depends on individual preferences and type of sexual activity (e.g., use of a vibrator that cannot be used with a silicone-based product; a

Table 5.6 Non-pharmacologic strategies for managing sexual problems

Management strategy	Sexual problems	Description	Comments
Education	Lack of knowledge regarding sexual impacts	Information about sexual impacts of cancer treatments and treatment-related hormonal changes	Available resources: American Cancer Society, "Sex and the Adult Female with Cancer" (http://www.cancer.org); Scientific Network on Female Sexual Health and Cancer resource page (http://cancersexnetwork.org/); MacMillan Cancer Support Community, Impacts of Cancer A to Z (http://www.macmillan.org.uk); Cancer Council of Australia resources (www.cancercouncil.com.au)
Moisturizers	Vulvovaginal dryness and associated symptoms	Used on a regular basis, independent of sexual activity, to maintain tissue integrity, elasticity, and pliability	Expert opinion suggesting that moisturizers should be used several times per week to daily to help maintain vaginal moisture and pH balance; Avoid products that contain potential irritants (e.g., parabens, glycerin, propylene glycol)
Lubricants	Reduce friction and discomfort during sexual activity	Water-, oil-, or silicone-based. Applied to genital area and involved body parts/items shortly before sexual activity with reapplication as needed	Silicone-based lubricants should not be used with items made from silicone; avoid products that contain potential irritants (e.g., parabens, glycerin, propylene glycol, warming agents); WHO recommends using a lubricant with osmolality <1200 mOsm/kg and a pH of 3.8 to 4.5
Gel or cream with hyaluronic acid	Vulvovaginal dryness and associated symptoms	Used on a regular basis, independent of sexual activity, to maintain tissue integrity, elasticity, and pliability	A schedule of 3 to 5 times per week may be effective for obtaining symptom relief in breast cancer survivors; additional research is needed to further examine use and outcomes for breast cancer survivors
Sexual devices	Decreased sensation, difficulty building arousal, sexual pain	Clitoral stimulators, vibrators for external and internal use, dildos, devices that preclude deep insertion	Can be used during partnered or unpartnered activity; can help to manage sexual problems or expand available sexual activities; devices should be made of nontoxic, nonporous materials (silicone, hypoallergenic metals); avoid items labeled for novelty use, made with porous materials, made of jelly latex, and scented items
Vaginal dilators	Dyspareunia, symptomatic vaginal atrophy, and fear of penetration	Systematic, graduated approach with a set of tapered devices that vary in size, and facilitate mechanical stretch of vaginal tissue	While data is limited, clinical guidelines suggest consistent use of dilators (e.g., 3 times per week for 10–15 minutes) and using dilators in a progressive fashion. Evaluation and support from a pelvic floor physical therapist is often helpful
Pelvic floor physical therapy	Dyspareunia, difficulty with arousal and orgasm, and urinary incontinence	Pelvic floor muscle training, manual therapies, biofeedback	Should be provided by a physical therapist specialized and trained in pelvic floor disorders. Provider listing available at https://ptl.womenshealthapta.org/
Counseling and sex therapy	Overall sexual response and functioning, sexual satisfaction, body image, intimacy and relationship issues, coping with pain	Specialized type of psychotherapy provided by a mental health professional that focuses on the psychological, behavioral, interpersonal, and health-related factors that impact sexual function and satisfaction	Sex therapy approaches often include cognitive-behavioral interventions, mindfulness techniques, couples-based psychotherapy interventions, and psycho-education. Several professional organizations (see Table 5.5) provide online resources to assist with identifying sex therapy providers by geographic location

Table 5.7 Pharmacologic and Medical Interventions for Managing Sexual Problems

Management strategy	Sexual problems	Description	Comments
Topical lidocaine	Pain with penetrative sexual activity	Topical applied as a compress to the vaginal vestibule prior to vaginal penetration	Limited data available. Demonstrated benefits for pain reduction in one pilot trial in breast cancer survivors
Local estrogen-based treatments	Vulvovaginal dryness, atrophy and associated symptoms	Vaginal cream, vaginal inserts, vaginal ring in consultation with oncologist regarding risk	Used for severe symptoms that have not responded to non-hormonal interventions; consultation and evaluation of risk with the breast survivor's oncologist is needed
Vaginal dehydroepiandrosterone (DHEA)	Moderate to severe dyspareunia caused by vulvovaginal atrophy	Vaginal cream not recommended for use in breast cancer survivors	FDA-approved vaginal DHEA has not been studied in breast cancer survivors, and its label includes a warning against using this product in breast cancer survivors; short- and long-term safety remains unknown for breast cancer survivors
Vaginal testosterone	Vaginal atrophy and associated symptoms	Intravaginal cream not recommended for use in breast cancer survivors	There are no FDA-approved formulations of local testosterone for use in women. Off-label use in breast cancer survivors is not recommended.
Vaginal estriol	Vulvovaginal atrophy and associated symptoms	Vaginal cream, gel, or suppositories not recommended for use in breast cancer survivors	Not FDA approved for any indication. Efficacy and safety has not been demonstrated for breast cancer survivors or women with no cancer history.
Selective Estrogen Receptor Modulators (SERM)	Vulvovaginal atrophy and associated dyspareunia	Oral medication; ospemifene (not used in the USA for breast cancer survivors)	Not FDA approved for use with breast cancer survivors in the USA. Safety and efficacy data for breast cancer survivors lacking. Impact on risk of recurrence unknown
Vaginal laser treatment	Vaginal dryness and associated dyspareunia	Nonablative erbium-doped yttrium aluminum garnet laser (FotonaSmooth®) or microablative CO_2 laser (MonaLisa Touch®)	Aim to stimulate vascularity and promote production of new collagen in vaginal tissue; not FDA approved for vaginal tissue; prospective randomized clinical trials needed to determine the efficacy and safety of these treatments
Bupropion	Desire and arousal disorders	Oral medication; antidepressant, belongs to the aminoketone class	Shown to improve sexual function in premenopausal women with hypoactive sexual desire disorder or SSRI-induced sexual dysfunction; limited data available for breast cancer survivors and caution may be needed for women taking tamoxifen; one small pilot study suggested potential benefits in breast cancer survivors.
Flibanserin	Hypoactive sexual desire disorder	Oral medication; multifunctional serotonin agonist antagonist	FDA approved for treatment of hypoactive sexual desire disorder in premenopausal women; currently administered under a Risk Evaluation and Mitigation Strategy program; common side effects include dizziness, somnolence, nausea, and headache; use of alcohol contraindicated; safety and efficacy unknown for breast cancer survivors

Table 5.7 (continued)

Management strategy	Sexual problems	Description	Comments
Bremelanotide	Hypoactive sexual desire disorder	Injection; activates melanocortin receptors	FDA approved for treatment of hypoactive sexual desire disorder in premenopausal women; women inject it under the skin of the abdomen or thigh at least 45 minutes before anticipated sexual activity; should not be used in women with uncontrolled high blood pressure or those with or at risk for cardiovascular disease; safety and efficacy has not been studied in breast cancer survivors
PDE5 inhibitors	Used for erectile disorder, with no evidence for female sexual dysfunction	Oral medication (sildenafil, tadalafil, and vardenafil); not recommended for use in women	Not FDA approved for the treatment of female sexual dysfunction; data regarding treatment for female sexual dysfunction inconsistent and largely unfavorable; no data regarding safety in breast cancer survivors

patient may prefer different types of lubricant for vaginal versus anal penetration). While water-based lubricants may dry out or evaporate during longer periods of sexual activity or require re-application during activity, water-based lubricants are generally compatible with latex, silicone vaginal dilators, and silicone sexual devices or toys (e.g., vibrators). Water-based lubricants are also unlikely to stain linens or fabrics. Silicone-based lubricants (e.g., dimethicone, cyclomethicone) do not evaporate and are longer lasting than water-based lubricants. While silicone-based lubricants are safe to use with latex condoms and can be used underwater, they should not be used with vaginal dilators, sexual devices, or toys made from silicone, as it will cause the surface to deteriorate and the material will degrade over time. Oil-based lubricants are long-lasting and do not wash away easily. However, these products should not be used with latex condoms as they can break down the material, and because they are long-lasting, they may increase the risk of infection [94]. Oil-based lubricants are also likely to stain linens and fabrics. Use of silicone-based and oil-based lubricants should be avoided on hard surfaces (e.g., tiled areas, showers, bathtubs) because they will make surfaces extremely slippery and can be difficult to remove, increasing the risk of falls. Petroleum or mineral oil-based products (e.g., Vaseline®, baby oil) should not be used in the vagina [88]. Use of petroleum jelly is associated with an increased risk of bacterial infection or bacterial vaginosis, and mineral oil-based products can increase the risk of yeast infection. Both petroleum and mineral oil-based products reduce the effectiveness of latex condoms.

The ingredients and chemical compositions of vaginal moisturizers and sexual lubricants vary widely, and many commercially available products may cause detrimental effects to vulvovaginal tissues due to additives, their osmolality (i.e., the concentration of dissolved particles per unit of water), and/or pH [80, 91, 95, 96]. Women with breast cancer should avoid using moisturizer and lubricant products that contain additives that are potential irritants, such as parabens, glycerin, and propylene glycol [88]. Additives such as warming agents, bactericides, microbicides, perfumes, and artificial colors and flavors can also further irritate the already sensitive vulvar region and vagina [88]. Depending on their chemical make-up and ingredients, moisturizers and lubricants have varying levels of osmolality. The World Health Organization (WHO) recommends that lubricants have an osmolality of <380 mOsm/kg; an osmolality of <1200 mOsm/kg is considered acceptable, while osmolality of >1200 mOsm/kg is associated with mucosal irritation [80]. Using a lubricant with high osmolality can dry out the vulvar and vaginal tissues, placing women at increased risk of abrasions, skin sloughing, and other cell damage. A 2018 study conducted by Ayehunie and colleagues [95] examined several widely available lubricants using a three-dimensional human vaginal epithelium tissue model and found that lubricants with osmolality >1500 mOsm/kg markedly reduced epithelial barrier properties and damaged the tissue structure. Products with pH levels in the normal range for healthy adult women (3.8–4.5) are considered acceptable, and those with pH levels of 3.0 or less are considered unacceptable due to risk for vaginal irritation [80]. In terms of osmolality and pH, breast cancer survivors should use products that are as "body-similar" as possible to vaginal secretions [96]. Unfortunately, most commercially available and widely used products have very high osmolality, with formulations that have high concentrations of glycerol, propylene glycol, or other ingredients that result in products with 4 to 30 times the osmolality of healthy vaginal fluid [95]. For example, in the study conducted by Ayehunie and colleagues [95], commercial products with high osmolality included RepHresh (1500 mOsm/kg; Lil' Drug Store Products, Inc., Cedar Rapids), K-Y Jelly Personal Lubricant (2200 mOsm/kg; Reckitt Benckiser LLC, Parsippany, NJ), ID Glide (2900 mOsm/kg; Westridge Laboratories, Inc., Newport Beach, CA), Astroglide (4500 mOsm/kg; Bio film, Inc., Vista, CA), and K-Y Warming Jelly (8600 mOsm/kg; Reckitt Benckiser, LLC., Parsippany, NJ). Non-irritant products with osmolality <1200 mOsm/kg examined in this study included Aloe Cadabra (118 mOsm/kg; Seven Oaks Farm, Ventura, CA), Good Clean Love (194 mOsm/kg; GCL, Eugene, OR), Pre-Seed (295 mOsm/kg; Lil' Drug Store Products, Inc., Cedar Rapids, IA), and Restore (340 mOsm/kg; GCL, Eugene, OR).

Many available moisturizers and lubricants do not list osmolality or pH on the product label, making it difficult for women to determine the safety of products. This lack of available information is further complicated by a rapidly changing marketplace, characterized by frequent introductions of new products, manufacturers changing/updating product formulations, and product relabeling.

Box 5.3 Important steps when selecting a sexual lubricant

1. Examine the label to check for ingredients that should be avoided including potential irritants such as parabens, glycerin, and propylene glycol. Additives such as warming agents, bactericides, microbicides, perfumes, and artificial colors and flavors should also be avoided.
2. Review the lists of lubricant testing results conducted by the WHO and other researchers. These lists include the brand name, osmolality, and pH level of each product. These lists are maintained and made available online by professional and women's health organizations. For example, at the time of writing this chapter, Women's Voices for the Earth (WVE) maintains a lubricant factsheet and listing of lubricant product information online (https://www.womensvoices.org/osmolality-ph-properties-commercial-lubricants/). Keep in mind that the WHO recommends using a lubricant with osmolality <1200 mOsm/kg and a pH of 3.8 to 4.5 [80].
3. If a product is not included in available lists, contact the manufacturer to obtain information about product ingredients, osmolality, and pH.
4. If any reactions or symptoms occur after using a product, stop using it immediately and try a different product.

Gel or Cream with Hyaluronic Acid

Vaginal creams or gels with hyaluronic acid are receiving growing attention for their potential to manage vaginal dryness and associated symptoms [97–102]. Several small studies have examined the use of products with hyaluronic acid and have found them to be safe and as effective as vaginal estrogen in reducing vulvovaginal symptoms (i.e., vaginal dryness, itching and dyspareunia) [97–99]. One small randomized pilot trial in breast cancer survivors starting aromatase inhibitors ($N = 57$) found that women who received a hyaluronic acid-based moisturizer reported less dyspareunia and sexual distress at 6 months compared to women who received usual care [102]. Further, women who received the hyaluronic acid-based moisturizer reported improved sexual function and well-being (as measured by the FSFI) compared to women who received a vaginal moisturizer without hyaluronic acid [102]. In a recent single-arm prospective, longitudinal pilot study, Carter and colleagues examined the use of hyaluronic acid gel over 24 weeks in 101 breast cancer survivors taking aromatase inhibitors [101]. Vulvovaginal health and sexual function improved over time, and the authors concluded that using hyaluronic acid gel on a schedule of 3–5 times per week may be effective for improving symptoms of vaginal dryness and dyspareunia in breast cancer survivors [101]. Similar findings were reported for women with endometrial cancer [100]. While products containing hyaluronic acid show promise for managing vulvovaginal symptoms, additional research is needed to further examine the safety, potential benefits, and longer-term outcomes for breast cancer survivors.

Sexual Devices

For breast cancer survivors who experience decreased sensation, difficulty building arousal, sexual pain, and other difficulties, sexual devices can be used to help manage these challenges or expand the repertoire of available sexual activities to accommodate changes in sexual function [14, 88]. Prior to starting a conversation with breast cancer survivors about the use of sexual devices, it is important to ask a few screening questions to determine individuals' familiarity, comfort level, and openness to discussing and using sexual devices (e.g., Have you ever or do you currently use a sexual device alone or with a partner?; Would you consider using a sexual device if it would improve your sexual health and wellness?) [103]. Because survivors may have a lack of knowledge or experience with sexual devices, providing descriptions or basic information about common types of sexual devices is often helpful (e.g., clitoral stimulator, vibrators for external and internal use).

As part of any discussion about sexual devices, breast cancer survivors should be given information regarding the importance of using safe and nontoxic materials [103]. Nonporous materials, such as silicone and hypoallergenic metals (e.g., stainless steel, titanium), are generally preferable as porous materials may prevent effective disinfection. If patients use glass materials, this should be done with extreme caution in the vagina in order to prevent lacerations. Borosilicate material is stronger than other glass materials with reduced risk of breakage. It is important to recognize that there are currently no organizations, boards, or coalitions that regulate the safety of commercially available sexual devices in the USA, Japan, Canada, or the European Union. Any product or device labeled as "For Novelty Use Only" should be avoided. Devices made with jelly latex (which contains polyvinyl chloride (PVC)) are common and should also be avoided, as this type of material may leak toxins especially as it ages. In general, products containing jelly latex are soft and have a plastic smell (e.g., smell like a new shower curtain). Products that are scented should also be avoided, because of risk of irritation.

For breast cancer survivors experiencing decreased sensation or difficulty building arousal, vibrators or self-stimulators may be helpful for providing extra or more intense stimulation to areas of the clitoris, vulva, and vagina [14, 88]. Stimulation with devices that promote blood flow and circulation in the pelvic region (i.e., vibrators, clitoral stimulators, clitoral vacuum devices) may be helpful for facilitating arousal and for reducing discomfort or pain [14, 76, 80]. Vibrators and stimulators are available in a wide range of types, and there are a range of available features (e.g., varying strengths, patterns, speeds, and types of stimulation; range of sizes and surfaces used for stimulation; ability to connect to apps or electronic devices; waterproof or water resistant). External vibrators and clitoral stimulators (including clitoral vacuum devices) are designed to be used externally for clitoral stimulation. Internal vibrators are designed to be used internally (e.g., inserted into the vagina) or externally and are typically shaped for insertion. Sexual devices that are specifically designed for use with a partner are also available (e.g., hands free clitoral stimulators, vibrators that attach to a partner's hand or a penis). In addition to seeking out products made with safe and non-toxic materials, factors to consider when selecting a vibrator or stimulator include intended use (i.e., external and/or internal stimulation; self-stimulation and/or partnered activity), type of stimulation (e.g., vibration, vacuum), preference for size and aesthetic (e.g., subtle, anatomically realistic), strength and patterns of stimulation available, and preferred special features (e.g., waterproof, ability to connect to apps or devices). The selection of sexual devices depends on individual preferences and desired sexual activity.

For women who have foreshortening of the vaginal canal or those experiencing deep vaginal/pelvic pain with penetrative sexual activity, the use of a sexual device that precludes deep insertion may be helpful. One such product is The Ohnut™, which includes four interlocking, soft rings that can be placed around the base of a penis, vaginal dilator, or sex toy to restrict the depth of penetration. The female breast cancer survivor can choose the number of rings to use based on the amount of depth that is comfortable during penetrative activity and when used with a male partner the rings provide stimulation to the partner. This product and similar available products are available without a prescription and can be ordered online.

Vaginal Dilators

Regular use of vaginal dilators has been recommended for the management of symptomatic vaginal atrophy and has been found to reduce pain with vaginal penetration by improving vaginal elasticity [80, 89]. Vaginal dilator protocols may also be helpful for women experiencing fear of pain or vaginal tightness due to resulting pelvic floor or bodily tension associated with fear of penetration [51]. Use of vaginal dilators involves a systematic, graduated approach with a set of tapered devices that vary in size and facilitate mechanical stretch of vaginal tissue and underlying pelvic floor muscles. While data regarding the effectiveness of specific vaginal dilator protocols is limited, general clinical guidelines suggest consistent use of dilators, using dilators in a progressive fashion (e.g., graduated sizes) and use of dilators at least three times per week for approximately 10–15 minutes per session [51]. If vaginal dilators are recommended, breast cancer survivors should be given clear instructions regarding how to use vaginal dilators in graduated sizes (either by themselves or with their partner) [80]. Physical therapists trained in pelvic floor physical therapy may be particularly helpful in providing women with education, clear protocols, and instructions for using vaginal dilators [104, 105]. After completing an external and internal evaluation (e.g., skin integrity, evidence of prolapse, pelvic floor contraction/relaxation and associated movement, reflex assessment, and pain or muscle spasm during palpation), a pelvic floor physical therapist can provide women with a vaginal dilator protocol and instructions to specifically address their presenting concerns. Providing ongoing support and instruction for women using vaginal dilators is essential for program adherence [106, 107].

Pelvic Floor Physical Therapy

The network of pelvic floor muscles and fascia play an important role in sexual function and continence [108, 109]. Pelvic floor muscle dysfunction can contribute to dyspareunia, difficulty with arousal and orgasm, and urinary incontinence [105, 109]. A study of 167 long-term breast cancer survivors found that 45% of women reported pain during sexual intercourse [110]. It is important to promptly address sexual pain as repeated or ongoing sexual experiences can lead to secondary vaginismus and chronically over-engaged pelvic floor muscles [14]. Pelvic floor physical therapy with a physical therapist specifically trained in the management of pelvic floor disorders is recommended for breast cancer survivors experiencing pain with sexual activity by the consensus guidelines of the North American Menopause Society and the International Society for the Study of Women's Sexual Health [80]. Pelvic floor physical therapy treats pelvic floor muscle dysfunction and has been found to improve sexual function as well as urinary symptoms [109, 111]. In women without a cancer history, pelvic floor physical therapy is effective in treating sexual pain and all types of incontinence, and women treated with pelvic floor physical therapy are more likely to report improvements in sexual and urinary symptoms as well as better quality of life than controls [104, 105, 112]. In a pilot study conducted by Juraskova and colleagues [113], 25 breast cancer survivors with dyspareunia received pelvic floor muscle relaxation training under the direction of a physical therapist. Women experienced significantly less dyspareunia and improvements in sexual function and quality of life, with 92% of women reporting that pelvic floor muscle training was helpful. Two pilot randomized controlled trials [111, 114] conducted with gynecologic cancer survivors found that after pelvic floor physical therapy women had better sexual function, decreased urinary incontinence, and improved quality of life, without adverse effects. While little research has examined the use of pelvic floor physical therapy in breast cancer survivors, pilot studies suggest that pelvic floor physical therapy is efficacious and acceptable, with no adverse effects [111, 113, 114].

Counseling and Sex Therapy

Psychological and behavioral interventions (i.e., counseling or psychotherapy, sex therapy) are key components of treating many of the sexual difficulties experienced by breast cancer survivors [51, 88, 115]. The American Society of Clinical Oncology (ASCO) Practice Guideline for addressing sexual problems in cancer survivors states that psychosocial and/or psychosexual counseling should be offered to all cancer survivors to improve sexual response, body image, intimacy and relationship issues, and overall sexual functioning and satisfaction [116].

Sex therapy (or psychosexual counseling) is a specialized type of psychotherapy provided by a trained mental health professional (e.g., psychologist, marital and family therapist, social worker) that focuses on addressing the psychological, behavioral, and interpersonal factors that impact sexual function and satisfaction. Sex therapy also focuses on helping individuals, and couples manage the sexual impacts of physical and functional sexual health changes. Sex therapy approaches often include cognitive-behavioral interventions, mindfulness techniques, couples-based psychotherapy interventions, and psycho-education. Sex therapy is frequently used in combination with medical and/or physical therapy interventions. When making recommendations for sex therapy, it is important to provide breast cancer survivors with a clear description of this treatment approach, as many individuals have preconceived, incorrect ideas about sex therapy (e.g., clarify that sex therapy is a form of psychotherapy and does not involve physical contact with the therapist) [117]. Several professional organizations (see Table 5.5) provide online resources to assist with identifying sex therapy providers by geographic location (e.g., the American Association of Sexuality Educators, Counselors, and Therapists).

Accumulating evidence supports the use of sex therapy interventions to address the sexual difficulties many women experience following cancer treatment [118–125]. Sex therapy interventions have yielded significant improvements in desire, arousal, satisfaction, and overall sexual function and well-being among breast cancer survivors [123, 125–128] and women treated for other cancers [118, 119, 124]. Sex therapy interventions can be provided in an individual or couples therapy context [14]. For example, Rowland and colleagues [127] conducted a randomized control trial of a 6 week group intervention for breast cancer survivors aimed at improving sexual well-being. Breast cancer survivors' partners were not included in the intervention. The intervention included psycho-education, communication training, and sex therapy using a sensate focus approach (i.e., a sex therapy intervention approach that utilizes structured touch-based home practice exercises). Intervention participants reported a general increase in sexual satisfaction, relationship adjustment, and communication compared to the control group (printed educational material), and 64% noted at least some improvement in their relationship, despite partners not being included in the intervention sessions.

Among partnered breast cancer survivors, couples-based counseling can help to address communication issues, relationship dynamics, and conflicts that negatively impact the sexual relationship [115]. Couples often struggle with communication about and approaching sexual intimacy after breast cancer [10, 122]. Challenges to intimacy that often arise include partners' reactions to the treatment-related and sexual changes women experience, fear of pain or hurting one's partner, uncertainty about touching the chest region or surgically altered breast, and changes in roles that occurred during treatment (e.g., shift from partner to caregiver) [10, 115, 126].

Couples-based counseling can help to improve communication, problem solving, and coping skills, as well as help to improve the breast cancer survivor's response to sexual activity and ability to manage body image concerns [42, 115, 126].

Individual psychotherapy or counseling should be considered to help address other underlying concerns that can negatively impact sexual function and well-being, such as depression, anxiety, or trauma-related symptoms [115]. Cognitive-behavioral therapies (e.g., systematic desensitization) can also be helpful for breast cancer survivors experiencing fear or anticipatory pain related to sexual activity, genital touch, or genital exam [51].

Pharmacologic and Medical Approaches

Topical Lidocaine

For women experiencing pain with penetrative sexual activity (i.e., insertional dyspareunia), the use of topical lidocaine applied to the vaginal vestibule prior to vaginal penetration may help to reduce pain. One pilot double-blind randomized trial of 4% aqueous lidocaine versus saline has been conducted in breast cancer survivors ($N = 46$) with severe vaginal dryness, atrophy, and dyspareunia [129]. In both the lidocaine and saline groups, women also used a silicone-based lubricant. Users of lidocaine (applied as a compress to the vaginal vestibule approximately three minutes prior to penetration) reported less pain during intercourse, less sexual distress, and improved sexual function, with no adverse effects. In addition, sexual partners did not report penile numbness.

Local Estrogen-Based Treatments

While international guidelines recommend against systemic hormone replacement therapy in breast cancer survivors [80], local estrogen-based treatments, with estradiol or estriol, for vaginal dryness and atrophy remain controversial, and the safety of vaginal estrogen has yet to be strongly established for breast cancer survivors [116, 130]. This book's chapter on the management of genitourinary symptoms of menopause provides a discussion of the available data regarding the safety and efficacy of local estrogen for breast cancer survivors. The first-line approach for managing vaginal dryness and atrophy in breast cancer survivors should include non-hormonal options [80]. For breast cancer survivors, whose symptoms remain severe with non-hormonal treatments, recommendations from the American College of Obstetricians and Gynecologists (ACOG), the North American Menopause Society, the International Society for the Study of Women's Sexual Health, and the ASCO advise that consideration of using local estrogen-based treatments should be individualized for each breast cancer survivor, involve close consultation with the survivor's oncologist, and take into account the uncertainties regarding risks [80, 116, 130]. When considering the use of local estrogen-based treatments for breast cancer survivors, the following steps should be taken.

- Determine the presence of symptoms that are severe, negatively impact quality of life and have not responded to non-hormonal interventions [116].
- Evaluate the factors that impact the potential risk of using local estrogen in breast cancer survivors including breast cancer stage and

subtype, endocrine therapy use, and time since diagnosis [80]. While data are limited, consensus opinion indicates that factors associated with lower risk for use of local estrogen-based treatments include Stage 0 to 2 disease, low or intermediate grade disease, no lymph node involvement, negative hormone-receptor status, use of tamoxifen vs. an aromatase inhibitor, low risk of recurrence, and longer-term survivorship [80].

- Discuss treatment options, provide patient education, and discuss the risks versus benefits of treatment using a shared decision-making approach with breast cancer survivors considering local estrogen-based treatment. This discussion should include information about mechanisms of action when known, data regarding safety, potential efficacy, and potential adverse effects of treatment options [80, 116]. Balancing the benefits of potential symptom reduction versus a breast cancer survivor's fears or concerns about breast cancer recurrence risk should be discussed and considered.
- Review recent, clinical guidelines to obtain guidance on products, dosages, and safety, as there are a range of local estrogen-based treatments available (e.g., creams, rings, inserts) and there is currently no strong evidence for the safety and efficacy of one vaginal estrogen product versus another [80, 130].
- In cases where local estrogen-based treatment is initiated, regular monitoring and follow-up care should be provided to assess impact on symptoms, adherence, and barriers to treatment [80].

Because estradiol is more potent than estriol, estradiol has been more commonly used as a vaginal preparation and is FDA approved in several preparations in the USA. Vaginal estriol (gels, creams, or suppositories) is also available in several countries outside the USA, but is not FDA approved for any indication in the USA. The efficacy and safety of vaginal estriol has not been demonstrated for breast cancer survivors or women with no cancer history. The use of vaginal estriol in breast cancer survivors is not recommended [80].

Vaginal Dehydroepiandrosterone (DHEA)

Vaginal DHEA has been approved by the FDA for postmenopausal women with moderate to severe dyspareunia caused by vulvovaginal atrophy. The FDA-approved vaginal DHEA has not been studied in breast cancer survivors, and its label includes a warning against using this product in women with a history of breast cancer. Clinical studies of women without cancer indicate that there may be a slight increase in plasma estradiol and testosterone after use of vaginal DHEA (i.e., prasterone) [131]. One clinical trial conducted with breast and gynecologic cancer survivors compared vaginal DHEA (3.25 mg and 6.5 mg) versus placebo over 12 weeks for the treatment of moderate vaginal dryness or dyspareunia [132, 133]. While DHEA (either dose) yielded no improvement in vaginal dryness or dyspareunia compared to placebo, women using 6.5 mg of DHEA reported significant improvement in sexual function on the FSFI [133]. Importantly, significantly increased hormone concentrations (i.e., circulating DHEA-S, testosterone, and estradiol) were found in women using 6.5 mg of DHEA, though levels remained in the lower half of the postmenopausal range and estrogen concentrations remained unchanged in women taking aromatase inhibitors [132]. In terms of the efficacy and safety of vaginal DHEA versus local estrogen-based treatments, there are no studies directly comparing these treatments in breast cancer survivors. The short- and long-term safety of vaginal DHEA remains largely unknown for breast cancer survivors, and caution should be used when considering vaginal DHEA for breast cancer survivors whose cancer is known to be androgen-receptor positive, whether they are taking tamoxifen or an aromatase inhibitor [80].

Vaginal Testosterone

The off-label use of vaginal testosterone for the treatment of vulvovaginal symptoms in breast cancer survivors is not recommended [80].

Currently, there are no FDA-approved formulations of local testosterone for use in women. Very little data is available regarding the use of vaginal testosterone in breast cancer survivors, and data is only available for breast cancer survivors taking aromatase inhibitors [134–136]. In one trial of breast cancer survivors taking aromatase inhibitors, 12% of women were found to have elevated estradiol levels after 4 weeks of treatment [136].

Selective Estrogen Receptor Modulators (SERM)

SERMs are estrogen receptor ligands that in some tissues, such as bone and cardiovascular system, act like estrogen but in other tissues, such as the breast and central nervous system, block the effects of estrogen. Different SERMs have varying effects on organs [137]. For instance, tamoxifen, the first SERM shown to effectively treat breast cancer, acts as an anti-estrogen on breast tissue, breast cancer cells, and the central nervous system, while having estrogenic effects on bone, the cardiovascular system, the endometrial lining, and the vaginal mucosa [138–140]. The estrogenic effect on the vaginal mucosa causes a vaginal discharge. Recognition of this side effect led to the study of SERMs and their potential benefit in alleviating vaginal dryness and its consequences [141].

Ospemifene is a SERM used to treat postmenopausal vulvovaginal atrophy and associated dyspareunia. Ospemifene was found to be effective for treating vulvovaginal atrophy in a Phase 3 trial with postmenopausal women with no cancer history [142], but this medication has not been adequately evaluated for use in breast cancer survivors [80]. Ospemifene's impact on breast cancer risk in women with no cancer history remains unclear, and its impact on risk of recurrence in breast cancer survivors has not been studied. While ospemifene is used in Europe for breast cancer survivors who have completed treatment, it is not FDA approved for use with breast cancer survivors in the USA [80].

Vaginal Laser Treatment

Vaginal laser therapies are increasingly being offered for the treatment of genitourinary symptoms of menopause [143, 144]. Vaginal laser treatments aim to induce changes in vaginal tissue to stimulate vascularity and promote production of new collagen, which could result in improved integrity and elasticity of vaginal tissue [80]. The FDA has approved laser treatment for other medical indications (e.g., dental procedures, cosmetic surgery, cataract removal), but to date these therapies have not been approved for treating vaginal tissue. Available data suggest that vaginal laser therapy with either the nonablative erbium-doped yttrium aluminum garnet laser (FotonaSmooth®) or the microablative CO_2 laser (MonaLisa Touch®) may reduce symptoms of vaginal dryness and dyspareunia in women with no cancer history [143, 144]. However, many of these studies have small samples, short duration of follow-up, and poor quality research designs or methodology and/or are device-sponsored. In breast cancer survivors, one retrospective study ($N = 26$) evaluated the effects of CO_2 laser treatment on vulvovaginal symptoms [145]. Women were treated with three cycles of laser therapy, with each cycle occurring every 30–40 days. Vulvovaginal symptoms significantly decreased over time regardless of type of adjuvant breast cancer therapy or age. Another small study prospectively evaluated the effects of CO_2 laser treatment in postmenopausal breast cancer survivors ($N = 20$) [146]. This study found significant reductions in vulvovaginal symptoms from baseline to 30 days after the second laser treatment and, importantly, non-significant changes in the vaginal microbiome suggesting that laser treatment may be safe for breast cancer survivors. One study evaluated Erbium laser treatment (three cycles occurring every 30 days) in post-menopausal breast cancer survivors ($N = 43$) [147]. Vaginal dryness and dyspareunia were reduced after the third treatment and up to 12 months after treatment, but effects were no longer present at 18 months. While these preliminary studies suggest that vaginal laser treatments could potentially improve vaginal dryness and dyspareunia in breast cancer survivors, prospective randomized clinical trials are needed to determine the efficacy and safety of these treatments. Further, the optimal number of treatment cycles, duration between cycles, and number of retreatments needed have yet to be determined. High-quality data describing the indications, safety, benefits, and appropriate treatment regimens for vaginal laser treatment in breast cancer survivors are needed before recommendations regarding the use of these therapies can be made [80].

Bupropion

The antidepressant bupropion has been increasingly used to treat sexual desire and arousal disorders [148]. Bupropion belongs to the aminoketone class of antidepressants and is not related to tricyclics or to serotonin reuptake inhibitors. It is generally well tolerated with common side effects that include difficulties with concentration, insomnia, and tremors. While the mechanism of action for bupropion has not been clearly defined, it may facilitate dopamine and norepinephrine neuro-transmission by inhibiting reuptake [149].

Bupropion, sustained-release at 300 to 400 mg daily dose, has been shown to improve sexual arousal, orgasm, and sexual satisfaction in premenopausal women with hypoactive sexual desire disorder, and women report being satisfied with the treatment [150, 151]. Bupropion has also been shown to increase sexual desire, arousal, orgasm intensity, and overall sexual satisfaction in premenopausal women experiencing selective serotonin reuptake inhibitor (SSRI)-induced sexual dysfunction [152]. Adding bupropion sustained-release 150 mg twice daily to the SSRI regimen decreases SSRI-induced sexual dysfunction [148]. One small open-label trial has been conducted to evaluate the relationship between bupropion and sexual function in breast cancer survivors ($N = 20$; age: $M = 50.6$ years, $SD = 2.7$) [153]. Women who had completed chemotherapy and were on adjuvant endocrine therapy (with tamoxifen or an aromatase inhibitor) were eligible to participate. Breast cancer survivors received oral bupropion 150 mg daily for 8 weeks. After 4 weeks of treatment, women reported improved sexual function that persisted until the end of the study (i.e., 8 weeks). Women reported significant improvements in sexual desire, arousal, vaginal lubrication, orgasm, and sexual satisfaction. While this study reported no serious adverse events during the course of its short duration, data regarding the long-term safety and efficacy of bupropion in breast cancer survivors, especially those taking tamoxifen, is lacking [153]. Some data suggest that bupropion may inhibit CYP2D6 and interfere with metabolism of tamoxifen [88], though the clinical impact of this pharmacologic interaction is likely negligible [154].

Flibanserin

The FDA approved flibanserin (Addyi®) 100 mg tablets in 2015 for the treatment of hypoactive sexual desire disorder (HSDD) in premenopausal women [155]. Flibanserin is a multifunctional serotonin agonist antagonist (a serotonin$_{1A}$ receptor agonist and a serotonin$_{2A}$ receptor antagonist). The reported mechanism of action is to increase the release of norepinephrine and dopamine and decrease the release of serotonin in the cortex of the brain, which is believed to enhance sexual desire [156]. Studies examining the safety of flibanserin for premenopausal and postmenopausal women with hypoactive sexual desire disorder have found that common side effects include dizziness, somnolence, nausea, and headache [155]. The use of alcohol is contraindicated with flibanserin due to an increased risk for severe hypotension, syncope, sedation, and somnolence. In order to inform patients about these risks, flibanserin is currently administered in the context of a Risk Evaluation and Mitigation Strategy (REMS) program. The safety and efficacy of flibanserin has not been studied in breast cancer survivors. One observational study is currently underway (estimated enrollment $N = 20$ with an estimated completion date in 2021) to examine the feasibility of using flibanserin in breast cancers survivors taking tamoxifen or aromatase inhibitors (ClinicalTrials.gov identifier NCT03707340). The ASCO Practice Guideline for addressing sexual problems in cancer survivors [116] states that clinicians may offer flibanserin to premenopausal women who are experiencing hypoactive sexual desire disorder. The Practice Guideline also includes an important Qualifying Statement noting that flibanserin has not been evaluated in women with a history of cancer or those on endocrine therapy, and the risk/benefit ratio for this medication is uncertain.

Bremelanotide

Bremelanotide (Vyleesi®) was approved by the FDA in June 2019 for the treatment of acquired, generalized HSDD in premenopausal women [155, 157]. Bremelanotide activates melanocortin receptors, but the mechanism by which it improves sexual desire is unknown. To use bremelanotide, women inject it under the skin of the abdomen or thigh at least 45 minutes before anticipated sexual activity. The optimal time to inject bremelanotide may vary based on the duration of benefit and side effects experienced. More than one dose of bremelanotide should not be used within 24 hours or more than eight doses per month. Common side effects include nausea, vomiting, flushing, injection site reactions, and headache. Bremelanotide should not be used in women with high blood pressure that is uncontrolled or in those with known cardiovascular disease, and it is not recommended for women at high risk for cardiovascular disease [157]. The safety and efficacy of bremelanotide has not been studied in breast cancer survivors, and there are no recommendations regarding its use in this population.

Phosphodiesterase Type 5 (PDE5) Inhibitors

While PDE5 inhibitors (e.g., sildenafil, tadalafil, and vardenafil) are used to treat male erectile dysfunction, these medications are not FDA approved for the treatment of female sexual dysfunction. Available data regarding the benefits of PDE5 inhibitor treatment for female sexual dysfunction are inconsistent and largely unfavorable [158]. The lack of efficacy for PDE5 inhibitor treatment in women may be due to the discordance between genital and subjective measures of sexual response commonly found in women. Importantly, there are no adequately sized studies with longer-term data regarding the safety of PDE5 Inhibitors in breast cancer survivors [88].

Herbs, Botanicals, and Other Products

Many breast cancer survivors express interest in supplements, natural remedies, botanicals, or herbal products for managing sexual difficulties [88]. Breast cancer survivors should be educated about the importance of carefully reading the ingredients and consulting with their oncology provider before using any such product [80]. There is no or very little data available regarding the safety and efficacy of these products for breast cancer survivors, and many of these products may be contraindicated for women with hormone-sensitive cancers. Table 5.8 summarizes information from important online resources [159–161] and provides key information for several commonly available products, including purpose used, ingredients, and any known contraindications.

Fertility Concerns

For women of reproductive age, treatments for breast cancer, including chemotherapies and endocrine therapies, may impact fertility (see Table 5.9) [11]. Organizations including the ASCO [162], ACOG [163, 164], American Society for Reproductive Medicine (ASRM) [165], NCCN [166], and International Consensus Conference for Breast Cancer in Young Women [167] recommend that, prior to treatment, providers discuss the potential impact of cancer treatment on fertility and provide rapid referral (e.g.,

Table 5.8 Herbs, botanicals, and other products

Product	Description	Purported uses	Warnings and contraindications	Comments
ArginMax	Dietary supplement containing gingko biloba, panax ginseng, American ginseng, damiana, L-arginine, vitamins A, C, E, B-complex, zinc, and selenium	Increase sexual satisfaction and improve sexual function	Possible estrogenic activity of ginseng; L-Arginine may affect blood sugar levels; L-Arginine may worsen asthma symptoms; do not use during pregnancy or breast feeding. Possible interactions with anticoagulants, antihypertensive, and hypoglycemic drugs	Thought to enhance blood circulation and muscle relaxation; study in breast cancer survivors found no benefit for sexual function [217]
Avlimil	Dietary supplement containing sage leaf, red raspberry leaf, kudzu root extract, red clover extract, capsicum pepper, licorice root, bayberry fruit, damiana leaf, valerian root, ginger root, and black cohosh root	Reduce symptoms of female sexual dysfunction including desire, arousal, and orgasm difficulties. Reduce pain with intercourse	Possible estrogenic effect of ingredients; Federal Trade Commission charged the marketers of Avlimil in making false and unsubstantiated claims	Thought to promote blood flow and muscle relaxation; No data available for formulation used in commercially available product; has not been studied in breast cancer survivors
Maca	Plant root used to make extracts, tablets, and capsules	Increase sexual desire; reduce symptoms of menopause; infertility	Possible estrogenic effect; safety unknown during pregnancy and breast feeding	Data regarding benefits for sexual dysfunction, menopausal symptoms and infertility are inconsistent and lacking [218, 219].
Yohimbe	Bark used to make extracts, tablets, and capsules	Increase sexual desire	Interacts with numerous drugs and can cause severe adverse effects. Contraindicated for those with high blood pressure, heart disease, arrhythmias, Parkinson's disease, seizure disorders, kidney, thyroid, or liver disease, sexual organ inflammatory disorders, ulcers, or psychiatric disorders. Do not use during pregnancy or breast feeding. Should not be taken with antidepressants, foods containing tyramine, decongestants, diet aids, or phenylpropanolamine-containing products	Products containing yohimbe have a large number of documented contraindications, are responsible for frequent toxic effects, and have severe events requiring hospitalization. Amount of yohimbe in commercially available products is often inaccurate or not reported
Zestra	Topical botanical formulation containing borage seed oil, evening primrose oil, angelica root extract, coleus forskohlii extract, ascorbyl palmitate, and di-alpha tocopherol	Reduce symptoms of female sexual dysfunction including desire, arousal, and orgasm difficulties. Reduce pain with intercourse	Contraindicated in women who are pregnant and breastfeeding and in those trying to conceive; not recommended for use in women with vaginal irritation, atrophy, or infection	Has not been studied in breast cancer survivors

Note: Information compiled from the Natural Medicines Comprehensive Database Consumer Version [159], National Center for Complementary and Integrative Health [160], and the Memorial Sloan Kettering Cancer Center online database on herbs, botanicals, and other products [161]

Table 5.9 Female level of risk for ovarian failure and infertility after chemotherapy. Adapted from the Pediatric Initiative Network [220]

Type of chemotherapy		Minimally increased risk	Significantly increased risk	High level of significantly increased risk
Alkylating agents by cyclophosphamide equivalent dose (CED, gm/m2) [221]		CED <4	4–8	>8
Heavy metals/platinum agents		Cisplatin Carboplatin		
Hematopoietic stem cell transplant (HSCT) conditioning				Alkylating agent +/− total body irradiation (TBI). Includes myeloablative and reduced intensity regimens
Radiation exposure	Ovary [221, 222]		<10 Gy	≥ 10 Gy
	Hypothalamus [223]	22–29.9 Gy	> 30–39.9 Gy	> 40 Gy

within 24 hours) for fertility preservation when possible. During this consultation, breast cancer patients should be provided with a personalized estimation of their risk of gonadal failure and infertility after their cancer treatment as well as information regarding available fertility preservation strategies, the timing of fertility preservation procedures in relation to the initiation of cancer treatments, success rates, costs, and possible ethical considerations (e.g., posthumous use of stored oocytes or embryos, the use of embryos in the event of separation or divorce) [11, 168]. Decisions related to fertility preservation are complex and, for many patients, can be associated with emotional distress. Fertility-related emotional distress may in fact increase over the course of treatment and, for some patients, may persist for several years following treatment completion [169–171]. Thus, patients may also benefit from referral to a mental health professional to assist with making fertility-related decisions, processing the long-term implications of these decisions, and managing uncertainty regarding fertility [166].

For breast cancer patients who are candidates for fertility preservation, possible options include oocyte or embryo cryopreservation, ovarian tissue cryopreservation, and ovarian transposition [172, 173]. ASCO guidelines recommend that ovarian suppression with gonadotropin-releasing hormone (GnRH) agonists only be offered when proven fertility preservation methods are not feasible [162]. Considerations for choice of preservation modality may include patient preference, partner status, age, cost, the time required to pursue preservation modalities, and potential side effects and toxicities associated with the preservation strategy. For example, cryopreservation of oocytes or embryos, long considered the "gold standard" for female fertility preservation, requires approximately 2 weeks of ovarian stimulation and egg retrieval, which may not be feasible for patients needing to start potentially gonadotoxic therapy emergently. Ovarian tissue cryopreservation (OTC) was previously considered experimental but was recently deemed non-experimental by the ASRM [174]. OTC is typically performed by laparoscopic removal of ovarian tissue (either part of an ovary or an entire ovary). This surgery can be performed urgently prior to initiation of potentially gonadotoxic therapy (i.e., does not require the two weeks of stimulation needed for oocyte cryopreservation), it allows the patient to attempt natural conception after reimplantation, and it also restores endocrine (ovarian) function in the majority of women who undergo reimplantation. However, it is not currently offered at every center providing fertility preservation care, and it has been found to be more successful in younger women, with little data on resultant live births if tissue harvesting is performed over age 36–40 [175, 176].

Reproductive care is an essential component of cancer survivorship and necessary for patients planning to use cryopreserved oocytes, embryos, or ovarian tissue. Of note, only ~7% of patients return to use their cryopreserved gametes [175]. This may be because some patients conceive on their own, others do not attempt to conceive, and current studies often lack the long-term follow-up necessary to determine cumulative use. Following completion of adjuvant treatment with chemotherapy and/or radiation, and in consultation with the patient's oncologist and maternal fetal medicine specialist to determine safety of attempting conception, a patient may decide to use her preserved oocytes, embryos, or tissue. When appropriate, fertilization of oocytes with sperm via intracytoplasmic sperm injection (ICSI) can be used for creation of embryos. Embryo transfer typically involves several weeks of hormone supplementation (versus utilization of the patient's natural cycle) followed by a non-invasive office procedure for placing the embryo into the patient's uterine cavity; this procedure can be performed regardless of the patient's ovarian function and menopausal status after her cancer therapy. Rates of pregnancy among cancer survivors following embryo or oocyte cryopreservation are currently unknown. In the general population, the cumulative pregnancy rates for embryo and oocyte cryopreservation are approximately 60% and 50%, respectively [177]. From the planned ovarian tissue cryopreservation literature (sometimes referred to as "elective" fertility preservation for typical ovarian aging), the success rate is highly dependent on patient age and oocyte yield [178] and averages 5–7% chance of live birth per cryopreserved oocyte [179]. Finally, ovarian suppression with gonadotropin releasing hormone (GnRH) analogs administered during cytotoxic therapy have been associated with reduced risk for subsequent premature ovarian failure (and possibly higher rates of post-treatment pregnancy) in breast cancer patients [180]. A randomized prospective trial (POEMS) conducted by the SWOG cancer research network demonstrated improved rates of pregnancy in triple negative breast cancer patients who received the GnRH analog goserelin during their chemotherapy compared to control group who did not (21% vs 11%, p0.03) [181].

While patients with hormone receptor positive disease may have concerns about the impact of pregnancy and/or early termination of endocrine therapy on cancer outcomes, data from retrospective studies suggests that pregnancy is not associated with increased risk of recurrence or reduced disease-free survival [182–184]. It is not yet known whether stopping endocrine therapy to become pregnant is associated with poor cancer outcomes. A large-scale prospective study is currently under way to examine the risk of breast cancer recurrence associated with temporary interruption of endocrine therapy for estrogen receptor positive women who wish to become pregnant (POSITIVE: Pregnancy Outcome and Safety of Interrupting Therapy for Women with Endocrine Responsive Breast Cancer; NCT02308085). Women with estrogen receptor positive disease who interrupt endocrine therapy for the purpose of pregnancy should resume treatment following the birth of the child. It is also important to note that women with hormone receptor positive cancer who choose to cryopreserve oocytes or embryos will likely be offered co-administration of hormonal suppression during ovarian stimulation (e.g., with an aromatase inhibitor to decrease estradiol levels). This technique has been shown to successfully decrease the peak hormone levels reached during ovarian stimulation and does not appear to affect oocyte yield or quality [185, 186]. At a median follow-up of 5 years, patients with hormone-receptor positive cancer who chose to undergo fertility preservation with co-treatment with ovarian stimulation and aromatase inhibitor had no increase in recurrence rates compared with patients who did not undergo fertility preservation [185, 186].

Despite the availability of fertility preservation options, not all women are able or choose to engage in fertility preservation prior to initiating treatment. For women experiencing premature ovarian failure as a result of their treatments, there remain several options for family building. Women may engage in IVF using a donated oocyte fertilized by sperm from a partner or a donor; donor egg IVF has high cumulative pregnancy rates and is typically an option regardless of patient's menopausal status. Alternatively, for women unable to carry a child or who do not wish to undertake the risks of pregnancy, the use of a gestational carrier or adoption may be options [172, 180].

Conclusions

Breast cancer and its treatments significantly impact survivors' sexual and reproductive health [2, 3], and these changes often result in emotional distress, decreased emotional well-being, lower overall quality of life, and negatively impacted relationships [10, 12–15]. Because sexual and reproductive health difficulties are often complex, a multidisciplinary approach is required to address the many facets that can impact and be impacted by sexual and reproductive health changes. Current guidelines highlight the importance of routinely assessing and treating sexual problems as part of high-quality breast cancer survivorship care [14, 80, 116]. For women of reproductive age, multiple organizations stress the importance of addressing fertility concerns at the time of diagnosis, during treatment, and in longer-term survivorship [162–167]. The information provided in this chapter can help providers who care for breast cancer survivors better understand the impacts of breast cancer treatments on sexual function, approaches for assessing sexual problems, strategies for managing sexual problems, and recommendations for managing fertility concerns among these patients. It is also extremely important to recognize that addressing the sexual and reproductive health problems experienced by breast cancer survivors often requires a collaborative multidisciplinary team [14]. A robust referral network for sexual and reproductive health care is essential for helping oncology teams and breast cancer survivors manage these concerns. Working with breast cancer survivors to address their sexual and reproductive health difficulties can lead to greater emotional well-being, healthier relationships, and improved quality of life in breast cancer survivorship.

References

1. World Health Organization. Defining sexual health: report of a technical consultation on sexual health, 28–31 January 2002, Geneva. Geneva, Switzerland. 2006.
2. Katz A. Breast cancer and women's sexuality. Am J Nurs. 2011;111(4):63–7.
3. Bredart A, Dolbeault S, Savignoni A, et al. Prevalence and associated factors of sexual problems after early-stage breast cancer treatment: results of a French exploratory survey. Psychooncology. 2011;20(8):841–50.
4. Boehmer U, Ozonoff A, Timm A, Winter M, Potter J. After breast cancer: sexual functioning of sexual minority survivors. J Sex Res. 2014;51(6):681–9.
5. Boquiren VM, Esplen MJ, Wong J, Toner B, Warner E, Malik N. Sexual functioning in breast cancer survivors experiencing body image disturbance. Psychooncology. 2016;25(1):66–76.
6. Lee M, Kim YH, Jeon MJ. Risk factors for negative impacts on sexual activity and function in younger breast cancer survivors. Psychooncology. 2015;24(9):1097–103.
7. Safarinejad MR, Shafiei N, Safarinejad S. Quality of life and sexual functioning in young women with early-stage breast cancer 1 year after lumpectomy. Psychooncology. 2013;22(6):1242–8.
8. Schover LR, Baum GP, Fuson LA, Brewster A, Melhem-Bertrandt A. Sexual problems during the first 2 years of adjuvant treatment with aromatase inhibitors. J Sex Med. 2014;11(12):3102–11.
9. Raggio GA, Butryn ML, Arigo D, Mikorski R, Palmer SC. Prevalence and correlates of sexual morbidity in long-term breast cancer survivors. Psychol Health. 2014;29(6):632–50.
10. Male DA, Fergus KD, Cullen K. Sexual identity after breast cancer: sexuality, body image, and relationship repercussions. Curr Opin Support Palliat Care. 2016;10(1):66–74.
11. Lambertini M, Ginsburg ES, Partridge AH. Update on fertility preservation in young women undergoing breast cancer and ovarian cancer therapy. Curr Opin Obstet Gynecol. 2015;27(1):98–107.
12. Sadovsky R, Basson R, Krychman M, et al. Cancer and sexual problems. J Sex Med. 2010;7(1 Pt 2):349–73.
13. Zhou ES, Frederick NN, Bober SL. Hormonal changes and sexual dysfunction. Med Clin North Am. 2017;101(6):1135–50.
14. Bober SL, Reese JB, Barbera L, et al. How to ask and what to do: a guide for clinical inquiry and intervention regarding female sexual health after cancer. Curr Opin Support Palliat Care. 2016;10(1):44–54.
15. Sanchez Varela V, Zhou ES, Bober SL. Management of sexual problems in cancer patients and survivors. Curr Probl Cancer. 2013;37(6):319–52.
16. Thomas HN, Thurston RC. A biopsychosocial approach to women's sexual function and dys-

function at midlife: a narrative review. Maturitas. 2016;87:49–60.
17. Basson R. Human sexual response. In: Handbook of clinical neurology, vol. 130. Edinburgh: Elsevier; 2015. p. 11–8.
18. Kaplan HS. Disorders of sexual desire and other new concepts and techniques in sex therapy, vol. 2. New York: Bruner Meisel U; 1979.
19. Masters WH, Johnson VE. Human sexual response. Bronx: Ishi Press International; 1966.
20. Ussher JM, Perz J, Gilbert E. Changes to sexual Well-being and intimacy after breast cancer. Cancer Nurs. 2012;35(6):456–65.
21. Lewis PE, Sheng M, Rhodes MM, Jackson KE, Schover LR. Psychosocial concerns of young African American breast cancer survivors. J Psychosoc Oncol. 2012;30(2):168–84.
22. Quintard B, Constant A, Lakdja F, Labeyrie-Lagardere H. Factors predicting sexual functioning in patients 3 months after surgical procedures for breast cancer: the role of the sense of coherence. Eur J Oncol Nurs. 2014;18(1):41–5.
23. Andrzejczak E, Markocka-Maczka K, Lewandowski A. Partner relationships after mastectomy in women not offered breast reconstruction. Psychooncology. 2013;22(7):1653–7.
24. Gilbert E, Ussher JM, Perz J. Sexuality after breast cancer: a review. Maturitas. 2010;66(4):397–407.
25. Bancroft J, Graham CA, Janssen E, Sanders SA. The dual control model: current status and future directions. J Sex Res. 2009;46(2–3):121–42.
26. Nagoski E. Come as you are: the surprising new science that will transform your sex life. New York: Simon and Schuster; 2015.
27. Schlenz I, Kuzbari R, Gruber H, Holle J. The sensitivity of the nipple-areola complex: an anatomic study. Plast Reconstr Surg. 2000;105(3):905–9.
28. Wilmoth MC. The aftermath of breast cancer: an altered sexual self. Cancer Nurs. 2001;24(4):278–86.
29. Girgis A, Stacey F, Lee T, Black D, Kilbreath S. Priorities for women with lymphoedema after treatment for breast cancer: population based cohort study. BMJ. 2011;342:d3442.
30. Emilee G, Ussher JM, Perz J. Sexuality after breast cancer: a review. Maturitas. 2010;66(4):397–407.
31. Pillai-Friedman S, Ashline JL. Women, breast cancer survivorship, sexual losses, and disenfranchised grief - a treatment model for clinicians. Sex Relatsh Ther. 2014;29(4):436–53.
32. Kiebert GM, de Haes JC, van de Velde CJ. The impact of breast-conserving treatment and mastectomy on the quality of life of early-stage breast cancer patients: a review. J Clin Oncol. 1991;9(6):1059–70.
33. Markopoulos C, Tsaroucha AK, Kouskos E, Mantas D, Antonopoulou Z, Karvelis S. Impact of breast cancer surgery on the self-esteem and sexual life of female patients. J Int Med Res. 2009;37(1):182–8.
34. Aerts L, Christiaens MR, Enzlin P, Neven P, Amant F. Sexual functioning in women after mastectomy versus breast conserving therapy for early-stage breast cancer: a prospective controlled study. Breast. 2014;23(5):629–36.
35. Falk SJ, Dizon DS. Sexual dysfunction in women with cancer. Fertil Steril. 2013;100(4):916–21.
36. Choi EK, Kim IR, Chang O, et al. Impact of chemotherapy-induced alopecia distress on body image, psychosocial Well-being, and depression in breast cancer patients. Psychooncology. 2014;23(10):1103–10.
37. DeSimone M, Spriggs E, Gass JS, Carson SA, Krychman ML, Dizon DS. Sexual dysfunction in female cancer survivors. Am J Clin Oncol. 2014;37(1):101–6.
38. Lemieux J, Maunsell E, Provencher L. Chemotherapy-induced alopecia and effects on quality of life among women with breast cancer: a literature review. Psychooncology. 2008;17(4):317–28.
39. Bober SL, Varela VS. Sexuality in adult cancer survivors: challenges and intervention. J Clin Oncol. 2012;30(30):3712–9.
40. Howard-Anderson J, Ganz PA, Bower JE, Stanton AL. Quality of life, fertility concerns, and behavioral health outcomes in younger breast cancer survivors: a systematic review. J Natl Cancer Inst. 2012;104(5):386–405.
41. Ochsenkuhn R, Hermelink K, Clayton AH, et al. Menopausal status in breast cancer patients with past chemotherapy determines long-term hypoactive sexual desire disorder. J Sex Med. 2011;8(5):1486–94.
42. Rosenberg SM, Partridge AH. Premature menopause in young breast cancer: effects on quality of life and treatment interventions. J Thorac Dis. 2013;5(Suppl 1):S55–61.
43. Anchan RM, Ginsburg ES. Fertility concerns and preservation in younger women with breast cancer. Crit Rev Oncol Hematol. 2010;74(3):175–92.
44. Farthmann J, Hanjalic-Beck A, Veit J, et al. The impact of chemotherapy for breast cancer on sexual function and health-related quality of life. Support Care Cancer. 2016;24(6):2603–9.
45. Schover LR. Premature ovarian failure and its consequences: vasomotor symptoms, sexuality, and fertility. J Clin Oncol. 2008;26(5):753–8.
46. Biglia N, Bounous VE, D'Alonzo M, et al. Vaginal atrophy in breast cancer survivors: attitude and approaches among oncologists. Clin Breast Cancer. 2017;17(8):611–7.
47. Nappi RE, Kokot-Kierepa M. Vaginal health: insights, views & attitudes (VIVA) - results from an international survey. Climacteric. 2012;15(1):36–44.
48. Ussher JM, Perz J, Gilbert E. Information needs associated with changes to sexual Well-being after breast cancer. J Adv Nurs. 2013;69(2):327–37.
49. Burstein HJ, Lacchetti C, Anderson H, et al. Adjuvant endocrine therapy for women with hormone receptor-positive breast cancer: ASCO clinical practice guideline focused update. J Clin Oncol. 2019;37(5):423–38.
50. Baumgart J, Nilsson K, Evers AS, Kallak TK, Poromaa IS. Sexual dysfunction in women on

adjuvant endocrine therapy after breast cancer. Menopause. 2013;20(2):162–8.
51. Sears CS, Robinson JW, Walker LM. A comprehensive review of sexual health concerns after cancer treatment and the biopsychosocial treatment options available to female patients. Eur J Cancer Care (Engl). 2018;27(2):e12738.
52. Ljungman L, Ahlgren J, Petersson LM, et al. Sexual dysfunction and reproductive concerns in young women with breast cancer: type, prevalence, and predictors of problems. Psychooncology. 2018;27(12):2770–7.
53. Mok K, Juraskova I, Friedlander M. The impact of aromatase inhibitors on sexual functioning: current knowledge and future research directions. Breast. 2008;17(5):436–40.
54. Cardoso F, Loibl S, Pagani O, et al. The European Society of Breast Cancer Specialists recommendations for the management of young women with breast cancer. Eur J Cancer. 2012;48(18):3355–77.
55. Baumgart J, Nilsson K, Stavreus-Evers A, et al. Urogenital disorders in women with adjuvant endocrine therapy after early breast cancer. Am J Obstet Gynecol. 2011;204(1):26 e21–7.
56. Cella D, Fallowfield L, Barker P, et al. Quality of life of postmenopausal women in the ATAC ("Arimidex", tamoxifen, alone or in combination) trial after completion of 5 years' adjuvant treatment for early breast cancer. Breast Cancer Res Treat. 2006;100(3):273–84.
57. Potter JE, Moore KA. Lichen sclerosus in a breast cancer survivor on an aromatase inhibitor: a case report. J Gen Intern Med. 2013;28(4):592–5.
58. Funaro D. Lichen sclerosus: a review and practical approach. Dermatol Ther. 2004;17(1):28–37.
59. Ribi K, Luo W, Bernhard J, et al. Adjuvant tamoxifen plus ovarian function suppression versus tamoxifen alone in premenopausal women with early breast cancer: patient-reported outcomes in the suppression of ovarian function trial. J Clin Oncol. 2016;34(14):1601–10.
60. Portman DJ, Gass ML, Vulvovaginal Atrophy Terminology Consensus Conference P. Genitourinary syndrome of menopause: new terminology for vulvovaginal atrophy from the International Society for the Study of Women's Sexual Health and the North American Menopause Society. Maturitas. 2014;79(3):349–54.
61. National Comprehensive Cancer Network. NCCN clinical practice guidelines in oncology: survivorship version 2.2020. NCCN2020.
62. Annon JS. The PLISSIT model: a proposed conceptual scheme for the behavioral treatment of sexual problems. J Sex Educ Ther. 1976;2(1):1–15.
63. Mick J, Hughes M, Cohen MZ. Using the BETTER model to assess sexuality. Clin J Oncol Nurs. 2004;8(1):84–6.
64. Bakewell RT, Volker DL. Sexual dysfunction related to the treatment of young women with breast cancer. Clin J Oncol Nurs. 2005;9(6):697–702.
65. Dow J, Kennedy SL. Breast cancer survivors and sexuality: a review of the literature concerning sexual functioning, assessment tools, and evidence-based interventions. Clin J Oncol Nurs. 2015;19(4):456–61.
66. Carter J, Stabile C, Seidel B, Baser RE, Goldfarb S, Goldfrank DJ. Vaginal and sexual health treatment strategies within a female sexual medicine program for cancer patients and survivors. J Cancer Surviv. 2017;11(2):274–83.
67. Santos-Iglesias P, Mohamed B, Walker LM. A systematic review of sexual distress measures. J Sex Med. 2018;15(5):625–44.
68. Hatzichristou D, Rosen RC, Broderick G, et al. Clinical evaluation and management strategy for sexual dysfunction in men and women. J Sex Med. 2004;1(1):49–57.
69. Rosen R, Brown C, Heiman J, et al. The Female Sexual Function Index (FSFI): a multidimensional self-report instrument for the assessment of female sexual function. J Sex Marital Ther. 2000;26(2):191–208.
70. Baser RE, Li Y, Carter J. Psychometric validation of the Female Sexual Function Index (FSFI) in cancer survivors. Cancer. 2012;118(18):4606–18.
71. Bartula I, Sherman KA. Screening for sexual dysfunction in women diagnosed with breast cancer: systematic review and recommendations. Breast Cancer Res Treat. 2013;141(2):173–85.
72. Flynn KE, Lin L, Cyranowski JM, et al. Development of the NIH PROMIS (R) sexual function and satisfaction measures in patients with cancer. J Sex Med. 2013;10(Suppl 1):43–52.
73. Flynn KE, Reeve BB, Lin L, Cyranowski JM, Bruner DW, Weinfurt KP. Construct validity of the PROMIS(R) sexual function and satisfaction measures in patients with cancer. Health Qual Life Outcomes. 2013;11:40.
74. Weinfurt KP, Lin L, Bruner DW, et al. Development and initial validation of the PROMIS((R)) sexual function and satisfaction measures version 2.0. J Sex Med. 2015;12(9):1961–74.
75. Clayton AH, Groth J. Etiology of female sexual dysfunction. Womens Health (Lond). 2013;9(2):135–7.
76. Faubion SS, Rullo JE. Sexual dysfunction in women: a practical approach. Am Fam Physician. 2015;92(4):281–8.
77. Szabo RA, Marino JL, Hickey M. Managing menopausal symptoms after cancer. Climacteric. 2019;22(6):572–8.
78. Basson R. Sexual function of women with chronic illness and cancer. Womens Health (Lond). 2010;6(3):407–29.
79. Kingsberg SA, Rezaee RL. Hypoactive sexual desire in women. Menopause. 2013;20(12):1284–300.
80. Faubion SS, Larkin LC, Stuenkel CA, et al. Management of genitourinary syndrome of menopause in women with or at high risk for breast cancer: consensus recommendations from The North American Menopause Society and The International

Society for the Study of Women's Sexual Health. Menopause. 2018;25(6):596–608.
81. Iverson KM, McLaughlin KA, Gerber MR, et al. Exposure to interpersonal violence and its associations with psychiatric morbidity in a U.S. National Sample: a gender comparison. Psychol Violence. 2013;3(3):273–87.
82. World Health Organization. Violence against women: A global health problem of epidemic proportions. http://www.who.int/mediacentre/news/releases/2013/violence_against_women_20130620/en/2013.
83. Ackerson K. A history of interpersonal trauma and the gynecological exam. Qual Health Res. 2012;22(5):679–88.
84. Huber JD, Pukall CF, Boyer SC, Reissing ED, Chamberlain SM. "Just relax": physicians' experiences with women who are difficult or impossible to examine gynecologically. J Sex Med. 2009;6(3):791–9.
85. Schnur JB, Dillon MJ, Goldsmith RE, Montgomery GH. Cancer treatment experiences among survivors of childhood sexual abuse: a qualitative investigation of triggers and reactions to cumulative trauma. Palliat Support Care. 2018;16(6):767–76.
86. Ades V. The trauma-informed examination. In: Ades V, editor. Sexual and gender-based violence: a complete clinical guide. Cham: Springer International Publishing; 2020. p. 129–46.
87. Latif EZ, Diamond MP. Arriving at the diagnosis of female sexual dysfunction. Fertil Steril. 2013;100(4):898–904.
88. Krychman ML, Katz A. Breast cancer and sexuality: multi-modal treatment options. J Sex Med. 2012;9(1):5–13; quiz 14-15.
89. Management of symptomatic vulvovaginal atrophy: 2013 position statement of the North American Menopause Society. Menopause. 2013;20(9):888–902; quiz 903-884.
90. Carter J, Goldfrank D, Schover LR. Simple strategies for vaginal health promotion in cancer survivors. J Sex Med. 2011;8(2):549–59.
91. Edwards D, Panay N. Treating vulvovaginal atrophy/genitourinary syndrome of menopause: how important is vaginal lubricant and moisturizer composition? Climacteric. 2016;19(2):151–61.
92. Mitchell CM, Guthrie KA, Larson J, et al. Sexual frequency and pain in a randomized clinical trial of vaginal estradiol tablets, moisturizer, and placebo in postmenopausal women. Menopause. 2019;26(8):816–22.
93. Mitchell CM, Reed SD, Diem S, et al. Efficacy of vaginal estradiol or vaginal moisturizer vs placebo for treating postmenopausal vulvovaginal symptoms: a randomized clinical trial. JAMA Intern Med. 2018;178(5):681–90.
94. Brown JM, Hess KL, Brown S, Murphy C, Waldman AL, Hezareh M. Intravaginal practices and risk of bacterial vaginosis and candidiasis infection among a cohort of women in the United States. Obstet Gynecol. 2013;121(4):773–80.
95. Ayehunie S, Wang YY, Landry T, Bogojevic S, Cone RA. Hyperosmolal vaginal lubricants markedly reduce epithelial barrier properties in a three-dimensional vaginal epithelium model. Toxicol Rep. 2018;5:134–40.
96. Potter N, Panay N. Vaginal lubricants and moisturizers: a review into use, efficacy, and safety. Climacteric. 2021;24(1):19–24. https://doi.org/10.1080/13697137.2020.1820478. Epub 2020 Sep 29. PMID: 32990054.
97. Jokar A, Davari T, Asadi N, Ahmadi F, Foruhari S. Comparison of the hyaluronic acid vaginal cream and conjugated estrogen used in treatment of vaginal atrophy of menopause women: a randomized controlled clinical trial. Int J Community Based Nurs Midwifery. 2016;4(1):69–78.
98. Chen J, Geng L, Song X, Li H, Giordan N, Liao Q. Evaluation of the efficacy and safety of hyaluronic acid vaginal gel to ease vaginal dryness: a multicenter, randomized, controlled, open-label, parallel-group, clinical trial. J Sex Med. 2013;10(6):1575–84.
99. Stute P. Is vaginal hyaluronic acid as effective as vaginal estriol for vaginal dryness relief? Arch Gynecol Obstet. 2013;288(6):1199–201.
100. Carter J, Goldfarb S, Baser RE, et al. A single-arm clinical trial investigating the effectiveness of a non-hormonal, hyaluronic acid-based vaginal moisturizer in endometrial cancer survivors. Gynecol Oncol. 2020;158(2):366–74. https://doi.org/10.1016/j.ygyno.2020.05.025. Epub 2020 Jun 8. PMID: 32522420. PMCID: PMC7423634.
101. Carter J, Baser RE, Goldfrank DJ, et al. A single-arm, prospective trial investigating the effectiveness of a non-hormonal vaginal moisturizer containing hyaluronic acid in postmenopausal cancer survivors. Support Care Cancer. 2020.
102. Advani P, Brewster AM, Baum GP, Schover LR. A pilot randomized trial to prevent sexual dysfunction in postmenopausal breast cancer survivors starting adjuvant aromatase inhibitor therapy. J Cancer Surviv. 2017;11(4):477–85.
103. Rubin ES, Deshpande NA, Vasquez PJ, Kellogg SS. A clinical reference guide on sexual devices for obstetrician-gynecologists. Obstet Gynecol. 2019;133(6):1259–68.
104. Capobianco G, Donolo E, Borghero G, Dessole F, Cherchi PL, Dessole S. Effects of intravaginal estriol and pelvic floor rehabilitation on urogenital aging in postmenopausal women. Arch Gynecol Obstet. 2012;285(2):397–403.
105. Faubion SS, Shuster LT, Bharucha AE. Recognition and management of nonrelaxing pelvic floor dysfunction. Mayo Clin Proc. 2012;87(2):187–93.
106. Bakker RM, Vermeer WM, Creutzberg CL, Mens JW, Nout RA, Ter Kuile MM. Qualitative accounts of patients' determinants of vaginal dilator use after pelvic radiotherapy. J Sex Med. 2015;12(3):764–73.

107. Bakker RM, ter Kuile MM, Vermeer WM, et al. Sexual rehabilitation after pelvic radiotherapy and vaginal dilator use: consensus using the Delphi method. Int J Gynecol Cancer. 2014;24(8):1499–506.
108. Bernard S, Ouellet MP, Moffet H, Roy JS, Dumoulin C. Effects of radiation therapy on the structure and function of the pelvic floor muscles of patients with cancer in the pelvic area: a systematic review. J Cancer Surviv. 2016;10(2):351–62.
109. Rosenbaum TY. Physiotherapy treatment of sexual pain disorders. J Sex Marital Ther. 2005;31(4):329–40.
110. Pumo V, Milone G, Iacono M, et al. Psychological and sexual disorders in long-term breast cancer survivors. Cancer Manag Res. 2012;4:61–5.
111. Yang EJ, Lim JY, Rah UW, Kim YB. Effect of a pelvic floor muscle training program on gynecologic cancer survivors with pelvic floor dysfunction: a randomized controlled trial. Gynecol Oncol. 2012;125(3):705–11.
112. Cacciari LP, Dumoulin C, Hay-Smith EJ. Pelvic floor muscle training versus no treatment, or inactive control treatments, for urinary incontinence in women: a cochrane systematic review abridged republication. Braz J Phys Ther. 2019;23(2):93–107.
113. Juraskova I, Jarvis S, Mok K, et al. The acceptability, feasibility, and efficacy (phase I/II study) of the OVERcome (Olive Oil, Vaginal Exercise, and MoisturizeR) intervention to improve dyspareunia and alleviate sexual problems in women with breast cancer. J Sex Med. 2013;10(10):2549–58.
114. Rutledge TL, Rogers R, Lee SJ, Muller CY. A pilot randomized control trial to evaluate pelvic floor muscle training for urinary incontinence among gynecologic cancer survivors. Gynecol Oncol. 2014;132(1):154–8.
115. Marsh S, Borges VF, Coons HL, Afghahi A. Sexual health after a breast cancer diagnosis in young women: clinical implications for patients and providers. Breast Cancer Res Treat. 2020;184(3):655–63. https://doi.org/10.1007/s10549-020-05880-3. Epub 2020 Sep 23. PMID: 32968951.
116. Carter J, Lacchetti C, Andersen BL, et al. Interventions to address sexual problems in people with cancer: American Society of Clinical Oncology Clinical Practice Guideline Adaptation of Cancer Care Ontario Guideline. J Clin Oncol. 2018;36(5):492–511.
117. Ramanathan V, Redelman M. Sexual dysfunctions and sex therapy: the role of a general practitioner. Aust J Gen Pract. 2020;49(7):412–5.
118. Brotto LA, Heiman JR, Goff B, et al. A psychoeducational intervention for sexual dysfunction in women with gynecologic cancer. Arch Sex Behav. 2008;37(2):317–29.
119. Brotto LA, Erskine Y, Carey M, et al. A brief mindfulness-based cognitive behavioral intervention improves sexual functioning versus wait-list control in women treated for gynecologic cancer. Gynecol Oncol. 2012;125(2):320–5.
120. Caldwell R, Classen C. Lagana' L, et al. changes in sexual functioning and mood among women treated for gynecological cancer who receive group therapy: a pilot study. J Clin Psychol Med Settings. 2003;10(3):149–56.
121. Scott JL, Halford WK, Ward BG. United we stand? The effects of a couple-coping intervention on adjustment to early stage breast or gynecological cancer. J Consult Clin Psychol. 2004;72(6):1122–35.
122. Scott JL, Kayser K. A review of couple-based interventions for enhancing women's sexual adjustment and body image after cancer. Cancer J (Sudbury, Mass). 2009;15(1):48–56.
123. Derzko C, Elliott S, Lam W. Management of sexual dysfunction in postmenopausal breast cancer patients taking adjuvant aromatase inhibitor therapy. Curr Oncol. 2007;14(Suppl 1):S20–40.
124. DuHamel K, Schuler T, Nelson C, et al. The sexual health of female rectal and anal cancer survivors: results of a pilot randomized psycho-educational intervention trial. J Cancer Surviv. 2016;10(3):553–63.
125. Hummel SB, van Lankveld J, Oldenburg HSA, et al. Efficacy of internet-based cognitive behavioral therapy in improving sexual functioning of breast cancer survivors: results of a randomized controlled trial. J Clin Oncol. 2017;35(12):1328–40.
126. Reese JB, Porter LS, Casale KE, et al. Adapting a couple-based intimacy enhancement intervention to breast cancer: a developmental study. Health Psychol. 2016;35(10):1085–96.
127. Rowland JH, Meyerowitz BE, Crespi CM, et al. Addressing intimacy and partner communication after breast cancer: a randomized controlled group intervention. Breast Cancer Res Treat. 2009;118(1):99–111.
128. Schover LR, Yuan Y, Fellman BM, Odensky E, Lewis PE, Martinetti P. Efficacy trial of an internet-based intervention for cancer-related female sexual dysfunction. J Natl Compr Cancer Netw. 2013;11(11):1389–97.
129. Goetsch MF, Lim JY, Caughey AB. A practical solution for dyspareunia in breast cancer survivors: a randomized controlled trial. J Clin Oncol. 2015;33(30):3394–400.
130. American College of O, Gynecologists' Committee on Gynecologic P, Farrell R. ACOG Committee opinion no. 659: the use of vaginal estrogen in women with a history of estrogen-dependent breast cancer. Obstet Gynecol. 2016;127(3):e93–6.
131. Martel C, Labrie F, Archer DF, et al. Serum steroid concentrations remain within normal postmenopausal values in women receiving daily 6.5mg intravaginal prasterone for 12 weeks. J Steroid Biochem Mol Biol. 2016;159:142–53.
132. Barton DL, Shuster LT, Dockter T, et al. Systemic and local effects of vaginal dehydroepiandrosterone (DHEA): NCCTG N10C1 (Alliance). Support Care Cancer. 2018;26(4):1335–43.

133. Barton DL, Sloan JA, Shuster LT, et al. Evaluating the efficacy of vaginal dehydroepiandosterone for vaginal symptoms in postmenopausal cancer survivors: NCCTG N10C1 (Alliance). Support Care Cancer. 2018;26(2):643–50.
134. Witherby S, Johnson J, Demers L, et al. Topical testosterone for breast cancer patients with vaginal atrophy related to aromatase inhibitors: a phase I/II study. Oncologist. 2011;16(4):424–31.
135. Dahir M, Travers-Gustafson D. Breast cancer, aromatase inhibitor therapy, and sexual functioning: a pilot study of the effects of vaginal testosterone therapy. Sex Med. 2014;2(1):8–15.
136. Melisko ME, Goldman ME, Hwang J, et al. Vaginal testosterone cream vs estradiol vaginal ring for vaginal dryness or decreased libido in women receiving aromatase inhibitors for early-stage breast cancer: a randomized clinical trial. JAMA Oncol. 2017;3(3):313–9.
137. Mirkin S, Pickar JH. Selective estrogen receptor modulators (SERMs): a review of clinical data. Maturitas. 2015;80(1):52–7.
138. Clemons M, Danson S, Howell A. Tamoxifen ("Nolvadex"): a review. Cancer Treat Rev. 2002;28(4):165–80.
139. Assikis VJ, Jordan VC. Risks and benefits of tamoxifen therapy. [Review] [13 refs]. Oncology. 1997;11(2 Suppl 1):21.
140. Robinson E, Kimmick GG, Muss HB. Tamoxifen in postmenopausal women a safety perspective. Drugs Aging. 1996;8(5):329–37.
141. Pinkerton JV, Stanczyk FZ. Clinical effects of selective estrogen receptor modulators on vulvar and vaginal atrophy. Menopause. 2014;21(3):309–19.
142. Bachmann GA, Komi JO, Ospemifene SG. Ospemifene effectively treats vulvovaginal atrophy in postmenopausal women: results from a pivotal phase 3 study. Menopause. 2010;17(3):480–6.
143. Hillard TC. Lasers in the era of evidence-based medicine. Climacteric. 2020;23(sup1):S6–S10.
144. Mounir DM, Hernandez N, Gonzalez RR. Update: the clinical role of vaginal lasers for the treatment of the genitourinary syndrome of menopause. Urology. 2021;151:2–7. https://doi.org/10.1016/j.urology.2020.09.012. Epub 2020 Sep 20. PMID: 32966821.
145. Pagano T, De Rosa P, Vallone R, et al. Fractional microablative CO2 laser for vulvovaginal atrophy in women treated with chemotherapy and/or hormonal therapy for breast cancer: a retrospective study. Menopause. 2016;23(10):1108–13.
146. Becorpi A, Campisciano G, Zanotta N, et al. Fractional CO2 laser for genitourinary syndrome of menopause in breast cancer survivors: clinical, immunological, and microbiological aspects. Lasers Med Sci. 2018;33(5):1047–54.
147. Gambacciani M, Levancini M. Vaginal erbium laser as second-generation thermotherapy for the genitourinary syndrome of menopause: a pilot study in breast cancer survivors. Menopause. 2017;24(3):316–9.
148. Taylor MJ, Rudkin L, Bullemor-Day P, Lubin J, Chukwujekwu C, Hawton K. Strategies for managing sexual dysfunction induced by antidepressant medication. Cochrane Database Syst Rev. 2013;5:CD003382.
149. Carroll FI, Blough BE, Mascarella SW, Navarro HA, Lukas RJ, Damaj MI. Bupropion and bupropion analogs as treatments for CNS disorders. Adv Pharmacol. 2014;69:177–216.
150. Segraves RT, Clayton A, Croft H, Wolf A, Warnock J. Bupropion sustained release for the treatment of hypoactive sexual desire disorder in premenopausal women. J Clin Psychopharmacol. 2004;24(3):339–42.
151. Safarinejad MR, Hosseini SY, Asgari MA, Dadkhah F, Taghva A. A randomized, double-blind, placebo-controlled study of the efficacy and safety of bupropion for treating hypoactive sexual desire disorder in ovulating women. BJU Int. 2010;106(6):832–9.
152. Clayton AH, Warnock JK, Kornstein SG, Pinkerton R, Sheldon-Keller A, McGarvey EL. A placebo-controlled trial of bupropion SR as an antidote for selective serotonin reuptake inhibitor-induced sexual dysfunction. J Clin Psychiatry. 2004;65(1):62–7.
153. Mathias C, Cardeal Mendes CM, Ponde de Sena E, et al. An open-label, fixed-dose study of bupropion effect on sexual function scores in women treated for breast cancer. Ann Oncol. 2006;17(12):1792–6.
154. Mayer SE, Weiss NS, Chubak J, et al. CYP2D6-inhibiting medication use and inherited CYP2D6 variation in relation to adverse breast cancer outcomes after tamoxifen therapy. Cancer Causes Control. 2019;30(1):103–12.
155. Kingsberg SA, Simon JA. Female hypoactive sexual desire disorder: a practical guide to causes, clinical diagnosis, and treatment. J Womens Health (Larchmt). 2020;29(8):1101–12.
156. Stahl SM. Mechanism of action of flibanserin, a multifunctional serotonin agonist and antagonist (MSAA), in hypoactive sexual desire disorder. CNS Spectr. 2015;20(1):1–6.
157. Mayer D, Lynch SE. Bremelanotide: new drug approved for treating hypoactive sexual desire disorder. Ann Pharmacother. 2020;54(7):684–90.
158. Chivers ML, Rosen RC. Phosphodiesterase type 5 inhibitors and female sexual response: faulty protocols or paradigms? J Sex Med. 2010;7(2 Pt 2):858–72.
159. Therapeutic Research Faculty. Natural medicines comprehensive database consumer version [Internet]. https://medlineplus.gov/druginfo. 2020.
160. National Center for Complementary and Integrative Health. Herbs at a glance. https://www.nccih.nih.gov/health/herbsataglance. 2020.
161. Memorial Sloan Kettering Cancer Center. About herbs, botanicals, and other products. https://www.mskcc.org/cancer-care/diagnosis-treatment/symptom-management/integrative-medicine/herbs. 2020.

162. Oktay K, Harvey BE, Partridge AH, et al. Fertility preservation in patients with cancer: ASCO clinical practice guideline update. J Clin Oncol. 2018;36(19):1994–2001.
163. ACOG Committee opinion no. 747 summary: gynecologic issues in children and adolescent cancer patients and survivors. Obstet Gynecol. 2018;132(2):535–6.
164. ACOG: committee opinion no. 584: oocyte cryopreservation. Obstet Gynecol. 2014;123(1):221–2.
165. Ethics Committee of American Society for Reproductive Medicine. Fertility preservation and reproduction in patients facing gonadotoxic therapies: a committee opinion. Fertil Steril. 2013;100(5):1224–31.
166. National Comprehensive Cancer Network. National comprehensive cancer center clinical practice guidelines in oncology (NCCN Guidelines): adolescent and young adult (AYA) oncology. 2019; Version 1.2020:https://www.nccn.org/professionals/physician_gls/pdf/aya.pdf.
167. Paluch-Shimon S, Pagani O, Partridge AH, et al. ESO-ESMO 3rd international consensus guidelines for breast cancer in young women (BCY3). Breast. 2017;35:203–17.
168. Lambertini M, Anserini P, Levaggi A, Poggio F, Del Mastro L. Fertility counseling of young breast cancer patients. J Thorac Dis. 2013;5 Suppl 1(Suppl 1):S68–80.
169. Logan S, Perz J, Ussher JM, Peate M, Anazodo A. Systematic review of fertility-related psychological distress in cancer patients: informing on an improved model of care. Psychooncology. 2019;28(1):22–30.
170. Hammond C, Abrams JR, Syrjala KL. Fertility and risk factors for elevated infertility concern in 10-year hematopoietic cell transplant survivors and case-matched controls. J Clin Oncol. 2007;25(23):3511–7.
171. Canada AL, Schover LR. The psychosocial impact of interrupted childbearing in long-term female cancer survivors. Psychooncology. 2012;21(2):134–43.
172. Waimey KE, Smith BM, Confino R, Jeruss JS, Pavone ME. Understanding fertility in young female cancer patients. J Womens Health (Larchmt). 2015;24(10):812–8.
173. Adrienne GW, Ann HP. Fertility preservation in patients with breast cancer: necessity, methods, and safety. J Natl Compr Canc Netw. 2016;14(3):355–63.
174. Practice Committee of the American Society for Reproductive Medicine. Fertility preservation in patients undergoing gonadotoxic therapy or gonadectomy: a committee opinion. Fertil Steril. 2019;112(6):1022–33.
175. Diaz-Garcia C, Domingo J, Garcia-Velasco JA, et al. Oocyte vitrification versus ovarian cortex transplantation in fertility preservation for adult women undergoing gonadotoxic treatments: a prospective cohort study. Fertil Steril. 2018;109(3):478–485. e472.
176. Oktay K. Evidence for limiting ovarian tissue harvesting for the purpose of transplantation to women younger than 40 years of Ageb. J Clin Endocrinol Metabol. 2002;87(4):1907–8.
177. Hudson JN, Stanley NB, Nahata L, Bowman-Curci M, Quinn GP. New promising strategies in oncofertility. Expert Rev Qual Life Cancer Care. 2017;2(2):67–78.
178. Donnez J, Dolmans M-M. Fertility preservation in women. N Engl J Med. 2017;377(17):1657–65.
179. Doyle JO, Richter KS, Lim J, Stillman RJ, Graham JR, Tucker MJ. Successful elective and medically indicated oocyte vitrification and warming for autologous invitro fertilization, with predicted birth probabilities for fertility preservation according to number of cryopreserved oocytes and age at retrieval. Fertil Steril. 2016;105(2):459–466.e452.
180. Lambertini M, Richard F, Nguyen B, Viglietti G, Villarreal-Garza C. Ovarian function and fertility preservation in breast cancer: should gonadotropin-releasing hormone agonist be administered to all premenopausal patients receiving chemotherapy? Clin Med Insights Reprod Health. 2019;13:1179558119828393.
181. Moore HCF, Unger JM, Phillips KA, et al. Final analysis of the prevention of early menopause study (POEMS)/SWOG intergroup S0230. J Natl Cancer Inst. 2019;111(2):210–3.
182. Azim HA Jr, Kroman N, Paesmans M, et al. Prognostic impact of pregnancy after breast cancer according to estrogen receptor status: a multicenter retrospective study. J Clin Oncol. 2013;31(1):73–9.
183. Lambertini M, Kroman N, Ameye L, et al. Safety of pregnancy in patients (pts) with history of estrogen receptor positive (ER+) breast cancer (BC): long-term follow-up analysis from a multicenter study. J Clin Oncol. 2017;35(15_suppl):LBA10066.
184. Lambertini M, Kroman N, Ameye L, et al. Long-term safety of pregnancy following breast cancer according to estrogen receptor status. JNCI: Journal of the National Cancer Institute. 2017;110(4):426–9.
185. Azim AA, Costantini-Ferrando M, Oktay K. Safety of fertility preservation by ovarian stimulation with Letrozole and gonadotropins in patients with breast cancer: a prospective controlled study. J Clin Oncol. 2008;26(16):2630–5.
186. Kim J, Turan V, Oktay K. Long-term safety of letrozole and gonadotropin stimulation for fertility preservation in women with breast cancer. J Clin Endocrinol Metab. 2016;101(4):1364–71.
187. Bitzer J, Giraldi A, Pfaus J. Sexual desire and hypoactive sexual desire disorder in women. Introduction and overview. Standard operating procedure (SOP Part 1). J Sex Med. 2013;10(1):36–49.
188. Maseroli E, Scavello I, Vignozzi L. Cardiometabolic risk and female sexuality-part I. risk factors and potential pathophysiological underpinnings for female Vasculogenic sexual dysfunction syndromes. Sex Med Rev. 2018;6(4):508–24.

189. Esposito K, Ciotola M, Maiorino MI, et al. Hyperlipidemia and sexual function in premenopausal women. J Sex Med. 2009;6(6):1696–703.
190. Maseroli E, Fanni E, Cipriani S, et al. Cardiometabolic risk and female sexuality: focus on clitoral vascular resistance. J Sex Med. 2016;13(11):1651–61.
191. Jaarsma T, Fridlund B, Martensson J. Sexual dysfunction in heart failure patients. Curr Heart Fail Rep. 2014;11(3):330–6.
192. Emami Zeydi A, Sharafkhani M, Armat MR, Gould KA, Soleimani A, Hosseini SJ. Women's sexual issues after myocardial infarction: a literature review. Dimens Crit Care Nurs. 2016;35(4):195–203.
193. Grenier-Genest A, Gerard M, Courtois F. Stroke and sexual functioning: a literature review. NeuroRehabilitation. 2017;41(2):293–315.
194. Rahmanian E, Salari N, Mohammadi M, Jalali R. Evaluation of sexual dysfunction and female sexual dysfunction indicators in women with type 2 diabetes: a systematic review and meta-analysis. Diabetol Metab Syndr. 2019;11:73.
195. Carosa E, Sansone A, Jannini EA. Management of endocrine disease: female sexual dysfunction for the endocrinologist. Eur J Endocrinol. 2020;182(6):R101.
196. Di Francesco S, Caruso M, Robuffo I, Militello A, Toniato E. The impact of metabolic syndrome and its components on female sexual dysfunction: a narrative mini-review. Curr Urol. 2019;12(2):57–63.
197. Wang Y, Wang H. Effects of hypothyroidism and subclinical hypothyroidism on sexual function: a meta-analysis of studies using the female sexual function index. Sex Med. 2020;8(2):156–67.
198. Newman AM. Arthritis and sexuality. Nurs Clin North Am. 2007;42(4):621–30;vii.
199. Rosenbaum TY. Musculoskeletal pain and sexual function in women. J Sex Med. 2010;7(2 Pt 1):645–53.
200. Cook DJ, Guyatt GH, Adachi JD, et al. Quality of life issues in women with vertebral fractures due to osteoporosis. Arthritis Rheum. 1993;36(6):750–6.
201. Sadeghi-Nejad H, Wasserman M, Weidner W, Richardson D, Goldmeier D. Sexually transmitted diseases and sexual function. J Sex Med. 2010;7(1 Pt 2):389–413.
202. La Rosa VL, Ciebiera M, Lin LT, et al. Multidisciplinary management of women with pelvic organ prolapse, urinary incontinence and lower urinary tract symptoms.A clinical and psychological overview. Prz Menopauzalny. 2019;18(3):184–90.
203. Pluchino N, Wenger JM, Petignat P, et al. Sexual function in endometriosis patients and their partners: effect of the disease and consequences of treatment. Hum Reprod Update. 2016;22(6):762–74.
204. Levy G, Lowenstein L. Overactive bladder syndrome treatments and their effect on female sexual function: a review. Sex Med. 2020;8(1):1–7.
205. Szydlarska D, Jakubowska A, Rydzewska G. Assessment of sexual dysfunction in patients with inflammatory bowel disease. Prz Gastroenterol. 2019;14(2):104–8.
206. Krysko KM, Graves JS, Dobson R, et al. Sex effects across the lifespan in women with multiple sclerosis. Ther Adv Neurol Disord. 2020;13:1756286420936166.
207. Polat Dunya C, Tulek Z, Uchiyama T, Haslam C, Panicker JN. Systematic review of the prevalence, symptomatology and management options of sexual dysfunction in women with multiple sclerosis. Neurourol Urodyn. 2020;39(1):83–95.
208. Meco G, Rubino A, Caravona N, Valente M. Sexual dysfunction in Parkinson's disease. Parkinsonism Relat Disord. 2008;14(6):451–6.
209. Oertel WH, Wachter T, Quinn NP, Ulm G, Brandstadter D. Reduced genital sensitivity in female patients with multiple system atrophy of parkinsonian type. Mov Disord. 2003;18(4):430–2.
210. Latella D, Maggio MG, De Luca R, et al. Changes in sexual functioning following traumatic brain injury: an overview on a neglected issue. J Clin Neurosci. 2018;58:1–6.
211. Rathore C, Henning OJ, Luef G, Radhakrishnan K. Sexual dysfunction in people with epilepsy. Epilepsy Behav. 2019;100(Pt A):106495.
212. Bossini L, Fagiolini A, Valdagno M, Polizzotto NR, Castrogiovanni P. Sexual disorders in subjects treated for mood and anxiety diseases. J Clin Psychopharmacol. 2007;27(3):310–2.
213. Cyranowski JM, Bromberger J, Youk A, Matthews K, Kravitz HM, Powell LH. Lifetime depression history and sexual function in women at midlife. Arch Sex Behav. 2004;33(6):539–48.
214. Cipriani A, Furukawa TA, Salanti G, et al. Comparative efficacy and acceptability of 12 new-generation antidepressants: a multiple-treatments meta-analysis. Lancet. 2009;373(9665):746–58.
215. Association of Reproductive Health Professionals. Women's sexual health in midlife and beyond. AHRP Clin Proc. 2005;5:8–12.
216. American Society of Health-System Pharmacists I. AHFS patient medication information database. https://medlineplus.gov/druginformation.html. 2020. Accessed 15 Oct 2020.
217. Greven KM, Case LD, Nycum LR, et al. Effect of ArginMax on sexual functioning and quality of life among female cancer survivors: resu lts of the WFU CCOP Research Base protocol 97106. J Community Support Oncol. 2015;13(3):87–94.
218. Lee MS, Shin BC, Yang EJ, Lim HJ, Ernst E. Maca (Lepidium meyenii) for treatment of menopausal symptoms: a systematic review. Maturitas. 2011;70(3):227–33.
219. Shin BC, Lee MS, Yang EJ, Lim HS, Ernst E. Maca (L. meyenii) for improving sexual function: a systematic review. BMC Complement Altern Med. 2010;10:44.

220. Meacham LR, Burns K, Orwig KE, Levine J. Standardizing risk assessment for treatment-related gonadal insufficiency and infertility in childhood adolescent and young adult cancer: the pediatric initiative network risk stratification system. J Adolesc Young Adult Oncol. 2020;9(6):662–6.
221. Levine JM, Whitton JA, Ginsberg JP, et al. Nonsurgical premature menopause and reproductive implications in survivors of childhood cancer: a report from the childhood cancer survivor study. Cancer. 2018;124(5):1044–52.
222. Chemaitilly W, Mertens AC, Mitby P, et al. Acute ovarian failure in the childhood cancer survivor study. J Clin Endocrinol Metabol. 2006;91(5):1723–8.
223. Green DM, Nolan VG, Kawashima T, et al. Decreased fertility among female childhood cancer survivors who received 22-27 Gy hypothalamic/pituitary irradiation: a report from the childhood cancer survivor study. Fertil Steril. 2011;95(6):1922–1927.e1921.

6 Arthralgias

Gretchen G. Kimmick, Rachel Anne Pienknagura, and Sophia C. Weinmann

Introduction

Arthralgia is defined as non-inflammatory joint pain, whereas arthritis describes inflammatory joint pain. This distinction is paramount in a breast cancer survivor, as the etiologies of non-inflammatory and inflammatory joint pain differ. In this chapter, we will review several causes of joint pain, both inflammatory and non-inflammatory, for the practicing oncologist and clinicians who are caring for breast cancer survivors. We will discuss recommended approaches to further evaluation, diagnosis, and treatment, with particular attention to treatment of aromatase inhibitor-associated arthralgia (AIAA). We also discuss cases when it is appropriate to refer to a rheumatologist for further evaluation and treatment. Expert overviews on arthritis and arthralgia are available elsewhere [1, 2].

Arthralgia in a Patient with a Breast Cancer History – Differential Diagnosis and Work-Up

- Figure 6.1 outlines our recommended approach to a patient who has a history of breast cancer and develops new joint pain. Although the algorithm flows as though the evaluation is sequential and the cause of joint pain can be clearly defined, care must be taken to consider multiple causes and approaches, since there may be more than one contributing factor.
- The differential diagnosis will help to guide the initial evaluation, which should include a detailed history, physical exam, and basic laboratory evaluation. Table 6.1 provides a broad list of possible causes of joint pain.
- Laboratory evaluation is often helpful in diagnosing inflammatory arthritis or secondary causes of joint pain, but should only be used to supplement clinical assessment by history and physical exam. Table 6.2 lists laboratory tests that should be considered in evaluation of suspected inflammatory joint pain.

G. G. Kimmick (✉)
Medical Oncology, Duke University School of Medicine/Duke Cancer Institute, Durham, NC, USA
e-mail: Gretchen.kimmick@duke.edu

R. A. Pienknagura
Medical Oncology, Duke University Medical Center/Duke Cancer Institute, Durham, NC, USA

S. C. Weinmann
Rheumatology and Immunology, Duke University Medical Center, Durham, NC, USA

G. G. Kimmick et al. (eds.), *Common Issues in Breast Cancer Survivors*,
https://doi.org/10.1007/978-3-030-75377-1_6

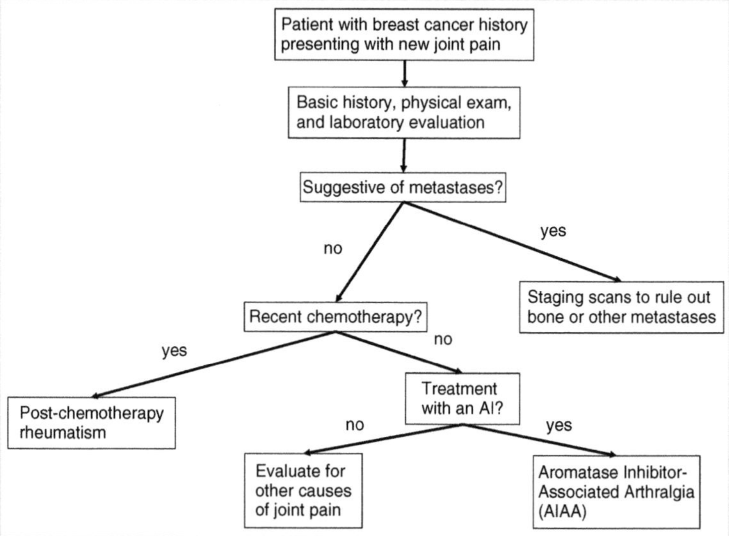

Fig. 6.1 Recommended approach to arthralgia in a woman with a breast cancer history

Table 6.1 Differential diagnosis for joint pain

Causes of arthralgia	History	Physical exam	Laboratory evaluation
Endocrine Estrogen deficiency Hypothyroidism Hyperparathyroidism Vitamin D deficiency Anemia	Cessation of menses; menopausal symptoms Weight gain, fatigue, hyporeflexia Abdominal pain Fatigue, proximal myopathy Fatigue	–	Estradiol, FSH, LH TSH, Free-T4, T3 Hypercalcemia, elevated PTH Low 25-hydroxyvitaminD Low hemoglobin and hematocrit
Drug-related Statins and other lipid-lowering drugs Aromatase inhibitors Selective estrogen receptor modulators Bisphosphonates (particularly IV) Thiazide diuretics	–	–	–
Metabolic Liver disease Renal disease	–	–	LFP RFP
Rheumatic Connective tissue disease (CTD; lupus, scleroderma, Sjogrens) Sarcoidosis Vasculitis Hyperuricemia Hypermobility Fibromyalgia	Fatigue, sleep disturbance, anxiety or depression, other pain syndromes	Rash, oral ulcers, other clinical features of CTD Joint hypermobility	Elevated ANA titer Elevated serum ACE ANCA positive Elevated serum urate

Table 6.1 (continued)

Causes of arthralgia	History	Physical exam	Laboratory evaluation
Infection Parvovirus Hepatitis B/C/HIV Ross River virus Brucellosis Whipple's disease Lyme disease	Viral symptoms Relevant exposure history History of insect bite	Rash Jaundice	Positive serology for infectious agent
Malignancy Bone metastases Paraneoplastic syndrome	Weight loss, bone pain, fever	Bone pain	Abnormal bone scan

ANA antinuclear antibody, *ACE* angiotensin converting enzyme, *ANCA* anti-neutrophil cytoplasmic antibodies, *FSH* follicular stimulating hormone, *LH* luteinizing hormone, *TSH* thyroid stimulating hormone, *PTH* parathyroid hormone, *LFP* liver function panel, *RFP* renal function panel

Table 6.2 Laboratory tests helpful for evaluation of joint pain

Complete blood count (CBC) and white blood cell differential
Biochemistry profile, to include liver function panel and renal function panel (includes electrolytes and calcium)
Urea
Acute phase reactants: c-reactive protein (CRP) and erythrocyte sedimentation rate (ESR)
Serum urate
Creatinine kinase
Thyroid function
Parathyroid hormone
Anemia work-up: iron studies, B12 (± methylmalonic acid level), RBC-folate
25-hydroxyvitamin D level
Autoantibodies (ANA, RF, anti-cyclic citrullinated peptide antibodies)
Viral or other serologic testing (ex. Parvovirus B19, hepatitis B, C, HIV)

LFP liver function panel, *RFP* renal function panel, *RBC* red blood cell, *RF* rheumatoid factor, *HIV* human immunodeficiency virus

Evaluation of Arthralgia (for the Non-rheumatologist)

Most breast cancer survivors will experience non-inflammatory arthralgia, but one must consider new-onset inflammatory arthritis as well (Fig. 6.2). The differences between non-inflammatory and inflammatory arthritis are presented side by side for comparison in Table 6.3. Rheumatoid arthritis is the most common inflammatory arthritis and presents in women in the 4th to 5th decade of life. The prevalence of rheumatoid arthritis is about 1% of the population [3]. Inflammatory arthritis is marked by joint pain with associated swelling, morning stiffness for 1 hour or greater, elevated inflammatory markers such as erythrocyte sedimentation rate (ESR) and c-reactive protein (CRP), autoantibody production in some cases, and radiographic changes of joint space narrowing, peri-articular osteopenia, and joint erosions [4]. Some patients with inflammatory arthritis will also have a mild anemia secondary to chronic inflammation.

Non-inflammatory joint pain is usually characterized by pain in the absence of swelling, morning stiffness that lasts up to 30 minutes, normal inflammatory markers, and radiographic changes of joint space narrowing and bone growth, such as osteophytes. There are several causes of non-inflammatory arthralgia in breast cancer survivors, including post-chemotherapy rheumatism, aromatase inhibitor associated arthralgia (AIAA), post-menopausal arthralgia, joint hypermobility syndrome (JHS), and osteoarthritis (OA). While osteoarthritis is the most common etiology for arthralgia in the general

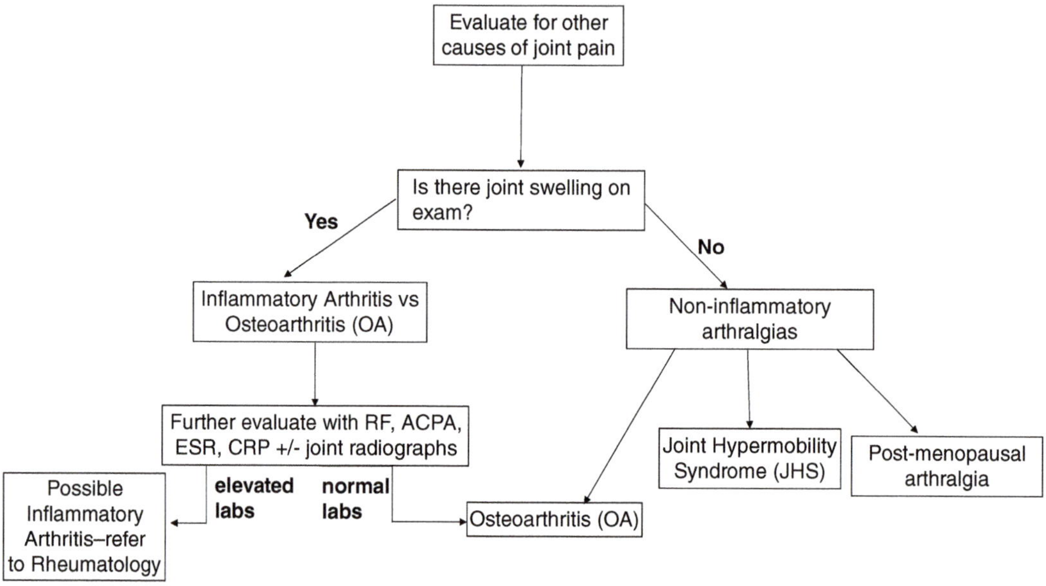

Fig. 6.2 Approach to evaluate for other causes of arthralgia

Table 6.3 Inflammatory Arthritis versus Non-inflammatory Arthralgia Comparison Chart

	Inflammatory Arthritis	Non-Inflammatory Arthralgia
History & Clinical Findings	Joint pain with associated swelling Morning stiffness ≥1 hour	Joint pain without swelling Morning stiffness ≤30 mins
Lab Test Abnormalities	Positive autoantibodies (RF, ACPA) Elevated inflammatory markers (ESR, CRP) Anemia (chronic inflammation)	Normal inflammatory markers (ESR, CRP)

population with about 250 million people affected worldwide, special consideration must be given to breast cancer survivors for these other types of non-inflammatory arthralgia [5]. Post-chemotherapy rheumatism and AIAA are discussed further in subsequent sections, but both are related to current or recent treatment regimens. Post-menopausal arthralgia results from changes in a woman's estrogen levels and should be highly suspected in breast cancer survivors who have undergone menopause via medical treatments or surgical treatments like bilateral oophorectomy [6]. Joint hypermobility syndrome (JHS) is a benign hypermobility syndrome that is sometimes referred to as a milder variant of Ehlers-Danlos syndrome (EDS) and can affect women of all ages. Joint hypermobility predisposes women to having earlier-onset osteoarthritis, making early recognition vital to begin lifestyle modification treatments to prevent injury and morbidity associated with JHS [7].

When screening for inflammatory arthritis in women with a history of breast cancer, checking a rheumatoid factor (RF) and an anti-citrullinated peptide antibody (ACPA) is necessary. While two-thirds of patients with rheumatoid arthritis will have positive auto-antibodies, one-third of patients will be "seronegative," meaning the rheumatoid factor and anti-citrullinated peptide antibody are both negative, despite the patient having a clinical diagnosis of rheumatoid arthritis [5]. Inflammatory markers ESR and CRP should also be checked in patients with swollen joints. A patient in whom inflammatory arthritis is suspected by history, physical, and laboratory evaluation, or in whom inflammatory arthritis cannot be ruled out with certainty, should be referred to rheumatology for further evaluation and treatment recommendations.

While evaluating for common and treatable causes of arthralgia, consideration should be given to the patient's breast cancer and treatment history (Fig. 6.1). If she had a cancer that was advanced stage and/or high risk of metastases, if there are findings on physical exam or laboratory evaluation that raise concern for metastases, then staging scans should be done to rule out metastatic disease as the cause of the new pain. If not, and she has recently completed chemotherapy, the onset of arthralgia may be due to post-chemotherapy rheumatism. If there is low suspicion for metastases and she has not had chemotherapy, and is on an AI, the AI may be contributing to the arthralgia. Referral to a rheumatologist should be considered if the arthralgia history raises the concern about the presence of a rheumatologic disorder and inflammatory arthritis or if the arthralgia is more severe and persistent than what would be expected for AIAA.

Post-chemotherapy Rheumatism

Post-chemotherapy rheumatism is a syndrome of arthralgia that arises within a few months after finishing chemotherapy, lasts for 3–4 months, and then subsides [8, 9]. The first published report of arthralgia after chemotherapy was published by Dr. Loprinzi and colleagues [8]. They suggested that symptoms generally occur within 1–2 months following the completion of chemotherapy. Subsequently, others have reported similar short intervals to the onset of arthralgia of about 3–8 months [9–11]. Loprinzi et al. identified cyclophosphamide/fluorouracil adjuvant chemotherapy as the most common regimen associated with post-chemotherapy rheumatism [8]. Since that first report, other regimens, such as standard adjuvant chemotherapy for patients with lung cancer and those containing cyclophosphamide for breast cancer patients, were also reported to be associated with the development of rheumatic symptoms [9, 10]. Another retrospective analysis of patients with post-treatment rheumatism, which included various cancer types, found that fluorouracil most commonly caused the syndrome, followed by cyclophosphamide and cisplatin [11]. Other case series reported post-chemotherapy rheumatic symptoms with many chemotherapeutic agents and not limited to a single agent or group of drugs [12].

Symptoms of post-chemotherapy rheumatism can involve many joints, most commonly toes, fingers, ankles, knees, and shoulders [10–13]. Symptoms are usually treated with common analgesics, but subside within a few months with or without treatment [8]. Patients in whom the onset of arthralgia is within 3–4 months of completing chemotherapy, therefore, likely have post-chemotherapy rheumatism and can be reassured that the symptom course is self-limited.

Post-chemotherapy Rheumatism

- Timing: onset a few months after chemotherapy, lasts 3–4 months and subsides with or without treatment
- Involved joints: many
- Treatment: analgesics

Aromatase Inhibitor-Associated Arthralgia

Aromatase inhibitors (AIs) are the mainstay of adjuvant treatment for hormone receptor positive breast cancer in postmenopausal women. Compared to tamoxifen in the adjuvant setting, AIs lead to better rates of relapse-free survival [14]. The safety of adjuvant AIs has been established in large, randomized trials including the Anastrozole, Tamoxifen Alone or in Combination (ATAC) [15], Breast International Group 1-98 (BIG 1-98) [16, 17], and Intergroup Exemestane Study (IES) [18]. Initially, the greater therapeutic benefit of AIs and lower risk of serious complications, such as thrombotic events and estrogenic effects on the endometrial lining leading to vaginal bleeding and endometrial cancer that have been associated with tamoxifen, led to great enthusiasm [19]. Subsequently, however, musculoskeletal side effects of AIs, including non-inflammatory joint pain, stiffness, and achiness, have proven very bothersome and highly prevalent [13, 20, 21].

The prevalence of AI-associated arthralgia (AIAA) spans 10–80% of women on AIs, depending on the population studied and the method of data collection [22–26]. In clinical trials, the incidence is up to 36% [27–30], while in clinical practice and where musculoskeletal side effects were the study focus, the rate is reported to be as high as 80% [22, 23, 26, 31–36].

The clinical presentation can vary considerably, but typical symptoms include symmetrical pain or stiffness in the joints that is not associated with inflammation or joint destruction [13]. Symptoms can appear anywhere from 6 weeks to 12 months after starting AI therapy, increase over time, cease upon discontinuation of AI therapy, and range from minor to moderate or severe, with almost 70% reporting symptoms as moderate to severe [22, 25, 34, 37–40]. Affected joints typically include the hands, wrists, ankles, knees, hips, pelvic bones, and spine [24, 26, 41]. Patients may describe soreness or stiffness in the joints, early morning stiffness, swelling, difficulty sleeping, difficulty completely closing or stretching the hand and/or fingers, and even difficulty performing daily activities, such as dressing, driving, or typing [32, 42, 43]. Ultrasound evaluation of the joints in AI users found that AI users have joint and tendon effusions and thicker tendons than non-AI users [32]. Carpal tunnel syndrome, trigger finger, and other tendinopathies are more common in women on AIs [44–47]. Symptoms can be severe enough to cause women to stop taking this potentially life-saving treatment. In fact, AIAA is the most common reason for noncompliance with AIs [24, 48, 49]. Both non-adherence to and early discontinuation of AIs are independent predictors of mortality [50].

The risk factors for AIAA are not well defined [22, 40, 51, 52]. In the absence of AI therapy, arthralgias are more prevalent in postmenopausal compared to pre- or perimenopausal women and in people with higher BMI and lower overall physical activity [53–55]. Described predictors of AIAA are listed in Table 6.4. In the ATAC trial, obesity (BMI >30 kg/m^2 versus <25 mg/m^2; OR 1.32 [1.14–1.53]), history of hormone replacement therapy (OR 1.72 [95%CI 1.53–1.93]), and taking anastrozole (versus tamoxifen; OR 1.25 [1.11–1.40]) and prior chemotherapy (OR 1.34 [95%CI 1.17–1.53]) significantly increased the risk of arthralgia [40]. Geographic region (i.e., living in North America versus United Kingdom) and hormone receptor positive cancer, versus negative, were also risk factors in the ATAC trial. In a cross-sectional analysis of joint symptoms among postmenopausal women taking AIs in an urban academic breast oncology clinic, arthralgia was less common among overweight (BMI 25–30 kg/m^2) women compared with those women with a normal BMI (<25 mg/kg^2) or those classified as obese (BMI > 30 mg/kg^2). Participants who had taken prior tamoxifen therapy also had less arthralgia, but prior taxane therapy increased the likelihood of arthralgias fourfold (odds ratio [OR] for joint pain = 4.08, 95% CI, 1.58–10.57 and OR for joint stiffness = 4.76; 95% CI, 1.84–12.28) [22]. A multivariable model among women initiating AI showed that baseline severity of menopausal symptoms and presence of joint-related comorbidity (OA, RA, psoriatic arthritis, lupus, gout, ankylosing spondylitis, fibromyalgia, osteoporosis, osteopenia, or Sjogren's syndrome) were associated with increased arthralgia severity over a year [39]. They did not see an association between arthralgia severity and use of radiotherapy or chemotherapy.

Table 6.4 Risk factors for aromatase inhibitor-associated arthralgia

History of hormone replacement therapy
Under weight (BMI <25) or obese (BMI >30)
Recent prior adjuvant chemotherapy
Prior taxane chemotherapy
Baseline severity of menopausal symptoms
The presence of joint-related comorbidity (OA, RA, psoriatic arthritis, lupus, gout, ankylosing spondylitis, fibromyalgia, osteoporosis, osteopenia, or Sjogren's syndrome)
Lower physical activity

Management of AIAA (Fig. 6.3)

Several reports have described potential algorithms to guide management of AIAA [24, 56–60]. Most of the algorithms are based on anecdotal evidence and evidence borrowed from other

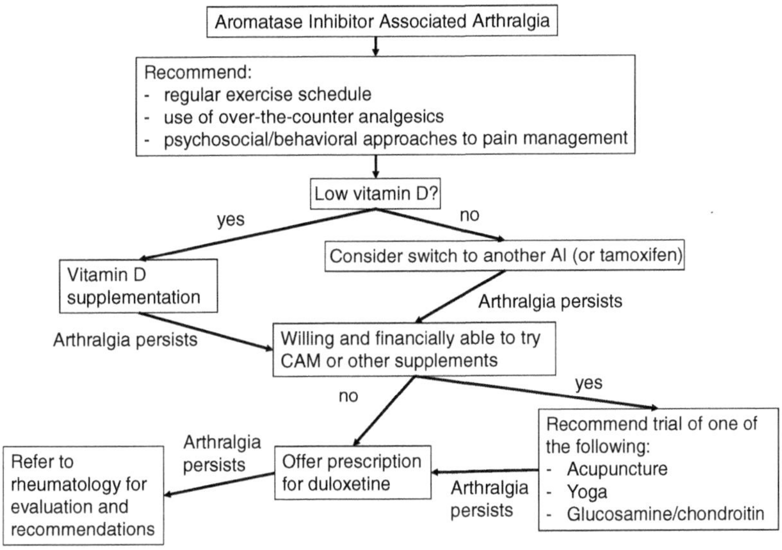

Fig. 6.3 Recommended management approach for aromatase inhibitor-associated arthralgia (AIAA)

fields of research, such as arthritis, rather than trials specific to AIAA. We propose an algorithm based on the data available for AIAA and that is supported by sound clinical principles. For instance, the effect size for pain improvement favors pharmacologic approaches, such as duloxetine, compared to physical exercise and vitamin D supplementation [61], but other health benefits of physical exercise and vitamin D supplementation led us to recommend those before a prescription for duloxetine.

Over-the-counter (OTC) pain relievers, including oral analgesics, such as acetaminophen, ibuprofen, and naproxen, and topical agents, such as capsaicin, salicylates, other anti-inflammatory agents, counterirritants, and anesthetics, can be helpful in alleviating minor joint pain. OTC pain relievers have been informally reported to be beneficial for AIAA in cross-sectional surveys [22, 23]. One cross-sectional study of arthralgias from AIs found that half of women used OTC pain medicines, most commonly acetaminophen and non-steroidal anti-inflammatory drugs (NSAIDs), and over three-quarters reported relief in arthralgia symptoms [22]. The use of stronger, prescription analgesics, such as NSAIDs, other pain modifiers, and sleep aids [21, 56, 57, 62], can be considered, but have not been studied in AIAA and may have more serious side effects. Given that OTC pain relievers are readily available, we recommend that management of AIAA starts with these and the recommendation to establish a regular exercise schedule.

Psychological and behavioral approaches, such as cognitive-behavioral therapy (CBT), mindfulness, Acceptance and Commitment (ACT)-based therapy, and relaxation techniques, have proven benefits for chronic pain, for arthritic pain [63], and for cancer-related pain [64–67] and are currently being studied for AIAA [68]. Cognitive-behavioral therapy is a short-term form of psychotherapy that focuses on modifying emotions, behaviors, and thoughts in order to find solutions to a problem. During CBT, patients learn how to increase awareness of thoughts and to modify thought patterns to reduce severity of symptoms. Based on the success of psychological and behavioral approaches for pain in general, we included it as an initial option for AIAA pain in our algorithm.

The presence of joint symptoms may indicate greater efficacy of AI therapy [69, 70]. Patients should be reassured by the following: (1) their symptoms are not due to permanent changes in the joints or joint destruction and are reversible upon AI withdrawal, (2) the exacerbation of joint symptoms may be a surrogate marker of the effectiveness of the endocrine therapy and may be associated with a reduced risk of breast cancer recurrence [70], and (3) the symptoms will likely improve with time, even on therapy.

Exercise

The benefit of regular physical activity in breast cancer survivors has been extensively studied. Exercise has been shown to decrease the severity of arthritis and AIAA [71–75], decrease the risk of cancer recurrence, decrease cancer morbidity (both breast cancer and all cause), decrease fatigue, and improve bone density [76, 77]. Greater exercise is also associated with weight maintenance, important because breast cancer survivors whose BMI increases by 0.5–2 points have a 40% greater risk of recurrence than those who maintain their weight [77]. Despite the substantial benefits, compliance with exercise recommendations poses a significant barrier. Studies have shown that only 20–30% of patients are active following a cancer diagnosis (mean time since diagnosis was 9.5 years). Approximately 20% of women gain between 10 and 20 kg during chemotherapy [78]. In order to increase patient participation in exercise, we recommend that an exercise prescription, outlining specific recommendations (see below), be given to every breast cancer survivor. It is important to review symptom management strategies with each patient and encourage them to increase activity as tolerated, as symptoms are a key barrier to exercise in this population. Additionally, it is important that a member of the health-care team inquire about compliance and progress at each follow-up visit.

The mechanisms underlying pain reduction due to regular exercise include (1) endogenous opioid production, (2) increased pain threshold, and (3) decreased excitation and increased inhibition of central nervous system pathways responsible for pain production [79]. In patients with chronic pain, there are alterations in the central nervous system that lead to impaired pain modulation. In animal models, for example, pain relief significant after 8 weeks of physical activity, but not after 5 days [80]. This suggests that patients are not likely to experience an immediate reduction in their pain and require repeated, regular physical activity in order to experience analgesia. We, as clinicians, must set this expectation with our patients in order to promote increased compliance.

The benefit of exercise in alleviating AIAA has been evaluated in the Hormones and Physical Exercise (HOPE) study, which examined the effects of a regimented exercise program versus standard of care on AIAA [71]. The study included 121 participants who had been on an AI for at least 6 months, reported less than 90 minutes of exercise per week, and ranked their arthralgia pain as 3/10 or greater (based on the Brief Pain Inventory Questionnaire). Participants were randomized into a standard of care group (no instruction about exercise from care team) or the exercise intervention group. Participants in the exercise intervention group participated in twice-weekly, supervised resistance training sessions with a certified cancer exercise trainer and 150 minutes of independently led cardiovascular exercise per week, which could include

Cardiovascular exercise	150 minutes/week of moderate-intensity aerobic exercise OR 75 minutes per week of high-intensity exercise OR a combination of both Try to spread sessions throughout the week	Examples of moderate- intensity: walking, gardening, treading water, riding a bike on flat terrain/stationary bike, cleaning/doing chores Examples of high- intensity: jogging, swimming, tennis, hiking, dancing, riding a bike on an incline, playing tag with your children or grandchildren
Strength Training	Moderate- to high-intensity muscle-strengthening activity (such as resistance or weights) on at least 2 days per week.	Research recommends 8–12 different exercises targeting the major muscle groups, for 1–3 sets Major muscle groups include quadriceps, hamstrings, calves, chest, back, shoulders, triceps, biceps, forearms, abdominal muscles These exercises can be done using free-weights, resistance bands, or machines

walking or biking inside or outside. In order to monitor adherence to the cardiovascular exercise, participants were given a heart rate monitor to wear during exercise, and they kept a log detailing the type, duration, and average heart rate during each work-out. The logs were reviewed by the exercise trainer on a weekly basis. Data was analyzed at 3, 6, 9, and 12 months. Results showed the most significant improvement at 12 months. After 12 months, the exercise intervention group showed a 1.6 point reduction in their worst pain, and a 1.1 point reduction in the severity of their pain and pain interference ($p < 0.001$). Notably, this study showed that there was not a dose-dependent effect: attending more frequent strength training sessions and increasing the amount of cardiovascular exercise did not improve pain from arthralgia. This raises the question about a plateau effect, whereby more frequent or intense exercise has little additional benefit.

Other studies have also established the benefit of regular physical activity on decreasing pain, but the frequency and duration required to achieve optimal benefits remains unclear [72, 73, 81]. It is apparent, however, that sustained compliance to any regular regimen yields benefit [71, 77]. It is vital that we help set individualized, attainable goals for our patients. During periodic assessments, we can titrate recommendations based on patient response. Additionally, we must set the expectation with our patients that meaningful pain relief may not be achieved for up to a year. In Table 6.5, we outline general exercise goals. Exercise recommendations will vary between patients, however, according to functional and psychosocial factors. There are many free or low-cost programs and exercise groups available to cancer survivors. We encourage each clinician to research local programs and share this information with patients.

Table 6.5 Recommendations for exercise

Goals	Examples
150 Minutes of Moderate-Intensity Aerobic Exercise Per Week	Walking Bicycling Dancing Water aerobics Housework
2 Strength Training Sessions Per Week	8–12 different exercises with 1–3 sets targeting major muscle groups (quadriceps, hamstrings, calves, chest, back, shoulders, triceps, biceps, forearms, abdominal muscles)
Periodic Assessments of Adherence and Progress	Phone call Verbal or written assessment at follow-up visits

Vitamin D

Vitamin D, through its metabolite, calcitriol, binding to the vitamin D receptor (VDR), is important to many body functions [82]. This includes not only its essential role in calcium and phosphate absorption in the kidneys, intestine, and bones that leads to normal bone mineralization and remodeling [83] but also its role in promoting normal, healthy cell proliferation in breast and other tissues. In fact, risk of breast cancer is increased when vitamin D level is low [84]. The symptoms of vitamin D deficiency vary broadly among patients. Patients may present endorsing generalized musculoskeletal stiffness/aches, peripheral neuropathy, muscle weakness, fatigue, and seasonal depression (particularly in the winter, secondary to decreased sun exposure manufacture of vitamin D by the skin) [85]. Vitamin D can be measured in the blood as its active metabolite, calcitriol (1,25-dihydroxyvitamin D), or as its relatively inactive precursor, calcidiol (25-hydroxyvitamin D [25-OHD]). Under most circumstances, vitamin D status is more accurately reflected by measuring 25-OHD, because it has a long half-life, is present in higher concentrations, and is not influenced by parathyroid hormone levels and other hormones. In unique cases, such as renal disease, 1,25 dihydroxyvitamin D level may be used to better determine vitamin D status. Vitamin D deficiency is defined as plasma levels of 25-hydroxyvitamin D (25-OHD) <20 ng/ml, and insufficiency as 21–31 ng/ml [86]. Studies have shown that 90% of women have baseline 25-OHD concentrations of <30 ng/ml. Due to the large amount of overlap between cancer, chemotherapy side effects, and vitamin D deficiency, we suggest that the testing of plasma concentrations of 25-OHD be added to the standard lab panel for any patient endorsing AIAA, every new patient, and at least once for any patient that has not been tested previously. Early implementation of vitamin D supplementation can be helpful in preventing and reducing the incidence of AIAA [86–88].

Several studies have looked into optimal plasma concentrations of 25-OHD needed in order to prevent/attenuate arthralgia in women on AI therapy. A prospective cohort study conducted in Barcelona, Spain, followed 260 postmenopausal women diagnosed with early-stage breast cancer who had 25-OHD concentrations <30 ng/ml and were started on an AI [87]. Patients with preexisting bone disorders (rheumatoid arthritis, metabolic/endocrine disorders, etc.) were excluded from this study. Results were adjusted for age, BMI, season when the 25-OHD sample was drawn, type of AI, prior tamoxifen therapy, and previous fracture. In assessing pain, participants were asked to exclude chronic back pain and post-operative pain; 30% of participants had preexisting joint pain. All participants scored the intensity of their joint pain using the visual analogic scale (VAS) at baseline and at 3 months. Additionally, plasma concentrations of 25-OHD were drawn at 0 and 3 months. All participants received calcium and 800 UI of vitamin D3 daily, with an additional 16,000 UI of vitamin D3 every 2 weeks. The median VAS for joint pain at 3 months increased by 1.5 units in the entire cohort ($p < 0.001$). Overall, women who achieved plasma threshold concentrations of 30 and 40 ng/ml had less increase in their joint pain ($p < 0.05$). Women who had a 25-OHD plasma concentration ≥ 40 ng/ml at the 3 month follow-up and no joint pain at baseline were significantly less likely to develop incident joint pain ($p = 0.003$).

The Aromatase Inhibitor Musculoskeletal Symptoms Study (AIMSS) was a Phase II, double-blind placebo-controlled randomized trial that aimed to determine if high-dose vitamin D2 supplementation in women receiving adjuvant anastrozole decreased the severity of arthralgia [89]. Women were stratified into two groups based on their baseline 25-OHD plasma concentrations: Group A 20–29 ng/ml and Group B 10–19 ng/ml. Group A received 50,000 IU of vitamin D2 (HDD) weekly for 8 weeks and then monthly for 4 months or placebo. Group B received HDD weekly for 16 weeks and then monthly for 2 months or placebo. Sixty women were enrolled, and symptoms were assessed using the Brief Pain Inventory-Short Form (BPI-SF), the Fibromyalgia Impact Questionnaire (FIQ), and the Health Assessment Questionnaire-Disability Index (HAQ-DI) at 0, 2, 4, and 6 months. There was a significant reduction in pain ($p = 0.0045$), worst pain ($p = 0.04$), average pain ($p = 0.0067$), pain severity ($p = 0.04$), and pain interference in daily life ($p = 0.034$) observed at the 2 month interval in both groups receiving HDD when compared to placebo. Group B experienced significantly less pain severity and pain interference across all time points when compared to placebo ($p < 0.05$), while statistically significant results were only observed at the 2-month mark in group A. This result may be due to the switch from HDD once weekly to monthly after 8 weeks in this cohort, suggesting that the monthly schedule is suboptimal dosing.

The ideal concentration of 25-OHD is widely debated. Exogenous supplementation with vitamin D can lead to side effects stemming from hypercalcemia and hyperphosphatemia [90]. Although intoxication is rare, it can lead to irreversible organ damage. Side effects are most commonly seen with prolonged use and large doses given annually. Signs and symptoms may include GI upset, peptic ulcers, pancreatitis, nephrolithiasis, changes in urine, arrhythmia, hypertension, cardiomyopathy, cardiac calcifications, psychological changes, musculoskeletal complaints, and changes in vision. A study conducted by Sanders et al. found that a single dose of 500,000 IU of vitamin D3 annually increased the risk of falls ($p = 0.003$) and fractures ($p = 0.047$) when compared to placebo in women 70 years of age and older [91]. A retrospective, observational cohort study conducted in Denmark involving 247,574 participants found a reverse J-shaped curve when looking at the association between all-cause mortality and 25-OHD levels.

They found that the lowest mortality risk was associated with levels ranging between 50 and 60 nmol/l [92].

Based on the AIMSS study discussed above, we recommend testing 25-OHD in all patients endorsing arthralgia. For patients with a serum concentration ≤ 40 ng/ml, we recommend 50,000 IU of vitamin D2 weekly for 12–24 weeks, followed by a daily supplement containing 800–1000 IU of vitamin D. If arthralgia recurs after discontinuing HDD, we recommend restarting HDD, with annual 25-OHD testing. Due to changes in organ function affecting vitamin D pharmacokinetics, special attention regarding dosing should be paid to patients age 70 years and older, as well as those with underlying renal, cardiovascular, or endocrine abnormalities.

Switch to Another Endocrine Therapy

Joint symptoms are common with menopause and are reported to occur with endocrine therapy in general, though arthralgias are about twice as likely with AIs than with tamoxifen [40, 93]. The three AIs – anastrozole, letrozole, and exemestane – have similar efficacy to each other and, as a drug family, are more effective than tamoxifen [18, 27, 29, 94], but each of these endocrine agents may be tolerated differently by individual patients. For instance, in one study comparing joint symptoms of letrozole and anastrozole, the frequency and severity of joint symptoms were similar between the two drugs, but more than half of patients with symptoms on one AI did not have the same symptoms when switched to another AI [41]. Switching among AIs is, therefore, a common AIAA management option [41, 95].

Support for switching between AIs also comes from a prospective trial. The Articular Tolerance of Letrozole (ATOLL) study was a prospective, single-arm study of 179 patients who had AIAA while on anastrozole [95]. In this study, women with AIAAs stopped anastrozole for 1 month and then were started on letrozole. Improvement in joint symptoms and good compliance with treatment were seen beyond 6 months. Mean Brief Pain Inventory (BPI) score, which assesses the severity of pain and the impact of pain on daily function, decreased from 4.9 ± 1.6 at baseline to 3.8 ± 2.4 at 6 months ($p < 0.01$). Quality of life (QOL), as assessed by the SF-12, a health-related QOL questionnaire consisting of 12 questions that measure eight domains to assess physical and mental health, also improved. As assessed by SF-12, there was significant improvement in both physical ($p < 0.001$) and mental ($p = 0.01$) QOL [95]. Importantly, this translated to good treatment adherence with 71.5% of patients remaining on letrozole at 6 months and only 28.5% discontinuing letrozole because of severe joint pain.

Switching to another AI, versus switching to tamoxifen, is the preferable first switch, given the superior efficacy of AIs over tamoxifen in preventing cancer recurrence. If intolerance to more than one AI is demonstrated, then tamoxifen, instead of an AI, should be offered as most patients who have significant arthralgias on an AI will have few joint symptoms when switched from the AI to tamoxifen [96].

Tamoxifen is also less likely than an AI to cause other joint issues, such as tenosynovial and weak grip strength [97, 98]. Joint symptoms and weakness associated with AIs may be particularly disabling in older patients [97, 99]. In the case of older patients on an AI, switching to tamoxifen, instead of another AI, may be preferable.

Complementary and Alternative Medicine (CAM) and Supplement Approaches

If arthralgia persists despite switching to another AI or to tamoxifen, then the benefits of nonprescription and/or use of nontraditional medicine approaches should be considered. We present these as a group because there may be practical barriers to their utilization. In general, insurance does not cover CAM and supplements, making their use cost-prohibitive to some and undesirable to others. It may also be difficult to find reputable and licensed providers for interventions, such as acupuncture. Nevertheless, these options may alleviate symptoms in some patients. The high prevalence of use of complementary therapies and supplements among women with breast cancer [100–102] warrants review of the data evaluating these alternatives.

Acupuncture Acupuncture is an ancient traditional Chinese medicine technique, dating back more than 3000 years, in which fine needles are inserted into selected body parts, called acupuncture points or acupoints, defined by the body's meridian system, through which our vital life energy, or "qi", flows [103]. This technique is commonly used to treat pain, though the mechanism of action is unclear; it may involve decreasing inflammation, increasing circulating opioid peptides, or improving blood flow [104, 105]. In a systematic review of 13 randomized clinical trials studying acupuncture versus placebo acupuncture versus no acupuncture to treat pain, there was minimal efficacy [106]. Only a small, questionable, analgesic effect was noted for acupuncture over placebo acupuncture; placebo acupuncture also had a small analgesic effect over no acupuncture. For knee arthritis, a systematic review of acupuncture found some benefit for pain, but no improvement of function [107]. Despite lack of scientific rationale and proof of efficacy, acupuncture has steadily gained acceptance and popularity, with more than 6% of Americans having used acupuncture at some point [108]. Several groups have studied acupuncture for AIAA.

In a pilot study, investigators at Columbia University in New York showed the promise of acupuncture for AIAA [109]. They then conducted a single-institution, randomized controlled trial (RCT) of acupuncture versus sham acupuncture in postmenopausal women taking adjuvant aromatase inhibitors [110]. In the RCT, 43 women who had AIAA were randomly assigned to receive acupuncture versus sham procedure, twice weekly for 6 weeks. Pain was assessed at baseline and 6 weeks using the Brief Pain Inventory-Short Form (BPI-SF). Patients in the acupuncture group received standard, full-body, manual acupuncture to standard acupoints, in addition to acupuncture to acupoints specific for the most painful joints. The sham acupuncture group had superficial needle insertion at non-acupoint locations. Compared to the sham procedure, acupuncture significantly reduced pain severity ($p = 0.003$), pain-related interference ($p = 0.002$), and stiffness ($p = 0.01$).

A RCT from the United Kingdom compared acupuncture to sham control [111]. For this study, 51 postmenopausal women with early-stage breast cancer and AIAA were randomized to receive acupuncture to 15 real acupoints versus acupuncture to sham acupoints. Sham acupoints were midpoints of the line between two real acupoints. Patients received acupuncture weekly for 8 weeks. In this study, both groups had improvements in functional ability and pain, but there was no significant difference between the groups with regard to endpoints ($p = 0.31$). In addition, inflammatory cytokines (interferon-γ, IL-1, IL-6, IL-8, and IL-10) did not change, but IL-17 decreased significantly ($p \leq 0.009$) in both groups. Neither estradiol nor β-endorphin levels changed.

The Southwest Oncology Group (SWOG) conducted a 3-arm RCT of acupuncture versus sham acupuncture, versus waitlist control for AIAA in women on adjuvant AIs for breast cancer [112]. Theirs was the largest trial to date ($n = 226$) and was multicenter. Patients were randomized 2:1:1 to three groups: acupuncture, sham acupuncture, or waitlist. Acupuncture was delivered at standard acupuncture points plus most painful joint-specific points. Sham acupuncture was given using shallow needles at non-acupuncture points and joint-specific and auricular points. Treatments were delivered twice weekly for 6 weeks and then once a week for 6 weeks. At 6 weeks, joint pain decreased in all 3 groups, but the magnitude of decrease was greater with acupuncture than sham ($p = 0.01$) or waitlist control ($p = 0.01$). Patients in the acupuncture group did experience significantly more grade 1 bruising compared to sham procedure (47% vs 25%, $p = 0.01$).

Acupuncture techniques may also include electrostimulation. After conducting a pilot study of electrostimulation delivered by transcutaneous electrical nerve stimulation (TENS) unit and showing promising results for AIAA [113], investigators at Abramson Cancer Center in

Philadelphia, PA, conducted an RCT [114]. They randomized 67 patients to one of three groups: electroacupuncture, sham electroacupuncture, or waitlist control. Acupuncture was delivered using a manualized protocol with 2 Hz electrostimulation delivered by a TENS unit. Sham procedure used non-penetrating needles at nontraditional acupuncture points and without electrostimulation. Acupuncture and sham procedures were delivered twice weekly for 2 weeks and then weekly for 6 weeks. Pain and interference were measured after 8 and 12 weeks by BPI. After 8 and 12 weeks, pain severity ($p = 0.004$ and $p < 0.0001$, respectively) and pain-related interference ($p = 0.0006$ and 0.003, respectively) improved more with the TENS unit compared to waitlist controls. The sham procedure produced similar benefit. Electroacupuncture and sham procedures were well tolerated, and there were only a few, minor adverse events.

Investigators from Australia conducted an RCT comparing standard electroacupuncture, which consisted of connecting needles through an electrode with bilateral rotation at various acupoints until de qi sensation, such as tingling or numbness, occurred, with a sham procedure, where the acupuncture needle did not penetrate the skin [115]. The study included 32 patients on adjuvant AI who had the procedure twice a week for 6 weeks. Using standardized scales (WOMAC and BPI-SF), they found no significant difference between the procedures with regard to joint pain, stiffness, or physical function. They also measured serum inflammatory markers, C-reactive protein, and erythrocyte sedimentation rate and found no significant reduction with acupuncture or sham procedures.

The results of the randomized trials are somewhat perplexing. Only one of the trials clearly showed that acupuncture was superior to sham acupuncture, and both procedures appeared to have similar benefits when compared to waitlist control. Likewise, a systematic review of four randomized trials published in 2015 described hopeful results, but encouraged further research due to bias in the studies [116], and a meta-analysis published in 2015 showed no statistically significant effect [117]. The extent of the placebo effect with both acupuncture and sham acupuncture is likely important. Despite the unclear physiology of acupuncture, its possible benefit, popularity, and lack of serious side effects make it a reasonable option for management of AIAA.

Yoga Yoga is a combined mental and physical approach to improve well-being and manage symptoms. It is widely available in the community and has been shown to improve quality of life in breast cancer survivors [118]. Several studies suggest a beneficial effect of yoga on joint pain in women with breast cancer [119, 120], including two prospective studies [121–123].

Galantino et al. studied a modified Iyengar yoga program, consisting of precise postures, breathing exercises, and meditation, in 10 postmenopausal women on an adjuvant AI with AIAA [121, 122]. They evaluated the effect of yoga on pain, functional outcomes, and health-related quality of life in women with AIAA [121]. Yoga classes were held for 90 minutes, twice per week for 8 weeks after which patients were instructed to continue a home-based yoga program. Participants experienced improvements in pain level ($p < 0.05$), balance ($p < 0.05$), and QOL ($p < 0.05$).

Peppone and colleagues did a secondary analysis of an RCT studying yoga for sleep in breast cancer patients on endocrine therapy with AI or tamoxifen [123]. This was a nationwide, multisite, randomized, controlled clinical trial. Participants were assigned to a 4-week yoga intervention involving 75 minute sessions twice a week or control. The yoga program consisted of breathing exercises, 18 gentle Hatha and restorative yoga postures, and meditation. At baseline, AI users ($n = 95$) reported higher levels of general pain, muscle aches, and total physical discomfort than tamoxifen users ($n = 72$) (all = <0.05). Patients in the yoga group were significantly more likely to have relief of total body aches ($p = 0.02$) and improvement in physical well-being (($p = 0.011$). There was no significant improvement in pain ($p = 0.094$) or muscle aches ($p = 0.352$). Measures specific to arthralgia and joint pain were not collected for this study.

Glucosamine Sulfate + Chondroitin Sulfate Glucosamine and chondroitin are natural compounds found in healthy cartilage and are hypothesized to have local anti-inflammatory effects within joints [124]. As such, the combination as a dietary supplement is available over-the-counter and is a popular remedy for non-inflammatory arthritis pain. Its use is supported by a large randomized, placebo-controlled trial of glucosamine sulfate and chondroitin sulfate for painful knee osteoarthritis. The Glucosamine/Chondroitin Arthritis Intervention Trial (GAIT), found that, in patients with moderate to severe pain at baseline, the rate of pain relief was significantly higher with glucosamine and chondroitin than with placebo (79.2% versus 54.3%, $p = -0.002$) [125].

Investigators at Columbia University in New York conducted a phase II study of glucosamine sulfate and chondroitin sulfate in 40 women with joint symptoms who were taking an adjuvant AI for hormone receptor-positive breast cancer [126]. A regimen of 1500 mg glucosamine plus 1200 mg chondroitin given daily over 24 weeks produced improvement in joint pain ($p = 0.02$). Overall, 46.2% of participants reported a clinically meaningful response within 6 months of treatment. Hand grip ($p = 0.00005$) was also improved. This regimen of glucosamine-sulfate and chondroidin-sulfate was also deemed safe, as there was no significant increase in estradiol level. There were minimal adverse effects at 12 weeks, most commonly headache (26%), dyspepsia (17%), and nausea (17%), all grade 1–2.

Duloxetine

Duloxetine (CymbaltaTM), a serotonin and norepinephrine reuptake inhibitor, was originally approved by the US Food and Drug Administration (FDA) for major depressive disorder, but has also been found efficacious for treatment of pain disorders. It is now FDA approved for treatment of fibromyalgia, diabetic peripheral neuropathic pain, and chronic musculoskeletal pain [127]. It is thought that duloxetine may alter central pain processing, but the exact mechanism by which it relieves pain is unclear.

Investigators from the University of Michigan Cancer Center studied duloxetine for treatment of AIAA. In a pilot study, after 8 weeks of duloxetine therapy, 21 of 29 (72%) evaluable patients reported at least 30% reduction in pain ($p < 0.001$) [128]. Furthermore, 18 of 23 (78.3%) who completed protocol therapy continued taking duloxetine. This work led to a larger, multicenter, placebo-controlled, RCT of duloxetine run by SWOG [129]. The RCT included 255, postmenopausal women with early-stage breast cancer who had AIAA at a level of 4 or greater on a 10 point scale. Patients were randomized 1:1 to receive duloxetine or placebo for 13 weeks. The average pain score decreased more with duloxetine than with placebo; pain with duloxetine was 0.82 points (95% CI 1.24–0.40, $p = 0.0002$) different than placebo. Compared to baseline, at 6 weeks, significantly more patients treated with duloxetine than placebo reached the prespecified clinically meaningful improvement in pain of two or greater points (68% vs 49%; $p = 0.03$), though rates of meaningful improvement were not significantly different at 2, 12, and 24 weeks. Adverse events were more common in the duloxetine than the placebo group (78% vs 50%, $p < 0.001$). The most common adverse events in the duloxetine-treated patients were fatigue, nausea, dry mouth, and headache. Most (78%) adverse events were grade 1–2.

Other Interventions with Minimal Evidence to Support Use in AIAA

There are a few reports claiming success with other supplements to alleviate AIAA. A complementary medicine regime including sodium selenite, plant enzymes (bromelaine and papain), and lens culinaris lectin has been studied in Germany [130–132]. These single-arm studies report benefit of this regime, but use an unvalidated self-assessment score of pain. Additional study of this regime will be needed. A case report describing relief of AIAA in a postmenopausal breast cancer patient treated with complementary regimen of Juzentaihoto followed by aconite root, which are elements of traditional Japanese Kampo medicine, provides very preliminary support that may lead to future studies [133]. Another pilot study from China, based on evidence that disturbance in immune cytokine balance may contribute to AIAA, administered thymosin α1, also called zadazin, a hormone produced by the thymus that increases immune function of cells, found benefit of thymosin α1 [134]. In this study, thymosin α1 was given to 16 participants by subcutaneous injection, 1.6 mg twice a week for 4 weeks. After 4 weeks, there were improvements in pain severity ($p = 0.014$), pain-related functional interference ($p = 0.001$), and physical well-being ($p = 0.001$) compared to baseline. This treatment, however, is not widely available so has limited use.

Low-dose steroids have also been studied. One report was a single-arm study of 27 patients given a short-course of low-dose prednisolone [135]. Prednisolone was given at a dose of 5 mg each morning for 1 week. Most (70%) of patients reported immediate relief in joint pain and 63% reported ongoing improvement at 1 month. Follow-up was only 2 months in this report. Given the fact that corticosteroids have significant side effects, their role in AIAA is limited.

Interventions that Are Not Indicated for AIAA Based on Available Literature

Tai-Chi Tai-Chi is focused on body awareness, deep breathing, and weight bearing. A study of 12 participants with early-stage breast cancer and AIAA who participated in Tai-Chi for 1 hour twice a week over 8 weeks showed no change in pain level ($p = 0.058$) or physical well-being ($p = 0.052$), but significant improvement in anxiety ($p = 0.003$), depression ($p = 0.02$), emotional well-being (0.027), and fatigue ($p = 0.03$) [136]. Though Tai-Chi likely improves quality of life, this study does not support its use to alleviate pain in patients with AIAA.

Omega-3 Fatty Acids Based on anti-inflammatory effects of omega-3 fatty acids [137] and benefits of use for rheumatoid arthritis [138] as well as acute and chronic back pain [139], they were studied in AIAA. Based on the RCT of the Southwest Oncology Group (SWOG), which studied omega-3 fatty acids versus placebo, omega-3 fatty acid supplements cannot be recommended for AIAA [140]. In this multicenter, RCT, those randomized to intervention received 3.3 g of omega-3 fatty acids, and those randomized to placebo received a blend of soybean and corn oil. Pills were taken daily for 24 weeks. Both placebo and omega-3 fatty acid groups had improvement in joint pain. There was no difference between groups with regard to change in pain level ($p = 0.66$), inflammation measured by C-reactive protein ($p = 0.71$), or lipid profiles, except for triglycerides.

Conclusions

Non-inflammatory joint pain, or arthralgia, is common among women, especially among women with recent diagnosis and treatment for breast cancer. Work-up should include a baseline evaluation with history, physical examination, and laboratory evaluation that focuses on general causes of joint pain and on causes of arthralgia specific to breast cancer treatment. If an inflammatory cause of joint pain is suspected, if pain does not fit a diagnosis of arthralgia related to breast cancer treatment, or if pain and discomfort persists despite standard/acceptable intervention, then a referral to a rheumatologist is warranted. Post-chemotherapy rheumatism is a time-limited syndrome that occurs within 3–4 months after completing chemotherapy, is typically unrelieved by standard approaches, and subsides within 3–4 months. AIAA is troublesome in postmenopausal women who are on adjuvant AIs because it interferes with full adherence to potentially life-saving treatment and negatively impacts quality of life. A regular exercise schedule and adequate levels of vitamin D intake demonstrated by appropriate blood levels can improve both arthralgia and breast cancer outcomes and are, therefore, recommended. Randomized trials have shown that switching to an alternative endocrine therapy, use of acupuncture techniques, yoga practice, glucosamine-sulfate and chondroitin sulfate, and duloxetine can also provide relief of AIAA. Attention to the onset of arthralgia in women with breast cancer will help lead to appropriate and effective therapies that will relieve symptoms and improve adherence to life-saving AI therapy.

References

1. Watt FE. Musculoskeletal pain and menopause. Post Reprod Health. 2018;24(1):34–43.
2. Alpay-Kanitez N, Celik S, Bes C. Polyarthritis and its differential diagnosis. Eur J Rheumatol. 2018;6(4):167–73.
3. Symmons DPM. Epidemiology of rheumatoid arthritis: determinants of onset, persistence and outcome. Best Pract Res Clin Rheumatol. 2002;16(5):707–22.
4. Grassi W, et al. The clinical features of rheumatoid arthritis. Eur J Radiol. 1998;27 Suppl 1:p. S18–S24.
5. Hunter DJ, Bierma-Zeinstra S. Osteoarthritis. Lancet. 2019;393(10182):1745–59.
6. Magliano M. Menopausal arthralgia: fact or fiction. Maturitas. 2010;67(1):29–33.
7. Kumar B, Lenert P. Joint hypermobility syndrome: recognizing a commonly overlooked cause of chronic pain. Am J Med. 2017;130(6):640–7.
8. Loprinzi CL, Duffy J, Ingle JN. Postchemotherapy rheumatism. J Clin Oncol. 1993;11:768.
9. Amiri AH, Rafiei A. Analysis of patients with post-chemotherapy arthralgia and arthritis in breast cancer. Indian J Med Sci. 2010;64(5):197–203.
10. Amiri AH, Jaferian S. Post-chemotherapy arthralgia and arthritis in lung cancer. South Asian J Cancer. 2012;1(2):72–5.
11. Kim MJ, et al. Chemotherapy-related arthropathy. J Rheumatol. 2006;33(7):1364–8.
12. Almoallim H, et al. Clinical characteristics and outcomes of cancer patients with post-chemotherapy arthritis: a retrospective case series report. Open Access Rheumatol. 2017;9:111–6.
13. Burstein HJ. Aromatase inhibitor-associated arthralgia syndrome. Breast. 2007;16(3):223–34.
14. Dowsett M, et al. Aromatase inhibitors versus tamoxifen in early breast cancer: patient-level meta-analysis of the randomised trials. Lancet. 2015;386(10001):1341–52.
15. Forbes JF, et al. Effect of anastrozole and tamoxifen as adjuvant treatment for early-stage breast cancer: 100-month analysis of the ATAC trial. Lancet Oncol. 2008;9(1):45–53.
16. Mouridsen H, et al. Letrozole therapy alone or in sequence with tamoxifen in women with breast cancer. N Engl J Med. 2009;361(8):766–76.
17. Coates AS, et al. Five years of letrozole compared with tamoxifen as initial adjuvant therapy for postmenopausal women with endocrine-responsive early breast cancer: update of study BIG 1-98. J Clin Oncol. 2007;25(5):486–92.
18. Coombes RC, et al. Survival and safety of exemestane versus tamoxifen after 2-3 years' tamoxifen treatment (Intergroup Exemestane Study): a randomised controlled trial. Lancet. 2007;369(9561):559–70.
19. Braithwaite RS, et al. Meta-analysis of vascular and neoplastic events associated with tamoxifen. J Gen Intern Med. 2003;18(11):937.
20. Henry NL, Giles JT, Stearns V. Aromatase inhibitor-associated musculoskeletal symptoms: etiology and strategies for management. Oncology (Williston Park). 2008;22(12):1401–8.
21. Coleman RE, et al. Aromatase inhibitor-induced arthralgia: clinical experience and treatment recommendations. Cancer Treat Rev. 2008;34(3):275–82.
22. Crew KD, et al. Prevalence of joint symptoms in postmenopausal women taking aromatase inhibitors for early-stage breast cancer. J Clin Oncol. 2007;25(25):3877–83.
23. Lombard JM, et al. Aromatase inhibitor induced musculoskeletal syndrome: a significant problem with limited treatment options. Support Care Cancer. 2016;24(5):2139–46.
24. Niravath P. Aromatase inhibitor-induced arthralgia: a review. Ann Oncol. 2013;24(6):1443–9.
25. Donnellan PP, et al. Aromatase inhibitors and arthralgia. J Clin Oncol. 2001;19(10):2767.
26. Presant CA, et al. Aromatase inhibitor-associated arthralgia and/ or bone pain: frequency and characterization in non-clinical trial patients. Clin Breast Cancer. 2007;7(10):775–8.
27. Howell A, et al. Results of the ATAC (arimidex, tamoxifen, alone or in combination) trial after completion of 5 years' adjuvant treatment for breast cancer. Lancet. 2005;365(9453):60.
28. Coombes RC, et al. A randomized trial of exemestane after two to three years of tamoxifen therapy in postmenopausal women with primary breast cancer. N Engl J Med. 2004;350(11):1081.
29. Thurlimann B, et al. A comparison of letrozole and tamoxifen in postmenopausal women with early breast cancer. N Engl J Med. 2005;353(26):2747–57.
30. Goss PE, et al. A randomized trial of letrozole in postmenopausal women after five years of tamoxifen therapy for early-stage breast cancer. N Engl J Med. 2003;349(19):1793.
31. Boonstra A, et al. Arthralgia during aromatase inhibitor treatment in early breast cancer patients: prevalence, impact, and recognition by healthcare providers. Cancer Nurs. 2013;36(1):52–9.
32. Dizdar O, et al. Sonographic and electrodiagnostic evaluations in patients with aromatase inhibitor-related arthralgia. J Clin Oncol. 2009;27(30):4955–60.
33. Friedman CF, et al. Functional disability and aromatase inhibitor-associated arthralgia in breast cancer survivors. J Clin Oncol. 2010;28(15S).

34. Mao JJ, et al. Patterns and risk factors associated with aromatase inhibitor-related arthralgia among breast cancer survivors. Cancer. 2009;115(16):3631–9.
35. Oberguggenberger A, et al. Is the toxicity of adjuvant aromatase inhibitor therapy underestimated? Complementary information from patient-reported outcomes (PROs). Breast Cancer Res Treat. 2011;128(2):553–61.
36. Kanematsu M, et al. The time since last menstrual period is important as a clinical predictor for non-steroidal aromatase inhibitor-related arthralgia. BMC Cancer. 2011;11:436.
37. Singer O, et al. Defining the aromatase inhibitor musculoskeletal syndrome: a prospective study. Arthritis Care Res (Hoboken). 2012;64(12):1910–8.
38. Kimmick GG, et al. Musculoskeletal side effects over time and association with adherence in women taking neoadjuvant letrozole for estrogen receptor positive DCIS: CALGB 40903 (Alliance). Breast Cancer Res Treat. 2019; SABCS 2019(P5-14-17).
39. Castel LD, et al. Time course of arthralgia among women initiating aromatase inhibitor therapy and a postmenopausal comparison group in a prospective cohort. Cancer. 2013;119(13):2375–82.
40. Sestak I, et al. Risk factors for joint symptoms in patients enrolled in the ATAC trial: a retrospective, exploratory analysis. Lancet Oncol. 2008;9(9):866–72.
41. Renshaw L, et al. Comparison of joint problems as reported by patients in a randomised adjuvant trial of anastrozole and letrozole. Breast Cancer Res Treat. 2007;106:S108–S109.
42. Morales L, et al. Debilitating musculoskeletal pain and stiffness with letrozole and exemestane: associated tenosynovial changes on magnetic resonance imaging. Breast Cancer Res Treat. 2007;104(1):87–91.
43. Laroche F, et al. Classification of and risk factors for estrogen deprivation pain syndromes related to aromatase inhibitor treatments in women with breast cancer: a prospective multicenter cohort study. J Pain. 2014;15(3):293–303.
44. Spagnolo F, et al. Anastrozole-induced carpal tunnel syndrome: results from the international breast cancer intervention study II prevention trial. J Clin Oncol. 2016;34(2):139–43.
45. Sestak I, Sapunar F, Cuzick J. Aromatase inhibitor-induced carpal tunnel syndrome: results from the ATAC trial. J Clin Oncol. 2009;27(30):4961–5.
46. Papadimitriou K, et al. Bilateral de quervain syndrome after aromatase inhibitor administration: a case report and review of the literature. Case Rep Med. 2012;2012:810428.
47. Lee JH, Kim JY, Kim CH. A case of bilateral trigger thumbs secondary to aromatase inhibitor. Yonsei Med J. 2015;56(4):1167–9.
48. Murphy CC, et al. Adherence to adjuvant hormonal therapy among breast cancer survivors in clinical practice: a systematic review. Breast Cancer Res Treat. 2012;134(2):459–78.
49. Fontein DB, et al. High non-compliance in the use of letrozole after 2.5 years of extended adjuvant endocrine therapy. Results from the IDEAL randomized trial. Eur J Surg Oncol. 2012;38(2):110–7.
50. Hershman DL, et al. Early discontinuation and non-adherence to adjuvant hormonal therapy are associated with increased mortality in women with breast cancer. Breast Cancer Res Treat. 2011;126(2):529–37.
51. Henry NL, et al. Prospective characterization of musculoskeletal symptoms in early stage breast cancer patients treated with aromatase inhibitors. Breast Cancer Res Treat. 2008;111(2):365–72.
52. Moy B, et al. Clinical outcomes of ethnic minority women in MA.17: a trial of letrozole after 5 years of tamoxifen in postmenopausal women with early stage breast cancer. Ann Oncol. 2006;17(11):1637–43.
53. Xu J, et al. Natural history of menopause symptoms in primary care patients: a MetroNet study. J Am Board Fam Pract. 2005;18(5):374–82.
54. Fuh JL, et al. Quality of life and menopausal transition for middle-aged women on Kinmen island. Qual Life Res. 2003;12(1):53–61.
55. Bingefors K, Isacson D. Epidemiology, comorbidity, and impact on health-related quality of life of self-reported headache and musculoskeletal pain--a gender perspective. Eur J Pain. 2004;8(5):435–50.
56. Thorne C. Management of arthralgias associated with aromatase inhibitor therapy. Curr Oncol. 2007;14(Suppl 1):S11–9.
57. Younus J, Kligman L. Management of aromatase inhibitor-induced arthralgia. Curr Oncol. 2010;17(1):87–90.
58. Din OS, et al. Current opinion of aromatase inhibitor-induced arthralgia in breast cancer in the UK. Clin Oncol (R Coll Radiol). 2011;23(10):674–80.
59. Menas P, et al. Incidence and management of arthralgias in breast cancer patients treated with aromatase inhibitors in an outpatient oncology clinic. J Oncol Pharm Pract. 2012;18(4):387–93.
60. Park SH, Knobf MT, Sutton KM. Etiology, assessment, and management of aromatase inhibitor-related musculoskeletal symptoms. Clin J Oncol Nurs. 2012;16(3):260–6.
61. Yang GS, et al. Interventions for the treatment of aromatase inhibitor-associated arthralgia in breast cancer survivors: a systematic review and meta-analysis. Cancer Nurs. 2017;40(4):E26–41.
62. Dent SF, et al. Aromatase inhibitor therapy: toxicities and management strategies in the treatment of postmenopausal women with hormone-sensitive early breast cancer. Breast Cancer Res Treat. 2011;126(2):295–310.
63. Somers TJ, Wren AA, Shelby RA. The context of pain in arthritis: self-efficacy for managing pain and other symptoms. Curr Pain Headache Rep. 2012;16(6):502–8.

64. Jerant A, Franks P, Kravitz RL. Associations between pain control self-efficacy, self-efficacy for communicating with physicians, and subsequent pain severity among cancer patients. Patient Educ Couns. 2011;85(2):275–80.
65. Johannsen M, et al. The efficacy of psychosocial intervention for pain in breast cancer patients and survivors: a systematic review and meta-analysis. Breast Cancer Res Treat. 2013;138(3):675–90.
66. Sheinfeld Gorin S, et al. Meta-analysis of psychosocial interventions to reduce pain in patients with cancer. J Clin Oncol. 2012;30(5):539–47.
67. Kelleher SA, et al. A behavioral cancer pain intervention: A randomized noninferiority trial comparing in-person with videoconference delivery. Psychooncology. 2019;28(8):1671–8.
68. Shelby RA, et al. Testing a behavioral intervention to improve adherence to adjuvant endocrine therapy (AET). Contemp Clin Trials. 2019;76:120–131.
69. Khan QJ, O'Dea AP, Sharma P, Musculoskeletal adverse events associated with adjuvant aromatase inhibitors. J Oncol. 2010;2010:1–8.
70. Cuzick, J, et al. Treatment-emergent endocrine symptoms and the risk of breast cancer recurrence: a retrospective analysis of the ATAC trial. Lancet Oncol. 2008;9(12):1143–8.
71. Irwin ML et al. Randomized exercise trial of aromatase inhibitor-induced arthralgia in breast cancer survivors. J Clin Oncol. 2015;33(10):1104–11.
72. DeNysschen CA et al. Exercise intervention in breast cancer patients with aromatase inhibitor-associated arthralgia: a pilot study. Eur J Cancer Care (ENgl). 2014; 23(4):493–501.
73. Baglia MS et al. Endocrine-related quality of life in a randomized trial of exercise on aromatase inhibitor-induced arthralgias in breast cancer survivors. Cancer. 2019;125(13):2262–71.
74. Sisto SA, Malanga G. Osteoarthritis and therapeutic exercise. Am J Phys Med Rehabil. 2006;85(11 Suppl):S69–78.
75. Thomas KS et al. Home based exercise programme for knee pain and knee osteoarthritis: randomised controlled trial. BMJ. 2002;325(7367):752.
76. Ballard-Barbash R et al. Physical activity, biomarkers, and disease outcomes in cancer survivors: a systematic review. J Natl Cancer Inst. 2012;104(11):815–40.
77. Rock CL et al. Nutrition and physical activity guidelines for cancer survivors. CA Cancer J Clin. 2012;62(4):243–74.
78. Demark-Wahnefried W et al. Results of a diet/exercise feasibility trial to prevent adverse body composition change in breast cancer patients on adjuvant chemotherapy. Clin Breast Cancer. 2008;8(1):70–9.
79. Lima LV, Abner TSS, Sluka KA. Does exercise increase or decrease pain? Central mechanisms underlying these two phenomena. J Physiol. 2017;595(13):4141–50.
80. Polaski AM et al. Exercise-induced hypoalgesia: A meta-analysis of exercise dosing for the treatment of chronic pain. PLoS One. 2019;14(1):e0210418.
81. Nyrop KA, et al. Feasibility and promise of a 6-week program to encourage physical activity and reduce joint symptoms among elderly breast cancer survivors on aromatase inhibitor therapy. J Geriatr Oncol. 2014;5(2):148–55.
82. Hasan N, Sonnenschein C, Soto AM. Vitamin D3 constrains estrogen's effects and influences mammary epithelial organization in 3D cultures. Sci Rep. 2019;9(1):7423.
83. Jurutka PW et al. Vitamin D receptor: key roles in bone mineral pathophysiology, molecular mechanism of action, and novel nutrient ligands. J Bone Miner Res. 2007;22 Suppl 2:V2–10.
84. Crew KD et al. Association between plasma 25-hydroxyvitamin D and breast cancer risk. Cancer Prev Res (Phila). 2009;2(6):598–604.
85. Arvold DS et al. Correlation of symptoms with vitamin D deficiency and symptom response to cholecalciferol treatment: a randomized controlled trial. Endocr Pract. 2009;15(3):203–12.
86. Khan QJ, et al. Effect of vitamin D supplementation on serum 25-hydroxy vitamin D levels, joint pain, and fatigue in women starting adjuvant letrozole treatment for breast cancer. Breast Cancer Res Treat. 2009;119(1):111–8.
87. Prieto-Alhambra D et al. Vitamin D threshold to prevent aromatase inhibitor-induced arthralgia: a prospective cohort study. Breast Cancer Res Treat. 2011;125(3):869–78.
88. Prieto-Alhambra D, Javaid MK. Aromatase inhibitor induced arthralgia: is vitamin D deficiency responsibible? Maturitas. 2011;69(1):3–4.
89. Rastelli AL et al. Vitamin D and aromatase inhibitor-induced musculoskeletal symptoms (AIMSS): a phase II, double-bline, placebo-controlled, randomized trial. Breast Cancer Res Treat. 2011;129(1):107–16.
90. Razzaque MS. Can adverse effects of excessive vitamin D supplementation occur without developing hypervitaminosis D? J Steroid Biochem Mol Biol. 2018;180:81–6.
91. Sanders KM et al. Annual high-dose oral vitamin D and falls and fractures in older women: a randomized controlled trial. JAMA. 2010;202(18):1815–22.
92. Durup D et al. A reverse J-shaped assocition of all-cause mortality with serum 25-hydroxyvitamin D in general practice: the CopD study. J Clin Endocrinol Metab. 2012;97(8):2644–52.
93. Kimmick G, et al. Medication taking behaviors among breast cancer patients on adjuvant endocrine therapy. Breast. 2015;24(5):630–6.
94. Group, B.I.G.C., et al. Letrozole therapy alone or in sequence with tamoxifen in women with breast cancer. N Engl J Med. 2009;361(8):766–76.
95. Briot K, et al. Effect of a switch of aromatase inhibitors on musculoskeletal symptoms in postmenopausal women with hormone-receptor-positive breast cancer: the ATOLL (articular tolerance of letrozole) study. Breast Cancer Res Treat. 2010;120(1):127–34.
96. Garreau JR, et al. Side effects of aromatase inhibitors versus tamoxifen: the patients' perspective. Am J Surg. 2006;192(4):496–8.

97. Sitlinger A, et al. Higher symptom burden is associated with lower function in women taking adjuvant endocrine therapy for breast cancer. J Geriatr Oncol. 2019;10(2):317–21.
98. Morales L et al. Prospective study to assess short-term intra-articular and tenosynovial changes in the aromatase inhibitorassociated arthralgia syndrome. J Clin Oncol. 2008;26(19):3147–52.
99. Kanesvaran R, White HK, Kimmick GG. (AI) Can't get off my chair. J Am Geriatr Soc. 2012;60(10):1978–9.
100. Neuhouser ML, et al. Use of complementary and alternative medicine and breast cancer survival in the Health, Eating, Activity, and Lifestyle Study. Breast Cancer Res Treat. 2016;160(3):539–46.
101. Cassileth BR, Vickers AJ. High prevalence of complementary and alternative medicine use among cancer patients: implications for research and clinical care. J Clin Oncol. 2005;23(12):2590–2.
102. Velicer CM, Ulrich CM. Vitamin and mineral supplement use among US adults after cancer diagnosis: a systematic review. J Clin Oncol. 2008;26(4):665–73.
103. Sierpina VS, Frenkel MA. Acupuncture: a clinical review. South Med J. 2005;98(3):330–7.
104. Lim HD, et al. Anti-inflammatory effects of acupuncture stimulation via the vagus nerve. PLoS One. 2016;11(3):e0151882.
105. Sandberg M, et al. Effects of acupuncture on skin and muscle blood flow in healthy subjects. Eur J Appl Physiol. 2003;90(1–2):114–9.
106. Madsen MV, Gotzsche PC, Hrobjartsson A. Acupuncture treatment for pain: systematic review of randomised clinical trials with acupuncture, placebo acupuncture, and no acupuncture groups. BMJ. 2009;338:a3115.
107. Ezzo J, et al. Acupuncture for osteoarthritis of the knee: a systematic review. Arthritis Rheum. 2001;44(4):819–25.
108. Zhang Y, et al. Acupuncture use among American adults: what acupuncture practitioners can learn from national health interview survey 2007? Evid Based Complement Alternat Med. 2012;2012:710750.
109. Crew KD, et al. Pilot study of acupuncture for the treatment of joint symptoms related to adjuvant aromatase inhibitor therapy in postmenopausal breast cancer patients. J Cancer Surviv. 2007;1(4):283–91.
110. Crew KD, et al. Randomized, blinded, sham-controlled trial of acupuncture for the management of aromatase inhibitor-associated joint symptoms in women with early-stage breast cancer. J Clin Oncol. 2010;28(7):1154–60.
111. Bao T, et al. A dual-center randomized controlled double blind trial assessing the effect of acupuncture in reducing musculoskeletal symptoms in breast cancer patients taking aromatase inhibitors. Breast Cancer Res Treat. 2013;138(1):167–74.
112. Hershman DL, et al. Effect of acupuncture vs sham acupuncture or waitlist control on joint pain related to aromatase inhibitors among women with early-stage breast cancer: a randomized clinical trial. JAMA. 2018;320(2):167–76.
113. Mao JJ, et al. Feasibility trial of electroacupuncture for aromatase inhibitor-related arthralgia in breast cancer survivors. Integr Cancer Ther. 2009;8(2):123–9.
114. Mao JJ, et al. A randomised trial of electro-acupuncture for arthralgia related to aromatase inhibitor use. Eur J Cancer. 2014;50(2):267–76.
115. Oh B, et al. Acupuncture for treatment of arthralgia secondary to aromatase inhibitor therapy in women with early breast cancer: pilot study. Acupunct Med. 2013;31(3):264–71.
116. Bae K, et al. Acupuncture for aromatase inhibitor-induced arthralgia: a systematic review. Integr Cancer Ther. 2015;14(6):496–502.
117. Chien TJ, et al. Acupuncture for treating aromatase inhibitor-related arthralgia in breast cancer: a systematic review and meta-analysis. J Altern Complement Med. 2015;21(5):251–60.
118. Culos-Reed SN, et al. A pilot study of yoga for breast cancer survivors: physical and psychological benefits. Psychooncology. 2006;15(10):891–7.
119. Carson JW, et al. Yoga of awareness program for menopausal symptoms in breast cancer survivors: results from a randomized trial. Support Care Cancer. 2009;17(10):1301–9.
120. Ulger O, Yagli NV. Effects of yoga on the quality of life in cancer patients. Complement Ther Clin Pract. 2010;16(2):60–3.
121. Galantino ML, et al. Impact of yoga on functional outcomes in breast cancer survivors with aromatase inhibitor-associated arthralgias. Integr Cancer Ther. 2012;11(4):313–20.
122. Galantino ML, et al. A qualitative exploration of the impact of yoga on breast cancer survivors with aromatase inhibitor-associated arthralgias. Explore (NY). 2012;8(1):40–7.
123. Peppone LJ, et al. The effect of YOCAS(c)(R) yoga for musculoskeletal symptoms among breast cancer survivors on hormonal therapy. Breast Cancer Res Treat. 2015;150(3):597–604.
124. Lippiello L, et al. In vivo chondroprotection and metabolic synergy of glucosamine and chondroitin sulfate. Clin Orthop Relat Res. 2000;381:229–40.
125. Clegg DO, et al. Glucosamine, chondroitin sulfate, and the two in combination for painful knee osteoarthritis. N Engl J Med. 2006;354(8):795–808.
126. Greenlee H, et al. Phase II study of glucosamine with chondroitin on aromatase inhibitor-associated joint symptoms in women with breast cancer. Support Care Cancer. 2013;21(4):1077–87.
127. Lunn MP, Hughes RA, Wiffen PJ. Duloxetine for treating painful neuropathy, chronic pain or fibromyalgia. Cochrane Database Syst Rev. 2014;1:CD007115.
128. Henry NL, et al. Pilot study of duloxetine for treatment of aromatase inhibitor-associated musculoskeletal symptoms. Cancer. 2011;117(24):5469–75.

129. Henry NL, et al. Randomized, multicenter, placebo-controlled clinical trial of duloxetine versus placebo for aromatase inhibitor-associated arthralgias in early-stage breast cancer: SWOG S1202. J Clin Oncol. 2018;36(4):326–32.
130. Uhlenbruck G, et al. Reduced side-effects of adjuvant hormone therapy in breast cancer patients by complementary medicine. In Vivo. 2010;24(5):799–802.
131. Beuth J, et al. Large-scale survey of the impact of complementary medicine on side-effects of adjuvant hormone therapy in patients with breast cancer. In Vivo. 2016;30(1):73–5.
132. Beuth J, et al. Complementary medicine on side-effects of adjuvant hormone therapy in patients with breast cancer. In Vivo. 2013;27(6):869–71.
133. Chino A, et al. A case of aromatase inhibitor (anastrozole)-induced side-effects successfully treated with Kampo medicines. J Altern Complement Med. 2011;17(11):1075–7.
134. Zhang Q, Tang D, Zhao H. Immunological therapies can relieve aromatase inhibitor-related joint symptoms in breast cancer survivors. Am J Clin Oncol. 2010;33(6):557–60.
135. Kubo M, et al. Short-term and low-dose prednisolone administration reduces aromatase inhibitor-induced arthralgia in patients with breast cancer. Anticancer Res. 2012;32(6):2331–6.
136. Galantino ML, et al. Tai chi for well-being of breast cancer survivors with aromatase inhibitor-associated arthralgias: a feasibility study. Altern Ther Health Med. 2013;19(6):38–44.
137. Leslie CA, et al. Dietary fish oil modulates macrophage fatty acids and decreases arthritis susceptibility in mice. J Exp Med. 1985;162(4):1336–49.
138. Goldberg RJ, Katz J. A meta-analysis of the analgesic effects of omega-3 polyunsaturated fatty acid supplementation for inflammatory joint pain. Pain. 2007;129(1–2):210–23.
139. Maroon JC, Bost JW. Omega-3 fatty acids (fish oil) as an anti-inflammatory: an alternative to nonsteroidal anti-inflammatory drugs for discogenic pain. Surg Neurol. 2006;65(4):326–31.
140. Hershman DL, et al. Randomized multicenter placebo-controlled trial of omega-3 fatty acids for the control of aromatase inhibitor-induced musculoskeletal pain: SWOG S0927. J Clin Oncol. 2015;33(17):1910–7.

Persistent Breast Pain

7

Tamara Somers, Sarah Kelleher, and Devon Check

Persistent breast pain (PBP) following treatment for breast cancer is common and can be highly distressing for breast cancer survivors. Each year in the United States alone, more than a quarter million women are diagnosed with breast cancer and receive curative-intent treatments that can result in PBP. Overall, there are more than 3.5 million breast cancer survivors in the United States, with estimates of 25–60% having PBP, with symptoms lasting from months to years following breast cancer diagnosis and treatment [1, 2]. PBP following a cancer diagnosis is typically, though not always, thought to be related to surgery. Pain defined as PBP following breast cancer is often localized to the thorax, axillary upper arm, and medial upper arm and has been characterized as pain that is shooting, burning, or causes pressure or numbness [3–5]. In some cases, pain may result from damage to the nerve fibers from treatment and can be neuropathic in nature [3]. There are several factors associated with the development of PBP following breast cancer, and the overall etiology is likely multifactorial [6].

PBP can have a profound negative impact on quality of life for breast cancer survivors [7]. First, the breast pain that survivors experience can interfere with their ability to participate in critical activities of daily living as well as decrease their participation in activities they enjoy. There is evidence that PBP is a contributing factor to upper limb dysfunction [2] which further contributes to inabilities to engage in daily activities. Second, there are negative emotional consequences of PBP for survivors. PBP can serve as a constant negative reminder of cancer diagnosis, and this reminder can lead to a high level of psychological distress [8]. Third, PBP can result in the long-term use of pain medications, including opioid medications that can negatively influence patients' physical and psychological health and often provides only limited pain relief [9, 10]. Following breast cancer, women who report persistent pain are much more likely to report higher pain medication use than women who do not report persistent pain [11]. Finally, PBP may also have high financial costs; persistent pain following surgery in the United States is estimated to have direct costs of $560 to $635 billion annually or about $5600 per person [12]. Though PBP following breast cancer diagnosis and treatment is common and has several detrimental consequences, it has been challeng-

T. Somers (✉)
Department of Psychiatry and Behavioral Sciences, Duke University School of Medicine, Durham, NC, USA
e-mail: tamara.somers@duke.edu

S. Kelleher
Department of Psychiatry and Behavioral Sciences, Duke University Medical Center, Durham, NC, USA

D. Check
Department of Population Health Sciences, Duke University School of Medicine, Durham, NC, USA

G. G. Kimmick et al. (eds.), *Common Issues in Breast Cancer Survivors*,
https://doi.org/10.1007/978-3-030-75377-1_7

ing to identify risk factors, conduct thorough assessment, and outline optimal strategies for interventions.

Risk Factors

There are a number of factors that may increase a woman's risk of experiencing PBP following a breast cancer diagnosis and treatment. In this section, treatment- and patient-related factors that have the potential to increase a woman's risk for developing PBP are reviewed. Figure 7.1 provides a summary of risk factors for persistent breast pain.

Treatment-Related Factors

Surgery Surgical procedures for breast cancer, including mastectomy, breast conserving surgery (BCS), and axillary surgery, improve cancer morbidity and mortality but are closely associated with the development of PBP following treatment [1, 2]. Several research studies have examined the association between specific surgical procedures and PBP.

Mastectomy is a common surgical procedure following breast cancer diagnosis, and it is performed in over 40% of women with breast cancer [13]. While mastectomy is associated with a decreased risk of local recurrence compared to BCS [14, 15], for an estimated one-third of women [16], mastectomy leads to PBP. BCS, also called lumpectomy, quadrantectomy, or partial or segmental mastectomy, however, can also result in PBP [17–19].

Research has examined the rates of pain following surgery in women who have undergone mastectomy or breast conserving surgery for breast cancer. An epidemiological study examined the rates of chronic pain in the area of breast surgery or ipsilateral arm in 258 breast cancer survivors about 1.5 years following cancer surgery (either mastectomy or lumpectomy) and similar pain by location in a reference group of 774 women, randomly selected from the same population but not having undergone breast cancer surgery [20]. Rate of post-mastectomy pain syndrome was 24% in the surgery group compared to similar pain in 10% of the reference group: having undergone prior surgery, tumor location in the upper lateral quarter, and younger age both predicted increased risk for pain [20]. In

Treatment related factors	Demographic & health related factors
• Surgery --Mastectomy --Breast conserving surgery --Axillary surgery --Breast reconstructive surgery • Radiation • Chemotherapy • Endorcrine therapy	• Younger age (under 50) • Race/Ethnicity (non-white) • Lower education level • Lower income level • Medical comorbidities • High body mass index
Psychosocial factors	**Behavioral factors**
• Anxiety • Pain catastrophizing • Self-efficacy for pain management • Depression	• Lack of physical activity • Poor nutrition • Smoking • Poor sleep

Fig. 7.1 Risk factors for persistent breast pain

another study comparing PBP among women who received breast conserving surgery for breast cancer and women without a history of breast cancer, PBP was reported by nearly half (46.5%) of breast cancer survivors compared to 12.7% of women without a breast cancer history ($p < 0.05$) [21]. In a study of 261 women who had undergone single mastectomy in the last 3 years, 38% reported persistent pain in the axilla, excised breast area, medial arm, ipsilateral thorax, and/or mastectomy scar area [22].

Lymph node biopsy is another common surgery that women diagnosed with breast cancer are likely to undergo. Lymph node biopsy is often done to determine the staging of breast cancer, either sentinel lymph node biopsy or axillary lymph node dissection. Either of these procedures can lead to increased PBP; however, several studies have suggested that axillary lymph node dissection rather than sentinel lymph node biopsy is more likely to increase a woman's risk of PBP [2, 23, 24]. Axillary web syndrome is a common specific side effect that can result following lymph node biopsy; it involves the development of scarring of connective tissue under the arm leading to cording in the subcutaneous tissue and can result in painful shoulder movements [25].

Breast reconstructive surgery following mastectomy or breast conserving surgery is elected by approximately 40% of women [26]. There are several options for reconstructive surgery, and generally women report that this type of surgery improves their overall quality of life and can alleviate some of the emotional effects of breast cancer treatment procedures. However, there is also some evidence that reconstructive surgery can result in PBP. In particular, a retrospective study of women who underwent breast cancer surgery found that pain interference, upper limb dysfunction, and psychological distress were significantly higher in women who underwent reconstruction compared to women who did not [23].

Radiation Radiation therapy is a treatment that some women receive to decrease risk of cancer recurrence in the breast area following surgery for breast cancer. Fields of radiation can include whole breast, partial breast, chest wall, and lymph nodes. Radiation can improve overall cancer outcomes, though it is also associated with treatment-related side effects (e.g., breast swelling, skin changes, malaise, and fatigue). Radiation can be associated with PBP, the degree of which depends on the radiation treatment history [2, 27]. Among women who receive radiation therapy, radiation dose appears to be an important risk factor in the development of PBP [28, 29].

Chemotherapy Chemotherapy, usually delivered intravenously, improves breast cancer outcomes. Chemotherapy can occur before (i.e., neoadjuvant) or after surgery (i.e., adjuvant) for breast cancer. Although chemotherapy is not a well-established risk factor for PBP after breast cancer, a small number of studies have described an association between receipt of chemotherapy and PBP and general pain among women who completed treatment for breast cancer [27, 30]. Pain related to chemotherapy is often neuropathic in nature, possibly resulting from nerve damage caused by taxane or platinum chemotherapy which is commonly used in adjuvant chemotherapy for breast cancer.

Endocrine Therapy Adjuvant endocrine therapy for breast cancer, including tamoxifen and aromatase inhibitors, is frequently recommended for women with hormone receptor-positive disease following initial treatments for breast cancer (i.e., surgery, radiation, chemotherapy) and can be prescribed for up to 10 years or more. Adjuvant endocrine therapies reduce the risk of cancer recurrence and death. They have also been associated with a number of side effects including muscle pain and joint pain or stiffness. At least one study has also linked the use of endocrine therapy following a breast cancer diagnosis to PBP [27]. Side effects, including pain, can negatively impact patients' adherence to endocrine therapy, increasing the likelihood of cancer recurrence [31].

Demographic Risk Factors

Following a breast cancer diagnosis and treatment, there are patient-related and demographic factors associated with PBP and pain. Based on available research, women who are younger, typically thought of as under 50, are consistently more likely to develop PBP following breast cancer treatment [2, 24, 27, 30, 32–36]. Younger age has been associated with persistent pain following breast cancer diagnosis and treatment in several studies [37]. One study found that, compared to women aged 60 to 69 years, women aged 18 to 39 years had three times, and women aged 40 to 49 years had two times, the risk of developing persistent pain [2]. Possible explanations for the association of younger age with higher risk include increased nerve sensitivity, higher anxiety level which lowers pain threshold, and the often more aggressive nature of the breast cancer and possibly more extensive surgical treatment in this age group [19, 34, 38].

Other demographic factors that have been associated with persistent pain in general following breast cancer include race/ethnicity, education level, and income level. Miaskowski and colleagues [27] found that risk for PBP following breast cancer treatment was related to patients who are non-white, have less education, and have lower income. Lower income [39] and education [40] are well-established risk factors for chronic pain in the general population, as well.

There are also a number of health-related factors that may increase a woman's risk for developing both PBP and general pain following breast cancer treatment. In particular, comorbidity burden has been linked to pain among patients with cancer, including breast cancer [27, 41, 42]. In addition, overweight or high body mass index (BMI) is consistently reported as a risk factor for PBP following breast surgery [22, 36, 38, 43, 44].

Psychosocial Risk Factors

There are several psychosocial factors that have been suggested to contribute to patients' experience of persistent pain following breast cancer diagnosis and treatment. Anxiety and factors closely related to anxiety are consistently identified as likely to increase a woman's risk of PBP following a breast cancer diagnosis [7, 16, 27]. In particular, pain catastrophizing, the tendency to maintain exaggerated negative thoughts in response to and in anticipation of pain [45], has emerged as an important risk factor for persistent pain after breast cancer. A study of breast cancer survivors found that women with PBP were more likely to have higher levels of pain catastrophizing than women without breast pain [8]. The same study found that pain catastrophizing mediated the relationship between PBP and emotional distress; that is, women who catastrophize about their breast pain were more likely to experience increased emotional distress.

Patients' confidence in their ability to manage their pain (i.e., self-efficacy for pain management) has also emerged as a critical psychosocial factor related to disease-related pain across several medical conditions. Self-efficacy for pain management refers to an individual's confidence in their ability to effectively manage their pain [46]. Women with higher levels of confidence in their ability to manage their PBP are likely to experience lower pain severity [47]. Although more research is needed to understand the relationship between depressive symptoms and PBP, several longitudinal studies of women after breast cancer surgery have identified preoperative depression as a potential risk factor for the development of persistent postsurgical pain [21, 27, 48, 49].

Health Behavior Risk Factors

Poor health behaviors, such as lack of activity or exercise, poor nutrition, smoking, and poor sleep have been associated with increased pain in the general population [50]. However, most of these factors have not been studied with respect to their impact on PBP specifically in the context of breast cancer. The exception is sleep disturbance, which has been consistently shown to be associated with persistent pain following breast surgery [7, 16, 27]. These behavioral health risk factors have not been extensively studied in their relationship with PBP following breast cancer diagnosis and surgery, but these are important factors that may influence breast pain.

Genetic and Epigenetic Factors

Genetic and epigenetic variations may also help to identify patients at risk for PBP after breast cancer surgery. In particular, variations in three single-nucleotide polymorphisms (SNPs) (i.e., interleukin 6 rs2069840, C-X-C motif chemokine ligand 8, tumor necrosis factor rs1800610) have been associated with the development and maintenance of mild PBP [51]. Langford and colleagues [52] identified additional SNPs across 5 genes (i.e., potassium voltage-gated channel, subfamily A, member 1 [KCNA1], potassium voltage-gated channel, subfamily D, member 2 [KCND2], potassium inwardly rectifying channel, subfamily J, members 3 and 6 (KCNJ3 and KCNJ6), potassium channel, subfamily K, member 9 [KCNK9]) associated with development of mild PBP. This study also identified 3 SNPs and 1 haplotype across 4 genes (i.e., KCND2, KCNJ3, KCNJ6, KCNK9) that were associated with developing severe breast pain. These findings suggest that variations in potassium channel genes are associated with both mild and severe PBP after breast cancer surgery.

Screening for PBP

Screening for PBP can be challenging due to the inherently private, subjective, and complex experience of pain. However, it is critical to appropriately assess patients to identify those who are currently experiencing or may be at risk for experiencing PBP in order to intervene early to reduce symptom severity and interference and to improve patient outcomes. Assessment should include clinical interview and physical examination, and consideration of important risk factors, including breast cancer treatment history (i.e., surgery, radiation, chemotherapy, hormonal therapy) and demographic, psychosocial, and behavioral characteristics. These risk factors can be assessed in

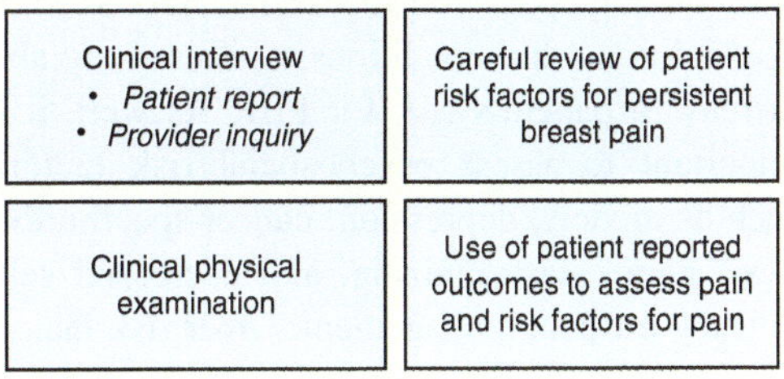

Fig. 7.2 Guide for assessment of persistent breast pain

several ways including clinical assessment at a provider appointment by either interview or questionnaires, evaluation of known risk factors using interview, questionnaires, and/or medical records, standardized patient reported outcome assessment measures, and/or a combination of these strategies. Figure 7.2 shows areas that are important in the assessment of PBP.

Provider Appointment

In the clinic setting with the health care provider, screening for PBP is multifaceted. PBP assessment should focus on clinical pain assessments that include provider assessment and exam and patient report, a brief standardized self-report pain assessment, and the provider's consideration of breast cancer treatment and demographic, psychosocial, and health behavioral risk factors. For the clinical pain assessment, the patient's qualitative report of PBP is a good starting point to provide context for the patient's pain symptoms, including location, onset and frequency/duration, severity, type of pain, and description. Providers are encouraged to ask the patient about breast pain, as it is not uncommon for patients either to not report or to underreport symptoms and side effects of cancer and its treatment. The provider's clinical assessment should include a careful physical examination to help identify the etiology of the breast pain, if possible, to rule out malignancy, and to inform treatment recommendations.

Providers should carefully assess patients' cancer treatment history to identify risk factors related to surgery, radiation, and chemotherapy and other therapies. Providers should also consider demographic and medical factors such as age and comorbid conditions, as these may also increase a patient's risk for PBP. As well, it is important to assess psychosocial risk factors, such as anxiety, depression, cancer-specific distress, pain catastrophizing, and decreased self-efficacy for pain management. Other risk factors such as lifestyle behaviors and genetic and epigenetic factors should be considered, as appropriate. Each of these treatment- and patient-related factors impact a patient's experience of pain and pain-related symptoms and inform treatment recommendations. Medical and demographic risk factor data can be identified based on medical chart review, and psychosocial risk factor data can be identified based on clinical interview and brief validated self-report tools commonly used in cancer patients.

Patient Reported Outcome Assessment Measures

Careful assessment of PBP following a breast cancer diagnosis and treatment includes the use of patient reported outcome (PRO) assessment measures. PRO assessment measures will typically include standardized survey tools with demonstrated strong psychometric properties. PROs for women with PBP should include assessment of pain and pain-related factors as well as variables known to be commonly associated with pain and/or PBP following a breast cancer diagnosis. Detailed information on the most widely used tools is provided below. Figure 7.3 provides a detailed overview of PROs that can be used to assess PBP. Figure 7.4 provides a quick guide to a brief battery of PROs that can be used in clinical practice [2, 16, 22, 53–69].

Pain The Brief Pain Inventory (BPI) [53] is one of the most frequently used PROs in the cancer setting and in patients with cancer. The BPI has several subscales, administration can be quick, and scoring is straightforward making it a reasonable tool for regular clinical practice. Pain severity is assessed with four BPI items, asking patients to rate their pain on a scale from 0 = no pain to 10 = worst pain imaginable, in response to "average pain," "worst pain," "least pain," and "pain right now," over the last 7 days. An average of the responses to these four items is used to create a single pain severity score. Pain interference is measured with seven items asking patients to rate how much pain has interfered with daily functioning (i.e., general activity, mood, walking ability, normal work, relations with other people, sleep, enjoyment of life) on a scale from 0 = does not interfere to 10 = completely interferes. The BPI also uses a body map to measure the location of pain and assesses pain

Patient reported outcome	# of Items	Brief description of assessment
Pain		
Brief Pain Inventory (53)	9–32	Pain severity, interference, location, medication
Breast Cancer Pain Questionnaire (16)	16	Pain frequency, location, intensity since surgery
McGill Pain Questionnaire (54)	15–2	Qualitative pain, body map, pain visual analog scale
Pain DETECT Questionnaire (55)	12	Neuropathic pain
Anxiety and depression		
Generalized Anxiety Disorder Scale (56)	2–7	Anxiety symptoms screening tool
Patient Health Questionnaire (59, 60)	2 or 9	Depression screening tool
Hospital Anxiety and Depression Scale (57)	14	Commonly used in medical setting for anxiety and depression
Pain catastrophizing		
Coping Strategies Questionnaire; Catastrophizing Subscale (64)	6	Focus on helplessness and pessimism related to pain coping
Pain Catastrophizing Scale (65)	13	Catastrophic thinking: rumination, magnification, and helplessness.
Self-efficacy for pain management		
Chronic Pain Self-Efficacy Scale (66, 67)	11–22	Self-efficacy for pain management, physical functioning, symptom coping
Pain Self-Efficacy Questionnaire (69)	2–10	Assesses level of confidence in coping with pain

Fig. 7.3 Patient reported outcome assessment tools for persistent breast pain

medications and the amount of pain relief in the past 24 hours or the past week. The short form BPI is 9 items and takes about 5 minutes for patients to complete, while the long form is 32 items and takes patients about 10 minutes to complete. The BPI has been shown to demonstrate change in response to behavioral pain management and pharmacological intervention for pain.

Anxiety The Generalized Anxiety Disorder 7 Item Scale (GAD-7) is a brief reliable, valid, and efficient clinical measure that is used for screening for Generalized Anxiety Disorder and assessing and monitoring its severity in clinical practice and research [56]. The GAD-7 includes 7 items assessing clinically significant anxiety and asks patients how often they have been bothered by each of the symptoms over the past 2 weeks. Responses are measured on a rating scale that ranges from 0 = not at all to 3 = nearly every day. Example items include the following: feeling nervous, anxious, or on edge; not being able to stop or control worrying; trouble relaxing; and being so restless that it is hard to sit still. Items are summed to reflect an anxiety severity score and range from 5 to 9 indicating mild anxiety, 10–14 indicating moderate anxiety, and >15 indicating severe anxiety. When used as a screening tool, further assessment and/or referral to a mental health professional is recommended for scores of 10 or greater. The GAD-7 is not only helpful for determining the severity of initial anxiety symptoms but also for monitoring change in symptoms and effects of treatment over time [56]. An ultra-brief 2-item version of the GAD-7 (GAD-2) has been created and has been shown to be accurate in detecting the four main types of anxiety (i.e., generalized anxiety, panic, social anxiety, and posttraumatic stress) [57, 58]. The GAD-2 is an ideal option for screening for anxiety in busy clinic settings.

Depression The Patient Health Questionnaire Depression Module (PHQ-9) is a brief reliable and valid self-report measure of depression severity that is commonly used in medical practice as both a clinical and research tool [60]. The PHQ-9 includes 9 items assessing each of the 9 DSM-V depression criteria and asks patients how often they have been bothered by each of the symptoms over the past 2 weeks. Responses are measured on a rating scale that ranges from 0 = not at all to 3 = nearly every day. Example items include the following: little interest or pleasure in doing things; feeling down, depressed, or hopeless; feeling tired or having little energy; and trouble concentrating on things, such as reading the newspaper or watching television. Items are summed to reflect a depression severity score and range from 0 to 4 indicating minimal or none, 5–9 indicating mild, 10–14 indicating moderate, 15–19 indicating moderately severe, and 20–27 indicating severe depression. The PHQ-9 is helpful for determining the severity of initial depressive symptoms as well as to monitor change in symptoms and effects of treatment over time [60]. Similar to the GAD-2 described above, a 2-item version of the PHQ-9 (PHQ-2) has been developed and has demonstrated good sensitivity and specificity for detecting depressive disorders [57, 59]. Similarly, the PHQ-2 is ideal for screening for depression in busy clinic settings.

Combined Anxiety and Depression The Hospital Anxiety and Depression Scale (HADS) is a simple yet reliable tool that is used by clinical providers in the medical setting to screen for and understand a patient's experience of anxiety and depression, which often coexist [61, 62]. The HADS is a popular screening tool and preferred by many medical providers because it is brief and easy to use. It is comprised of 14 total items – 7 anxiety items and 7 depression items – and takes 2–5 minutes to complete. Items are scored on a response scale with four alternatives ranging from 0 to 3. Example items include the following: I feel tense or "wound up"; I still enjoy the things I used to enjoy; worrying thoughts go through my mind; and, I look forward with enjoyment to things. After adjusting for six items that are reverse scored, responses are summed to obtain the two subscale total scores. Recommended cut-off scores allow for quantification of mild (8–10), moderate (11–14), and severe (15–21) symptoms.

Pain Catastrophizing Pain catastrophizing in oncology patients is commonly measured with the

Coping Strategies Questionnaire's Pain Catastrophizing subscale [63, 64]. The 6-item catastrophizing subscale reflects elements of helplessness and pessimism in relation to one's ability to deal with pain. Items are rated on a scale ranging from 0 = never do to 6 = always do when in pain. Example items include the following: It's terrible and it's never going to get any better; I worry all the time about whether the pain will end; and I feel like I can't go on. There is also a 2-item version of this scale that can be used and has shown validity [70]. Research has shown that individuals who demonstrate high levels of pain catastrophizing experience high levels of physical and emotional distress associated with their pain.

The Pain Catastrophizing Scale (PCS) is another widely used measure of catastrophic pain-related thinking [65]. The PCS is a brief 13-item instrument, taking less than 5 minutes to complete and score, that assesses three dimensions of catastrophic thinking including rumination, magnification, and helplessness. The PCS asks individuals to reflect on past painful experiences and indicate the degree to which they experienced each of 13 thoughts or feelings when experiencing pain. Responses are measured on a 5-point scale ranging from 0 = not at all to 4 = all the time. Example items include the following: I can't stop thinking about how much it hurts; I worry that something serious may happen; and, It's awful and I feel that it overwhelms me. PCS items are summed to create three subscale scores as well as a total score. Research has shown that a total PCS score of 30 represents a clinically relevant level of catastrophizing. The PCS has demonstrated excellent internal consistency and validity [65].

Self-Efficacy The self-efficacy for pain management subscale of the Chronic Pain Self-Efficacy Scale [66, 67] is a brief questionnaire measuring patients' confidence in their ability to cope with the consequences of chronic pain. Specifically, this subscale contains 5 items that inquire about patients' certainty about degree of pain control, pain during daily activities, and making pain reductions without extra medication. Items are rated on a 10-point scale ranging from 10 = very uncertain to 100 = very certain. Example items include the following: How confident are you that you could decrease your pain quite a bit?; How certain are you that you can continue most of your daily activities?; and How certain are you that you can keep your pain from interfering with your sleep?. Items are averaged to provide an overall self-efficacy for pain control score. This scale has shown good reliability [66] and has often been used in patients with cancer [71].

The Pain Self-Efficacy Questionnaire (PSEQ) [68, 72] is another established measure of pain self-efficacy that is used with chronic pain patients in clinical and research settings. The PSEQ gets at an important element of self-efficacy – persistence in the face of obstacles and aversive experiences – by measuring an individual's level of confidence in performing activities in the context of pain. The PSEQ contains 10 items that ask an individual to rate their confidence that they can do various things at present, despite the pain. Items are rated on a scale ranging from 0 = not at all confident to 6 = very confident. Example items include the following: I can enjoy things, despite the pain; I can do most of the household chores, despite the pain; I can cope with my pain in most situations; and I can live a normal lifestyle, despite the pain. The PSEQ has strong psychometric properties, including a high degree of reliability and validity [68]. More recently, a 2-item short form of the PSEQ (PSEQ-2) has been developed to reduce patient and provider burden [69]. The PSEQ-2 has been shown to be valid and reliable, and can save valuable time in busy clinical settings [69].

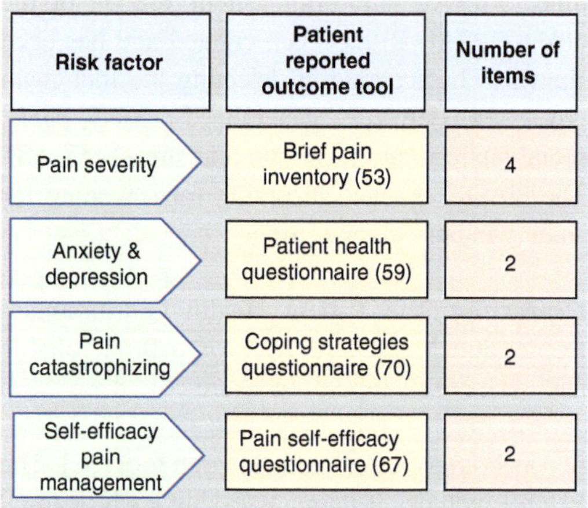

Fig. 7.4 Quick guide to brief assessment of psychosocial risk factors for persistent breast pain

Treatment of PBP

With high survival rates and longer survivorship, breast cancer is being considered within a chronic disease framework. There is increasing attention given to comprehensive post-treatment intervention strategies to address the impact of breast cancer. When recommending treatments, providers should consider all patient risk factors and patient's individual interest to determine the most appropriate and targeted intervention. For example, exercise interventions may be particularly beneficial for patients with PBP and comorbid obesity. Further, patients with PBP who are experiencing anxiety and depression may be particularly good candidates for a mindfulness-based behavioral treatment due to its known benefits on emotional and physical health (e.g., reduced stress, improved sleep, reduced fatigue). Here we provide an overview of potential treatments for women with PBP. Figure 7.5 provides an overview of treatment options for PBP.

Medication

Medications commonly used for pain, such as acetaminophen or non-steroidal anti-nflammatory drugs, may provide some pain relief and can be considered for PBP. The use of medication specifically for PBP following breast cancer diagnosis and surgery has not been well studied, though some work has identified several medications that may be useful in treating PBP. Gabapentin and venlafaxine have shown some success in decreasing pain following mastectomy and lumpectomy [73, 74]. Amitriptyline escalated from 25 mg to 100 mg per day over 4 weeks has also been shown to provide greater relief than placebo for neuropathic pain following breast cancer surgery in a randomized trial; however, there was some concern among study participants related to adverse effects of the active medication [75]. The use of medications for PBP following surgery should be considered ensuring a careful assessment of a patient's pain and consideration of other risk factors with particular attention paid to the duration, severity, and description of pain as well as side effects of medication. Also see discussion about post-mastectomy pain syndrome elsewhere in this volume, in Chap. 8 (Neuropathy).

Exercise, Physical Activity, and Physical Therapy

Exercise and physical activity show strong benefits in the treatment of general pain as well as mobility, fatigue, and quality of life in women following a breast cancer diagnosis and treatment [76]. Historically, a common concern has been the safety of exercise or physical activity in patients during and after cancer treatment; however, a growing body of research suggests that most exercise- or activity-based programs are safe, well tolerated, and effective in providing physical and psychological health benefits to women with breast cancer [77–81]. There is evi-

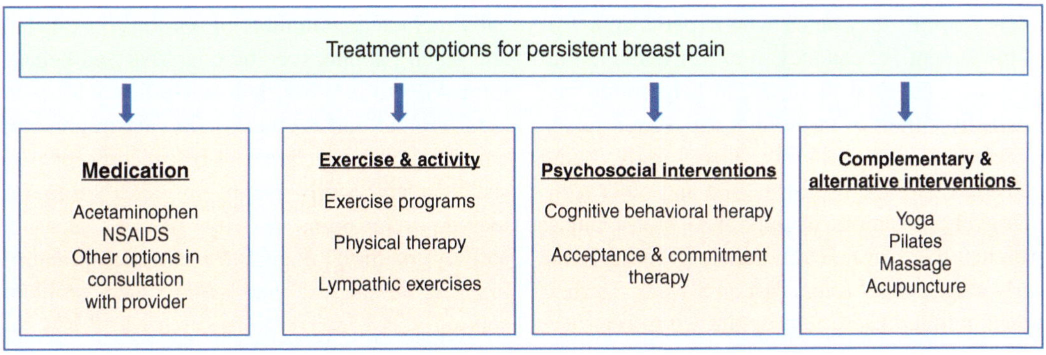

Fig. 7.5 Treatment options for persistent breast pain

dence in several disease populations that exercise can reduce anxiety and depression and improve self-efficacy and cognitive function. In a study of older breast cancer survivors undergoing aromatase inhibitor therapy, a 9-month combined resistance and aerobic exercise program lead to decreased bodily pain along with other positive outcomes [82]. It is always strongly recommended that patients consult their physician prior to starting any type of exercise program.

While exercise programs appear to provide a number of benefits for women following a breast cancer diagnosis [83], less work has been done on how exercise specifically impacts PBP following a breast cancer diagnosis and treatment. A systematic review found that programs including stretching and active exercises are effective for treating postoperative pain and limited range of motion following breast cancer treatment [84]. One study examined the use of physical therapy or physical therapy combined with manual lymphatic drainage in 41 women with axillary web syndrome following lymph node biopsy [85]. Axillary web syndrome is a side effect of surgery that involves scarring or connective tissue under the arm; it can cause pain and impact movement. This 4-week program included 3 weekly sessions of physical therapy for both conditions, and the condition with lymphatic drainage received 5 manual lymphatic drainage sessions weekly. Compared to the physical therapy-only group, the combined treatment group demonstrated significantly greater changes in pain and arm volume improvements in quality of life, pain, strength, and other important outcomes were seen in all participants [85]. Physical therapy may be especially helpful for women who experience a fear of movement or hesitancy to exercise due to fear of injury; physical therapy can help safely and gradually introduce movement and exercise.

Exercise programs are increasingly being delivered with the use of mobile and other technology. For example, a study of 81 breast cancer patients who completed adjuvant therapy for early-stage cancer found that an 8-week internet-based, tailored exercise program led to improvements in arm symptoms and reductions in participants' rating of pain severity and interference. In addition, House et al. [83] examined the use of an 8-week virtual robotic rehabilitation system that engaged breast cancer patients in upper body bimanual exercises while also providing cognitive training and affective relief; they found that pain tended to decrease and depression improved. Other researchers are actively developing mobile programs for exercise following breast cancer diagnosis and treatment. For example, Fu and colleagues [86] have developed and are evaluating a mobile-based system to promote the completion of daily routine exercises to increase lymph flow and drainage using a web-based and mobile system targeting lymphatic pain.

Psychosocial Interventions

Psychosocial interventions have shown benefits for a number of distressing symptoms following breast cancer, including pain, and are desirable because they are associated with minimal side effects. Systematic reviews and meta-analyses have found that psychosocial interventions reduce pain following breast cancer and also have positive impacts on many outcomes, including quality of life [87, 88]. Psychosocial interventions have most commonly targeted general pain, in contrast to breast pain specifically. As these do show benefits for pain in general, this suggests that there will also be benefits for patients with PBP.

Cognitive-behavioral therapy (CBT) is a common psychosocial intervention used to improve outcomes in patients with disease-related chronic pain including cancer. CBT interventions typically include a set number of sessions (i.e., 4–12) and teach patients specific cognitive and behavioral skills to improve their self-efficacy for pain management and decrease pain catastrophizing, which are two psychosocial risk factors for persistent pain. Skills taught in CBT protocols include relaxation, activity pacing, pleasant activity planning, cognitive restructuring, calming self-statements, goal setting, and problem solving. CBT interventions often use PROs for assessment, and the therapist and the patient can review improvements in pain symptoms and problem solve around symptoms that may not be improving. In a study that included women with breast cancer, a 4-session CBT protocol delivered by both in-person sessions at the medical center and videoconferencing in the patient's home (a highly accessible intervention) was found to improve pain severity and interference [89] as well as increase self-efficacy for pain. Other work has found that a similar protocol delivered to women with breast cancer and persistent pain in a medically underserved area at their oncology community clinic led to decreased pain and improved self-efficacy [90].

Mindfulness-based psychosocial interventions, particularly Acceptance and Commitment Therapy (ACT), have demonstrated benefits for reducing pain as well as improving sleep and reducing fatigue in women following a breast cancer diagnosis [91]. Mindfulness-based interventions focus on increasing mindfulness and pain acceptance and improving overall emotional functioning. One study, in a group of women undergoing breast cancer surgery ($N = 54$), compared a single session ACT intervention to usual care and found positive effects of ACT on post-surgical pain and anxiety up to 3 months following surgery [92].

Complementary and Alternative Interventions

Complementary and alternative interventions may have some positive effects on pain as well as other symptoms following a breast cancer diagnosis. Complementary and alternative interventions include the use of natural products, mind-body medicine, manipulative body-based practices (e.g., massage), mindfulness-based interventions (e.g., yoga), and acupuncture. Evidence for these approaches in reducing PBP remains limited due to a lack of high-quality research and represents an area for further study to broaden potential treatment options for patients with PBP.

Yoga is another treatment option for women with PBP that has grown in popularity over recent years due to increasing interest in mind-body practices. Yoga teaches strategies that promote strength, balance, and flexibility; breathing techniques that have relaxing and energizing effects; and meditation for mental and emotional calm and clarity [93]. Yoga is also considered gentle and low impact, which is particularly important for cancer patients who experience PBP and fatigue. Research suggests yoga that takes a gentle approach (i.e., modified poses with meditation and breathing techniques) can reduce the number of side effects of treatment (e.g., pain, fatigue, nausea) and be effective in managing pain as well as fatigue and sleep problems [94, 95]. One study showed that an 8-week yoga program focused on gentle postures, meditation, and breathing significantly lessened pain and fatigue in women with metastatic breast cancer [93, 96]. Practicing yoga has also been shown to be beneficial in decreasing symptoms of anxiety and depression, which increase breast pain following treatment [97]. Other complementary and alternative practices, such as Pilates and acupuncture [98], may also provide benefits for decreasing PBP [99, 100].

Summary

PBP following a breast cancer diagnosis is distressing and has a significant negative impact on quality of life. Surgery for breast cancer, including mastectomy, breast conserving surgery, and lymph node surgery, can lead to PBP. Radiation, chemotherapy, and endocrine therapies can also contribute to the development of PBP in women following a breast cancer diagnosis. In addition to these treatment-related factors, younger age, minority racial status, lower education, lower income, and increased BMI are also related to PBP. Psychosocial factors such as anxiety, depression, pain catastrophizing, and decreased self-efficacy for pain management further contribute to the maintenance of PBP. Routine assessment for PBP in breast cancer survivors is recommended and can include provider clinical interview and patient clinical report, review of medical records to assess risk factors (e.g., surgical history, medical comorbidities), and use of standardized PROs. Once PBP has been diagnosed, treatment options include exercise and psychosocial interventions in addition to or in lieu of medications.

References

1. Langford DJ, Paul SM, West C, Levine JD, Hamolsky D, Elboim C, et al. Persistent breast pain following breast cancer surgery is associated with persistent sensory changes, pain interference, and functional impairments. J Pain. 2014;15(12):1227–37.
2. Gartner R, Jensen MB, Nielsen J, Ewertz M, Kroman N, Kehlet H. Prevalence of and factors associated with persistent pain following breast cancer surgery. JAMA. 2009;302(18):1985–92.
3. Jung BF, Ahrendt GM, Oaklander AL, Dworkin RH. Neuropathic pain following breast cancer surgery: proposed classification and research update. Pain. 2003;104(1–2):1–13.
4. Stubblefield MD, Custodio CM. Upper-extremity pain disorders in breast cancer. Arch Phys Med Rehabil. 2006;87(3 Suppl 1):S96–9; quiz S100–1.
5. Carpenter JS, Andrykowski MA, Sloan P, Cunningham L, Cordova MJ, Studts JL, et al. Postmastectomy/postlumpectomy pain in breast cancer survivors. J Clin Epidemiol. 1998;51(12):1285–92.
6. Andersen KG, Kehlet H. Persistent pain after breast cancer treatment: a critical review of risk factors and strategies for prevention. J Pain. 2011;12(7):725–46.
7. Schreiber KL, Martel MO, Shnol H, Shaffer JR, Greco C, Viray N, et al. Persistent pain in postmastectomy patients: comparison of psychophysical, medical, surgical, and psychosocial characteristics between patients with and without pain. Pain. 2013;154(5):660–8.
8. Bovbjerg DH, Keefe FJ, Soo MS, Manculich J, Van Denburg A, Zuley ML, et al. Persistent breast pain in post-surgery breast cancer survivors and women with no history of breast surgery or cancer: associations with pain catastrophizing, perceived breast cancer risk, breast cancer worry, and emotional distress. Acta Oncol. 2019;58(5):763–8.
9. Chou R, Turner JA, Devine EB, Hansen RN, Sullivan SD, Blazina I, et al. The effectiveness and risks of long-term opioid therapy for chronic pain: a systematic review for a National Institutes of Health Pathways to Prevention Workshop. Ann Intern Med. 2015;162(4):276–86.
10. Garland EL, Brintz CE, Hanley AW, Roseen EJ, Atchley RM, Gaylord SA, et al. Mind-body therapies for opioid-treated pain: a systematic review and meta-analysis. JAMA Intern Med. 2020;180(1):91–105.
11. Peuckmann V, Ekholm O, Rasmussen NK, Groenvold M, Christiansen P, Moller S, et al. Chronic pain and other sequelae in long-term breast cancer survivors: nationwide survey in Denmark. Eur J Pain. 2009;13(5):478–85.
12. (U.S.). IoM. Committee on Advancing Pain Research Care and Education. Relieving pain in America: a blueprint for transforming prevention, care, education, and research, vol. xvii. Washington, DC: National Academies Press; 2011. p. 364.
13. Katipamula R, Degnim AC, Hoskin T, Boughey JC, Loprinzi C, Grant CS, et al. Trends in mastectomy rates at the Mayo Clinic Rochester: effect of surgical year and preoperative magnetic resonance imaging. J Clin Oncol. 2009;27(25):4082–8.
14. Veronesi U, Cascinelli N, Mariani L, Greco M, Saccozzi R, Luini A, et al. Twenty-year follow-up of a randomized study comparing breast-conserving surgery with radical mastectomy for early breast cancer. N Engl J Med. 2002;347(16):1227–32.
15. Jatoi I, Proschan MA. Randomized trials of breast-conserving therapy versus mastectomy for primary breast cancer: a pooled analysis of updated results. Am J Clin Oncol. 2005;28(3):289–94.
16. Belfer I, Schreiber KL, Shaffer JR, Shnol H, Blaney K, Morando A, et al. Persistent postmastectomy pain in breast cancer survivors: analysis of clinical, demographic, and psychosocial factors. J Pain. 2013;14(10):1185–95.
17. Classification of chronic pain. Descriptions of chronic pain syndromes and definitions of pain terms. Prepared by the International Association for the Study of Pain, Subcommittee on Taxonomy. Pain Suppl. 1986;3:S1–226.
18. Frassica DA, Bajaj GK, Tsangaris TN. Treatment of complications after breast-conservation therapy. Oncology (Williston Park). 2003;17(8):1118–28. discussion 31–6, 41.
19. Kokosis G, Chopra K, Darrach H, Dellon AL, Williams EH. Re-visiting post-breast surgery pain syndrome: risk factors, peripheral nerve associations and clinical implications. Gland Surg. 2019;8(4):407–15.
20. Vilholm OJ, Cold S, Rasmussen L, Sindrup SH. The postmastectomy pain syndrome: an epidemiological study on the prevalence of chronic pain after surgery for breast cancer. Br J Cancer. 2008;99(4):604–10.
21. Edmond SN, Shelby RA, Keefe FJ, Fisher HM, Schmidt JE, Soo MS, et al. Persistent breast pain among women with histories of breast-conserving surgery for breast cancer compared with women without histories of breast surgery or cancer. Clin J Pain. 2017;33(1):51–6.
22. Juhl AA, Christiansen P, Damsgaard TE. Persistent pain after breast cancer treatment: a questionnaire-based study on the prevalence, associated treatment variables, and pain type. J Breast Cancer. 2016;19(4):447–54.
23. Chiang DLC, Kluger MT, Helsby NA, Somogyi AA, Kluger MT. The prevalence, impact, and risk factors for persistent pain after breast cancer surgery in a New Zealand population. Pain Med. 2019;20(9):1803–14.
24. Mejdahl MK, Andersen KG, Gartner R, Kroman N, Kehlet H. Persistent pain and sensory disturbances after treatment for breast cancer: six year nationwide follow-up study. BMJ. 2013;346:f1865.

25. Koehler LA, Haddad TC, Hunter DW, Tuttle TM. Axillary web syndrome following breast cancer surgery: symptoms, complications, and management strategies. Breast Cancer (Dove Med Press). 2019;11:13–9.
26. Bennett KG, Qi J, Kim HM, Hamill JB, Pusic AL, Wilkins EG. Comparison of 2-year complication rates among common techniques for postmastectomy breast reconstruction. JAMA Surg. 2018;153(10):901–8.
27. Miaskowski C, Cooper B, Paul SM, West C, Langford D, Levine JD, et al. Identification of patient subgroups and risk factors for persistent breast pain following breast cancer surgery. J Pain. 2012;13(12):1172–87.
28. Fekrmandi F, Panzarella T, Dinniwell RE, Helou J, Levin W. Predictive factors for persistent and late radiation complications in breast cancer survivors. Clin Transl Oncol. 2020;22(3):360–9.
29. Hille-Betz U, Vaske B, Bremer M, Soergel P, Kundu S, Klapdor R, et al. Late radiation side effects, cosmetic outcomes and pain in breast cancer patients after breast-conserving surgery and three-dimensional conformal radiotherapy : risk-modifying factors. Strahlenther Onkol. 2016;192(1):8–16.
30. Bell RJ, Robinson PJ, Nazeem F, Panjari M, Fradkin P, Schwarz M, et al. Persistent breast pain 5 years after treatment of invasive breast cancer is largely unexplained by factors associated with treatment. J Cancer Surviv. 2014;8(1):1–8.
31. Milata JL, Otte JL, Carpenter JS. Oral endocrine therapy nonadherence, adverse effects, decisional support, and decisional needs in women with breast cancer. Cancer Nurs. 2018;41(1):E9–E18.
32. Langford DJ, Schmidt B, Levine JD, Abrams G, Elboim C, Esserman L, et al. Preoperative breast pain predicts persistent breast pain and disability after breast cancer surgery. J Pain Symptom Manag. 2015;49(6):981–94.
33. Lundstedt D, Gustafsson M, Steineck G, Malmstrom P, Alsadius D, Sundberg A, et al. Risk factors of developing long-lasting breast pain after breast cancer radiotherapy. Int J Radiat Oncol Biol Phys. 2012;83(1):71–8.
34. Couceiro TC, Valenca MM, Raposo MC, Orange FA, Amorim MM. Prevalence of post-mastectomy pain syndrome and associated risk factors: a cross-sectional cohort study. Pain Manag Nurs. 2014;15(4):731–7.
35. Alves Nogueira Fabro E, Bergmann A, do Amaral ESB, Padula Ribeiro AC, de Souza Abrahao K, da Costa Leite Ferreira MG, et al. Post-mastectomy pain syndrome: incidence and risks. Breast. 2012;21(3):321–5.
36. Smith WC, Bournea D, Squair J, Phillips DO, Chambers WA. A retrospective cohort study of post mastectomy pain syndrome. Pain. 1999;83(1):91–5.
37. Poleshuck EL, Katz J, Andrus CH, Hogan LA, Jung BF, Kulick DI, et al. Risk factors for chronic pain following breast cancer surgery: a prospective study. J Pain. 2006;7(9):626–34.
38. Couceiro TC, Menezes TC, Valenca MM. Postmastectomy pain syndrome: the magnitude of the problem. Rev Bras Anestesiol. 2009;59(3):358–65.
39. Cimmino MA, Ferrone C, Cutolo M. Epidemiology of chronic musculoskeletal pain. Best Pract Res Clin Rheumatol. 2011;25(2):173–83.
40. Krueger AB, Stone AA. Assessment of pain: a community-based diary survey in the USA. Lancet. 2008;371(9623):1519–25.
41. Langford DJ, Paul SM, Tripathy D, West C, Dodd MJ, Schumacher K, et al. Trajectories of pain and analgesics in oncology outpatients with metastatic bone pain during participation in a psychoeducational intervention study to improve pain management. J Pain. 2011;12(6):652–66.
42. Utne I, Miaskowski C, Bjordal K, Paul SM, Jakobsen G, Rustoen T. Differences in the use of pain coping strategies between oncology inpatients with mild vs. moderate to severe pain. J Pain Symptom Manag. 2009;38(5):717–26.
43. Wallace MS, Wallace AM, Lee J, Dobke MK. Pain after breast surgery: a survey of 282 women. Pain. 1996;66(2–3):195–205.
44. Ding YY, Yao P, Wu L, Han ZK, Hong T, Zhu YQ, et al. Body mass index and persistent pain after breast cancer surgery: findings from the women's healthy eating and living study and a meta-analysis. Oncotarget. 2017;8(26):43332–43.
45. Sullivan MJ, Thorn B, Haythornthwaite JA, Keefe F, Martin M, Bradley LA, et al. Theoretical perspectives on the relation between catastrophizing and pain. Clin J Pain. 2001;17(1):52–64.
46. Somers TJ, Wren AA, Shelby RA. The context of pain in arthritis: self-efficacy for managing pain and other symptoms. Curr Pain Headache Rep. 2012;16(6):502–8.
47. Jerant A, Franks P, Kravitz RL. Associations between pain control self-efficacy, self-efficacy for communicating with physicians, and subsequent pain severity among cancer patients. Patient Educ Couns. 2011;85(2):275–80.
48. Ozalp G, Sarioglu R, Tuncel G, Aslan K, Kadiogullari N. Preoperative emotional states in patients with breast cancer and postoperative pain. Acta Anaesthesiol Scand. 2003;47(1):26–9.
49. Tasmuth T, Estlanderb A-M, Kalso E. Effect of present pain and mood on the memory of past postoperative pain in women treated surgically for breast cancer. Pain. 1996;68(2–3):343–7.
50. van Hecke O, Torrance N, Smith BH. Chronic pain epidemiology – where do lifestyle factors fit in? Br J Pain. 2013;7(4):209–17.
51. Stephens KE, Levine JD, Aouizerat BE, Paul SM, Abrams G, Conley YP, et al. Associations between genetic and epigenetic variations in cytokine genes and mild persistent breast pain in women following breast cancer surgery. Cytokine. 2017;99:203–13.
52. Langford DJ, Paul SM, West CM, Dunn LB, Levine JD, Kober KM, et al. Variations in potassium channel genes are associated with distinct trajectories of persistent breast pain after breast cancer surgery. Pain. 2015;156(3):371–80.

53. Cleeland CS, Ryan KM. Pain assessment: global use of the Brief Pain Inventory. Ann Acad Med Singap. 1994;23(2):129–38.
54. Melzack R. The McGill Pain Questionnaire: major properties and scoring methods. Pain. 1975;1(3): 277–99.
55. Freynhagen R, Baron R, Gockel U, Tolle TR. painDETECT: a new screening questionnaire to identify neuropathic components in patients with back pain. Curr Med Res Opin. 2006;22(10):1911–20.
56. Spitzer RL, Kroenke K, Williams JB, Lowe B. A brief measure for assessing generalized anxiety disorder: the GAD-7. Arch Intern Med. 2006;166(10):1092–7.
57. Tsaras K, Papathanasiou IV, Mitsi D, Veneti A, Kelesi M, Zyga S, et al. Assessment of depression and anxiety in breast cancer patients: prevalence and associated factors. Asian Pac J Cancer Prev. 2018;19(6):1661–9.
58. Kroenke K, Spitzer RL, Williams JB, Monahan PO, Lowe B. Anxiety disorders in primary care: prevalence, impairment, comorbidity, and detection. Ann Intern Med. 2007;146(5):317–25.
59. Kroenke K, Spitzer RL, Williams JB. The Patient Health Questionnaire-2: validity of a two-item depression screener. Med Care. 2003;41(11):1284–92.
60. Kroenke K, Spitzer RL, Williams JB. The PHQ-9: validity of a brief depression severity measure. J Gen Intern Med. 2001;16(9):606–13.
61. Zigmond AS, Snaith RP. The hospital anxiety and depression scale. Acta Psychiatr Scand. 1983;67(6):361–70.
62. Snaith RP. The hospital anxiety and depression scale. Health Qual Life Outcomes. 2003;1:29.
63. Rosenstiel AK, Keefe FJ. The use of coping strategies in chronic low back pain patients: relationship to patient characteristics and current adjustment. Pain. 1983;17(1):33–44.
64. Keefe FJ, Brown GK, Wallston KA, Caldwell DS. Coping with rheumatoid arthritis pain: catastrophizing as a maladaptive strategy. Pain. 1989;37(1): 51–6.
65. Sullivan MB, Bishop SR, Pivik J. The pain catastrophizing scale: development and validation. Psychol Assess. 1995;7:524–32.
66. Anderson KO, Dowds BN, Pelletz RE, Edwards WT, Peeters-Asdourian C. Development and initial validation of a scale to measure self-efficacy beliefs in patients with chronic pain. Pain. 1995;63(1):77–84.
67. Cheng ST, Chen PP, Chow YF, Chung JWY, Law ACB, Lee JSW, et al. Developing a short multidimensional measure of pain self-efficacy: the chronic pain self-efficacy scale-short form. Gerontologist. 2020;60(3):e127–e36.
68. Nicholas MK. The pain self-efficacy questionnaire: taking pain into account. Eur J Pain. 2007;11(2): 153–63.
69. Nicholas MK, McGuire BE, Asghari A. A 2-item short form of the Pain Self-efficacy Questionnaire: development and psychometric evaluation of PSEQ-2. J Pain. 2015;16(2):153–63.
70. Jensen MP, Keefe FJ, Lefebvre JC, Romano JM, Turner JA. One- and two-item measures of pain beliefs and coping strategies. Pain. 2003;104(3):453–69.
71. Porter LS, Keefe FJ, Garst J, McBride CM, Baucom D. Self-efficacy for managing pain, symptoms, and function in patients with lung cancer and their informal caregivers: associations with symptoms and distress. Pain. 2008;137(2):306–15.
72. Huang FF, Yang Q, Want AN, Zhang JP. Psychometric propoerties and performance of existing self-efficacy instruments in cancer populations: a systematic review. Health Qual Life Outcomes. 2018;16(1):241.
73. Patarica-Huber E, Boskov N, Pjevic M. Multimodal approach to therapy-related neuropathic pain in breast cancer. J BUON. 2011;16(1):40–5.
74. Tasmuth T, Hartel B, Kalso E. Venlafaxine in neuropathic pain following treatment of breast cancer. Eur J Pain. 2002;6(1):17–24.
75. Kalso E, Tiina T, Neuvonen PJ. Amitriptyline effectively relieves neuropathic pain following treatment of breast cancer. Pain. 1996;64(2):293–302.
76. Olsson Moller U, Beck I, Ryden L, Malmstrom M. A comprehensive approach to rehabilitation interventions following breast cancer treatment - a systematic review of systematic reviews. BMC Cancer. 2019;19(1):472.
77. Schmitz K. Physical activity and breast cancer survivorship. Recent Results Cancer Res. 2011;186: 189–215.
78. Pekmezi DW, Demark-Wahnefried W. Updated evidence in support of diet and exercise interventions in cancer survivors. Acta Oncol. 2011;50(2):167–78.
79. Ahmed RL, Thomas W, Yee D, Schmitz KH. Randomized controlled trial of weight training and lymphedema in breast cancer survivors. J Clin Oncol. 2006;24(18):2765–72.
80. Campbell A, Mutrie N, White F, McGuire F, Kearney N. A pilot study of a supervised group exercise programme as a rehabilitation treatment for women with breast cancer receiving adjuvant treatment. Eur J Oncol Nurs. 2005;9(1):56–63.
81. Duijts SF, Faber MM, Oldenburg HS, van Beurden M, Aaronson NK. Effectiveness of behavioral techniques and physical exercise on psychosocial functioning and health-related quality of life in breast cancer patients and survivors--a meta-analysis. Psycho-Oncology. 2011;20(2):115–26.
82. Paulo TRS, Rossi FE, Viezel J, Tosello GT, Seidinger SC, Simoes RR, et al. The impact of an exercise program on quality of life in older breast cancer survivors undergoing aromatase inhibitor therapy: a randomized controlled trial. Health Qual Life Outcomes. 2019;17(1):17.
83. House G, Burdea G, Grampurohit N, Polistico K, Roll D, Damiani F, et al. A feasibility study to determine the benefits of upper extremity virtual rehabilitation therapy for coping with chronic pain post-cancer surgery. Br J Pain. 2016;10(4):186–97.

84. De Groef A, Van Kampen M, Dieltjens E, Christiaens MR, Neven P, Geraerts I, et al. Effectiveness of post-operative physical therapy for upper-limb impairments after breast cancer treatment: a systematic review. Arch Phys Med Rehabil. 2015;96(6):1140–53.
85. Cho Y, Do J, Jung S, Kwon O, Jeon JY. Effects of a physical therapy program combined with manual lymphatic drainage on shoulder function, quality of life, lymphedema incidence, and pain in breast cancer patients with axillary web syndrome following axillary dissection. Support Care Cancer. 2016;24(5): 2047–57.
86. Fu MR, Axelrod D, Guth A, Scagliola J, Rampertaap K, El-Shammaa N, et al. A web- and Mobile-based intervention for women treated for breast cancer to manage chronic pain and symptoms related to lymphedema: randomized clinical trial rationale and protocol. JMIR Res Protoc. 2016;5(1):e7.
87. Johannsen M, Farver I, Beck N, Zachariae R. The efficacy of psychosocial intervention for pain in breast cancer patients and survivors: a systematic review and meta-analysis. Breast Cancer Res Treat. 2013;138(3):675–90.
88. Sheinfeld Gorin S, Krebs P, Badr H, Janke EA, Jim HS, Spring B, et al. Meta-analysis of psychosocial interventions to reduce pain in patients with cancer. J Clin Oncol. 2012;30(5):539–47.
89. Kelleher SA, Winger JG, Dorfman CS, Ingle KK, Moskovich AA, Abernethy AP, et al. A behavioral cancer pain intervention: a randomized noninferiority trial comparing in-person with videoconference delivery. Psycho-Oncology. 2019;28(8):1671–8.
90. Dorfman CS, Kelleher SA, Winger JG, Shelby RA, Thorn BE, Sutton LM, et al. Development and pilot testing of an mHealth behavioral cancer pain protocol for medically underserved communities. J Psychosoc Oncol. 2019;37(3):335–49.
91. Mosher CE, Secinti E, Li R, Hirsh AT, Bricker J, Miller KD, et al. Acceptance and commitment therapy for symptom interference in metastatic breast cancer patients: a pilot randomized trial. Support Care Cancer. 2018;26(6):1993–2004.
92. Hadlandsmyth K, Dindo LN, Wajid R, Sugg SL, Zimmerman MB, Rakel BA. A single-session acceptance and commitment therapy intervention among women undergoing surgery for breast cancer: a randomized pilot trial to reduce persistent postsurgical pain. Psychooncology. 2019;28(11):2210–7.
93. Carson JW, Carson KM, Olsen MK, Sanders L, Porter LS. Mindful yoga for women with metastatic breast cancer: design of a randomized controlled trial. BMC Complement Altern Med. 2017;17(1):153.
94. Cramer H, Lauche R, Klose P, Lange S, Langhorst J, Dobos GJ. Yoga for improving health-related quality of life, mental health and cancer-related symptoms in women diagnosed with breast cancer. Cochrane Database Syst Rev. 2017;1:CD010802.
95. Kumar N, Bhatnagar S, Velpandian T, Patnaik S, Menon G, Mehta M, et al. Randomized controlled trial in advance stage breast Cancer patients for the effectiveness on stress marker and pain through Sudarshan Kriya and Pranayam. Indian J Palliat Care. 2013;19(3):180–5.
96. Carson JW, Carson KM, Porter LS, Keefe FJ, Shaw H, Miller JM. Yoga for women with metastatic breast cancer: results from a pilot study. J Pain Symptom Manag. 2007;33(3):331–41.
97. Hardoerfer K, Jentschke E. Effect of yoga therapy on symptoms of anxiety in cancer patients. Oncol Res Treat. 2018;41(9):526–32.
98. Chien TJ, Liu CY, Fang CJ. The effect of acupuncture in breast Cancer-related Lymphoedema (BCRL): a systematic review and meta-analysis. Integr Cancer Ther. 2019;18:1534735419866910.
99. Zengin Alpozgen A, Razak Ozdincler A, Karanlik H, Yaman Agaoglu F, Narin AN. Effectiveness of Pilates-based exercises on upper extremity disorders related with breast cancer treatment. Eur J Cancer Care (Engl). 2017:26(6).
100. Pinto-Carral A, Molina AJ, de Pedro A, Ayan C. Pilates for women with breast cancer: a systematic review and meta-analysis. Complement Ther Med. 2018;41:130–40.

8 Neuropathy

Heather Moore, Carey Anders, Mallika P. Patel,
Anne Marie Fras, and Kimberly Slawson

Abbreviations

AE	Adverse event
ALA	Alpha-lipoic acid
ALC	Acetyl-L-carnitine
ALND	Axillary lymph node dissection
ANA	Antinuclear antibodies
BMI	Body mass index
Ca	Calcium
CIPN	Chemotherapy-induced peripheral neuropathy
CTCAE	Common terminology criteria for adverse events
EMG	Electromyography
EORTC	European organization for research and treatment of cancer
ESR	Erythrocyte sedimentation rate
FACT-G	Functional assessment of cancer therapy (general) questionnaire
FACT-GOG-Ntx	functional assessment of cancer therapy/gynecologic oncology group-neurotoxicity
IASP	International Association for the Study of Pain
ICBN	Intercostobrachial nerve
IFE	Immunofixation
IV	Intravenous
Mg	Magnesium
MGUS	Monoclonal gammopathy of undetermined significance
NCI	National cancer institute
NCI-CTC	National Cancer Institute Common Toxicity Criteria
NCS	Nerve conduction study
PMPS	Post-mastectomy pain syndrome
PPMP	Persistent post-mastectomy pain
QOL	Quality of life
RF	Rheumatoid factor
ROS	Reactive oxygen species
SLNB	Sentinel lymph node biopsy
SPEP	Serum protein electrophoresis
TCAs	Tricyclic antidepressants
TNS	Total neuropathy score
UPEP	Urine protein electrophoresis
VAS	Visual analog score

H. Moore (✉) · M. P. Patel
Department of Pharmacy – Oncology, Duke University Hospital, Durham, NC, USA
e-mail: Heather.N.Moore@Duke.edu; Mallika.Patel@Duke.edu

C. Anders
Department of Medicine – Oncology, Duke University Hospital, Durham, NC, USA
e-mail: Carey.Anders@Duke.edu

A. M. Fras
Department of Anesthesiology, Duke University Hospital, Durham, NC, USA
e-mail: Anne.Marie.Fras@Duke.edu

K. Slawson
Department of Cancer Center Support and Survivorship, Duke University Hospital, Durham, NC, USA
e-mail: Kimberly.Slawson@Duke.edu

G. G. Kimmick et al. (eds.), *Common Issues in Breast Cancer Survivors*,
https://doi.org/10.1007/978-3-030-75377-1_8

Introduction

Peripheral neuropathy is a very common side effect of breast cancer treatment that can arise from both surgical treatment and systemic treatment with chemotherapy agents. This can be a life-altering side effect during and after cancer treatment. Long-term neurotoxicity can have a substantial impact on quality of life and overall survivorship. This chapter on neuropathy within the breast cancer patient population will review different types or origins of treatment-induced neuropathy, identify risk factors, and summarize available literature regarding prevention and treatment. While the information provided on chemotherapy-induced peripheral neuropathy (CIPN) is somewhat generalizable to a variety of patients that have received chemotherapy or have certain risk factors, this is especially pertinent to breast cancer survivors, given the high percentage of patients that experience CIPN following disease treatment.

Origin

Post-mastectomy Pain

Persistent pain sometimes follows surgical treatment for breast cancer and has a negative impact on quality of life for cancer survivors [1]. Surgical treatment of breast cancer can be divided into two surgical procedures on the breast (lumpectomy and mastectomy) and two in the axilla (sentinel lymph node biopsy (SLNB) and axillary lymph node dissection (ALND)). The term postmastectomy pain syndrome (PMPS) has been used to describe a neuropathic pain syndrome in and around the site of surgery originally attributed to intercostobrachial nerve (ICBN) damage during surgical dissection [2]. The International Association for the Study of Pain (IASP) defines PMPS as persistent pain soon after mastectomy or lumpectomy affecting the anterior thorax, axilla, and/or upper arm [3]. PMPS has a variable prevalence ranging from 25% to 60% [4]. This wide prevalence range is likely due to inconsistent definitions across studies. Studies focusing on the narrower category of neuropathic pain tend to place the incidence at a lower rate (e.g., 23.9%) [5] than those including a broader range of post-mastectomy pain symptoms, such as musculoskeletal pain, phantom breast pain, or lymphedema (e.g., 47%) [1]. This broader range of pain syndromes has been characterized as persistent post-mastectomy pain (PPMP) to differentiate from the classic PMPS [1].

There are pre-, intra-, and postoperative risk factors associated with the development of persistent pain after breast cancer surgery [1]. Preoperative risk factors associated with PPMP include age under 40 years, minority race/ethnicity, the presence of preoperative breast or other pain, and the presence of a psychiatric diagnosis [1, 4]. The higher risk with younger age may be related to the more aggressive nature of the disease and more aggressive surgical treatment in the younger population [6]. The effect of race/ethnicity may be the consequences of minority patients receiving a diagnosis at a more advanced stage which would require more extensive surgical intervention, which is an independent risk factor for the development of PPMP [1]. Pain, whether at the breast or in distant areas of the body such as headache or low back pain [4, 7], predisposes to the development of PPMP. The mechanisms responsible for this vulnerability are unclear, but are thought to be related to central sensitization facilitating development of postoperative pain [1]. Multiple studies have confirmed the association of chronic postsurgical pain with depression, stress, and psychologic vulnerability [8]. Similarly, there is evidence of the association of anxiety, catastrophizing (the tendency to exaggerate the negative consequences of events or decisions), sleep disturbance, and somatization with the development of PPMP [9].

Intraoperative risk factors for the development of PPMP include the type of axillary surgery.

Having an ALND, vs SLNB, is associated with a higher risk of PPMP; of note, SLNB is the current standard of care for assessment in the presence of lymph node metastatic disease [4, 10]. Some, but not all, studies suggest that damage to the ICBN during axillary dissection leads to the development of PPMP [4, 11, 12]. In contrast, use of a preincisional paravertebral block has been reported to decrease the prevalence and the intensity of PPMP [13].

Postoperative risk factors for the development of PPMP include higher levels of acute postoperative pain (pain begets pain) [4, 12] and receipt of radiation therapy [14]. Adjuvant regional radiotherapy increases risk of the development of PPMP (OR = 1.5, 95% CI = 1.08–2.07, $p = 0.03$), likely due to associated tissue fibrosis, nerve entrapment, and limited range of motion of the shoulder [1, 15].

Taxane Therapy

Taxane chemotherapy agents, such as docetaxel (Taxotere™) and paclitaxel (Taxol™), are common chemotherapies utilized in the treatment of both early-stage and metastatic breast cancer [16]. Taxanes are antineoplastics that act as microtubule stabilizers, promoting the assembly of microtubules by enhancing the action of tubulin dimers and thereby inhibiting disassembly. This inhibits cell replication by interfering with the G2 mitotic phase. Additionally, chromosome breakage can result from mitotic spindle distortion [17]. Incidence of chemotherapy-induced peripheral neuropathy (CIPN) from taxanes can be as high as 87% and is more commonly seen with paclitaxel [18] than other taxanes. Because small-diameter sensory fibers are primarily affected, sensory dominant neuropathy is the primary presentation of taxane-induced neuropathy and includes paresthesias, dysesthesias, numbness, reduced proprioception, and loss of dexterity in fingers and toes, though other areas may also be impacted. Symptoms are dose-dependent and can start as early as days after the initial dose and can persist for up to 1–3 years after therapy is completed. In some cases, however, taxane-induced neuropathy does not subside with discontinuation of treatment and is a lifelong issue [18].

The causative mechanism for taxane-induced neurotoxicity is both complex and multifactorial and driven by the following: microtubule disruption, mitochondrial dysfunction, axon degeneration, altered calcium homeostasis, alterations in peripheral nerve excitability, and neuroinflammation and immune processes. The disruption of microtubules through aggregation and bundling impairs axonal transport of synaptic vesicles that contain lipids, proteins, and ion channels. Compromised transport to distal neuronal parts of these essential cellular components and of mRNA lead to increased production of reactive oxygen species (ROS). Increased levels of ROS result in apoptotic activation, demyelinization, and cell structure disruption that ultimately leads to signal transmission impairment, immune activation, and pro-inflammatory cytokine production that drives additional mitochondrial damage [18]. Additionally, axonal transport impairment leads to distal nerve segment degeneration and axonal membrane remodeling. Calcium homeostasis dysregulation may also contribute to chemotherapy-induced peripheral neuropathy as paclitaxel can cause mitochondrial calcium release and may incite endoplasmic reticulum calcium release. Ion channel expression and function alteration is perhaps another contributory mechanism as decreased voltage-gated potassium channels and increased voltage-gated sodium channels have been correlated to peripheral neuropathy development from paclitaxel. Finally, paclitaxel drives increased production of pro-inflammatory cytokines and decreases anti-inflammatory cytokines which leads to immune cell activation and neuroinflammation [18].

Risk and Baseline Workup

Peripheral neuropathy is a common and painful complication from treatment for breast cancer. Neuropathy can develop weeks or months after the initiation of chemotherapy and last for months to years after completion. One of the most common risk factors is the receipt of taxane- or platinum-based chemotherapy, as discussed above. Another treatment-related risk factor is having undergone mastectomy. Clinical risk factors for having neuropathy after cancer treatment include older age, higher body mass index (BMI), and the presence of neuropathy at baseline [19].

Diabetes is also a risk factor for CIPN. Patients with diabetes are already predisposed to developing peripheral neuropathy due to nerve endings being exposed to high levels of glucose. When combined with taxane therapy, diabetic patients tend to develop peripheral neuropathy at a greater rate. Diabetic patients with or without complications had a two-thirds greater chance of developing CIPN [20].

The importance of a thorough medical history should not be underestimated in the initial workup for breast cancer survivors with peripheral neuropathy. A workup for underlying and potentially treatable causes of peripheral neuropathy is indicated. Table 8.1 lists causes of peripheral neuropathy and how they are diagnosed or excluded.

Table 8.1 Neuropathy differential and workup

Risk factors	Diagnosis
Vitamin deficiencies	Check for deficiencies in vitamins such as B12, folate, copper, vitamin E, thiamine Check for excess vitamin B6
Toxin exposure	Alcohol consumption/ alcoholism (thiamine deficiency) Heavy metal screen – 24-hour urine specimen (lead, arsenic, mercury, industrial agents)
Infection	HIV testing Hepatitis serologies Lyme disease
Hypothyroidism	Thyroid function testing
Monoclonal gammopathy of undetermined significance (MGUS) Amyloidosis	SPEP UPEP Immunofixation
Autoimmune disorders (i.e., Guillain-Barre Syndrome)	Antinuclear antibodies (ANA), erythrocyte sedimentation rate (ESR) Rheumatoid factor (RF)
Diabetes	Hemoglobin A1c, fasting blood glucose

Lesser recognized risk factors for peripheral neuropathy include vitamin deficiencies and toxin exposure. Other causes of predominantly axonal neuropathy include long-standing HIV infection, chronic renal insufficiency, amyloidosis, hypothyroidism, Lyme disease, and monoclonal gammopathy of undetermined significance (MGUS). Peripheral neuropathy associated with autoimmune disorders are more commonly demyelinating, including Guillain-Barre Syndrome. While rare, there are known hereditary causes of neuropathy, including Charcot-Marie-Tooth, mitochondrial disorders, and leukodystrophies. These potentially undiagnosed conditions should be ruled out in patients with CIPN.

One significant risk factor for peripheral neuropathy after breast cancer treatment is obesity. Obesity is defined as a body mass index (BMI) greater than 30 kg/m^2. The study at Cleveland Clinic conducted by Ali et al. showed that obese patients were two times more likely to suffer from peripheral neuropathy than underweight or normal weight patients [21]. Obesity has also been reported to increase the incidence of diabetic-induced peripheral neuropathy [19]. This is due to increased insulin resistance and obesity-related complications such as dyslipidemia. Another possible cause of increased risk of peripheral neuropathy is that obese patients receive increased doses of chemotherapy due to higher body surface area.

Peripheral neuropathy symptoms prior to diagnosis/treatment of breast cancer are prognostic for peripheral neuropathy after treatment is complete. One study showed that there was no difference in reporting of peripheral neuropathy symptoms in these patients even if scheduling of paclitaxel is changed to every 2–3 weeks compared to weekly treatment [21]. Previous peripheral neuropathy symptoms can also be linked to a history of diabetes as stated above.

Older age is perhaps associated with increased incidence of CIPN. One study conducted at Memorial Sloan Kettering showed that, out of 296 study participants, 67.6% of participants who were older than 65 years old experienced neuropathy compared to 55.4% of participants who were younger than 65 [19]. This observation, however, was not noted across the board. Another study at Cleveland Clinic looking at 650 patients from 2009 to 2016 showed that older age was associated with lower risk of peripheral neuropathy ($p < 0.05$) [21]. Furthermore, there was another study where variables such as obesity, treatment schedule, and age were assessed. In this study, age was not an independent risk factor for CIPN [22]. Further research needs to be performed on this variable as the evidence is inconclusive.

Vitamin-related causes of peripheral neuropathy include deficiencies in vitamin B12, copper, vitamin E, and thiamine, and excess vitamin B6. Vitamin B12 deficiency can result from extreme strict veganism, pernicious anemia, gastric bypass, and/or prolonged antacid use with proton pump inhibitors or histamine-2 receptor antagonists. Copper competes with zinc absorption, so excessive zinc supplementation can cause copper deficiency and lead to peripheral neuropathy. Excessive vitamin B6, resulting from doses greater than 2 g per day or taking lower doses, such as 50 mg per day over an extended period of time, may also contribute to peripheral neuropathy [23].

Alcohol and toxin exposures are associated with peripheral neuropathy. Alcoholism, for instance, is associated with vitamin deficiencies such as thiamine and folate. Therefore, inquiring about alcohol use is important because patients who are heavy drinkers are at risk for peripheral neuropathy. Potential heavy metal toxins include lead, arsenic, mercury, and industrial agents. These are not particularly common in developed countries but could still be seen with industrial pesticides or well water. Exposure to these toxins is known to cause neurotoxicity. Testing for heavy metal toxins includes a 24-hour urine specimen [23].

The baseline workup for neuropathy in breast cancer survivors involves a series of investigations including history and physical exam, laboratory data (as in Table 8.1), and electrodiagnostic testing. In some cases, a referral to neurology is also encouraged. As initial history, it is important to gain a clear understanding of the duration and degree of chronic illnesses that may be associated with neuropathy (i.e., diabetes mellitus, monoclonal gammopathy) and duration of these illnesses. Patients should also be queried about recent viral illnesses, new medications, toxin exposures, current alcohol use, and family history of disease that may be associated with neuropathy. In addition to a full physical and neurologic exam, the neurologic exam should include assessment of upper and lower extremity reflexes, distal sensation, and assessment of distal muscle strength and atrophy [24]. As guided by the history and physical exam, there are laboratory studies that can help determine the underlying cause of neuropathy. Initial serum testing should include fasting glucose, hemoglobin A1c, vitamin B12 and folate, SPEP, thyroid function tests, antinuclear antibodies (ANA), and erythrocyte sedimentation rate (ESR). Baseline urine testing should include UPEP with immunofixation (IFE). Pending the history and physical exam, other tests to consider might include HIV, hepatitis serologies, rheumatoid factor (RF), heavy metal screen, porphyrin screen, and testing for Lyme disease, among others.

In addition to history/physical exam and laboratory testing, electrodiagnostic testing including either a nerve conduction study (NCS) or electromyography (EMG) should be considered to determine severity of neuropathy and type (i.e., demyelinating vs axonal vs both). The results can help narrow down the differential diagnosis in concert with laboratory findings. As an example, results that show a predominant axonal neuropathy would point toward a systemic disorder, toxin, or medication as underlying cause of neuropathy. On the other hand, results illustrating a demyelinating process would indicate an autoimmune or hereditary disorder. In some cases, where there is either a mixed picture, additional diagnostic testing is needed to make a diagnosis, such as a lumbar puncture or peripheral nerve biopsy.

Once a diagnosis of neuropathy is established, there are tools to help determine severity of the disease and/or how the symptoms may be impairing a patient's function and/or quality of life; see

Table 8.2. The Common Terminology Criteria for Adverse Events (CTCAE) was developed by the National Cancer Institute (NCI) as descriptive terminology which can be utilized for Adverse Event (AE) reporting in the context of clinical trials. A grading (severity) scale is provided for each AE term, in this case sensory peripheral neuropathy, from grade 1 (asymptomatic) to grade 4 (life-threatening consequences where urgent intervention is necessary). The European Organization for Research and Treatment of Cancer (EORTC) has developed a 20 question, self-reported, quality of life (QOL) questionnaire to assess chemotherapy-induced peripheral neuropathy termed the Cancer Quality of Life Questionnaire-Chemotherapy-Induced Peripheral Neuropathy (QLQ-CIPN20) [25]. This questionnaire supplements the core EORTC QOL assessment and provides information specific to severity and impact of CIPN to guide appropriate interventions. The Total Neuropathy Score (TNS) is another tool that has been developed to assess chemotherapy-induced neuropathy and has been directly compared with National Cancer Institute Common Toxicity Criteria (NCI-CTC) with high correlation between assessment scores; however, the TNS did show a higher sensitivity to CIPN changes than the NCI-CTC [26]. Finally, the Functional Assessment of Cancer Therapy/Gynecologic Oncology Group-Neurotoxicity (FACT-GOG-Ntx) questionnaire includes an 11-item subscale in addition to the FACT-G (general) questionnaire [27]. This validated tool reliably evaluates symptoms and concerns associated with CIPN. Each of these tools can be used to assess neuropathy in clinical breast cancer care and/or incorporated into the design of clinical trials devoted to this patient population.

Table 8.2 Neuropathy assessment tools

Neuropathy tools
CTCAE (common terminology criteria for adverse events)
QLQ-CIPN20 questionnaire
The Total neuropathy score (TNS)
FACT-GOG-Ntx (functional assessment of cancer therapy/gynecologic oncology group-neurotoxicity) questionnaire

Approaches to Treatment

Treatment of Post-mastectomy Pain Syndrome

Persistent post-mastectomy pain is a complex syndrome leading to pain and psychosocial and physical dysfunction. Therefore, consideration of a multidisciplinary approach may be beneficial for management [28]. Like many neuropathic pain syndromes, there is limited research on the treatment of PMPS and PPMP, and no consensus on treatment exists. Pharmacologic strategies are aimed at reducing overall disease burden and, therefore, should also be supplemented by non-pharmacologic strategies. A thorough patient assessment will identify the psychological factors (depression, anxiety, catastrophizing) discussed above that predispose to development of and complicate management of PPMP. Use of pharmacologic agents that target multiple aspects of the patient's presentation (e.g., use of duloxetine or venlafaxine to treat depression, anxiety, and neuropathic and musculoskeletal pain) may improve patient response [1].

The existing treatment modalities for PMPS that have randomized, controlled trials with evidence to support their efficacy include several small studies. Kalso et al. studied amitriptyline 25–100 mg/day and found reduced neuropathic pain ($p < 0.05$) with eight of 15 patients experiencing more than 50% reduction in pain intensity [29]. Tasmuth et al. showed venlafaxine 75 mg/day significantly ($p < 0.05$) reduced average pain and maximum pain intensity, but not average daily pain intensity compared to placebo [30]. Levetiracetam titrated to 3000 mg/day was not found to have an effect on PMPS [31]. Caviggiolo et al. studied autologous fat grafting in 72 study patients compared with 41 controls with PMPS and severe scar retractions following mastectomy and radiotherapy. A statistically significant 3.2 point decrease in visual analog score (VAS) ($p = 0.0005$) was found in the patients treated with autologous fat grafting [32].

Because of the lack of prospective randomized, controlled trials for the treatment of PMPS, guidelines published for the pharmacologic treatment of neuropathic pain are used to select agents. The systematic review and meta-analysis published by Finnerup provides guidance in selecting first-, second-, and third-line agents for neuropathic pain treatment. First-line agents include gabapentinoids, serotonin-norepinephrine reuptake inhibitors, and tricyclic antidepressants. Second-line agents include capsaicin 8% patches, lidocaine patches, and tramadol. Third-line agents with limited evidence or increased potential risks include botulinum toxin A and strong opioids, respectively [33]. Prospective studies evaluating standard neuropathic pain treatments to address their effectiveness in PPMP specifically are necessary to provide guidance on effective evidence-based treatment.

Treatment of CIPN

Herbal Supplements

Alpha-Lipoic Acid (ALA)

Alpha-lipoic acid (ALA) is an antioxidant compound with efficacy in patients with diabetic neuropathy, theorized to be due to oxidative stress and free-radical formation [34]. Due to its benefit in this type of neuropathy, investigators have studied its use for treatment of CIPN. In a small study of 14 patients who had received docetaxel and cisplatin chemotherapy, investigators tried to determine benefit from ALA on neurological symptoms [35]. Patients received treatment with ALA 600 mg IV once per week for 3–5 weeks, followed by 1800 mg orally once daily until symptom recovery or a maximum of 6 months. Neurologic symptoms were evaluated and eight patients were found to have symptom improvement [34]. Other results include a median time to response of 4 weeks and median duration of treatment with ALA of 2 months, and investigators did not find any significant adverse effects other than mild gastric pain and Grade I/II nausea/vomiting [35]. These studies include small sample sizes, and the authors conclude that larger, randomized studies are needed to better evaluate the role of ALA in treatment of CIPN.

L-Carnitine/ALC (Acetyl-L-Carnitine)

Acetyl-L-carnitine (ALC) is a compound that plays an important role in neuronal protection. In animal models, ALC has been shown to improve sensory neuropathy and reduce severity of neuropathy [34]. In a large, randomized, double-blind trial, investigators compared 409 patients receiving either ALC 3000 mg per day or placebo, to determine benefit in prevention of CIPN [36]. After 12 weeks, use of ALC provided no evidence of benefit compared to placebo. Concerningly, at further follow-up of 24 weeks, investigators noted that use of ALC was associated with a statistically significant increase in CIPN. This was the first study to provide evidence that a nutritional supplement increases neuropathy [37]. Maestri and colleagues performed a small pilot study of 27 patients to determine the effect of ALC on CIPN [38]. The primary objective of this study was to investigate the activity of ALC in reversing peripheral neuropathy. Patients were treated with ALC 1 g IV/day for at least 10 days. The majority (73%) of the patients showed at least one grade of reduction in severity of peripheral neuropathy [38]. While there was one case of insomnia reported from ALC, it was otherwise well-tolerated. ALC may provide some benefit for treatment of CIPN after chemotherapy cessation, but should not be used for prevention [39]; further studies are still needed to fully determine its role in treatment.

Prescription Medications

Many pharmacologic agents such as anticonvulsants including carbamazepine, gabapentinoids like gabapentin and pregabalin, as well as antidepressants such as amitriptyline have not been studied as preventatives for CIPN. Because of lack of evidence, these agents are not currently recommended for the prevention of CIPN [39]. As the majority of evidence is found in the CIPN treatment setting, the following will focus on current literature and recommendations for the treatment versus prevention of CIPN. A list of supplements and medications to be considered for the treatment of neuropathy in breast cancer survivors can be found in

Table 8.3 Supplements and medications for the treatment of neuropathy

	Dosing	Strength of recommendation
Herbal supplements		
Alpha-lipoic acid (ALA)	600 mg IV once weekly for 3–5 weeks, followed by 1800 mg/day orally until symptom recovery or a max of 6 months	Inconclusive, further larger, randomized trials are needed
Acetyl-L-carnitine (ALC)	1 g IV once daily for at least 10 days	Inconclusive, further larger studies still needed
Anticonvulsants		
Gabapentin	Incrementally escalated over 3 weeks to target dose of 2700 mg daily	Inconclusive data, but a reasonable option in select patients with CIPN
Pregabalin	75 mg twice daily with dose ranges of 150 mg to 450 mg daily	Limited data, but a reasonable option in select patients with CIPN
Lamotrigine	25 mg incrementally escalated every 2 weeks to maximum dose of 150 mg twice daily	Lack of evidence. Not recommended given concern for Stephens-Johnson syndrome
Tricyclic antidepressants		
Nortriptyline	Target maximum dose of 100 mg daily	Inconclusive data, but a reasonable option in select patients with CIPN
Amitriptyline	10 mg daily with dose escalation of 10 mg per week to maximum of 50 mg daily	Inconclusive data, but a reasonable option in select patients with CIPN
SNRIs/SSRIs		
Duloxetine	30 mg daily for 1 week then increased to 60 mg daily	Inconclusive data, but a reasonable option in select patients with CIPN
Topical		
Topical analgesic gel (amitriptyline/ketamine ± baclofen)	Varying doses due to compounded formulations, including: baclofen 10 mg, amitriptyline 40 mg (3%), ketamine 20 mg (1.5%) applied twice per day for up to 4 weeks	Inconclusive data, but a reasonable option in select patients with CIPN

Table 8.3, and our recommended management approach for patients who develop CIPN is outlined in Fig. 8.1.

Antidepressants

Duloxetine

Serotonin and norepinephrine are neurotransmitters that may inhibit input to neurons in the spinal dorsal horn resulting in suppression of transmission of painful peripheral stimuli [40]. Because serotonin-norepinephrine reuptake inhibitors have shown benefit in the treatment of neuropathy-related pain, they were hypothesized to potentially treat CIPN as well. CIPN benefit with duloxetine was demonstrated in a double-blind, crossover trial that included 231 patients with CIPN secondary to receiving a taxane or platinum. Patients assigned to duloxetine received 30 mg once daily for 1 week and then increased to 60 mg daily for an additional 4 weeks. The implementation of duloxetine resulted in improvement in functional and quality of life scores, pain, as well as improved numbness and tingling in feet, although no change in hands [41]. The benefit of duloxetine on CIPN is also supported by a small, randomized crossover Japanese trial in patients that had previously received oxaliplatin, paclitaxel, vincristine, or bortezomib. The trial included 34 patients in which patients were randomized to receive duloxetine 20 mg daily for 1 week and then increased to 40 mg daily for 3 weeks or vitamin B12 at 1.5 mg daily for 4 weeks [42]. Of note, patients were allowed to continue other analgesics including opioids, pregabalin, acetamino-

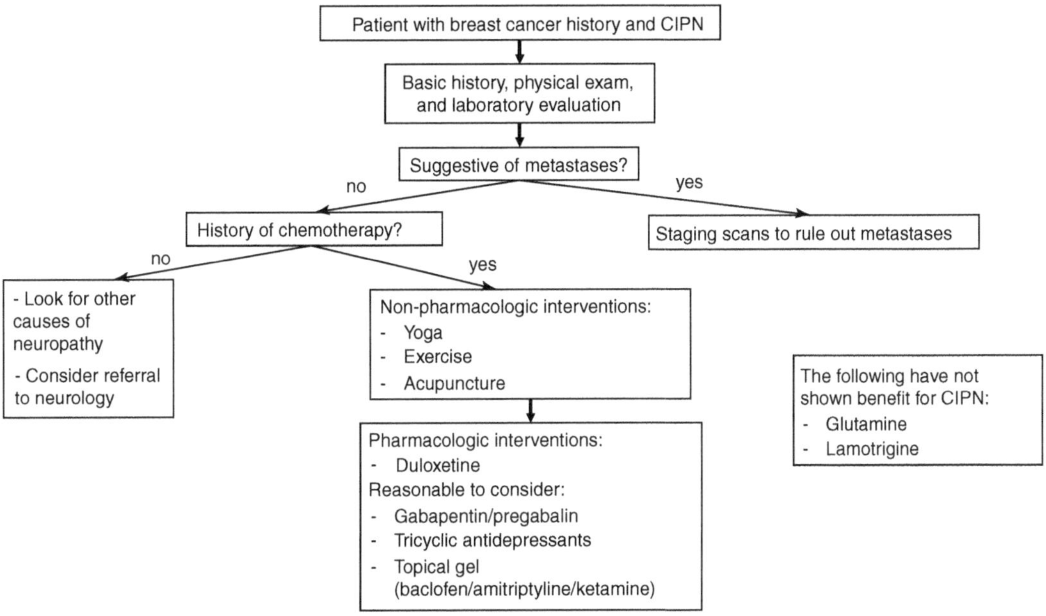

Fig. 8.1 Recommended approach chemotherapy-induced peripheral neuropathy (CIPN) in a breast cancer survivor

phen, and nonsteroidal anti-inflammatory agents though no new analgesic agents were allowed during the study. There was an improvement in severity of numbness and pain using a visual analog scale in patients that received duloxetine suggesting a beneficial effect on CIPN [42]. While potential benefit has been shown with the use of duloxetine for CIPN, additional prospective, randomized trials are needed to determine overall benefit and provide support for this recommendation. Duloxetine is provided as a recommendation for CIPN within the ASCO guidelines [39].

Tricyclic Antidepressants (TCAs): Nortriptyline and Amitriptyline

The analgesic effect of TCAs is thought to be related to increased serotonin and norepinephrine in pain modulating systems in the central nervous system [43]. In a randomized, double-blind, crossover study to determine the benefit of nortriptyline in CIPN, specifically with cisplatin, patients randomized to nortriptyline received a target maximum dose of 100 mg daily versus placebo. A total of 51 patients were included within the study. There was no significant difference with regard to quality of life or paresthesia between groups though there was potential effect in the second period of the crossover design which may have been due to carryover effect. Patients receiving nortriptyline did experience increased dry mouth, dizziness, and constipation [43].

The impact of another TCA, amitriptyline, on CIPN was also explored in a double-blind, randomized trial that included 44 patients that had previously received chemotherapy containing a platinum, taxane, or vinca alkaloid. Patients in the treatment arm were initially treated with amitriptyline 10 mg daily with a dose escalation of 10 mg per week, up to 50 mg per day, for a total of 8 weeks. While there was a trend toward improved quality of life and global improvement with patients receiving amitriptyline, sensory neuropathic symptoms were not improved, and no statistical significance was reached [44]. Despite lack of evidence supporting efficacy, the current CIPN ASCO guidelines report it is reasonable to consider TCAs given current limited treatment options [39].

Anticonvulsants: Gabapentin, Pregabalin, and Lamotrigine

After nerve injury, neuronal excitability is hypothesized to be caused by $\alpha 2\delta 1$ subunit upregulation of the voltage-dependent calcium channels in the dorsal nerve root ganglia. Gabapentin inhibits this subunit and thereby reduces calcium influx and neurotransmitter release from hyperexcited neurons, reducing nociception [45]. Given gabapentin's ability to relieve peripheral neuropathy in other settings, it was studied in a double-blind, placebo-controlled, randomized, crossover trial in 115 patients with symptomatic CIPN who had previously received chemotherapy to include taxanes, platinums, or vinca alkaloids. Patients were prescribed gabapentin (300 mg capsules), and the dose of gabapentin was incrementally escalated over 3 weeks with a target dose of 2700 mg daily for 6 weeks total of gabapentin. Overall, there was no difference in symptom severity between groups, and adverse events were similar, suggesting no benefit to the utilization of gabapentin for CIPN [46].

The benefit of pregabalin use for the treatment of CIPN was reviewed in two similar retrospective studies in which patients had been treated with oxaliplatin or paclitaxel chemotherapy. Pregabalin doses ranged from 150 mg to 450 mg daily. The administration of pregabalin was associated with a significant decrease in CIPN, suggesting pregabalin may be beneficial for reducing severity of CIPN. Of note, both studies are retrospective in nature [47, 48]. In a prospective, randomized trial, 46 patients diagnosed with breast cancer receiving paclitaxel 80 mg/m2 for 12 weeks were randomized to pregabalin or placebo. Patients receiving pregabalin were initiated on 75 mg twice daily starting on the first night of chemotherapy and continuing for 12 weeks. The pregabalin dose was decreased during the 13th week to once daily at bedtime, after which patients concluded the study. There was no difference seen between arms with regard to pain scores, which limited enthusiasm for conducting a phase II trial [49]. Although there is lack of evidence for benefit, the CIPN ASCO guidelines do provide gabapentin and pregabalin as reasonable treatment options for CIPN given current limited treatment options and established efficacy for other types of neuropathic pain [39].

Lamotrigine acts to inhibit neuronal sodium channel function, decreasing excitatory neurotransmitter release, such as glutamate and aspartate. Because increased activity of sodium channels may lead to hyperalgesia and based on lamotrigine's mechanism, lamotrigine has been studied as a possible treatment option for CINV. Lamotrigine was studied in 131 patients with symptomatic CIPN that had previously received chemotherapy with a taxane, platinum, or vinca alkaloid agent in a randomized, double-blind trial. Patients received lamotrigine 25 mg at bedtime for 2 weeks, 25 mg twice daily for 2 weeks, 50 mg twice daily for 2 weeks, 100 mg twice daily for 2 weeks, and then final dose escalation to 150 mg twice daily for 2 weeks. There was no statistical difference found between groups with regard to pain scores, suggesting no benefit of lamotrigine in the treatment of CINV [50]. Given lack of evidence of efficacy and the risk of Stephens-Johnson syndrome associated with lamotrigine, it is not recommended for the treatment of CIPN by the ASCO guidelines [37, 39].

Topical Analgesic Gel: Amitriptyline/Ketamine ± Baclofen

Topical analgesic agents have been studied in treatment of neuropathy, primarily in the setting of diabetic neuropathy [34]. Topical formulations have an advantage over oral agents in minimizing systemic absorption and therefore widespread toxicity and may be an innovative approach to management of CIPN. Based on data in other types of pain, a topical formulation of amitriptyline and ketamine with or without baclofen has been investigated for treatment of CIPN. These three agents were selected due to their unique mechanisms of action. In a double-blind, randomized, placebo-controlled trial of 208 patients, investigators sought to evaluate a compounded topical analgesic gel for treatment of CIPN [51]. Patients were randomized to receive 1.31 g of compounded gel containing baclofen 10 mg, amitriptyline 40 mg (3%), and ketamine 20 mg (1.5%) in a base of organogel versus an identical placebo gel; patients were instructed to apply one level spoonful of gel to each area of pain, numbness, and/or tingling twice/day for 4 weeks. The authors found a trend toward improvement in sensory ($p = 0.053$) and motor ($p = 0.021$) symptoms over placebo [51]. The compounded topical formulation appeared to be well-tolerated without systemic toxicities. However, further investigation is needed as this compound is not FDA approved and long-term safety has not been established. Another consideration is that compounded products are typically not covered by prescription insurance plans, leading to excessive costs. A larger phase III randomized, placebo-controlled study of amitriptyline and ketamine was evaluated in 462 cancer survivors with CIPN [52]. Patients were instructed to apply up to 4 g of a topical gel containing amitriptyline 4% and ketamine 2% twice/day to each area with pain, numbness, and/or tingling versus placebo. Results from this study did not show a benefit in use of amitriptyline/ketamine topical gel for decreasing CIPN in cancer patients [52]. Providers should be aware that there is limited scientific evidence for these topical gel formulations. The most recent ASCO Practice Guidelines panel suggests that there is declining interest in their use (Loprinzi et al. 2020).

Non-pharmacologic Treatment Options

Most research has focused on pharmacological therapies which are aimed at pain control, but this does not address the problem of motor weakness due to loss of sensation. This can cause significant problems with walking and balance which in turn impairs quality of life. Yoga elevates mood and improves balance. When yoga is practiced by cancer patients, flexibility and balance improve. They also demonstrate decreased pain severity which decreases stress and improves sleep quality [53].

Exercise, in general, has potent anti-inflammatory effects. Multiple biological pathways are affected during exercise. IL-6 is released during exercise which exerts anti-inflammatory properties. Both low to moderate intensity walking and resistance training are recommended with benefits for neuropathy as well as quality of life [54]. If a patient has difficulty with stability, water aerobics and a stationary bike are alternatives. If peripheral neuropathy affects the patient's hands, padded gloves are recommended [55].

Acupuncture has been an integral part of traditional Chinese medicine for over 2000 years. A small retrospective study of 18 patients showed that weekly acupuncture over 6 weeks resulted in symptomatic improvement in 82% of patients [56]. The acupuncture used needling Jing-Well points in both the hands and feet. Further research was performed to add reflexology to the protocol. Thirty breast cancer patients were treated with acupuncture of 20 minute sessions 1–2 times/week in addition to reflexology lasting 30–40 minutes. Reflexology included deep massage of the hands and feet including foot cushions in addition to rotating of the wrists, hands, ankles, and feet and rubbing the arms and ankles. Seven patients with grades 3–4 neuropathy reported grade 1–2 at 3 months and no symptoms at the 6 months evaluation. All of the patients completed the protocol without any significant adverse events [56]. This study demonstrates benefit for chemotherapy-induced peripheral neuropathy but is limited by small sample size.

Additional Considerations on Prevention

Chemotherapy treatments utilized for patients with breast cancer often result in untoward adverse effects, including neuropathy. When considering a management approach, prevention with various supplements may be helpful to minimize or prevent CIPN from occurring and affecting patients' quality of life. Dietary supplements are commonly used as an adjunct to traditional therapies in the breast cancer population [57]. Here we will review data to examine supplement use for prevention and treatment of CIPN. A summary of supplements for the prevention of CIPN is provided in Table 8.4.

Supplements

Calcium/Magnesium

IV infusions of calcium and magnesium (Ca/Mg) supplementation are a well-researched option for

Table 8.4 Supplements for the prevention of neuropathy

	Role	Dosing	Strength of recommendation
Calcium/ magnesium infusions	Prevention of CIPN	1 g calcium gluconate, 1 g magnesium sulfate	Moderate against use
Glutathione	Prevention of CIPN	1.5 g/m2 glutathione IV over 15 minutes before chemotherapy	Inconclusive for use with cisplatin/ oxaliplatin; moderately against use with paclitaxel/carboplatin
Glutamine	Prevention of CIPN	30 g divided daily for 4–7 days; initiate after chemotherapy infusion	Inconclusive, further placebo-controlled studies needed
Vitamin E	Prevention of CIPN	600–800 mg per day divided daily during chemotherapy and up to 3 months after cessation	Moderate against use

prevention of oxaliplatin-induced peripheral neuropathy. When utilized, common dosing of each agent consists of 1 g of calcium gluconate and 1 g of magnesium sulfate [34]. Oxaliplatin is associated with two phases of neurotoxicity, including acute and chronic, which are hypothesized to be mediated through different mechanisms [34]. In initial small studies, IV Ca/Mg infusions were shown to decrease incidence and severity of CIPN symptoms [58]. Several placebo-controlled trials were initiated to further support previous data; however, these were prematurely terminated due to inaccurate reports from one of these studies that showed a decreased antitumor activity from patients receiving Ca/Mg infusions [37]. In a large phase III, placebo-controlled, double-blind trial of 346 patients who received oxaliplatin, patients received IV infusions of Ca/Mg to prevent CIPN [59]. The study included three treatment groups and patients received a) Ca/Mg infusions before and after oxaliplatin, b) Ca/Mg before oxaliplatin with placebo after, and c) placebo infusions before and after oxaliplatin. Unfortunately, findings by Loprinzi and colleagues confirm no differences exist in neuropathy among the three study arms and therefore no benefit to use of Ca/Mg infusions to decrease CIPN from oxaliplatin therapy. Findings from this study were further investigated by Pachman and colleagues, which helped to describe patterns of oxaliplatin-induced peripheral neuropathy and also supported the idea that presence of acute neuropathy projects progression to chronic neurotoxicity. Researchers report that patients with increased severity of acute CIPN with the first cycle of chemotherapy were found to experience further chronic sensory neurotoxicity ($P < 0.0001$) [60]. While we now have a better understanding of oxalipatin-induced neurotoxicity, Ca/Mg infusions do not have consistent evidence of benefit, and providers should not recommend this supplement for prevention of CIPN.

Glutathione

Glutathione is a natural and potent antioxidant supplement with a high affinity for heavy metals [34]. A related compound, N-acetylcysteine, activates glutathione peroxidase, which also results in an increased serum concentration of glutathione [61]. The mechanism of benefit of glutathione is thought to be due to prevention of platinum adducts in the dorsal root ganglia [61]. Further neuroprotective benefit of glutathione is through inhibiting the activation of p53 [61]. Several small studies have tried to evaluate the neuroprotective effects of glutathione, as well as N-acetylcysteine, against CIPN. In initial smaller studies, glutathione effectively prevented cisplatin-induced peripheral neuropathy without blunting effects of the chemotherapy on the tumor [34]. Based on these positive results, a randomized, double-blind trial of 151 patients with ovarian cancer was conducted to study the efficacy of cisplatin with placebo (normal saline) versus cisplatin with glutathione to decrease CIPN. Investigators found that there was a statistically significant difference in peripheral neurotoxicity in patients treated with glutathione compared to control; other quality of life measures were also improved [62]. The investigators concluded that the addition of glutathione to cisplatin-based regimens allows for further treatment with cisplatin due to decreased peripheral neuropathy as well as improvement in patient's quality of life. In contrast to the above data, however, Leal and colleagues performed a phase III, randomized, double-blind, placebo-controlled study of 185 patients on a paclitaxel and carboplatin regimen. Patients received either glutathione 1.5 g/m^2 IV over 15 minutes before chemotherapy or placebo. The study findings did not support the benefit of glutathione to prevent CIPN from this regimen [63]. As carboplatin is the least neurotoxic of the platinum compounds, investigators concluded that the majority of the neurotoxicity from this regimen was due to paclitaxel. Therefore, glutathione was ineffective in prevention of taxane-induced peripheral neuropathy [37]. Due to conflicting data, the recommendation for use of glutathione for prevention of CIPN from cisplatin and oxaliplatin remains inconclusive, and further larger studies are recommended. ASCO Practice Guidelines recommend moderately against the use of glutathione for prevention of CIPN with paclitaxel/carboplatin containing regimens [39].

Glutamine

Glutamine is an amino acid theorized to have neuroprotective effects [34]. This has only been studied in small trials to date with use of oral glutamine. In one small study of 46 patients, 17 received glutamine at a dose of 10 g three times/day for 4 days, starting 24 hours after completion of high-dose paclitaxel chemotherapy [64]. The investigators found that patients who received glutamine had significantly less weakness, less loss of vibratory sensation, and less toe numbness than the control group. However, this study was not randomized or blinded leading to possible bias. Another small study evaluated use of glutamine to prevent oxaliplatin-induced neuropathy in 86 patients [65]. Patients were randomized to receive glutamine 15 g twice/day for 7 days, starting after oxaliplatin infusion ($n = 42$) or not receive glutamine ($n = 44$). Patients who received glutamine had a significantly lower incidence of Grade III–IV peripheral neuropathy than the control group without any effect on response to treatment [65]. While these small studies may support use of oral glutamine to reduce CIPN, further investigation with randomized, placebo-controlled trials are recommended to elucidate if any benefit exists. Additionally, further standardization of appropriate dose of oral glutamine is necessary to monitor for possible adverse effects.

Vitamin E

In a small open label, randomized, controlled trial of breast cancer patients who received cisplatin, paclitaxel, or a combination regimen, subjects were randomized to supplementation with oral vitamin E (600 mg/day) during chemotherapy and 3 months after cessation compared to patients who received no supplementation [66]. Investigators found a statistically significant difference in the incidence and severity of CIPN in the subjects who received vitamin E supplementation compared to the control group. The authors conclude that vitamin E supplementation may have a neuroprotective effect; however, limitations include a small study sample without a placebo arm. These researchers expanded their 2005 study and looked in detail at neuropathy specifically from taxane chemotherapy, including safety profile [67]. They report that vitamin E is safe, well-tolerated, and easy to obtain since it is oral, thereby making it a cost-effective option for prevention of CIPN. A large, randomized, phase III study of 207 patients sought to better understand the role of vitamin E in prevention of CIPN [68]. Patients were randomized to receive oral vitamin E 400 mg twice/day or placebo; study subjects were on the following chemotherapy agents: taxanes ($n = 109$), cisplatin ($n = 8$), carboplatin ($n = 2$), oxaliplatin ($n = 50$), or combination ($n = 20$). There was no difference in incidence of grade 2+ neuropathy or time to onset of neuropathy between the two arms. Investigators found that vitamin E did not reduce CIPN; however, it was well-tolerated. ASCO Practice Guidelines further support that providers should not recommend vitamin E supplementation due to a lack of consistent evidence that it decreases peripheral neuropathy [39]. Moreover, data substantiates that use of antioxidants, such as vitamin E, during treatment worsens prognosis [69, 70].

N-Acetylcysteine

N-Acetylcysteine (NAC) is another supplement which has been considered for prevention of CIPN. NAC is considered to have a protective effect against CIPN through reduced oxidative stress and free-radical destruction [71]. Further, cysteine promotes production of glutathione, a potent antioxidant. In a small prospective, randomized controlled, open label study of breast cancer patients ($n = 75$) receiving paclitaxel for adjuvant therapy, investigators tried to determine the incidence of different grades of peripheral neuropathy [71]. Patients received either low-dose NAC therapy (1200 mg daily) or high-dose therapy (1200 mg twice daily) or were in the control group. At study conclusion (12 weeks), the incidence of grade 2 and 3 peripheral neuropathy was lower in the high-dose group (28.6%) than in the other two arms, including the low-dose group (61.9%) and control group (100%); this observation was statistically significant ($p < 0.001$) [71]. The authors concluded that oral NAC dosed at 1200 mg twice daily may reduce incidence and severity of peripheral neuropathy from paclitaxel therapy and improve patient's quality of life. However, due to limited data, the ASCO Practice Guidelines state that providers should not recommend NAC for prevention of CIPN [39].

Cryotherapy

Although not beneficial in the survivor setting posttreatment, a noteworthy strategy used for the possible prevention of chemotherapy-induced neuropathy that may be helpful for patients actively receiving chemotherapy has been cryotherapy. Cryotherapy is the incorporation of cold therapy, such as wearing frozen mitts and socks or applying ice to the hands and feet, prior, during, and after taxane infusions. The general principle behind this is due to vasoconstriction within these localized areas (hands and feet) which ultimately will reduce chemotherapy exposure to these areas and thus minimize associated toxicities such as neuropathy. Cryotherapy has been utilized with some success in reducing chemotherapy toxicities such as alopecia and oral mucositis [72]. The literature supporting cryotherapy is minimal and inconclusive as there have been both positive and negative trials; therefore, given this uncertainty, it has not been implemented within clinical guideline recommendations. A review of the clinical trials that have investigated the implementation of cryotherapy can be found in Table 8.5. Despite uncertainty of clinical benefit, the use of cryotherapy can be considered for some patients especially as overall it is considered a low-risk intervention as the primary adverse event, if reported, was poor cold tolerability. The majority of clinical data is within the breast cancer patient population receiving weekly paclitaxel. Cryotherapy is not recommended for every patient and should not be used in some, i.e., patients with Raynaud's disease. Of note, exclusion criteria were variable among trials but included: history of peripheral neuropathy, diabetes, peripheral vascular disease, Raynaud's disease, peripheral artery disease, hand-foot syndrome, and absence of a finger or toe. Consideration for cryotherapy should be made for each individual patient.

Conclusion

Due to both surgical interventions and systemic treatment, breast cancer survivors may be affected by peripheral neuropathy that can continue long after treatment concludes and can substantially impact quality of life and overall survivorship. While many potential treatment and

Table 8.5 Cryotherapy clinical trials with peripheral neuropathy outcomes

Study	Design	Intervention	Peripheral neuropathy outcome
Eckhoff et al., 2013	1725 breast cancer patients receiving docetaxel 100 mg/m^2 × 6 or 75 mg/m^2 × 3	Frozen gloves and socks 15 minutes before, during, and 15 minutes after treatment	Decreased
Griffiths et al., 2018	29 breast cancer patients treated with paclitaxel 175 mg/m^2 × 4	Elastogel gloves 15 minutes before, during, and 15 minutes after treatment	No change
Hanai et al., 2018	36 breast cancer patients treated with weekly paclitaxel 80 mg/m^2 × 12	Elastogel gloves 15 minutes before, during, and 15 minutes after treatment	Decreased
Kanbayashi et al., 2019	43 breast cancer patients receiving nab-paclitaxel 260 mg/m^2	Frozen gloves for 60 minutes	No change
Ruddy et al., 2019	46 patients receiving weekly paclitaxel 80 mg/m^2 × 12	Crushed ice 15 minutes before, during, and 15 minutes after treatment	No change
Sundar et al., 2017	20 breast cancer patients receiving weekly paclitaxel 80 mg/m^2 × 12	Continuous-flow hypothermia boots for 2.5 to 3 hours	Decreased
Wilkinson et al., 2016	41 breast cancer patients receiving weekly paclitaxel 80 mg/m^2 × 12	Hypothermia mitts and slippers 15 minutes before, during, and 15 minutes after treatment	Decreased

preventative measures have been investigated and outlined within this chapter, there continues to be a lack of literature support to provide strong recommendations. Additional clinical trials and supportive evidence are needed in this unique patient population.

References

1. Tait RC, Zoberi K, Ferguson M, Levenhagen K, Luebbert RA, Rowland K, et al. Persistent post-mastectomy pain: risk factors and current approaches to treatment. J Pain. 2018;19(12):1367–83.
2. Granek I, Ashikari R, Foley K. The post-mastectomy pain syndrome: clinical and anatomical correlates. Proc A Soc Clin Oncol. 1984;3:122.
3. Merskey. Classification of chronic pain: descriptions of chronic pain syndromes and definitions of pain terms. Pain. 1986:226.
4. Andersen KG, Kehlet H. Persistent pain after breast cancer treatment: a critical review of risk factors and strategies for prevention. J Pain. 2011;12(7):725–46.
5. Vilholm OJ, Cold S, Rasmussen L, Sindrup SH. The postmastectomy pain syndrome: an epidemiological study on the prevalence of chronic pain after surgery for breast cancer. Br J Cancer. 2008;99(4):604–10.
6. Kokosis G, Chopra K, Darrach H, Dellon AL, Williams EH. Re-visiting post-breast surgery pain syndrome: risk factors, peripheral nerve associations and clinical implications. Gland Surg. 2019;8(4):407–15.
7. Meretoja TJ, Leidenius MHK, Tasmuth T, Sipila R, Kalso E. Pain at 12 months after surgery for breast cancer. JAMA. 2014;311(1):90–2.
8. Hinrichs-Rocker A, Schulz K, Jarvinen I, Lefering R, Simanski C, Neugebauer EA. Psychosocial predictors and correlates for chronic post-surgical pain (CPSP) – a systematic review. Eur J Pain. 2009;13(7):719–30.
9. Belfer I, Schreiber KL, Shaffer JR, Shnol H, Blaney K, Morando A, et al. Persistent postmastectomy pain in breast cancer survivors: analysis of clinical, demographic, and psychosocial factors. J Pain. 2013;14(10):1185–95.
10. Mansel RE, Fallowfield L, Kissin M, Goyal A, Newcombe RG, Dixon JM, et al. Randomized multicenter trial of sentinel node biopsy versus standard axillary treatment in operable breast cancer: the ALMANAC trial. J Natl Cancer Inst. 2006;98(9):599–609.
11. Andersen KG, Aasvang EK, Kroman N, Kehlet H. Intercostobrachial nerve handling and pain after axillary lymph node dissection for breast cancer. Acta Anaesthesiol Scand. 2014;58(10):1240–8.
12. Andersen KG, Duriaud HM, Jensen HE, Kroman N, Kehlet H. Predictive factors for the development of persistent pain after breast cancer surgery. Pain. 2015;156(12):2413–22.
13. Kairaluoma PM, Bachmann MS, Rosenberg PH, Pere PJ. Preincisional paravertebral block reduces the prevalence of chronic pain after breast surgery. Anesth Analg. 2006;103(3):703–8.
14. Gartner R, Jensen M-B, Nielsen J, Ewertz M, Kroman N, Kehlet H. Prevalence of and risk factors associated with persistent pain following breast cancer surgery. JAMA. 2009;302:1985–92.
15. Poleshuck EL, Katz J, Andrus CH, Hogan LA, Jung BF, Kulick DI, et al. Risk factors for chronic pain following breast cancer surgery: a prospective study. J Pain. 2006;7(9):626–34.
16. NCCN. Breast Cancer Version 3.2020 2020.

17. Paclitaxel(Taxol)[packageinsert]. Paclitaxel (Taxol) [package insert]. 2011.
18. Zajaczkowska R, Kocot-Kepska M, Leppert W, Wrzosek A, Mika J, Wordliczek J. Mechanisms of chemotherapy-induced peripheral neuropathy. Int J Mol Sci. 2019;20(6):1451.
19. Bao T, Basal C, Seluzicki C, Li SQ, Seidman AD, Mao JJ. Long-term chemotherapy-induced peripheral neuropathy among breast cancer survivors: prevalence, risk factors, and fall risk. Breast Cancer Res Treat. 2016;159(2):327–33.
20. Hershman DL, Till C, Wright JD, Awad D, Ramsey SD, Barlow WE, et al. Comorbidities and risk of chemotherapy-induced peripheral neuropathy among participants 65 years or older in southwest oncology group clinical trials. J Clin Oncol. 2016;34(25):3014–22.
21. Mustafa Ali M, Moeller M, Rybicki L, Moore HCF. Long-term peripheral neuropathy symptoms in breast cancer survivors. Breast Cancer Res Treat. 2017;166(2):519–26.
22. Barginear M, Dueck AC, Allred JB, Bunnell C, Cohen HJ, Freedman RA, et al. Age and the risk of paclitaxel-induced neuropathy in women with early-stage breast cancer (Alliance A151411): results from 1,881 patients from cancer and leukemia group B (CALGB) 40101. Oncologist. 2019;24(5):617–23.
23. Staff NP, Windebank AJ. Peripheral neuropathy due to vitamin deficiency, toxins, and medications. Continuum (Minneap Minn). 2014;20:1293–306.
24. England J, Gronseth GS, Franklin G, Miller R, Asbury A, Carter G, et al. Distal symmetric polyneuropathy: a definition for clinical research: report of the American Academy of Neurology, the American Association of Electrodiagnostic Medicine, and the American Academy of Physical Medicine and Rehabilitation. Neurology. 2005;64:199–207.
25. Postma T, Aaronson NK, Heimans J, Muller M, Hildebrand J, Delattre J, et al. The development of an EORTC quality of life questionnaire to assess chemotherapy-induced peripheral neuropathy: the QLQ-CIPN20. Eur J Cancer. 2005;41:1135–9.
26. Cavaletti G, Frigeni B, Lanzani F, Piatti M, Rota S, Briani C, et al. The Total Neuropathy Score as an assessment tool for grading the course of chemotherapy-induced peripheral neurotoxicity: comparison with the National Cancer Institute-Common Toxicity Scale. J Peripher Nerv Syst. 2007;12:210–5.
27. Calhoun E, Welshman E, Chang C, Lurain J, Fishman D, Hunt T, et al. Psychometric evaluation of the Functional Assessment of Cancer Therapy/Gynecologic Oncology Group—neurotoxicity (Fact/GOG-Ntx) questionnaire for patients receiving systemic chemotherapy. Int J Gynecol Cancer. 2003;13:741–8.
28. Scascighini L, Toma V, Dober-Spielmann S, Sprott H. Multidisciplinary treatment for chronic pain: a systematic review of interventions and outcomes. Rheumatology (Oxford). 2008;47(5):670–8.
29. Kalso E, Tiina T, Neuvonen PJ. Amitriptyline effectively relieves neuropathic pain following treatment of breast cancer. Pain. 1996;64:293–302.
30. Tasmuth T, Hartel B, Kalso E. Venlafaxine in neuropathic pain following treatment of breast cancer. Eur J Pain. 2002;6(1):17–24.
31. Vilholm OJ, Cold S, Rasmussen L, Sindrup SH. Effect of levetiracetam on the postmastectomy pain syndrome. Eur J Neurol. 2008;15(8):851–7.
32. Caviggioli F, Maione L, Forcellini D, Klinger F, Klinger M. Autologous fat graft in postmastectomy pain syndrome. Plast Reconstr Surg. 2011;128(2):349–52.
33. Finnerup NB, Attal N, Haroutounian S, McNicol E, Baron R, Dworkin RH, et al. Pharmacotherapy for neuropathic pain in adults: a systematic review and meta-analysis. Lancet Neurol. 2015;14(2):162–73.
34. Pachman DR, Barton DL, Watson JC, Loprinzi CL. Chemotherapy-induced peripheral neuropathy: prevention and treatment. Clin Pharmacol Ther. 2011;90(3):377–87.
35. Gedlicka C, Kornek GV, Schmid K, Scheithauer W. Amelioration of docetaxel/cisplatin induced polyneuropathy by α-lipoic acid. Ann Oncol. 2003;14:339–40.
36. Hershman DL, Unger JM, Crew KD, Minasian LM, Awad D, Moinpour CM, et al. Randomized double-blind placebo-controlled trial of acetyl-L-carnitine for the prevention of taxane-induced neuropathy in women undergoing adjuvant breast cancer therapy. J Clin Oncol. 2013;31(20):2627–33.
37. Hershman DL, Lacchetti C, Dworkin RH, Lavoie Smith EM, Bleeker J, Cavaletti G, et al. Prevention and management of chemotherapy-induced peripheral neuropathy in survivors of adult cancers: American Society of Clinical Oncology clinical practice guideline. J Clin Oncol. 2014;32(18):1941–67.
38. Maestri A, Ceratti ADP, Cundari S, Zanna C, Cortesi E, Crinò L. A pilot study on the effect of acetyl-L-carnitine in paclitaxel-and cisplatin-induced peripheral neuropathy. Tumori J. 2005;91:135–8.
39. Loprinzi C, Lacchetti C, Bleeker J, Cavaletti G, Chauhan C, Hertz D. Prevention and Management of Chemotherapy-Induced Peripheral Neuropathy in Survivors of Adult Cancers: ASCO Guideline Update J Clin Oncol. (ascopubs.org) 2020;38(38):3325–50
40. Willis WD, Westlund KN. Neuroanatomy of the pain system and of the pathways that modulate pain. J Clin Neurophysiol. 1997;14:2–31.
41. Smith EM, Pang H, Cirrincione C, Fleishman S, Paskett ED, Ahles T, et al. Effect of duloxetine on pain, function, and quality of life among patients with chemotherapy-induced painful peripheral neuropathy: a randomized clinical trial. JAMA. 2013;309(13):1359–67.
42. Hirayama Y, Ishitani K, Sato Y, Iyama S, Takada K, Murase K, et al. Effect of duloxetine in Japanese patients with chemotherapy-induced peripheral neuropathy: a pilot randomized trial. Int J Clin Oncol. 2015;20(5):866–71.

43. Hammack J, Michalak JC, Loprinzi C, Sloan J, Novotny P, Soori G, et al. Phase III evaluation of nortriptyline for alleviation of symptoms of cis-platinum-induced peripheral neuropathy. Pain. 2002;98:195–203.
44. Kautio A, Haanpää M, Saarto T, Kalso E. Amitriptyline in the treatment of chemotherapy-induced neuropathic symptoms. J Pain Symptom Manag. 2008;35:31–9.
45. Luo Z, Chaplan SR, Higuera E, Sorkin L, Stauderman K, Williams M, et al. Upregulation of dorsal root ganglion α2δ calcium channel subunit and its correlation with allodynia in spinal nerve-injured rats. The Journal of Neuroscience. 2001;21(6):1868–75.
46. Rao RD, Michalak JC, Sloan JA, Loprinzi CL, Soori GS, Nikcevich DA, et al. Efficacy of gabapentin in the management of chemotherapy-induced peripheral neuropathy: a phase 3 randomized, double-blind, placebo-controlled, crossover trial (N00C3). Cancer. 2007;110(9):2110–8.
47. Nihei S, Sato J, Kashiwaba M, Itabashi T, Kudo K, Takahashi K. Efficacy and safety of pregabalin for oxaliplatin- and paclitaxel-induced peripheral neuropathy. Gan To Kagaku Ryoho. 2013;40:1189.
48. Nagahara H, Noda E, Maeda K, Inoue T, Hirakawa T, Hasegawa T, et al. Promising effects of pregabalin in the treatment of oxaliplatin-induced sensory neuropathy in patients with colorectal carcinoma. Gan To Kagaku Ryoho. 2013;40:1181.
49. Shinde S, Seisler D, Soori G, Atherton P, Pachman D, Lafky J. Can pregabalin prevent paclitaxel-associated neuropathy? – an ACCRU pilot trial. Support Care Cancer. 2015;24:547–53.
50. Rao RD, Flynn PJ, Sloan JA, Wong GY, Novotny P, Johnson DB, et al. Efficacy of lamotrigine in the management of chemotherapy-induced peripheral neuropathy: a phase 3 randomized, double-blind, placebo-controlled trial, N01C3. Cancer. 2008;112(12):2802–8.
51. Barton DL, Wos EJ, Qin R, Mattar BI, Green NB, Lanier KS, et al. A double-blind, placebo-controlled trial of a topical treatment for chemotherapy-induced peripheral neuropathy: NCCTG trial N06CA. Support Care Cancer. 2011;19(6):833–41.
52. Gewandter JS, Mohile SG, Heckler CE, Ryan JL, Kirshner JJ, Flynn PJ, et al. A phase III randomized, placebo-controlled study of topical amitriptyline and ketamine for chemotherapy-induced peripheral neuropathy (CIPN): a University of Rochester CCOP study of 462 cancer survivors. Support Care Cancer. 2014;22(7):1807–14.
53. Galantino ML, Tiger R, Brooks J, Jang S, Wilson K. Impact of somatic yoga and meditation on fall risk, function, and quality of life for chemotherapy-induced peripheral neuropathy syndrome in cancer survivors. Integr Cancer Ther. 2019;18:1–16.
54. Kleckner IR, Dunne RF, Asare M, Cole C, Fleming F, Fung C, et al. Exercise for toxicity management in cancer – a narrative review. Oncol Hematol Rev. 2018;14:28–37.
55. Brami C, Bao T, Deng G. Natural products and complementary therapies for chemotherapy-induced peripheral neuropathy: a systematic review. Crit Rev Oncol Hematol. 2016;98:325–34.
56. Ben-Horin I, Kahan P, Ryvo L, Inbar M, Lev-Ari S, Geva R. Acupuncture and reflexology for chemotherapy-induced peripheral neuropathy in breast cancer. Integr Cancer Ther. 2017;16:258–62.
57. Zirpoli GR, McCann SE, Sucheston-Campbell LE, Hershman DL, Ciupak G, Davis W, et al. Supplement use and chemotherapy-induced peripheral neuropathy in a cooperative group trial (S0221): the DELCaP study. J Natl Cancer Inst. 2017;109(12):djx098.
58. Gamelin L, Boisdron-Celle M, Delva R, Guérin-Meyer V, Ifrah N, Morel A, et al. Prevention of oxaliplatin-related neurotoxicity by calcium and magnesium infusions: a retrospective study of 161 patients receiving oxaliplatin combined with 5-fluorouracil and leucovorin for advanced colorectal cancer. Clin Cancer Res. 2004;10:4055–61.
59. Loprinzi CL, Qin R, Dakhil SR, Fehrenbacher L, Flynn KA, Atherton P, et al. Phase III randomized, placebo-controlled, double-blind study of intravenous calcium and magnesium to prevent oxaliplatin-induced sensory neurotoxicity (N08CB/Alliance). J Clin Oncol. 2014;32(10):997–1005.
60. Pachman DR, Qin R, Seisler DK, Smith EM, Beutler AS, Ta LE, et al. Clinical course of Oxaliplatin-induced neuropathy: results from the randomized phase III trial N08CB (alliance). J Clin Oncol. 2015;33(30):3416–22.
61. Hu LY, Mi WL, Wu GC, Wang YQ, Mao-Ying QL. Prevention and treatment for chemotherapy-induced peripheral neuropathy: therapies based on CIPN mechanisms. Curr Neuropharmacol. 2019;17(2):184–96.
62. Smyth J, Bowman A, Perren T, Wilkinson P, Prescott R, Quinn K, et al. Glutathione reduces the toxicity and improves quality of life of women diagnosed with ovarian cancer treated with cisplatin: results of a double-blind, randomised trial. Ann Oncol. 1997;8:569–73.
63. Leal AD, Qin R, Atherton PJ, Haluska P, Behrens RJ, Tiber CH, et al. North Central Cancer Treatment Group/Alliance trial N08CA-the use of glutathione for prevention of paclitaxel/carboplatin-induced peripheral neuropathy: a phase 3 randomized, double-blind, placebo-controlled study. Cancer. 2014;120(12):1890–7.
64. Stubblefield M, Vahdat LT, Balmaceda C, Troxel A, Hesdorffer C, Gooch C. Glutamine as a neuroprotective agent in high-dose paclitaxel-induced peripheral neuropathy: a clinical and electrophysiologic study. Clin Oncol. 2005;17:271–6.
65. Wang WS, Lin JK, Lin TC, Chen WS, Jiang JK, Wang HS, et al. Oral glutamine is effective for preventing oxaliplatin-induced neuropathy in colorectal cancer patients. Oncologist. 2007;12(3):312–9.
66. Argyriou A, Chroni E, Koutras A, Ellul J, Papapetropoulos S, Katsoulas G, et al. Vitamin E

for prophylaxis against chemotherapy-induced neuropathy – a randomized controlled trial. Neurology. 2005;64:26–31.
67. Argyriou A, Chroni E, Koutras A, Iconomou G, Papapetropoulos S, Polychronopoulos P, et al. Preventing paclitaxel-induced peripheral neuropathy: a phase II trial of vitamin E supplementation. J Pain Symptom Manag. 2006;32:237–44.
68. Kottschade LA, Sloan JA, Mazurczak MA, Johnson DB, Murphy BP, Rowland KM, et al. The use of vitamin E for the prevention of chemotherapy-induced peripheral neuropathy: results of a randomized phase III clinical trial. Support Care Cancer. 2011;19(11):1769–77.
69. Jung AY, Cai X, Thoene K, Obi N, Jaskulski S, Behrens S, et al. Antioxidant supplementation and breast cancer prognosis in postmenopausal women undergoing chemotherapy and radiation therapy. Am J Clin Nutr. 2019;109(1):69–78.
70. Ambrosone C, Zirpoli G, Hutson A, McCann W, McCann S, Barlow W, Kelly K, et al. Dietary supplement use during chemotherapy and survival outcomes of patients with breast Cancer enrolled in a cooperative group clinical trial (SWOG S0221). J Clin Oncol. 2020;38:804–14.
71. Khalefa HG, Shawki MA, Aboelhassan R, El Wakeel LM. Evaluation of the effect of N-acetylcysteine on the prevention and amelioration of paclitaxel-induced peripheral neuropathy in breast cancer patients: a randomized controlled study. Breast Cancer Res Treat. 2020;183(1):117–25.
72. Peyton L, Fischer-Cartlidge E. Extremity cooling: a synthesis of cryotherapy interventions to reduce peripheral neuropathy and nail changes from taxane-based chemotherapy. Clin J Oncol Nurs. 2019;23:522–8.

Cancer-Related Cognitive Impairment

9

Austin Wesevich, Karen S. Johnson, and Ivy Altomare

Introduction

There is growing subjective and objective evidence to support the hypothesis that cancer itself, independent of or together with chemotherapy, can have a lasting negative impact on cognition. Cancer-related cognitive impairment (CRCI) is a broad term which refers to cognitive deficits caused by either cancer, cancer treatment, or both, and it is often difficult if not impossible to pinpoint the exact cause in an affected patient. Colloquially, this condition is often called "chemobrain." CRCI can be one of the most frustrating aspects of cancer diagnosis, treatment, and survivorship for both patients and providers. Defining this impairment, estimating the risk, testing for deficits, and managing symptoms are extremely challenging. Though it is widely recognized that many cancer patients and survivors experience a decline in cognitive function associated with cancer and/or treatment, there is a relative paucity of data as analyses are limited by inconsistent definitions, varying tumor types and treatment regimens, disparate screening tools, and non-randomized studies. The largest body of evidence studying CRCI exists among patients with breast cancer. Here we summarize the available data as it applies to breast cancer patients for CRCI epidemiology, pathogenesis, screening, and treatment.

A. Wesevich
Departments of Medicine and Pediatrics, Duke University Medical Center, Durham, NC, USA

K. S. Johnson
Physical Therapy and Occupational Therapy Department, Duke University Hospital, Durham, NC, USA

I. Altomare (✉)
Department of Medicine, Division of Medical Oncology, Duke University Medical Center, Durham, NC, USA
e-mail: ivy.altomare@duke.edu

Definition and Pathophysiology

CRCI describes mild to moderate cognitive impairment any time after cancer diagnosis or treatment in one or more of the eight cognitive domains: sensation, perception, motor skills, attention and concentration, memory, executive functioning, processing speed, and verbal skills (Table 9.1) [1]. In studies of chemotherapy-related cognitive decline, the domains related to the cerebral frontosubcortical circuit, namely, memory, processing speed, and executive function, are most commonly affected [2]. Yet the nature and magnitude of deficits are highly variable among patients, and even the designation of cognitive fields varies among studies. One cross-sectional study of 28 early-stage breast cancer patients most frequently identified decreased attention, concentration, memory, mental flexibility, motor function, and visuospatial ability

G. G. Kimmick et al. (eds.), *Common Issues in Breast Cancer Survivors*,
https://doi.org/10.1007/978-3-030-75377-1_9

Table 9.1 Cognitive domains and subdomains [1]

Cognitive domain	Subdomain I	Subdomain II	Subdomain III
Sensation	Multisensory		
Perception	Object recognition Organizational strategies		
Motor skills and construction	Copying Drawing Other praxic skills		
Attention and concentration	Selective attention Sustained attention/vigilance		
Memory	Working memory Central executive Maintenance Manipulation Episodic/declarative Procedural Semantic Prospective	Verbal Spatial Object Location Time-based Event-based	Encoding Storage Retrieval (free, cued, forced-choice)
Executive functioning	Reasoning Problem-solving Component skills management		
Processing speed	Fluency Coding and tracking		
Language/verbal skills	Naming Fluency Reading and comprehension		

compared to matched controls [3]. A longitudinal study of 18 breast cancer patients receiving adjuvant FAC (5-fluorouracil, doxorubicin, and cyclophosphamide) chemotherapy found the most common domains involved in cognitive decline at 3 weeks post-chemotherapy were attention, learning, and processing speed [4].

As mentioned above, CRCI describes the mental deficits caused by the cancer itself as well as any effects on cognition by chemotherapy or other anti-neoplastic therapies such as radiation, endocrine therapy, and targeted therapy. Notably, up to one-third of cancer patients may have neurocognitive deficits at baseline, even before they receive cancer treatment [5]. Hypotheses for the etiologies of CRCI have centered upon the cancer itself, the treatment received, or risk factors shared between developing cancer and developing cognitive problems. For example, impairment can be caused by direct DNA damage by cytotoxic therapy leading to neurodegeneration, DNA repair impairment, cytokine elevation, neurotransmitter depletion, reduced antioxidant capacity, or thrombosis within CNS microvasculature. We will focus on data examining the specifically proposed mechanisms of genetic susceptibility, underlying inflammation or immune dysfunction, neural toxicity, and hormonal alterations [6–8].

Host Characteristics and Genetic Susceptibility

One of the theories for CRCI pathogenesis is that the genetic risk factors for developing cancer itself and for cognitive problems after treatment are shared. Risk factors include the presence of low-efficiency efflux pumps, deficits in DNA-repair mechanisms, deregulated immune responses and functioning of cytokines, inherently compromised blood-brain barrier efficiency, and genetically modulated reductions in neural repair capacity and neurotransmitter activity [9]. Specifically, one study assessed the role of the E4 allele of apolipoprotein E, as it is associated with higher risk of Alzheimer's disease and worse cognitive outcomes for those with brain injury, and found that lymphoma and breast cancer survivors treated with standard chemotherapy who had at least one copy of the allele had worse visual memory and spatial ability than those without any copies of the E4 allele [10, 11].

Inflammation and Immune Dysfunction

Several studies have assessed various cytokine levels in breast cancer patients to determine their potential roles in CRCI. One study focused on elucidating the role of inflammation since it is a process that could be modified. Breast cancer survivors who received post-surgical radiotherapy and cyclophosphamide, methotrexate, and 5-fluorouracil (CMF) chemotherapy had a lower global cognitive performance on average than a population-based sample of similarly aged cancer-free women. There was a statistically significant association between higher levels of inflammatory markers and lower general cognitive factor scores, even when stratifying to cancer survivors [6]. Another analysis attempted to determine the relationship between circulating cytokines and cognitive performance prior to starting cancer treatment. Post-menopausal patients with newly diagnosed breast cancer had lower memory performance and higher levels of IL-1ra than age-matched controls, while cytokines explained 6% of the total variance in memory performance in cancer patients but not control patients, after adjusting for demographics and cognitive factors [5]. Measurement of cytokine levels prior to chemotherapy and then 12 weeks after initiating chemotherapy in 99 breast cancer patients demonstrated statistically significant associations to change in cognitive performance from baseline before chemotherapy over the same time period for IL-1β and IL-6 with an inverse relationship, and for IL-4 with a direct relationship [12]. Lastly, another study measured 17 different cytokines in 75 early-stage breast cancer patients at five different time points over 2 years and found the most variability over time in IL-6, IL-12, IL-17, G-CSF, MIPS-1β, and MCP-1. At baseline, patients with faster psychomotor speed also had higher G-CSF and lower IL-17. At the conclusion of the study, IL-7 and MCP-1 were inversely associated with psychomotor speed and complex attention, while MIPS-1β correlated to better complex attention [13].

Neural Toxicity

A variety of neuroimaging studies demonstrate pervasive gray and white matter volume loss, reduced white matter connectivity and integrity, and altered brain activation for patients with CRCI, with changes both existing prior to treatment and/or exacerbated by chemotherapy [7, 14, 15]. One study sought to evaluate associations between brain imaging and cytokine levels for breast cancer patients who had completed initial treatment and found that metabolism within the medial prefrontal and anterior temporal cortices on PET/CT brain imaging corresponded to pro-inflammatory cytokine levels (IL-1ra and sTNF-RII) and memory complaints at baseline, after treatment, and 1 year after chemotherapy [16]. Another study used MRI to measure bilateral hippocampal volumes in breast cancer survivors and healthy female controls and compared measurements to various cytokine levels. The results suggest that cytokine levels and left hippocampal volumes for both groups were associated with verbal memory performance, and that changes in hippocampal volume and in verbal memory after chemotherapy could be mediated by TNF-α and IL-6 [17]. A prospective study of breast cancer patients and healthy controls demonstrated increased bifrontal and decreased left parietal activation than controls prior to treatment; this resulted in decreased frontal hyperactivation after completing chemotherapy and increased hyperactivation 1 year after completing chemotherapy [15].

Hormonal Alterations

Both animal and human studies allude to a role that estrogen might play in cognitive function. Estrogen receptors are located throughout the brain in the hypothalamus, pituitary gland, limbic system, and cerebral cortex. Estrogen has been found to have a variety of positive effects in oophorectomized rats: improved synapse formation, promoted cholinergic activity, and reduced β-amyloid deposition [18, 19]. A variety of observational studies demonstrate the possible negative effects of estrogen absence after oophorectomy, including increased risk of cognitive impairment, dementia, and parkinsonism, and those effects were directly correlated with worse outcomes for oophorectomy at an earlier age, regardless of indication [19–23]. However, a meta-analysis of 36 randomized trials confirmed a negative impact of oophorectomy but concluded that estrogen replacement therapy may have a stronger and more lasting negative effect on cognition over time [24].

Several studies have looked at the role of hormone therapy on cognition. A randomized trial of over 2000 post-menopausal women determined there were small decreases in global cognitive functioning when receiving conjugated equine estrogen therapies that persisted even after stopping therapy [25, 26]. Similarly, estrogen receptor modulators tamoxifen and raloxifene both seem to lead to small negative effects in cognitive function in postmenopausal women [27, 28]. Various other studies demonstrate a possible relationship between antiestrogen medications and cognitive deficits [18, 29, 30]. However, a longitudinal study of 101 breast cancer patients determined that there were no significant adverse effects of aromatase inhibitors or tamoxifen with regard to cognitive function [31]. Thus, the true impact of oophorectomy and anti-estrogen hormonal therapy on CRCI is, as yet, unclear.

Epidemiology

Prevalence rates of CRCI in breast cancer patients and survivors vary greatly depending on the study. One systematic review concluded a prevalence of 17–75% of breast cancer survivors having deficits in various cognitive domains, occurring from 6 months to 20 years after being exposed to chemotherapy [32]. A different paper cited an incidence of 19–78% of CRCI [2]. The wide range of reported CRCI rates may relate to inconsistent definitions of cognitive impairment across the studies [33]. Therefore, the lack of a clear definition of CRCI causes inherently wide variations of prevalence rates, making it difficult to counsel patients on the risk of this sometimes debilitating condition.

As mentioned previously, cognitive deficits may pre-exist before ever being treated with chemotherapy, with 20–30% of breast cancer patients having lower cognitive performance than age- and education-matched controls at baseline [32]. Assessing cognitive function at baseline is problematic, however, as performance may be affected by emotional distress due to the recent cancer diagnoses, introducing bias [34]. A study of 101 breast cancer patients administered 12 standardized cognitive tests prior to starting chemotherapy and after completion; at baseline prior to chemotherapy, patients were below test norms for 5 of the 12 tests, but patients showed significant improvement overall at the second assessment that occurred roughly 5 months later ($p < 0.001$). Performance was independent of anxiety, depression, or self-reported cognitive problems [33].

Some studies question whether "chemobrain" is a true phenomenon. A meta-analysis of 30 studies outlined a negative relationship between cognitive domains and chemotherapy for 20 of 21 average weighted effect sizes, and a nonsignificant association between chemotherapy and cognitive scores when comparing cognitive performance to a patient's own baseline score [35]. Two follow-up meta-analyses suggested diminishing relationships between chemotherapy and cognitive impairment, especially when taking into consideration whether study design was prospective and longitudinal [36, 37]. By following the same patients over time instead of comparing them to controls or test score norms, the relationship between chemotherapy and cognitive impairment becomes less and less clear [33]. It is unclear if this is because the relationship does not exist or if the effects attenuate over time.

A longitudinal study of 18 breast cancer patients was designed to evaluate the aforementioned meta-analysis' claim and found that 6 patients had cognitive impairment at baseline, 11 patients had relative impairment compared to baseline in at least one domain shortly after chemotherapy, and of those 11, 5 remained stable long-term, 5 showed improvement, and 1 showed mixed results [4]. A larger longitudinal study later compared 50 breast cancer patients on adjuvant chemotherapy to 43 healthy controls and demonstrated that patients receiving chemotherapy were more likely to show cognitive decline over time than controls (34% vs 19%, OR 2.25) [38]. A third longitudinal study of 71 breast cancer patients demonstrated declines in visuospatial skill, attention, delayed memory, and motor function from pre-chemotherapy baseline to 1 week after completing chemotherapy that then improved by 6 months post-chemotherapy, but it did not find any changes in immediate memory, language, and executive function scores [39]. A fourth longitudinal study of 42 breast cancer patients demonstrated that 21% had cognitive dysfunction at baseline and that a majority of patients had cognitive decline during and shortly after chemotherapy that continued declining 1 year after completing chemotherapy, while a subset demonstrated new delayed cognitive decline [40].

Summarizing data from these reports and others, it seems that up to 30% of breast cancer patients have a cognitive deficit prior to chemotherapy, as high as 75% experience CRCI during treatment, and up to 35% continue to experience CRCI for many years after completing treatment [7, 41, 42]. A subgroup of patients, roughly 17–34%, suffer from persistent long-term cognitive changes after completing chemotherapy [9]. A case-cohort study compared 196 breast cancer patients with prior CMF therapy to 1509 healthy women aged 50–80 years old, and demonstrated worse immediate and delayed verbal memory, processing speed, executive functioning, and psychomotor speed more than 20 years after completing chemotherapy [43].

Chemotherapy Type

For cognitive deficits occurring during treatment, there does seem to be a dose-response relationship with chemotherapy [14]. This could be related to direct neurotoxicity from higher doses of chemotherapy or multi-agent chemotherapy [2]. A workshop in 2003 comprised of oncologists, psychologists, radiologists, basic scientists, and patient advocates published a report that discussed how patients who received CMF had greater cognitive dysfunction than those who received anthracycline-based chemotherapy [34]. A different study compared rates of CRCI among patients receiving cyclophosphamide, thiotepa, and carboplatin (CTC), FEC, and healthy controls. While there were no differences at baseline, the CTC group had worse cognitive performance 6 months after completing chemotherapy than the control group, but a significant difference was not observed between FEC and controls or between no chemotherapy and controls [44].

Symptom Burden and Comorbid Conditions

Patients experiencing chemobrain may report multiple symptoms regarding their thinking ability, fatigue, and mood. Fatigue may play a role in cognitive performance, as one study of 75 women with early-stage breast cancer demonstrated that fatigue severity worsened during chemotherapy and resolved close to baseline by 2 years after chemotherapy, and fatigue severity and impact correlated with slower processing speed and reduced complex attention performance [45]. Several studies comment on the relationship between psychological distress, such as depression or anxiety, and measured cognitive deficits. In one study, the subset of breast cancer patients who reported symptoms of depression or anxiety that met the definition of "clinically significant distress-impaired" (CSD-I) were significantly more likely to be cognitively impaired [46]. In contrast, a study comparing breast cancer patients and healthy controls showed no differences between those with cognitive deficits and normal cognitive performance with regard to depression, anxiety, or fatigue [47]. Finally, a recent longitudinal study comparing 581 breast cancer patients to 364 age-matched non-cancer controls found significant increases in self-reported cognitive difficulties for patients immediately post-chemotherapy and at 6 months follow-up compared to controls, and baseline anxiety and depression as well as decreased cognitive reserve were associated with lower scores [41].

When looking longitudinally, some of the symptom burden might improve more for cancer patients over subsequent years than for controls. Fatigue, menopausal symptoms, and cognitive dysfunction all showed greater improvement at 1 and 2 years post-chemotherapy than the relative changes for healthy controls in a study of 100 pairs of patients with patient-nominated age-matched controls [48]. Patients treated with CMF therapy had fewer symptoms of depression 20 years after chemotherapy than controls even if their memory complaints were more severe and not entirely explained by their cognitive test performance [43].

Work-Up and Cognitive Assessments

Various tools exist to identify cognitive impairment, yet a concise validated screening assessment is lacking. Methods include objective functioning tests, neuropsychological testing, magnetic resonance imaging (MRI), and questionnaires and interviews. The lack of validated and universally accepted assessments makes clinical diagnosis challenging and complicates interpretation of research in this field. The following is a discussion of available tools and recommendations for clinical work-up (Fig. 9.1).

Screening for Comorbid Conditions and Medication Review

Comorbid medical and psychiatric conditions can exacerbate cognitive dysfunction, and therefore diagnosing such conditions should be part of the initial work-up for CRCI. The physician or care team should screen for depression, anxiety, substance use/abuse, and sleep disorders. Fatigue and pain syndromes should be identified. Limited laboratory tests are useful to evaluate for vitamin deficiencies, thyroid imbalance, hepatic or renal insufficiency, and/or anemia and may be checked at the provider's discretion. The Mini-Mental State Examination is not sensitive enough to detect subtle declines in cognitive performance but can be deployed to screen for underlying dementia [49]. A full review of the patient's medications, herbal supplements, and over-the-counter medicines should be conducted in order to eliminate and/or adjust medications which can impair cognition as much as is possible.

Neuroimaging

Neuroimaging can reveal structural brain changes among patients during or after chemotherapy treatment, supporting a neural basis for cognitive changes when compared with baseline imaging or healthy controls. One prospective study performed sequential structural MRIs to assess voxel-based morphometry (VBM) in 55 breast cancer patients treated with and without chemotherapy and compared them to matched healthy controls. VBM is a neuroimaging technique that investigated associations between gray and white matter [50]. Decreased white matter density was found among chemotherapy patients, which correlated to self-reported difficulties in executive functioning [51]. In a similar MRI study among breast cancer survivors, decreased gray matter was shown in the frontal lobes, temporal lobes, and cerebellar regions 1 month after chemotherapy with partial recovery after 1 year [52]. A more recent assessment measured VBM in 28 breast cancer patients and 29 matched controls, and found decreased gray matter density in various areas of the frontal cortex and cerebellum after chemo. Furthermore, the number of chemotherapy cycles was negatively associated with verbal fluency, digit span performance, and general cognitive capacity [53]. Despite the objective evidence of brain changes, it is neither feasible nor cost-effective to perform complex neuroimaging in clinical practice to diagnose CRCI, and therefore these modalities remain methods of research.

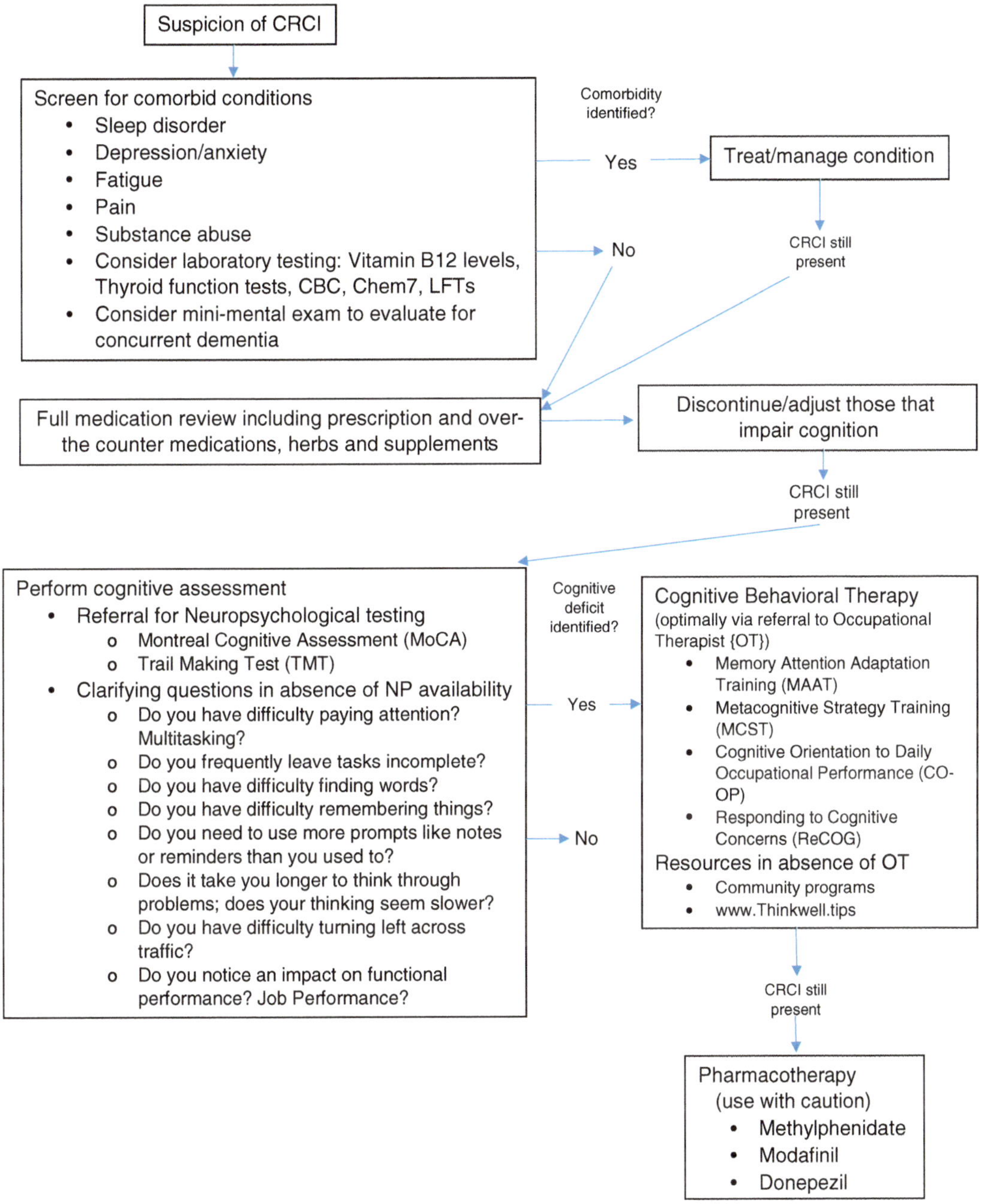

Fig. 9.1 Assessment and management of CRCI

Neuropsychological Testing

Neuropsychological testing is comprised of robust, comprehensive, and complex assessments typically performed by a neuropsychologist, neurologist, or geriatric psychiatrist, usually taking at least 4 hours to complete. Neuropsychological testing consists of a thorough battery of tests to assess eight functional domains [1] and can be helpful to clarify specific areas of cognitive dysfunction [49]. As mentioned previously, the number, classification, and description of the various domains and subdomains are generally agreed upon, though there are inconsistencies in the clinical and research literature, with some sources indicating fewer or more domains and varying definitions, further complicating research and interpretation of outcomes in this field [1]. Functional assessments are not standardized and can vary by practitioner, but usually include evaluation of motivation, IQ, attention, information processing, language functioning, visual spatial function, executive functioning, memory, and behavioral and emotional functioning [54]. One study used neuropsychological testing to measure cognitive function in 50 breast cancer patients before and after chemotherapy treatments and 43 healthy controls. The neuropsychological testing used in the study measured visual memory, verbal memory, executive functioning, working memory, and processing speed along with two questionnaires related to psychological morbidity and everyday cognitive problems [38]. The study found that chemotherapy patients were more likely to show cognitive decline than the controls. These findings were confirmed in another study of 60 newly diagnosed breast cancer patients and 45 healthy controls where neuropsychological testing of verbal memory, visual memory, processing speed, simple vigilance, distractibility, executive functioning, and verbal ability was measured several times over a year. The findings reliably detected moderate to large cognitive changes, with limited ability to detect more subtle cognitive changes. Even with differences among testing methods used by investigators, these studies support supports neuropsychological testing as the gold standard for assessing CRCI [54].

Occupational therapists often perform the Montreal Cognitive Assessment (MoCA), Trail Making Test (TMT), and other functional assessments as part of their evaluation for patients referred for therapy. Therefore a referral accomplishes both screening and treatment (discussed below), ensuring a thorough assessment, insight into scope of impairments, impact of occupations, and establishment of client-centered goals for optimized improvements. Working in conjunction with rehabilitation services can give better insight than relying on screening measures such as the MOCA or TMT alone [55].

Treatment

Treatments to address CRCI include acknowledgment of the problem, addressing comorbid issues, behavioral and/or occupational therapy, and pharmacologic treatments (Fig. 9.1). The most important first step in treatment is to acknowledge that CRCI is a real syndrome. For many survivors, validation of impairments can be therapeutic and helpful on its own [49]. Optimal treatment of CRCI requires a team approach. "A proactive inter-disciplinary team approach comprising the oncology medical staff and allied health professionals is essential to ensure a holistic partnership to provide better care, and to address the participation needs of cancer patients" [56].

Comorbid Conditions and Medication Review

If one of the aforementioned comorbidities is identified such as sleep disorder, depression, thyroid imbalance, vitamin deficiency, anemia, anxiety, pain, and/or fatigue, aggressive management should be initiated. Substance use and/or abuse should be identified and addressed. A thorough medication review, including over-the-counter medications, vitamins, and supplements, should be conducted to minimize use of medications which impair cognition. If there is concern for concurrent dementia, a referral to a neurologist may be warranted for management.

Cognitive Behavioral Therapy

Cognitive Behavioral Therapy (CBT) is perhaps the best way to address CRCI which persists after comorbid condition management and medication reconciliation, though large randomized trials confirming efficacy are limited. One small prospective randomized study compared 32 breast cancer survivors to a wait list control group of 16 patients. Patients were eligible if they had stage I–III breast cancer, completed treatment 18 months to 5 years earlier, and had documented cognitive complaints and poor scores on neuropsychological testing. CBT was delivered over 5 weeks for 2 hours per week via group interventions targeting attention over the first 2 weeks, executive functioning in week 3, memory in week 4, and functions and review in week 5. Education included instruction, in-class and homework exercises, and goal-setting. The patients receiving CBT showed immediate and sustained improvements at 2 months post treatment in self-reported cognitive complaints, memory functioning, and neurocognitive testing [57].

Another form of CBT, Memory and Attention Adaptation Training (MAAT), has been successfully used to treat cognitive impairment in breast cancer survivors. MAAT consists of four cognitive-behavioral components: (1) education on memory and attention; (2) self-awareness training; (3) self-regulation emphasizing arousal reduction through relaxation training, activity scheduling, and pacing; and (4) cognitive compensatory strategies training [58]. MAAT was implemented in 29 patients with stage I or II breast cancer and CRCI an average of 8 years post chemotherapy. For the intervention, each participant received a workbook, four individual monthly visits, and seven phone contacts between visits for support. The visits were 30–50 minutes and included reviewing the participants' current knowledge of chemo-associated memory problems, strategies to identify "at risk" situations where memory failures occur, and learned and rehearsed compensatory strategies specific to their difficulties. Telephone contact provided support and assistance for applying strategies. Assessment of self-reported cognitive function, quality of life, and standard neuropsychological testing was performed post treatment, 2 months and 6 months after treatment. Significant improvements were noted in self-reporting of daily cognitive function, quality of life measures, and neuropsychological test performance [58]. Another study of MAAT was conducted consisting of 40 stage I and II female breast cancer survivors with CRCI. Participants were assessed at baseline, and post-intervention at 2-month follow-up on measures of self-reported daily cognitive failures, quality of life, and neuropsychological performance as well as satisfaction with MAAT. Treatments consisted of four biweekly individual office visits with phone contacts between visits. The visits were 30–50 minutes in duration and included review of present findings and knowledge about cognitive effects of chemotherapy, strategies to improve awareness of times when cognitive failures might occur, education, and rehearsal for compensatory strategies to prevent or lessen negative consequences of cognitive failure. MAAT participants made significant improvements on the spiritual well-being subscale of the quality of life measure and on verbal memory; statistical significance was not achieved on self-reporting of daily cognitive complaints. Participants rated MAAT with high satisfaction [59].

Occupational Therapy

Occupational therapy (OT) is a highly skilled patient-centered practice focused on improving health, well-being, and functional abilities [60]. OT has the potential to limit and/or reverse cancer-related disability through client-centered therapy interventions. Treatments for CRCI address cognitive deficits related to function and might include remedial as well as compensatory strategies to improve a patient's ability to engage in activities that are meaningful to them. Occupational therapists work with patients to find strategies that work best for their life and might include setting alarms, using written reminders for appointment or medications, strategies for improving safety with cooking, and money and home management. Additionally, occupational therapists address patients' continuing engagement in the community including safety with shopping, driving, wayfinding, and use of public transportation [61]. Occupational therapists are trained and able to use CBT with good results. Improvements in cognitive outcomes result from metacognitive strategy training (MCST), another form of CBT that facilitates improvements in cognitive dysfunction. The MCST treatment approach, led by an occupational therapist using Cognitive Orientation to Daily Occupational Performance (CO-OP), incorporates seven key features: (1) cognitive strategy use, (2) patient-chosen goals, (3) dynamic performance analysis, (4) guided discovery, (5) enabling principles, (6) parent/significant other involvement, and (7) intervention. The process for creating goals, working through, and attaining goals is a dynamic process between the client and the therapist. This approach was tested in 17 female breast cancer survivors with CRCI. Fourteen of the 17 women completed the CO-OP treatment, which was implemented over 12 sessions with reassessment at 4 weeks after completion. The program resulted in a medium to very large effect on primary cognitive outcomes with the exception of sleep function [62]. In another study of 27 breast cancer survivors with CRCI at least 6–60 months out from completing primary treatment, Cognitive Rehab (CR) led by occupational therapists was evaluated. Responding to Cognitive Concerns (ReCog) is a method used by trained OTs and/or CBT psychologists which involves skills training, compensatory strategies, group discussion, and, between sessions, homework to reinforce practice and understanding of the group-taught techniques over 4 weeks in groups of 3–9 participants. Session topics included aging, health, cancer and cognitive function, memory, attention fatigue, emotions, and cognition. Four sessions were completed weekly for 2 hours and co-facilitated by two occupational therapists or an occupational therapist and an occupational therapy student. Participants reported improved perception of cognitive impairments, improved impact on their quality of life, improved working memory, decreased impulsivity, and decreased psychological distress. Objective improvements were seen in information processing and executive functioning [63].

Community Programs

Unfortunately, not all breast cancer survivors with CRCI will have access to OT or CBT but might benefit from community programs (available locally or accessed via the Internet). Community programs can reach a broader base including breast cancer survivors and family members and improve overall brain health literacy. An example of this includes The Think Well program which provides face-to-face educational seminars and extension via their website (www.ThinkWell.tips) [64]. The goals of the program are to impact broad areas known to influence brain health and cognition including physical exercise/activity, intellectual exercise/activity, sleep hygiene, substance use, mood support, social engagement, and nutrition. Materials are supplied to leverage other free or low-cost local resources. This program was able to reach 666 attendees comprised of cancer survivors and family or friends of breast cancer survivors over a span of 4 years. Attendees reported high satisfaction with the program reporting that their goals were met for attending, the material was relevant for cognitive needs, relevant to their cultural beliefs, and useful for coping and to communicate cognitive concerns [64].

In summary, CBT is the most promising therapy for CRCI, and when paired with individualized or group care led by an occupational therapist, patients have reported high satisfaction. Additionally, occupational therapists can address any other impairments such as pain, fatigue, and peripheral neuropathy that may impact daily skills such as bathing, dressing, cooking, writing, and medication management [61]. OT focuses on effective strategies to decrease limitations and optimize function and quality of life [49]. Though data supports use of CBT and OT, improvements are admittedly modest, with improvements in perceptions of function by the survivor with compensatory strategies rather than full restoration of premorbid cognitive functioning.

Pharmacological Treatments

Pharmacological treatments may be an option after non-pharmacologic interventions have not been successful. Drugs such as methylphenidate, modafinil, and donepezil have shown a very limited positive impact on cognitive functioning, only in a minority of cognitive domains tested, with results of studies detailed below. Data is sparse, and cumulative side effects of these medications must be weighed against any perceived benefit.

CNS Stimulants

The central nervous system (CNS) stimulant methylphenidate commonly used for attention deficit hyperactivity disorder (ADHD) and narcolepsy has demonstrated limited benefit with regard to CRCI among child cancer survivors [65]. One placebo-controlled randomized trial of 122 children in remission from acute lymphocytic leukemia (ALL) assessed attention, memory, and academic achievement via neuropsychiatric testing before and after study drug administration [65]. Significant improvement was seen in selective attention, impulsivity, and cognitive flexibility, but no improvement in global attention, concentration, or memory. Studies evaluating methylphenidate among breast cancer survivors have been even more disappointing [66]. In a randomized placebo controlled trial of 57 breast cancer patients undergoing neuropsychiatric testing at baseline and 6 months after treatment completion, there was no difference in quality of life or neuropsychology testing results at any time point among patients taking methylphenidate [66]. Another CNS stimulant, modafinil, is used in narcolepsy and works by binding to the dopamine transporter, inhibiting dopamine reuptake. It's utility for CRCI was tested in a randomized placebo controlled trial of 4 weeks treatment in 82 breast cancer survivors [67]. This study was designed primarily to assess the impact of modafinil on fatigue, though a secondary analysis evaluated cognitive function. After a brief 4-week exposure to modafinil, patients experienced significant improvement in the speed of memory, quality of memory, and continuity of attention but no improvements in the quality of working memory or power of attention [67]. Modafinil may be helpful for fatigue, and may enhance some attention skills, but has limited ability to impact global cognitive functioning.

Cholinesterase Inhibitors

Donepezil is a cholinesterase inhibitor which has been used for years to improve memory and cognitive functioning in patients with Alzheimer's disease and other forms of dementia. Unfortunately, use in CRCI shows little benefit to date [68]. A prospective randomized placebo controlled trial of 62 breast cancer survivors, 1–5 years after treatment completion, was conducted. Patients were given donepezil or placebo for 24 weeks with dose escalation, and neuropsychological testing via the Hopkins Verbal Learning Test and self-reported quality of life was assessed at baseline and after treatment. The parameters of attention, memory, language, visuomotor skills, processing speed, executive function, and motor dexterity were analyzed. The results were disappointing, and showed an improvement in only two of seven categories – recall and word discrimination – and no difference in any other functioning measures, quality of life, or subjective cognitive function [68].

In summary, the aforementioned pharmacologic therapies have been tested with disappointing or limited results and often no measurable benefit in cognitive function and/or quality of life, and therefore cannot be universally recommended.

Summary and Recommendations

It is clear that CRCI, or chemobrain, is a real medical issue affecting breast cancer survivors. Defining, studying, and testing this problem is challenging. Trials are small and sometimes poor quality, chemotherapy regimens may be outdated, and the amount of chemotherapy exposure, timing of assessment, and duration of follow-up vary among trials, limiting applicability of findings and comparison of data. Validated neuropsychological testing tools are lacking, use is inconsistent among trials, and many of these are not feasible in clinical practice. Indeed, performance on neuropsychological testing may not even reflect the degree of the patient's perceived deficit. Thes available dsata suggest that prevalence of long-term CRCI is 35%. Risk factors are unclear, though age and cognitive deficit at baseline seem important. The magnitude of deficit will vary widely among patients, with longer chemotherapy duration correlating with more profound deficits, and impairment may or may not improve over time. Brain imaging supports organic injury and the mechanism of damage is clearly complex. Screening is recommended, but informal, and useful tools include referral for extensive neuropsychological testing or in-office use of the MOCA and/or TMT tests. Care teams should identify and address comorbid conditions such as depression, anxiety, substance use/abuse, pain, and sleep disturbance. Referral to a cognitive or occupational therapist is likely the best and most comprehensive way to identify and impact CRCI, though availability of and reimbursement for these services restricts widespread implementation. Small trials of brief exposure to CNS stimulants or anti-dementia medications offer slight subjective and/or objective benefit, and can be helpful for some patients. There is vast opportunity for further research in this burdensome condition.

References

1. Harvey PD. Domains of cognition and their assessment. Dialogues Clin Neurosci. 2019;21:227–37.
2. Wefel JS, Schagen SB. Chemotherapy-related cognitive dysfunction. Curr Neurol Neurosci Rep. 2012;12:267–75.
3. Wieneke MH, Dienst ER. Neuropsychological assessment of cognitive functioning following chemotherapy for breast cancer. Psychooncology. 1995;4:61–6.
4. Wefel JS, Lenzi R, Theriault RL, Davis RN, Meyers CA. The cognitive sequelae of standard-dose adjuvant chemotherapy in women with breast carcinoma: results of a prospective, randomized, longitudinal trial. Cancer. 2004;100:2292–9.
5. Patel SK, et al. Inflammatory biomarkers, comorbidity, and neurocognition in women with newly diagnosed breast cancer. JNCI J Natl Cancer Inst. 2015;107(8):djv131.
6. van der Willik KD, et al. Inflammation markers and cognitive performance in breast cancer survivors 20 years after completion of chemotherapy: a cohort study. Breast Cancer Res BCR. 2018;20(1):135.
7. Janelsins MC, Kesler SR, Ahles TA, Morrow GR. Prevalence, mechanisms, and management of cancer-related cognitive impairment. Int Rev Psychiatry Abingdon Engl. 2014;26:102–113.
8. Ahles TA, et al. Longitudinal assessment of cognitive changes associated with adjuvant treatment for breast cancer: impact of age and cognitive reserve. J Clin Oncol. 2010;28:4434–40.
9. Ahles TA, Saykin AJ. Candidate mechanisms for chemotherapy-induced cognitive changes. Nat Rev Cancer. 2007;7:192–201.
10. Ahles TA, et al. The relationship of APOE genotype to neuropsychological performance in long-term cancer survivors treated with standard dose chemotherapy. Psychooncology. 2003;12:612–9.
11. Vardy J, Wefel JS, Ahles T, Tannock IF, Schagen SB. Cancer and cancer-therapy related cognitive dysfunction: an international perspective from the Venice cognitive workshop. Ann Oncol. 2008;19:623–9.
12. Cheung YT, et al. Association of proinflammatory cytokines and chemotherapy-associated cognitive impairment in breast cancer patients: a multi-centered, prospective, cohort study. Ann Oncol. 2015;26:1446–51.
13. Lyon DE, et al. Relationship of systemic cytokine concentrations to cognitive function over two years in women with early stage breast cancer. J Neuroimmunol. 2016;301:74–82.
14. Wefel JS, Kesler SR, Noll KR, Schagen SB. Clinical characteristics, pathophysiology, and management of noncentral nervous system cancer-related cognitive impairment in adults. CA Cancer J Clin. 2015;65:123–38.
15. McDonald BC, Conroy SK, Ahles TA, West JD, Saykin AJ. Alterations in brain activation during working memory processing associated with breast cancer and treatment: a prospective functional magnetic resonance imaging study. J Clin Oncol. 2012;30:2500–8.
16. Pomykala KL, et al. The association between pro-inflammatory cytokines, regional cerebral

metabolism, and cognitive complaints following adjuvant chemotherapy for breast cancer. Brain Imaging Behav. 2013;7:511–23.
17. Kesler S, et al. Reduced hippocampal volume and verbal memory performance associated with interleukin-6 and tumor necrosis factor-alpha levels in chemotherapy-treated breast cancer survivors. Brain Behav Immun. 2013;30:S109–16.
18. Phillips K-A, Bernhard J. Adjuvant breast cancer treatment and cognitive function: current knowledge and research directions. JNCI J Natl Cancer Inst. 2003;95:190–7.
19. Rocca WA, et al. Increased risk of cognitive impairment or dementia in women who underwent oophorectomy before menopause. Neurology. 2007;69:1074–83.
20. Rocca WA, Grossardt BR, Shuster LT. Oophorectomy, estrogen, and dementia: a 2014 update. Mol Cell Endocrinol. 2014;389:7–12.
21. Rocca WA, Grossardt BR, Maraganore DM. The long-term effects of oophorectomy on cognitive and motor aging are age dependent. Neurodegener Dis. 2008;5:257–60.
22. Rocca WA, et al. Increased risk of parkinsonism in women who underwent oophorectomy before menopause. Neurology. 2008;70:200–9.
23. Rocca WA, et al. Bilateral oophorectomy and accelerated aging: cause or effect? J Gerontol A Biol Sci Med Sci. 2017;72:1213–7.
24. Hogervorst E, Bandelow S. Sex steroids to maintain cognitive function in women after the menopause: a meta-analyses of treatment trials. Maturitas. 2010;66:56–71.
25. Resnick SM, et al. The Women's Health Initiative Study of Cognitive Aging (WHISCA): a randomized clinical trial of the effects of hormone therapy on age-associated cognitive decline. Clin Trials. 2004;1:440–50.
26. Espeland MA, et al. Long term effects of conjugated equine estrogens therapies on domain-specific cognitive function: results from the Women's Health Initiative Study of Cognitive Aging (WHISCA) extension. J Am Geriatr Soc. 2010;58:1263–71.
27. Espeland MA, et al. Relative effects of tamoxifen, raloxifene, and conjugated equine estrogens on cognition. J Women's Health. 2010;19:371–9.
28. Legault C, et al. Effects of tamoxifen and raloxifene on memory and other cognitive abilities: cognition in the study of tamoxifen and raloxifene. J Clin Oncol. 2009;27:5144–52.
29. Castellon SA, et al. Neurocognitive performance in breast cancer survivors exposed to adjuvant chemotherapy and tamoxifen. J Clin Exp Neuropsychol. 2004;26:955–69.
30. Palmer JL, Trotter T, Joy AA, Carlson LE. Cognitive effects of tamoxifen in pre-menopausal women with breast cancer compared to healthy controls. J Cancer Surviv. 2008;2:275–82.
31. Hermelink K, et al. Short-term effects of treatment-induced hormonal changes on cognitive function in breast cancer patients. Cancer. 2008;113:2431–9.
32. Ahles TA, Root JC, Ryan EL. Cancer- and cancer treatment–associated cognitive change: an update on the state of the science. J Clin Oncol. 2012;30:3675–86.
33. Hermelink K, et al. Cognitive function during neoadjuvant chemotherapy for breast cancer. Cancer. 2007;109:1905–13.
34. Tannock IF, Ahles TA, Ganz PA, van Dam FS. Cognitive impairment associated with chemotherapy for cancer: report of a workshop. J Clin Oncol. 2004;22:2233–9.
35. Anderson-Hanley C, Sherman ML, Riggs R, Agocha VB, Compas BE. Neuropsychological effects of treatments for adults with cancer: a meta-analysis and review of the literature. J Int Neuropsychol Soc. 2003;9:967–82.
36. Jansen CE, Miaskowski C, Dodd M, Dowling G, Kramer J. A metaanalysis of studies of the effects of cancer chemotherapy on various domains of cognitive function. Cancer. 2005;104:2222–33.
37. Falleti MG, Sanfilippo A, Maruff P, Weih L, Phillips K-A. The nature and severity of cognitive impairment associated with adjuvant chemotherapy in women with breast cancer: a meta-analysis of the current literature. Brain Cogn. 2005;59:60–70.
38. Shilling V, Jenkins V, Morris R, Deutsch G, Bloomfield D. The effects of adjuvant chemotherapy on cognition in women with breast cancer—preliminary results of an observational longitudinal study. Breast. 2005;14:142–50.
39. Jansen CE, Cooper BA, Dodd MJ, Miaskowski CA. A prospective longitudinal study of chemotherapy-induced cognitive changes in breast cancer patients. Support Care Cancer. 2011;19:1647–56.
40. Wefel JS, Saleeba AK, Buzdar AU, Meyers CA. Acute and late onset cognitive dysfunction associated with chemotherapy in women with breast cancer. Cancer. 2010;116:3348–56.
41. Janelsins MC, et al. Cognitive complaints in survivors of breast cancer after chemotherapy compared with age-matched controls: an analysis from a nationwide, multicenter, prospective longitudinal study. J Clin Oncol. 2017;35:506–14.
42. Janelsins MC, et al. An update on cancer- and chemotherapy-related cognitive dysfunction: current status. Semin Oncol. 2011;38:431–8.
43. Koppelmans V, et al. Neuropsychological performance in survivors of breast cancer more than 20 years after adjuvant chemotherapy. J Clin Oncol. 2012;30:1080–6.
44. Schagen SB, Muller MJ, Boogerd W, Mellenbergh GJ, van Dam FSAM. Change in cognitive function after chemotherapy: a prospective longitudinal study in breast cancer patients. JNCI J Natl Cancer Inst. 2006;98:1742–5.

45. Gullett JM, et al. Relationship of fatigue with cognitive performance in women with early-stage breast cancer over 2 years. Psychooncology. 2019;28:997–1003.
46. Wefel JS, et al. 'Chemobrain' in breast carcinoma? Cancer. 2004;101:466–75.
47. Ahles TA, et al. Cognitive function in breast cancer patients prior to adjuvant treatment. Breast Cancer Res Treat. 2008;110:143–52.
48. Fan HGM, et al. Fatigue, menopausal symptoms, and cognitive function in women after adjuvant chemotherapy for breast cancer: 1- and 2-year follow-up of a prospective controlled study. J Clin Oncol. 2005;23:8025–32.
49. Denlinger CS, et al. Survivorship: cognitive function, version 1.2014. J Natl Compr Canc Netw. 2014;12:976–86.
50. Nemoto K. Understanding voxel-based morphometry. Brain Nerve Shinkei Kenkyu No Shinpo. 2017;69:505–11.
51. McDonald BC, Conroy SK, Smith DJ, West JD, Saykin AJ. Frontal gray matter reduction after breast cancer chemotherapy and association with executive symptoms: a replication and extension study. Brain Behav Immun. 2013;30:S117–25.
52. McDonald BC, Conroy SK, Ahles TA, West JD, Saykin AJ. Gray matter reduction associated with systemic chemotherapy for breast cancer: a prospective MRI study. Breast Cancer Res Treat. 2010;123:819.
53. Li M, Caeyenberghs K. Longitudinal assessment of chemotherapy-induced changes in brain and cognitive functioning: a systematic review. Neurosci Biobehav Rev. 2018;92:304–17.
54. Andreotti C, et al. Reliable change in neuropsychological assessment of breast cancer survivors. Psychooncology. 2016;25:43–50.
55. Ryan EL, Miskovitz G, Sutton D, Ahles T. A tailored occupational therapy approach to cognitive rehabilitation of chemotherapy-related cognitive side effects in breast cancer survivors: two case studies of premenopausally affected women. Psicooncología Madr. 2011;8:315–42.
56. Selamat MH, Loh SY, Mackenzie L, Vardy J. Chemobrain experienced by breast cancer survivors: a meta-ethnography study investigating research and care implications. PLoS One San Franc. 2014;9:e108002.
57. Ercoli LM, et al. Cognitive rehabilitation group intervention for breast cancer survivors: results of a randomized clinical trial. Psychooncology. 2015;24:1360–7.
58. Ferguson RJ, et al. Cognitive-behavioral management of chemotherapy-related cognitive change. Psychooncology. 2007;16:772–7.
59. Ferguson RJ, et al. Development of CBT for chemotherapy-related cognitive change: results of a waitlist control trial. Psychooncology. 2012;21:176–86.
60. The American Occupational Therapy Association [AOTA]. Occupational therapy practice framework: Domain and Process (3rd Edition). Am J Occup Ther. 2014;68:S1–S48.
61. Pergolotti M, Williams GR, Campbell C, Munoz LA, Muss HB. Occupational therapy for adults with cancer: why it matters. Oncologist. 2016;21:314–9.
62. Wolf TJ, et al. The feasibility of using metacognitive strategy training to improve cognitive performance and neural connectivity in women with chemotherapy-induced cognitive impairment. Oncology. 2016;91:143–52.
63. Green HJ, Tefay M, Mihuta ME. Feasibility of small group cognitive rehabilitation in a clinical cancer setting. Psychooncology. 2018;27:1341–3.
64. Vo JB, et al. Thinking well beyond diagnosis: a four-year evaluation of a cognitive changes education for breast cancer survivors. Nurs Res Rev. 2019;21–9.
65. Conklin HM, et al. Acute neurocognitive response to methylphenidate among survivors of childhood cancer: a randomized, double-blind, cross-over trial. J Pediatr Psychol. 2007;32:1127–39.
66. Mar Fan HG, et al. A randomised, placebo-controlled, double-blind trial of the effects of d-methylphenidate on fatigue and cognitive dysfunction in women undergoing adjuvant chemotherapy for breast cancer. Support Care Cancer. 2008;16:577–83.
67. Kohli S, et al. The effect of modafinil on cognitive function in breast cancer survivors. Cancer. 2009;115:2605–16.
68. Lawrence JA, et al. A study of donepezil in female breast cancer survivors with self-reported cognitive dysfunction 1 to 5 years following adjuvant chemotherapy. J Cancer Surviv. 2016;10:176–84.

Cancer-Related Fatigue 10

Po-Ju Lin, Elizabeth K. Belcher, Nikesha J. Gilmore, Sara J. Hardy, Huiwen Xu, and Karen M. Mustian

Cancer-Related Fatigue in Survivors of Breast Cancer: Definition, Prevalence, and Impact

Cancer-related fatigue (CRF) is a distressing, persistent, and subjective sense of physical, emotional, and/or cognitive tiredness or exhaustion related to cancer or cancer treatment that is not proportional to recent activity and interferes with usual functioning [1, 2]. CRF is more persistent and severe than common physical or mental tiredness and is less likely to be relieved by adequate sleep or rest. CRF is multidimensional; patients with CRF may experience generalized weakness, diminished concentration and attention, decreased motivation, or no interest in engaging in usual activities, and emotional instability. The relationship between CRF and depression is complex. Some of the symptoms of CRF overlap with those of depression. Furthermore, higher levels of depression are associated with higher levels of CRF, and depression has been shown to be one of the strongest predictors of CRF [3–5]. While there is an overlap in characteristics of CRF and depression, data suggests that they have different correlates and different courses over time [6–8].

CRF can occur as a consequence of breast cancer itself [9] and/or its treatments (e.g., chemotherapy, radiation therapy, hormonal and biological therapies) [9–13]. CRF is among the most commonly reported and troublesome symptoms in patients with breast cancer receiving active treatments and survivors after the completion of treatments [14, 15]. Up to 90% of patients with breast cancer experience CRF during chemotherapy and/or radiation therapy. CRF can persist after the completion of treatments and up to 10 years post-diagnosis. Approximately 33% of survivors of breast cancer still report CRF post-treatment [3, 16–23].

CRF has a host of deleterious effects on long-term health outcomes and can have multiple manifestations including physical, mental, and emotional problems. These effects ultimately result in limiting survivors' ability to perform essential daily activities and engage socially, disrupting their quality of life, and reducing survival [3, 13, 24–29]. Survivors of breast cancer report more severe fatigue compared to age-matched healthy controls. This greater level of fatigue is associated with increased depression, pain, and sleep disturbance [3]. Depression and pain are among the strongest predictors of CRF while sleep disturbance serves as a possible mediator

P.-J. Lin (✉) · E. K. Belcher · N. J. Gilmore
S. J. Hardy · H. Xu · K. M. Mustian
The University of Rochester Medical Center, Rochester, NY, USA
e-mail: po-ju_lin@urmc.rochester.edu; elizabeth_belcher@urmc.rochester.edu; nikesha_gilmore@urmc.rochester.edu; sara_hardy@urmc.rochester.edu; huiwen_xu@urmc.rochester.edu; karen_mustian@urmc.rochester.edu

G. G. Kimmick et al. (eds.), *Common Issues in Breast Cancer Survivors*,
https://doi.org/10.1007/978-3-030-75377-1_10

[3, 30]. Furthermore, it has been shown that CRF intensifies menopausal symptoms [3].

Possible Mechanisms Associated with Cancer-Related Fatigue

Understanding the biological mechanisms of CRF can help identify treatment options. Several biological mechanisms may contribute to CRF in patients and survivors of breast cancer, including inflammation, hypothalamic-pituitary-adrenal (HPA) axis dysregulation, and serotonin dysregulation. Additionally, the relative contributions of disease, treatment, and comorbid conditions to CRF in patients with cancer are unclear.

One of the most studied mechanisms of CRF is inflammation [25, 31, 32]. Both cancer and its treatments can lead to the release of pro-inflammatory cytokines from tumors and somatic cells [33–37]. Elevated levels of circulating pro-inflammatory markers, including tumor necrosis factor-alpha (TNF-α), interleukin-6 (IL-6), interleukin-1β (IL-1β), C-reactive protein (CRP), and monocyte chemoattractant protein-1 (MCP-1), are associated with CRF in patients with breast cancer [31, 32, 38–40]. Pro-inflammatory marker levels may remain elevated years after the completion of treatment for breast cancer and contribute to long-lasting CRF [40, 41]. Genomic studies suggest that polymorphisms in the promoter regions of pro-inflammatory cytokines may predispose some patients to greater inflammation and CRF in response to cancer and its treatment [42, 43].

The central nervous system has multiple points of contact with the rest of the body to detect systemic inflammation. Cytokines in the blood can be transported directly into the brain. Additionally, circulating pro-inflammatory cytokines stimulate vagal afferent nerve fibers, the circumventricular organs of the brain that lie outside the blood-brain barrier, and receptors on perivascular macrophages and endothelial cells. Together, these mechanisms of detecting systemic inflammation lead to a variety of local central nervous system responses, including responses that result in CRF.

Another proposed mechanism of CRF is dysregulation of the HPA axis, which regulates the basal and stress-induced release of cortisol. Reduced cortisol and adrenocorticotropic hormone (ACTH) release in response to stress, flatter diurnal cortisol slopes, and elevated evening cortisol levels have been shown to be associated with CRF in patients with cancer [44–47]. However, whether altered cortisol regulation is a result or a cause of CRF is yet to be determined [48, 49]. Genetic and social-behavioral factors such as early life stress and coping mechanisms affect the activity of the HPA axis and may play a role in increasing the severity of CRF [48].

Serotonin dysregulation is theorized to play a role in the pathogenesis of CRF based on 1) the co-occurrence of CRF and depression in patients with cancer, 2) the relationship of serotonin to sleep disturbances, and 3) the mutual feedback between the serotonin system, inflammation, and the HPA axis [12]. Although serotonin cannot be measured non-invasively in the human central nervous system, it is hypothesized that CRF may be related to increased or decreased levels of serotonin [49, 50]. However, clinical trials have failed to show that the use of antidepressants, including selective serotonin reuptake inhibitors, reduce CRF in patients with breast cancer, suggesting that serotonin dysregulation may not be a major contributing factor to CRF [51, 52].

Importantly, proposed mechanisms causing CRF have multiple points of overlap and feedback. For example, elevated levels of pro-inflammatory cytokines can alter cortisol release, serotonin regulation, and vagal nerve activation, which in turn can alter inflammatory cytokine regulation. Similarly, serotonin neurotransmission, HPA axis activity, and vagal nerve stimulation can influence each other [12]. These proposed mechanisms of CRF are not fully understood, and further investigation of the role of endocrine mechanisms in the etiology of CRF is needed [49, 53].

Other factors that may contribute to CRF, including anemia, endocrine dysregulation, physical impairment or other cancer-related symptoms, sleep disturbances, stress, and energy/nutritional deficits and imbalance [25, 54, 55], will be discussed in the later section "Ruling Out Treatable Causes of Fatigue".

Screening and Treatments of Cancer-Related Fatigue

Screening for and treating CRF are priorities of major professional societies and have prompted the development of consensus statements on the topic. In Fig. 10.1, we provide a simplified and practical algorithm based on the ASCO [1, 56], National Comprehensive Cancer Network (NCCN) [57, 58], and Pan-Canadian Clinical Practice Guidelines [59]. We also incorporate information from the Oncology Nursing Society [60] and the best available clinical evidence. This algorithm covers the recommendations on screening, comprehensive and focused assessment, and treatment options for mild, moderate, and severe fatigue.

Screening

Health providers should routinely screen for CRF at the time of initial diagnosis and on subsequent visits, including after the completion of primary treatment. CRF is a subjective sense of tiredness or exhaustion; therefore, patient-reported outcome tools are the most common reliable and validated methods to screen for and assess CRF. CRF can be assessed as one component of a medical outcome survey, quality of life scale, or profile of mood states or by instruments designed specifically to measure multiple dimensions of fatigue. Two systematic reviews identified 40 instruments (3 unidimensional, 37 multidimensional) to assess CRF in patients and survivors with cancer [61, 62]. These instruments vary by the number of items, rating scales, fatigue dimensions/domains, types of cancer population studied, and psychometric properties. They also have different levels of validity and reliability, evalu-

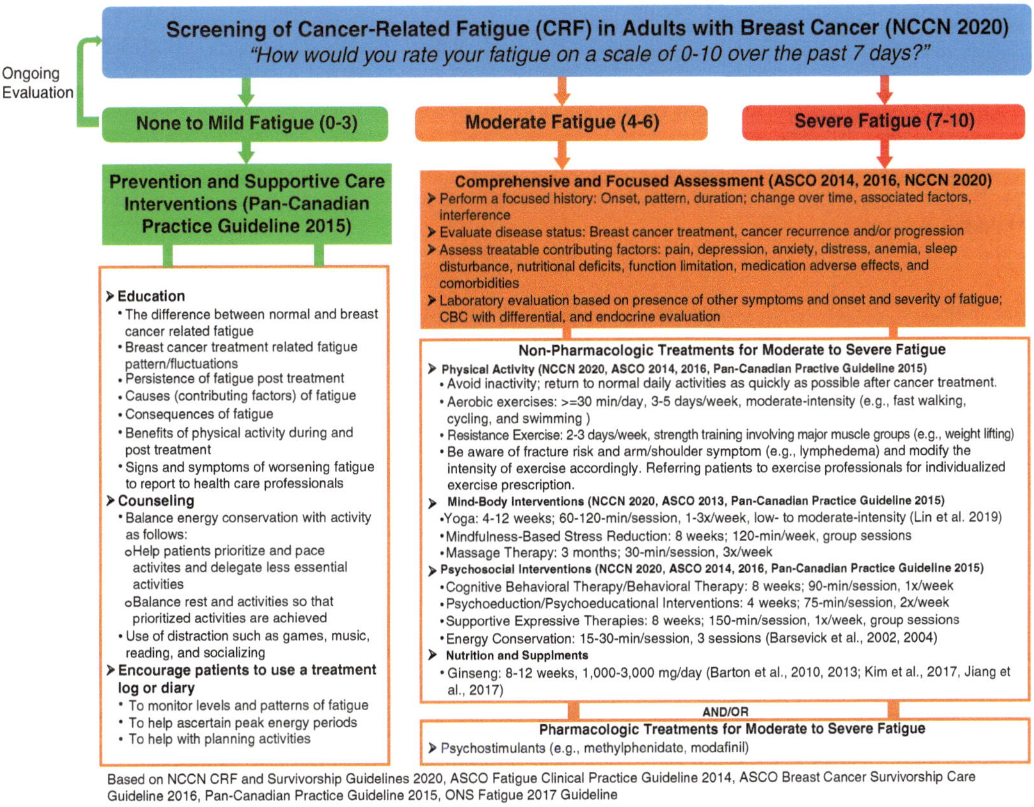

Fig. 10.1 Practical algorithm of screening, assessment, and treatment of cancer-related fatigue

ated by internal consistency, test-retest reliability, and convergent validity, depending on the population studied. According to the systematic reviews, of the 40 instruments available, the following have optimal validity and reliability: the Brief Fatigue Inventory (BFI) [63], the Cancer Fatigue Scale (CFS) [64], the European Organization for Research and Treatment of Cancer Quality-of-Life Questionnaire Core 30 Fatigue Scale (EORTC QLQ C30 FA) [65], the Functional Assessment of Chronic Illness Therapy-Fatigue subscale (FACIT-F) [66], and the Multidimensional Fatigue Symptom Inventory-Short Form (MFSI-SF) [67].

CRF instruments are not universally standardized, and some instruments are more commonly used than others. Table 10.1 lists some commonly used instruments for CRF assessment in patients and survivors with breast cancer [68–70]. A stepwise approach can be used to detect and define CRF. A unidimensional instrument (e.g., EORTC QLQ C30 FA, VAS) is often used as a screening tool for identifying the presence and the severity of CRF. The NCCN guidelines recommend screening for CRF based on the patient's rating of symptoms on an 11-point scale in response to this question: "How would you rate your fatigue on a scale of 0–10 over the past 7 days?" (0 = no fatigue, and 10 = worst fatigue) [58]. The fatigue is then categorized to none to mild (0–3), moderate (4–6), or severe (7–10) based on the scale rating. Some multidimensional instru-

Table 10.1 Commonly used instruments to screen for and assess cancer-related fatigue

Instruments	Number of items	Rating scales	Fatigue dimensions/domains	Evaluation period
Unidimensional				
EORTC QLQ C30 FA [65]	3	4-point (1–4) Likert	Severity of fatigue	Past week
FACIT-F [66]	13	5-point (0–4) Likert	Severity of fatigue	Past week
POMS-F [72]	7	5-point (0–4) Likert	Severity of fatigue	Past week and right now
SF-36 Vitality [73]	4	6-point (1–6) Likert	Severity of fatigue	Past 4 weeks
VAS [74]	1	Analogue	Severity of fatigue	Current
Multidimensional				
BFI [63]	9	11-point (0–10) Likert	Severity and interference of fatigue	Past 24 hours
CFS [64]	15	5-point (1–5) Likert	Physical, affective, and cognitive fatigue	Current
CFQ [75]	14	4-point (0–3) Likert	Physical and mental fatigue	Current
FSI [76]	13	11-point (0–10) Likert	Intensity, duration, and interference of fatigue	Past week, current
MFI-20 [77]	20	5-point (1–5) Likert	Cognitive, physical, and emotional fatigue, reduced activity, reduced motivation	Current
MFSI-SF [67]	30	5-point (0–4) Likert	General, physical, mental, and emotional fatigue, vigor	Past week
PFS [78]	22	11-point (0–10) Likert	Behavioral/severity of fatigue, affective meaning, sensory, cognitive/mood	Now or today
SCFS-6 [79]	6	5-point (1–5) Likert	Physical and perceptual fatigue	Past 2–3 days

EORTC QLQ C30 FA European Organization for Research and Treatment of Cancer Quality-of-Life Questionnaire Core 30 Fatigue Scale, *FACIT-F* Functional Assessment of Chronic Illness Therapy-Fatigue subscale, *POMS-F* Profile of Mood Sates-Fatigue subscale, *SF-36* Short Form 36-item Health Survey Vitality Scale, *VAS* Visual Analogue Scale, *BFI* Brief Fatigue Inventory, *CFS* Cancer Fatigue Scale, *CFQ* Chalder Fatigue Scale, *FSI* Fatigue Symptom Inventory, *MFI-20* Multidimensional Fatigue Inventory-20 items, *MFSI-SF* Multidimensional Fatigue Symptom Inventory-Short Form, *PFS* Piper Fatigue Scale, *SCFS-6* Schwartz Cancer Fatigue Scale-6

ments can further characterize CRF into different domains: physical, emotional (affective), and cognitive. Once CRF is detected, a multidimensional instrument should be employed to identify the most problematic domain(s) of CRF to prescribe an optimal intervention for patients receiving treatment and survivors' post-treatment. In addition, the time required to complete the CRF instrument should be considered, particularly for patients with advanced cancer. The BFI is a reasonable instrument to choose because it is short, has optimal psychometric properties, and is sensitive to changes of CRF over time [61]. The 3-item fatigue scale of the EORTC QLQ C30 has also been used in patients with advanced cancer [61] and validated with good test-retest reliability [71].

If CRF is detected by screening, the severity should then be defined as "None to Mild," "Moderate," or "Severe" (Fig. 10.1). Recommendations for management are then based on the severity of CRF (Fig. 10.1).

Recommendations for None to Mild Cancer-Related Fatigue

For patients with none to mild fatigue, prevention and supportive care are recommended [59]. Clinicians should educate patients about CRF (e.g., its pattern, causes, consequences), especially those features related to breast cancer, advise patients to self-monitor fatigue levels, and provide general strategies for CRF management [1]. Patients are encouraged to use a treatment log or diary for tracking the progress of CRF. Patients can also learn how to use distractions, such as games, music, and exercise, to demote CRF.

Recommendations for Moderate to Severe Cancer-Related Fatigue

For patients with moderate or severe CRF, clinicians should perform a comprehensive and focused assessment including fatigue history (e.g., onset, pattern, duration), assessment of disease status (breast cancer treatment, cancer recurrence and/or progression), and evaluation for the presence of other treatable contributing factors, such as anemia, sleep disturbance, endocrine dysfunction, anxiety, depression, nutritional deficiency, and medications [1, 56, 58]. Laboratory evaluation (e.g., CBC with differential and endocrine evaluation) may be performed, if indicated.

Ruling Out Treatable Causes of Fatigue

Patients who manifest symptoms of CRF should first be evaluated for treatable conditions that may be contributing to or causing the fatigue. These include anemia, deconditioned status, sleep disturbance, endocrine dysfunction (hypothyroidism), anxiety, depression, nutritional deficiencies, electrolyte disturbance, and medications (Table 10.2). Appropriately managing other contributing conditions may alleviate CRF symptoms.

Many patients with cancer are at risk for anemia, which can contribute to symptoms of fatigue. A thorough history can help to identify reversible causes of anemia, including blood loss, hemolysis, iron or vitamin deficiency, or renal disease. Iron and vitamins (folate, B12) supplements might be suggested for patients with iron and vitamin deficiency to help red blood cells grow. Red blood cell transfusions can also be used in appropriate patients; however, further studies are needed to evaluate efficacy in this patient population [80]. Appropriate management of physical symptoms such as pain, nausea, or shortness of breath can improve fatigue in cancer patients. For patients with advanced cancer, a randomized controlled trial evaluated monitoring and protocolized treatment of physical symptoms and the impact on fatigue symptoms. There were 152 patients randomized to either standard care or an intervention, including meeting with a nurse specialist, treatments to alleviate physical symptoms, and education. Significant improvement in general fatigue as well as in secondary endpoints such as interference of fatigue with daily life and anxiety was observed in the intervention group [81].

Insomnia occurs frequently in cancer patients (also see Chap. 11, Sleep Issues and Insomnia).

Table 10.2 Treatable causes of cancer-related fatigue, risk factors, and screening tests

Treatable causes	Risk factors	Suggested screening tests
Anemia	Nutritional deficiency, prior exposure to chemotherapy, renal disease	CBC with diff, peripheral blood smear, iron studies, B12, folate, FACT-anemia subscale
Anxiety/depression	History of prior mood disorder, family history	Patient health questionnaires 2 (PHQ-2) and 9 (PHQ-9), generalized anxiety disorder 7-item (GAD-7)
Comorbidities	Presence of comorbid conditions including congestive heart failure, chronic obstructive pulmonary disease, human immunodeficiency syndrome, multiple sclerosis, rheumatologic conditions	Focused history
Deconditioning	Poor social support, comorbidities	Focused history of daily activities
Electrolyte disturbance	Poor nutrition, brain tumor, paraneoplastic conditions such as SIADH, nausea, vomiting, diarrhea, or bowel obstruction	A complete metabolic panel including sodium, potassium, calcium, magnesium
Endocrine dysfunction: hypothyroidism	Radiation impacting the hypothalamus, immunotherapy (hypophysitis)	Hypothyroidism: serum free T4 and thyroid-stimulating hormone
Medications	Sedating medications including benzodiazepines, opioids, beta-blockers, first-generation antihistamines	Focused history
Nutritional deficiency	Mild cognitive impairment or dementia, poor social support, esophagitis related to cancer treatment, thrush, older age	Focused nutritional history, weight changes, iron levels, B12 and folate, nutritional assessment, and registered dietitian consultant
Physical symptoms	Uncontrolled pain, dyspnea, nausea	Focused history, quantification can include scales and interference with daily activities
Sleep disturbance	For sleep apnea, elevated BMI, untreated/undertreated pain	Sleep history including symptoms of sleep apnea
Substance use	Use of alcohol, marijuana, opioids, cocaine, or other stimulants	Focused history describing the quantity and frequency of substance use

Fifty-one to 90% of cancer survivors have some type of sleep disturbance, such as difficulty falling asleep and staying asleep, early and frequent awakenings, and excessive daytime sleepiness, which can cause daytime dysfunction [82–84]. For patients with insomnia or other sleep disturbance, treatments to improve sleep may mitigate fatigue symptoms. Cognitive behavioral therapy for insomnia (CBT-I) and behavioral interventions involving sleep management/hygiene education sessions are effective approaches for improving insomnia and sleep disturbance in patients and survivors with breast cancer [85–89]. Berger et al. compared an intervention, using an individualized sleep management plan with components of sleep hygiene, relaxation therapy, stimulus control, and sleep restriction techniques, with a "healthy eating" control in 219 patients with breast cancer. Patients in the intervention arm reported significant improvements in global sleep quality assessed via Pittsford Sleep Quality Index [86]. Another study of a sleep management program including relaxation techniques, sleep hygiene, cognitive techniques, and stimulus control advice also demonstrated improvements in sleep latency, sleep duration, sleep efficiency, sleep quality, and daytime dysfunction [87]. Yoga is another effective approach to improve sleep disturbance in patients and survivors with cancer [89–91]. Mustian et al. demonstrated that cancer survivors who participated in a standardized 4-week yoga program (Yoga for Cancer Survivors, YOCAS©®) had improved sleep quality, reduced daytime dysfunction, and decreased sleep medication use compared to the usual care controls [90]. The authors further reported that improvements in sleep significantly mediated the positive effect of yoga on CRF in cancer survivors [30]. Physical symptoms, such as pain, anxiety, and depression, are associated with the severity of insomnia in patients with breast cancer [92–94]. Relief of pain, anxiety, and/or depression may help to alleviate sleep disturbance in breast cancer patients suffering from insomnia. If patients do not respond to education or behavioral interventions, medications such as benzodiazepines, antihistamines, melatonin, or non-benzodiazepine hypnotics are suggested. Overall, there are a variety of pharmacologic and non-pharmacologic means to improve sleep in patients with cancer.

Preexisting endocrinopathies or treatment that impairs the function of endocrine organs can lead to fatigue. Radiation, if fields include the thyroid or pituitary, increases the risk of hypothyroidism [95, 96]. Adjuvant endocrine therapy, prescribed for up to 10 years to decrease the risk of cancer recurrence, causes symptoms similar to menopause. Greater than 50% of patients taking aromatase inhibitors report moderate to severe fatigue [97]. For patients on immunotherapy, immune-related adverse events can include hypophysitis, thyroid dysfunction, and insulin-dependent diabetes mellitus [98]. Patients with risk factors for endocrine dysfunction should be screened with appropriate laboratory tests (Table 10.2). If hypothyroidism is present, it should be treated.

Non-Pharmacologic and Pharmacologic Treatments for CRF

If the initial work-up is negative for treatable causes of fatigue, there are proven non-pharmacologic and pharmacologic treatment options for directly managing CRF. Non-pharmacologic options include physical activity interventions (aerobic, anaerobic/strength, or both), mind-body approaches (yoga, mindfulness, acupuncture), psychosocial interventions (cognitive behavioral therapy, psycho-educational interventions.), and nutritional supplements. Pharmacologic options include psychostimulants, antidepressants, and glucocorticoids. Treatment decisions should consider patients' and their caregivers' preferences, physical and mental condition, resource availability, financial burden, and potential harm. A meta-analysis of 113 randomized trials of exercise (aerobic, resistance, or both), psychological interventions, exercise plus psychological interventions, and pharmacologic interventions demonstrated that exercise, psychological interventions, and exercise plus psychological interventions were significantly more effective than pharmacologic interventions [99]. For this reason, non-pharmacologic interventions should be considered first-line treatments.

Non-Pharmacologic Treatments

Physical Activity

Many systematic reviews and meta-analyses have demonstrated a significant and consistent beneficial effect of exercise on CRF among patients and survivors with breast cancer [68–70, 100–102]. Studies have evaluated different types of exercise including walking [103], bicycling [104], resistance training [105, 106], aquatic exercise [107], a combined approach [108], or others in which patients could choose the type of exercise [109]. Exercise interventions have been carried out during [69, 70, 110, 111] and after treatment [100, 110, 112, 113]. The duration of the studied exercise program has varied in studies from 6 weeks to 6 months. Most data support aerobic exercise [114], but resistance exercise also has a significant impact and possibly a larger effect size [115]. ASCO guidelines recommend 150 minutes of moderate or 75 minutes of vigorous aerobic exercise per week with 2–3 sessions of strength training [1, 56].

Breast cancer survivors with known cardiovascular (CVD), metabolic (type 1 and 2 diabetes mellitus), or renal disease or who have any signs or symptoms suggestive of CVD, DM, or renal disease are recommended to obtain medical clearance to start or continue an exercise program. Otherwise, routine cardiac screening is not necessary before starting an exercise program for survivors without known CVD [116]. The type of exercise program undertaken depends not only on preexisting comorbidity, including cardiovascular disease, but also on conditions resulting from previous cancer treatment, such as chemotherapy-induced peripheral neuropathy (CIPN), cardiomyopathy, osteoporosis, arthralgia, and lymphedema. Breast cancer survivors with CIPN may be prone to falls or dropping things, which may impact safety during an exercise program. The presence of balance issues requires greater stability during exercise, such as using a stationary bike rather than walking or running [117]. Past use of chemotherapy or endocrine therapy increases the risk of bone loss, so patients should be monitored using dual-energy x-ray absorptiometry scans to determine fracture risk [117]. Evaluation for arm/shoulder morbidity is recommended before prescribing upper body exercises for breast cancer survivors with lymphedema. Active exercise may be carried out while wearing a compression sleeve on the affected side [118]. Studies have shown that carefully designed exercise programs with progressive upper extremity strength training are safe for women at risk for lymphedema [119, 120]. Exercise prescriptions should be individualized according to the individual's health status, disease trajectory, previous treatment, symptom burden, current fitness level, past and present exercise participation, and individual preferences to ensure safety and effectiveness [121].

Mind-Body Interventions

Mind-body approaches for CRF include mindfulness, meditation, acupuncture, and yoga [30, 122–131]. Rooted in Buddhist and Hindu teaching, mindfulness focuses on attention, awareness, and nonjudgmental acceptance to optimize one's ability to be fully present in the moment. Multiple randomized trials indicate that mindfulness-based approaches are effective in reducing stress in patients with breast cancer [132, 133]. The practice of yoga, which originated in ancient India, involves a group of physical, mental, and spiritual disciplines. Considerable data indicate that yoga reduces CRF [30, 123, 131]. A recent study by Lin et al. suggests that YOCAS©® yoga (gentle Hatha and Restorative yoga-based yoga program) significantly improves CRF and that 22% to 37% of the improvement in CRF from yoga therapy results from improvement in sleep quality and daytime dysfunction [30]. Yoga also leads to decreases in inflammatory mediators, such as IL-6 and IL-1β [131]. Acupuncture originated in traditional Chinese medicine and involves the insertion of very thin needles through the skin at strategic points on the body, thought to stimulate nerves, muscles, and connective tissue in a therapeutic way. The benefits of acupuncture with regard to CRF have been more controversial; some studies have suggested that acupuncture significantly improves CRF [134–136], but other studies did not see additional benefits of acupuncture on CRF when compared to sham acupuncture [137] or to massage only intervention [138].

Psychosocial Interventions

Psychosocial interventions include cognitive behavioral therapy (CBT), psychoeducational therapy, and other supportive therapies. CBT is a type of psychological therapy in which patients work with an experienced CBT therapist; the focus is on modifying dysfunctional thoughts, emotions, and behaviors. Psycho-educational interventions involve providing information, counseling, and strategies for survivors. Many small trials and multiple meta-analyses have shown small to moderate benefits with psychosocial interventions for CRF [99, 139–148]. The design of these interventions has varied by trials, some focusing on energy conservation and activity management interventions [141, 149], while others providing supportive interventions such as emotional and social support and self-care coaching [139]. Studies have shown that CBT may be more effective than other psychosocial approaches in reducing fatigue symptoms [150], with effects maintained at 2 years [151]. For the treatment of CRF, clinicians can refer breast cancer survivors to a provider who can provide CBT-based therapy.

Nutrition and Supplements

Nutritional supplements are commonly used to manage symptoms. Though meta-analyses and overviews regarding nutritional supplements and CRF describe no clear effect [152, 153], several are worthy of mention. A pilot study of breast cancer survivors by Zick et al. [154], for instance, showed a significant reduction in CRF with a diet rich in fruit, vegetables, whole grains, and omega-3 fatty acid-rich foods. Nutritional supplements, such as omega-3 or omega-6 fatty acids, coenzyme Q10, guaraná, and ginseng, have also been studied for their effects on CRF, due to their antioxidant and/or anti-inflammatory properties. Peppone et al. conducted a 3-arm study comparing omega-3 fatty acids, a combination of omega-3 and omega-6 fatty acids, and omega-6 fatty acid supplements on CRF in 108 breast cancer survivors. Although all participants showed improvement from baseline in their level of CRF, the improvements were significantly greater in those receiving omega-6 fatty acid supplements alone than in the other two arms [155].

Current evidence is insufficient and inconsistent to conclude the effects of coenzyme Q10 and guaraná supplements on CRF. Coenzyme Q10 is a nutrient that occurs naturally in the body. It acts as an antioxidant to protect cells from damage, plays an important role in metabolism, and has a side effect of mild insomnia. Coenzyme Q10 was shown reducing CRF in breast cancer patients receiving chemotherapy when supplementing it with L-carnitine and branched-chain amino acids [156] but did not reduce CRF when supplementing it with vitamin E [157]. Guaraná, derived from the seed of a Brazilian plant native to the Amazon basin, is touted to be helpful for weight loss, enhanced athletic performance, as a stimulant, and to reduce mental and physical fatigue. Stimulant properties of guaraná are likely due to its high caffeine content, which is among the highest of any plant. Compared to coffee which contains 2% caffeine by weight, guaraná contains 3.6–5.8% caffeine by weight. Effects of 2–3 weeks guaraná supplements on CRF in breast cancer patients receiving chemotherapy were also inconsistent [158–160].

Ginseng, used for centuries in Chinese medicine, is derived from the root of a plant and has antioxidant and anti-inflammatory properties. Ginseng appears to have some effects on reducing CRF [161–164]; however, the potential herbal-drug interactions need to be considered, particularly in patients undergoing chemotherapy [165]. A patient developed liver toxicity during chemotherapy when concurrent use of a ginseng supplement [166]. Another case report indicated that the ginseng supplement might lower a patient's response to chemotherapy [167].

Pharmacologic Treatments

Only limited data support the efficacy of pharmacologic treatment for CRF, but a therapeutic trial of medication can be tried if non-pharmacologic interventions are not helpful. Studies to date have evaluated psychostimulants (methylphenidate, dexmethylphenidate, and modafinil), antidepressants (paroxetine, sertraline), and glucocorticoids [51, 168–172]. Of the psychostimulants studied, the most data is available for methylphenidate and modafinil. A 2010 Cochrane review and 2018 meta-analysis both report improvement in CRF with the use of methylphenidate [169, 172]. However, the 2018 meta-analysis did not find that modafinil had any efficacy, and the magnitude of the effect of methylphenidate was of questionable clinical significance [169]. Data for the use of antidepressants for CRF has been disappointing. In the absence of depression, clinical trials have demonstrated no impact of antidepressants on fatigue in cancer survivors [51, 90, 170]. Glucocorticoids can alleviate CRF in cancer patients. In a randomized study of 84 patients with advanced cancer, significant improvements in the level of CRF and physical distress were seen after 15 days of dexamethasone, 4 mg twice daily, versus placebo. No significant increase in adverse events occurred during the short follow-up of this study [168]. Nonetheless, the risk of side effects of glucocorticoid use limits its application for CRF in cancer survivors.

Future Research

Many gaps exist in the area of CRF research. The negative impact of CRF on other outcomes such as healthcare utilization, cost, and survival needs to be studied. Despite studies consistently demonstrating the benefits of physical activity interventions in CRF, the optimal dose and intensity of exercise remain unclear. Given the multidimensional nature of CRF, a one-size-fits-all approach is likely not sufficient. Combinations of various strategies such as exercise and other non-pharmacologic interventions (e.g., psychological therapies, behavioral modifications) need to be further investigated. With an increasing emphasis on personalized medicine in oncology, an understanding of the biobehavioral mechanisms associated with CRF is necessary to develop individualized care plans and to know which treatment is most effective for whom. Finally, dissemination of the clinical practice guidelines into clinical settings is essential to identify patients with CRF and implement individualized treatment plans.

Conclusion

CRF is a commonly reported, debilitating toxicity experienced by patients surviving after breast cancer diagnosis and treatment and can persist for many years. Screening for CRF should be incorporated into routine cancer care. Non-pharmacologic interventions (e.g., physical activity, mind-body interventions, cognitive-behavioral interventions) can effectively treat CRF and should be prescribed prior to pharmacologic approaches into the care plan for breast cancer survivors with CRF.

References

1. Bower JE, Bak K, Berger A, Breitbart W, Escalante CP, Ganz PA, et al. Screening, assessment, and management of fatigue in adult survivors of cancer: an American Society of Clinical oncology clinical practice guideline adaptation. J Clin Oncol. 2014;32(17):1840–50.
2. National Comprehensive Cancer Network. Cancer-Related Fatigue (Version 2.2020). Available from: https://www.nccn.org/professionals/physician_gls/pdf/fatigue.pdf.
3. Bower JE, Ganz PA, Desmond KA, Rowland JH, Meyerowitz BE, Belin TR. Fatigue in breast cancer survivors: occurrence, correlates, and impact on quality of life. J Clin Oncol. 2000;18(4):743–53.
4. Oh HS, Seo WS. Systematic review and meta-analysis of the correlates of cancer-related fatigue. Worldviews Evid-Based Nurs. 2011;8(4):191–201.
5. Seo YM, Oh HS, Seo WS, Kim HS. Comprehensive predictors of fatigue for cancer patients. Taehan Kanho Hakhoe Chi. 2006;36(7):1224–31.
6. Brown LF, Kroenke K. Cancer-related fatigue and its associations with depression and anxiety: a systematic review. Psychosomatics. 2009;50(5):440–7.
7. Kim SH, Son BH, Hwang SY, Han W, Yang JH, Lee S, et al. Fatigue and depression in disease-free breast cancer survivors: prevalence, correlates, and association with quality of life. J Pain Symptom Manag. 2008;35(6):644–55.
8. Ruiz-Casado A, Alvarez-Bustos A, de Pedro CG, Mendez-Otero M, Romero-Elias M. Cancer-related fatigue in breast Cancer survivors: a review. Clin Breast Cancer. 2020.
9. Hofman M, Ryan JL, Figueroa-Moseley CD, Jean-Pierre P, Morrow GR. Cancer-related fatigue: the scale of the problem. Oncologist. 2007;12(Suppl 1):4–10.
10. Hickok JT, Roscoe JA, Morrow GR, Mustian K, Okunieff P, Bole CW. Frequency, severity, clinical course, and correlates of fatigue in 372 patients during 5 weeks of radiotherapy for cancer. Cancer. 2005;104(8):1772–8.
11. Henry DH, Viswanathan HN, Elkin EP, Traina S, Wade S, Cella D. Symptoms and treatment burden associated with cancer treatment: results from a cross-sectional national survey in the U.S. Support Care Cancer. 2008;16(7):791–801.
12. Morrow GR, Andrews PL, Hickok JT, Roscoe JA, Matteson S. Fatigue associated with cancer and its treatment. Support Care Cancer. 2002;10(5):389–98.
13. Jacobsen PB, Hann DM, Azzarello LM, Horton J, Balducci L, Lyman GH. Fatigue in women receiving adjuvant chemotherapy for breast cancer: characteristics, course, and correlates. J Pain Symptom Manag. 1999;18(4):233–42.
14. Rotonda C, Guillemin F, Bonnetain F, Conroy T. Factors correlated with fatigue in breast cancer patients before, during and after adjuvant chemotherapy: the FATSEIN study. Contemp Clin Trials. 2011;32(2):244–9.
15. de Ligt KM, Heins M, Verloop J, Ezendam NPM, Smorenburg CH, Korevaar JC, et al. The impact of health symptoms on health-related quality of life in early-stage breast cancer survivors. Breast Cancer Res Treat. 2019;178(3):703–11.
16. Bower JE. Cancer-related fatigue: links with inflammation in cancer patients and survivors. Brain Behav Immun. 2007;21(7):863–71.
17. Bower JE, Ganz PA, Desmond KA, Bernaards C, Rowland JH, Meyerowitz BE, et al. Fatigue in long-term breast carcinoma survivors: a longitudinal investigation. Cancer. 2006;106(4):751–8.
18. Ganz PA, Goodwin PJ. Breast Cancer survivorship: where are we today? Adv Exp Med Biol. 2015;862:1–8.

19. Garabeli Cavalli Kluthcovsky AC, Urbanetz AA, de Carvalho DS, Pereira Maluf EM, Schlickmann Sylvestre GC, Bonatto Hatschbach SB. Fatigue after treatment in breast cancer survivors: prevalence, determinants and impact on health-related quality of life. Support Care Cancer. 2012;20(8):1901–9.
20. Servaes P, Gielissen MF, Verhagen S, Bleijenberg G. The course of severe fatigue in disease-free breast cancer patients: a longitudinal study. Psychooncology. 2007;16(9):787–95.
21. Bardwell WA, Ancoli-Israel S. Breast Cancer and fatigue. Sleep Med Clin. 2008;3(1):61–71.
22. Abrahams HJ, Gielissen MF, Schmits IC, Verhagen CA, Rovers MM, Knoop H. Risk factors, prevalence, and course of severe fatigue after breast cancer treatment: a meta-analysis involving 12 327 breast cancer survivors. Ann Oncol. 2016;27(6):965–74.
23. Ganz PA, Bower JE. Cancer related fatigue: a focus on breast cancer and Hodgkin's disease survivors. Acta Oncol. 2007;46(4):474–9.
24. Andrykowski MA, Curran SL, Lightner R. Off-treatment fatigue in breast cancer survivors: a controlled comparison. J Behav Med. 1998;21(1):1–18.
25. Bower JE. Cancer-related fatigue--mechanisms, risk factors, and treatments. Nat Rev Clin Oncol. 2014;11(10):597–609.
26. Visser MR, Smets EM. Fatigue, depression and quality of life in cancer patients: how are they related? Support Care Cancer. 1998;6(2):101–8.
27. Broeckel JA, Jacobsen PB, Horton J, Balducci L, Lyman GH. Characteristics and correlates of fatigue after adjuvant chemotherapy for breast cancer. J Clin Oncol. 1998;16(5):1689.
28. Groenvold M, Petersen MA, Idler E, Bjorner JB, Fayers PM, Mouridsen HT. Psychological distress and fatigue predicted recurrence and survival in primary breast cancer patients. Breast Cancer Res Treat. 2007;105(2):209–19.
29. Quinten C, Maringwa J, Gotay CC, Martinelli F, Coens C, Reeve BB, et al. Patient self-reports of symptoms and clinician ratings as predictors of overall Cancer survival. Jnci-J Natl Cancer I. 2011;103(24):1851–8.
30. Lin PJ, Kleckner IR, Loh KP, Inglis JE, Peppone LJ, Janelsins MC, et al. Influence of yoga on Cancer-related fatigue and on mediational relationships between changes in sleep and Cancer-related fatigue: a Nationwide. Multicenter Randomized Controlled Trial of Yoga in Cancer Survivors Integr Cancer Ther. 2019;18:1534735419855134.
31. Saligan LN, Kim HS. A systematic review of the association between immunogenomic markers and cancer-related fatigue. Brain Behav Immun. 2012;26(6):830–48.
32. Schubert C, Hong S, Natarajan L, Mills PJ, Dimsdale JE. The association between fatigue and inflammatory marker levels in cancer patients: a quantitative review. Brain Behav Immun. 2007;21(4):413–27.
33. Coussens LM, Werb Z. Inflammation and cancer. Nature. 2002;420(6917):860–7.
34. Edwardson DW, Boudreau J, Mapletoft J, Lanner C, Kovala AT, Parissenti AM. Inflammatory cytokine production in tumor cells upon chemotherapy drug exposure or upon selection for drug resistance. PLoS One. 2017;12(9):e0183662.
35. Kawaguchi K, Sakurai M, Yamamoto Y, Suzuki E, Tsuda M, Kataoka TR, et al. Alteration of specific cytokine expression patterns in patients with breast cancer. Sci Rep. 2019;9(1):2924.
36. Lyon DE, McCain NL, Walter J, Schubert C. Cytokine comparisons between women with breast cancer and women with a negative breast biopsy. Nurs Res. 2008;57(1):51–8.
37. Stone HB, Coleman CN, Anscher MS, McBride WH. Effects of radiation on normal tissue: consequences and mechanisms. Lancet Oncol. 2003;4(9):529–36.
38. Cohen RA, Gullett JM, Woods AJ, Porges EC, Starkweather A, Jackson-Cook CK, et al. Cytokine-associated fatigue prior to, during, and post-chemotherapy for breast cancer. J Neuroimmunol. 2019;334:577001.
39. Liu L, Mills PJ, Rissling M, Fiorentino L, Natarajan L, Dimsdale JE, et al. Fatigue and sleep quality are associated with changes in inflammatory markers in breast cancer patients undergoing chemotherapy. Brain Behav Immun. 2012;26(5):706–13.
40. Orre IJ, Reinertsen KV, Aukrust P, Dahl AA, Fosså SD, Ueland T, et al. Higher levels of fatigue are associated with higher CRP levels in disease-free breast cancer survivors. J Psychosom Res. 2011;71(3):136–41.
41. van der Willik KD, Koppelmans V, Hauptmann M, Compter A, Ikram MA, Schagen SB. Inflammation markers and cognitive performance in breast cancer survivors 20 years after completion of chemotherapy: a cohort study. Breast Cancer Res. 2018;20(1):135.
42. Bower JE, Ganz PA, Irwin MR, Castellon S, Arevalo J, Cole SW. Cytokine genetic variations and fatigue among patients with breast cancer. J Clin Oncol. 2013;31(13):1656–61.
43. Miaskowski C, Dodd M, Lee K, West C, Paul SM, Cooper BA, et al. Preliminary evidence of an association between a functional interleukin-6 polymorphism and fatigue and sleep disturbance in oncology patients and their family caregivers. J Pain Symptom Manag. 2010;40(4):531–44.
44. Bower JE, Ganz PA, Aziz N. Altered cortisol response to psychologic stress in breast cancer survivors with persistent fatigue. Psychosom Med. 2005;67(2):277–80.
45. Bower JE, Ganz PA, Dickerson SS, Petersen L, Aziz N, Fahey JL. Diurnal cortisol rhythm and fatigue in breast cancer survivors. Psychoneuroendocrinology. 2005;30(1):92–100.
46. Schmidt ME, Semik J, Habermann N, Wiskemann J, Ulrich CM, Steindorf K. Cancer-related fatigue shows a stable association with diurnal cortisol dysregulation in breast cancer patients. Brain Behav Immun. 2016;52:98–105.

47. Tell D, Mathews HL, Janusek LW. Day-to-day dynamics of associations between sleep, napping, fatigue, and the cortisol diurnal rhythm in women diagnosed as having breast cancer. Psychosom Med. 2014;76(7):519–28.
48. Bower JE, Lamkin DM. Inflammation and cancer-related fatigue: mechanisms, contributing factors, and treatment implications. Brain, behavior, and immunity. 2013;30(Suppl(0)):S48-S57.
49. Jager A, Sleijfer S, van der Rijt CCD. The pathogenesis of cancer related fatigue: could increased activity of pro-inflammatory cytokines be the common denominator? Eur J Cancer. 2008;44(2):175–81.
50. Ryan JL, Carroll JK, Ryan EP, Mustian KM, Fiscella K, Morrow GR. Mechanisms of Cancer-related fatigue. Oncologist. 2007;12(S1):22–34.
51. Morrow GR, Hickok JT, Roscoe JA, Raubertas RF, Andrews PLR, Flynn PJ, et al. Differential effects of paroxetine on fatigue and depression: a randomized, double-blind trial from the University of Rochester Cancer Center Community Clinical Oncology Program. J Clin Oncol. 2003;21(24):4635–41.
52. Roscoe JA, Morrow GR, Hickok JT. Effect of paroxetine hydrochloride on fatigue and depression in breast cancer patients receiving chemotherapy. Breast Cancer Res Treat. 2005;89:243–9.
53. Alexander S, Stone P, White S, Andrews P, Nussey S, Bano G. Evaluation of central serotonin sensitivity in breast Cancer survivors with Cancer-related fatigue syndrome. J Pain Symptom Manag. 2010;40(6):892–8.
54. Aistars J. Fatigue in the cancer patient: a conceptual approach to a clinical problem. Oncol Nurs Forum. 1987;14(6):25–30.
55. Barsevick A, Frost M, Zwinderman A, Hall P, Halyard M. I'm so tired: biological and genetic mechanisms of cancer-related fatigue. Qual Life Res. 2010;19(10):1419–27.
56. Runowicz CD, Leach CR, Henry NL, Henry KS, Mackey HT, Cowens-Alvarado RL, et al. American Cancer Society/American Society of Clinical Oncology breast Cancer survivorship care guideline. J Clin Oncol. 2016;34(6):611–35.
57. Denlinger CS, Sanft T, Baker KS, Broderick G, Demark-Wahnefried W, Friedman DL, et al. Survivorship, version 1.2020, NCCN clinical practice guidelines in oncology. 2020.
58. Berger AM, Mooney K, Alvarez-Perez A, Breitbart WS, Carpenter KM, Cella D, et al. Cancer-related fatigue, version 1.2020, NCCN clinical practice guidelines in oncology. 2020.
59. Howell D, Keshavarz H, Broadfield L, Hack T, Hamel M, Harth T, et al. A Pan Canadian practice guideline for screening, assessment, and Management of Cancer-Related Fatigue in adults (version 2). 2015.
60. Mitchell SA, Hoffman AJ, Clark JC, DeGennaro RM, Poirier P, Robinson CB, et al. Putting evidence into practice: an update of evidence-based interventions for cancer-related fatigue during and following treatment. Clin J Oncol Nurs. 2014;18(Suppl):38–58.
61. Seyidova-Khoshknabi D, Davis MP, Walsh D. Review article: a systematic review of cancer-related fatigue measurement questionnaires. Am J Hosp Palliat Care. 2011;28(2):119–29.
62. Minton O, Stone P. A systematic review of the scales used for the measurement of cancer-related fatigue (CRF). Ann Oncol. 2009;20(1):17–25.
63. Mendoza TR, Wang XS, Cleeland CS, Morrissey M, Johnson BA, Wendt JK, et al. The rapid assessment of fatigue severity in cancer patients: use of the brief fatigue inventory. Cancer. 1999;85(5):1186–96.
64. Okuyama T, Akechi T, Kugaya A, Okamura H, Shima Y, Maruguchi M, et al. Development and validation of the cancer fatigue scale: a brief, three-dimensional, self-rating scale for assessment of fatigue in cancer patients. J Pain Symptom Manag. 2000;19(1):5–14.
65. Aaronson NK, Ahmedzai S, Bergman B, Bullinger M, Cull A, Duez NJ, et al. The European Organization for Research and Treatment of Cancer QLQ-C30: a quality-of-life instrument for use in international clinical trials in oncology. J Natl Cancer Inst. 1993;85(5):365–76.
66. Yellen SB, Cella DF, Webster K, Blendowski C, Kaplan E. Measuring fatigue and other anemia-related symptoms with the functional assessment of cancer therapy (FACT) measurement system. J Pain Symptom Manag. 1997;13(2):63.
67. Stein KD, Jacobsen PB, Blanchard CM, Thors C. Further validation of the multidimensional fatigue symptom inventory-short form. J Pain Symptom Manag. 2004;27(1):14–23.
68. Juvet LK, Thune I, Elvsaas I, Fors EA, Lundgren S, Bertheussen G, et al. The effect of exercise on fatigue and physical functioning in breast cancer patients during and after treatment and at 6 months follow-up: a meta-analysis. Breast. 2017;33:166–77.
69. Lipsett A, Barrett S, Haruna F, Mustian K, O'Donovan A. The impact of exercise during adjuvant radiotherapy for breast cancer on fatigue and quality of life: a systematic review and meta-analysis. Breast. 2017;32:144–55.
70. van Vulpen JK, Peeters PH, Velthuis MJ, van der Wall E, May AM. Effects of physical exercise during adjuvant breast cancer treatment on physical and psychosocial dimensions of cancer-related fatigue: a meta-analysis. Maturitas. 2016;85:104–11.
71. Pater JL, Zee B, Palmer M, Johnston D, Osoba D. Fatigue in patients with cancer: results with National Cancer Institute of Canada clinical trials group studies employing the EORTC QLQ-C30. Support Care Cancer. 1997;5(5):410–3.
72. Baker F, Denniston M, Zabora J, Polland A, Dudley WN. A POMS short form for cancer patients: psychometric and structural evaluation. Psychooncology. 2002;11(4):273–81.
73. Ware JE Jr, Sherbourne CD. The MOS 36-item short-form health survey (SF-36). I. Conceptual framework and item selection. Med Care. 1992;30(6):473–83.

74. Glaus A. Assessment of fatigue in cancer and non-cancer patients and in healthy individuals. Support Care Cancer. 1993;1(6):305–15.
75. Chalder T, Berelowitz G, Pawlikowska T, Watts L, Wessely S, Wright D, et al. Development of a fatigue scale. J Psychosom Res. 1993;37(2):147–53.
76. Hann DM, Denniston MM, Baker F. Measurement of fatigue in cancer patients: further validation of the fatigue symptom inventory. Qual Life Res. 2000;9(7):847–54.
77. Smets EM, Garssen B, Bonke B, De Haes JC. The multidimensional fatigue inventory (MFI) psychometric qualities of an instrument to assess fatigue. J Psychosom Res. 1995;39(3):315–25.
78. Piper BF, Dibble SL, Dodd MJ, Weiss MC, Slaughter RE, Paul SM. The revised Piper fatigue scale: psychometric evaluation in women with breast cancer. Oncol Nurs Forum. 1998;25(4):677–84.
79. Schwartz A, Meek P. Additional construct validity of the Schwartz Cancer fatigue scale. J Nurs Meas. 1999;7(1):35–45.
80. Preston NJ, Hurlow A, Brine J, Bennett MI. Blood transfusions for anaemia in patients with advanced cancer. Cochrane Database Syst Rev. 2012;(2):Cd009007.
81. de Raaf PJ, de Klerk C, Timman R, Busschbach JJ, Oldenmenger WH, van der Rijt CC. Systematic monitoring and treatment of physical symptoms to alleviate fatigue in patients with advanced cancer: a randomized controlled trial. J Clin Oncol. 2013;31(6):716–23.
82. Schultz PN, Klein MJ, Beck ML, Stava C, Sellin RV. Breast cancer: relationship between menopausal symptoms, physiologic health effects of cancer treatment and physical constraints on quality of life in long-term survivors. J Clin Nurs. 2005;14(2):204–11.
83. Otte JL, Carpenter JS, Russell KM, Bigatti S, Champion VL. Prevalence, severity, and correlates of sleep-wake disturbances in long-term breast cancer survivors. J Pain Symptom Manag. 2010;39(3):535–47.
84. Savard J, Simard S, Blanchet J, Ivers H, Morin CM. Prevalence, clinical characteristics, and risk factors for insomnia in the context of breast cancer. Sleep. 2001;24(5):583–90.
85. Quesnel C, Savard J, Simard S, Ivers H, Morin CM. Efficacy of cognitive-behavioral therapy for insomnia in women treated for nonmetastatic breast cancer. J Consult Clin Psychol. 2003;71(1):189–200.
86. Berger AM, Kuhn BR, Farr LA, Von Essen SG, Chamberlain J, Lynch JC, et al. One-year outcomes of a behavioral therapy intervention trial on sleep quality and cancer-related fatigue. J Clin Oncol. 2009;27(35):6033–40.
87. Simeit R, Deck R, Conta-Marx B. Sleep management training for cancer patients with insomnia. Support Care Cancer. 2004;12(3):176–83.
88. Aricò D, Raggi A, Ferri R. Cognitive behavioral therapy for insomnia in breast Cancer survivors: a review of the literature. Front Psychol. 2016;7:1162.
89. Zeichner SB, Zeichner RL, Gogineni K, Shatil S, Ioachimescu O. Cognitive behavioral therapy for insomnia, mindfulness, and yoga in patients with breast Cancer with sleep disturbance: a literature review. Breast cancer : basic and clinical research. 2017;11:1178223417745564.
90. Mustian KM, Sprod LK, Janelsins M, Peppone LJ, Palesh OG, Chandwani K, et al. Multicenter, randomized controlled trial of yoga for sleep quality among cancer survivors. J Clin Oncol. 2013;31(26):3233–41.
91. Cohen L, Warneke C, Fouladi RT, Rodriguez MA, Chaoul-Reich A. Psychological adjustment and sleep quality in a randomized trial of the effects of a Tibetan yoga intervention in patients with lymphoma. Cancer. 2004;100(10):2253–60.
92. Galiano-Castillo N, Arroyo-Morales M, Ariza-Garcia A, Fernández-Lao C, Fernández-Fernández AJ, Cantarero-Villanueva I. Factors that explain the Cancer-related insomnia. Breast J. 2017;23(4):387–94.
93. Overcash J, Tan A, Patel K, Noonan AM. Factors associated with poor sleep in older women diagnosed with breast Cancer. Oncol Nurs Forum. 2018;45(3):359–71.
94. Bardwell WA, Profant J, Casden DR, Dimsdale JE, Ancoli-Israel S, Natarajan L, et al. The relative importance of specific risk factors for insomnia in women treated for early-stage breast cancer. Psychooncology. 2008;17(1):9–18.
95. Hardy S, Ismat S, Michael M, Edward V, Constine Louis S. Hypopituitarism. In: Chang EL, Brown P, Lo SS, Sahgal A, Suh J, editors. Adult CNS radiation oncology. Springer; 2018.
96. Wolny-Rokicka E, Tukiendorf A, Wydmański J, Roszkowska D, Staniul BS, Zembroń-Łacny A. Thyroid function after postoperative radiation therapy in patients with breast Cancer. Asian Pac J Cancer Prev. 2016;17(10):4577–81.
97. Mao H, Bao T, Shen X, Li Q, Seluzicki C, Im EO, et al. Prevalence and risk factors for fatigue among breast cancer survivors on aromatase inhibitors. Eur J Cancer. 2018;101:47–54.
98. Girotra M, Hansen A, Farooki A, Byun DJ, Min L, Creelan BC, et al. The Current Understanding of the Endocrine Effects From Immune Checkpoint Inhibitors and Recommendations for Management. JNCI Cancer Spectrum. 2018;2(3):pky021.
99. Mustian KM, Alfano CM, Heckler C, Kleckner AS, Kleckner IR, Leach CR, et al. Comparison of pharmaceutical, psychological, and exercise treatments for Cancer-related fatigue: a meta-analysis. JAMA Oncol. 2017;3(7):961–8.
100. Meneses-Echavez JF, Gonzalez-Jimenez E, Ramirez-Velez R. Effects of supervised exercise on cancer-related fatigue in breast cancer survivors: a systematic review and meta-analysis. BMC Cancer. 2015;15:77.
101. Lahart IM, Metsios GS, Nevill AM, Carmichael AR. Physical activity for women with breast cancer

after adjuvant therapy. Cochrane Database Syst Rev. 2018;1(1):Cd011292.
102. Singh B, Spence RR, Steele ML, Sandler CX, Peake JM, Hayes SC. A systematic review and meta-analysis of the safety, feasibility, and effect of exercise in women with stage II+ breast Cancer. Arch Phys Med Rehabil. 2018;99(12):2621–36.
103. Mock V, Dow KH, Meares CJ, Grimm PM, Dienemann JA, Haisfield-Wolfe ME, et al. Effects of exercise on fatigue, physical functioning, and emotional distress during radiation therapy for breast cancer. Oncol Nurs Forum. 1997;24(6):991–1000.
104. Courneya KS, Mackey JR, Bell GJ, Jones LW, Field CJ, Fairey AS. Randomized controlled trial of exercise training in postmenopausal breast cancer survivors: cardiopulmonary and quality of life outcomes. J Clin Oncol. 2003;21(9):1660–8.
105. Steindorf K, Schmidt ME, Klassen O, Ulrich CM, Oelmann J, Habermann N, et al. Randomized, controlled trial of resistance training in breast cancer patients receiving adjuvant radiotherapy: results on cancer-related fatigue and quality of life. Ann Oncol. 2014;25(11):2237–43.
106. Schmidt ME, Wiskemann J, Armbrust P, Schneeweiss A, Ulrich CM, Steindorf K. Effects of resistance exercise on fatigue and quality of life in breast cancer patients undergoing adjuvant chemotherapy: a randomized controlled trial. Int J Cancer. 2015;137(2):471–80.
107. Cantarero-Villanueva I, Fernandez-Lao C, Cuesta-Vargas AI, Del Moral-Avila R, Fernandez-de-Las-Penas C, Arroyo-Morales M. The effectiveness of a deep water aquatic exercise program in cancer-related fatigue in breast cancer survivors: a randomized controlled trial. Arch Phys Med Rehabil. 2013;94(2):221–30.
108. Milne HM, Wallman KE, Gordon S, Courneya KS. Effects of a combined aerobic and resistance exercise program in breast cancer survivors: a randomized controlled trial. Breast Cancer Res Treat. 2008;108(2):279–88.
109. Segal R, Evans W, Johnson D, Smith J, Colletta S, Gayton J, et al. Structured exercise improves physical functioning in women with stages I and II breast cancer: results of a randomized controlled trial. J Clin Oncol. 2001;19(3):657–65.
110. Minton O, Jo F, Jane M. The role of behavioural modification and exercise in the management of cancer-related fatigue to reduce its impact during and after cancer treatment. Acta Oncol. 2015;54(5):581–6.
111. Meneses-Echavez JF, Gonzalez-Jimenez E, Ramirez-Velez R. Effects of supervised multimodal exercise interventions on Cancer-related fatigue: systematic review and meta-analysis of randomized controlled trials. Biomed Res Int. 2015;2015:328636.
112. Tian L, Lu HJ, Lin L, Hu Y. Effects of aerobic exercise on cancer-related fatigue: a meta-analysis of randomized controlled trials. Support Care Cancer. 2016;24(2):969–83.
113. Dennett AM, Peiris CL, Shields N, Prendergast LA, Taylor NF. Moderate-intensity exercise reduces fatigue and improves mobility in cancer survivors: a systematic review and meta-regression. J Physiother. 2016;62(2):68–82.
114. Cramp F, Byron-Daniel J. Exercise for the management of cancer-related fatigue in adults. Cochrane Database Syst Rev. 2012;11:CD006145.
115. Brown JC, Huedo-Medina TB, Pescatello LS, Pescatello SM, Ferrer RA, Johnson BT. Efficacy of exercise interventions in modulating cancer-related fatigue among adult cancer survivors: a meta-analysis. Cancer Epidemiol Biomark Prev. 2011;20(1):123–33.
116. Kenjale AA, Hornsby WE, Crowgey T, Thomas S, Herndon JE 2nd, Khouri MG, et al. Pre-exercise participation cardiovascular screening in a heterogeneous cohort of adult cancer patients. Oncologist. 2014;19(9):999–1005.
117. Wolin KY, Schwartz AL, Matthews CE, Courneya KS, Schmitz KH. Implementing the exercise guidelines for cancer survivors. J Support Oncol. 2012;10(5):171–7.
118. de Fatima Guerreiro Godoy M, Pereira de Godoy AC, Pereira de Godoy JM. Effect of exercise while utilizing a device with an arm compression sleeve to reduce lymphedema. Clin Exp Obstet Gynecol. 2017;44(1):17–9.
119. Schmitz KH, Troxel AB, Cheville A, Grant LL, Bryan CJ, Gross CR, et al. Physical activity and lymphedema (the PAL trial): assessing the safety of progressive strength training in breast cancer survivors. Contemp Clin Trials. 2009;30(3):233–45.
120. Ahmed RL, Thomas W, Yee D, Schmitz KH. Randomized controlled trial of weight training and lymphedema in breast cancer survivors. J Clin Oncol. 2006;24(18):2765–72.
121. Mustian KM, Sprod LK, Janelsins M, Peppone LJ, Mohile S. Exercise recommendations for Cancer-related fatigue, cognitive impairment, sleep problems, depression, pain, anxiety, and physical dysfunction: a review. Oncol Hematol Rev. 2012;8(2):81–8.
122. Banasik J, Williams H, Haberman M, Blank SE, Bendel R. Effect of Iyengar yoga practice on fatigue and diurnal salivary cortisol concentration in breast cancer survivors. J Am Acad Nurse Pract. 2011;23(3):135–42.
123. Bower JE, Garet D, Sternlieb B, Ganz PA, Irwin MR, Olmstead R, et al. Yoga for persistent fatigue in breast cancer survivors: a randomized controlled trial. Cancer. 2012;118(15):3766–75.
124. Bower JE, Greendale G, Crosswell AD, Garet D, Sternlieb B, Ganz PA, et al. Yoga reduces inflammatory signaling in fatigued breast cancer survivors: a randomized controlled trial. Psychoneuroendocrinology. 2014;43:20–9.
125. Johns SA, Brown LF, Beck-Coon K, Talib TL, Monahan PO, Giesler RB, et al. Randomized controlled pilot trial of mindfulness-based stress reduction compared to psychoeducational support for persistently fatigued breast and colorectal cancer survivors. Support Care Cancer. 2016;24(10):4085–96.

126. Johns SA, Brown LF, Beck-Coon K, Monahan PO, Tong Y, Kroenke K. Randomized controlled pilot study of mindfulness-based stress reduction for persistently fatigued cancer survivors. Psychooncology. 2015;24(8):885–93.
127. Lotzke D, Wiedemann F, Rodrigues Recchia D, Ostermann T, Sattler D, Ettl J, et al. Iyengar-yoga compared to exercise as a therapeutic intervention during (neo)adjuvant therapy in women with stage I-III breast Cancer: health-related quality of life, mindfulness, spirituality, life satisfaction, and Cancer-related fatigue. Evidence-based complementary and alternative medicine : eCAM. 2016;2016:5931816.
128. Sprod LK, Fernandez ID, Janelsins MC, Peppone LJ, Atkins JN, Giguere J, et al. Effects of yoga on cancer-related fatigue and global side-effect burden in older cancer survivors. J Geriatr Oncol. 2015;6(1):8–14.
129. Stan DL, Croghan KA, Croghan IT, Jenkins SM, Sutherland SJ, Cheville AL, et al. Randomized pilot trial of yoga versus strengthening exercises in breast cancer survivors with cancer-related fatigue. Support Care Cancer. 2016;24(9):4005–15.
130. Danhauer SC, Addington EL, Cohen L, Sohl SJ, Van Puymbroeck M, Albinati NK, et al. Yoga for symptom management in oncology: a review of the evidence base and future directions for research. Cancer. 2019;125(12):1979–89.
131. Kiecolt-Glaser JK, Bennett JM, Andridge R, Peng J, Shapiro CL, Malarkey WB, et al. Yoga's impact on inflammation, mood, and fatigue in breast cancer survivors: a randomized controlled trial. J Clin Oncol. 2014;32(10):1040–9.
132. Lengacher CA, Reich RR, Post-White J, Moscoso M, Shelton MM, Barta M, et al. Mindfulness based stress reduction in post-treatment breast cancer patients: an examination of symptoms and symptom clusters. J Behav Med. 2012;35(1):86–94.
133. Hoffman CJ, Ersser SJ, Hopkinson JB, Nicholls PG, Harrington JE, Thomas PW. Effectiveness of mindfulness-based stress reduction in mood, breast- and endocrine-related quality of life, and Well-being in stage 0 to III breast cancer: a randomized, controlled trial. J Clin Oncol. 2012;30(12):1335–42.
134. Molassiotis A, Bardy J, Finnegan-John J, Mackereth P, Ryder WD, Filshie J, et al. A randomized, controlled trial of acupuncture self-needling as maintenance therapy for cancer-related fatigue after therapist-delivered acupuncture. Ann Oncol. 2013;24(6):1645–52.
135. Molassiotis A, Sylt P, Diggins H. The management of cancer-related fatigue after chemotherapy with acupuncture and acupressure: a randomised controlled trial. Complement Ther Med. 2007;15(4):228–37.
136. Zhang Y, Lin L, Li H, Hu Y, Tian L. Effects of acupuncture on cancer-related fatigue: a meta-analysis. Support Care Cancer. 2018;26(2):415–25.
137. Deng G, Chan Y, Sjoberg D, Vickers A, Yeung KS, Kris M, et al. Acupuncture for the treatment of post-chemotherapy chronic fatigue: a randomized, blinded, sham-controlled trial. Support Care Cancer. 2013;21(6):1735–41.
138. Dilaveri CA, Croghan IT, Mallory MJ, Dion LJ, Fischer KM, Schroeder DR, et al. Massage compared with massage plus acupuncture for breast Cancer patients undergoing reconstructive surgery. J Altern Complement Med. 2020;26(7):602–9.
139. Ream E, Richardson A, Alexander-Dann C. Supportive intervention for fatigue in patients undergoing chemotherapy: a randomized controlled trial. J Pain Symptom Manag. 2006;31(2):148–61.
140. Armes J, Chalder T, Addington-Hall J, Richardson A, Hotopf M. A randomized controlled trial to evaluate the effectiveness of a brief, behaviorally oriented intervention for cancer-related fatigue. Cancer. 2007;110(6):1385–95.
141. Barsevick AM, Dudley W, Beck S, Sweeney C, Whitmer K, Nail L. A randomized clinical trial of energy conservation for patients with cancer-related fatigue. Cancer. 2004;100(6):1302–10.
142. Yates P, Aranda S, Hargraves M, Mirolo B, Clavarino A, McLachlan S, et al. Randomized controlled trial of an educational intervention for managing fatigue in women receiving adjuvant chemotherapy for early-stage breast cancer. J Clin Oncol. 2005;23(25):6027–36.
143. Lotfi-Jam K, Carey M, Jefford M, Schofield P, Charleson C, Aranda S. Nonpharmacologic strategies for managing common chemotherapy adverse effects: a systematic review. J Clin Oncol. 2008;26(34):5618–29.
144. Goedendorp MM, Gielissen MF, Verhagen CA, Bleijenberg G. Psychosocial interventions for reducing fatigue during cancer treatment in adults. Cochrane Database Syst Rev. 2009;(1):Cd006953.
145. Kwekkeboom KL, Abbott-Anderson K, Cherwin C, Roiland R, Serlin RC, Ward SE. Pilot randomized controlled trial of a patient-controlled cognitive-behavioral intervention for the pain, fatigue, and sleep disturbance symptom cluster in cancer. J Pain Symptom Manag. 2012;44(6):810–22.
146. Montgomery GH, David D, Kangas M, Green S, Sucala M, Bovbjerg DH, et al. Randomized controlled trial of a cognitive-behavioral therapy plus hypnosis intervention to control fatigue in patients undergoing radiotherapy for breast cancer. J Clin Oncol. 2014;32(6):557–63.
147. Jacobsen PB, Donovan KA, Vadaparampil ST, Small BJ. Systematic review and meta-analysis of psychological and activity-based interventions for cancer-related fatigue. Health Psychol. 2007;26(6):660–7.
148. Cillessen L, Johannsen M, Speckens AEM, Zachariae R. Mindfulness-based interventions for psychological and physical health outcomes in cancer patients and survivors: a systematic review and meta-analysis of randomized controlled trials. Psychooncology. 2019;28(12):2257–69.

149. Barsevick AM, Whitmer K, Sweeney C, Nail LM. A pilot study examining energy conservation for cancer treatment-related fatigue. Cancer Nurs. 2002;25(5):333–41.
150. Kangas M, Bovbjerg DH, Montgomery GH. Cancer-related fatigue: a systematic and meta-analytic review of non-pharmacological therapies for cancer patients. Psychol Bull. 2008;134(5):700–41.
151. Gielissen MF, Verhagen CA, Bleijenberg G. Cognitive behaviour therapy for fatigued cancer survivors: long-term follow-up. Br J Cancer. 2007;97(5):612–8.
152. Baguley BJ, Skinner TL, Wright ORL. Nutrition therapy for the management of cancer-related fatigue and quality of life: a systematic review and meta-analysis. Br J Nutr. 2019;122(5):527–41.
153. Inglis JE, Lin PJ, Kerns SL, Kleckner IR, Kleckner AS, Castillo DA, et al. Nutritional interventions for treating Cancer-related fatigue: a qualitative review. Nutr Cancer. 2019;71(1):21–40.
154. Zick SM, Colacino J, Cornellier M, Khabir T, Surnow K, Djuric Z. Fatigue reduction diet in breast cancer survivors: a pilot randomized clinical trial. Breast Cancer Res Treat. 2017;161(2):299–310.
155. Peppone LJ, Inglis JE, Mustian KM, Heckler CE, Padula GDA, Mohile SG, et al. Multicenter randomized controlled trial of omega-3 fatty acids versus omega-6 fatty acids for the control of cancer-related fatigue among breast cancer survivors. JNCI cancer spectrum. 2019;3(2):pkz005.
156. Iwase S, Kawaguchi T, Yotsumoto D, Doi T, Miyara K, Odagiri H, et al. Efficacy and safety of an amino acid jelly containing coenzyme Q10 and L-carnitine in controlling fatigue in breast cancer patients receiving chemotherapy: a multi-institutional, randomized, exploratory trial (JORTC-CAM01). Support Care Cancer. 2016;24(2):637–46.
157. Lesser GJ, Case D, Stark N, Williford S, Giguere J, Garino LA, et al. A randomized, double-blind, placebo-controlled study of oral coenzyme Q10 to relieve self-reported treatment-related fatigue in newly diagnosed patients with breast cancer. J Support Oncol. 2013;11(1):31–42.
158. da Costa MV, Trufelli DC, Santos J, Campos MP, Nobuo M, da Costa MM, et al. Effectiveness of guaraná (Paullinia cupana) for postradiation fatigue and depression: results of a pilot double-blind randomized study. J Altern Complement Med. 2009;15(4):431–3.
159. Sette CVM. Ribas de Alcântara BB, Schoueri JHM, Cruz FM, Cubero DIG, Pianowski LF, et al. purified dry Paullinia cupana (PC-18) extract for chemotherapy-induced fatigue: results of two double-blind randomized clinical trials. Journal of dietary supplements. 2018;15(5):673–83.
160. de Oliveira Campos MP, Riechelmann R, Martins LC, Hassan BJ, Casa FB, Del Giglio A. Guarana (Paullinia cupana) improves fatigue in breast cancer patients undergoing systemic chemotherapy. J Altern Complement Med. 2011;17(6):505–12.
161. Barton DL, Liu H, Dakhil SR, Linquist B, Sloan JA, Nichols CR, et al. Wisconsin ginseng (Panax quinquefolius) to improve cancer-related fatigue: a randomized, double-blind trial, N07C2. J Natl Cancer Inst. 2013;105(16):1230–8.
162. Barton DL, Soori GS, Bauer BA, Sloan JA, Johnson PA, Figueras C, et al. Pilot study of Panax quinquefolius (American ginseng) to improve cancer-related fatigue: a randomized, double-blind, dose-finding evaluation: NCCTG trial N03CA. Support Care Cancer. 2010;18(2):179–87.
163. Jiang SL, Liu HJ, Liu ZC, Liu N, Liu R, Kang YR, et al. Adjuvant effects of fermented red ginseng extract on advanced non-small cell lung cancer patients treated with chemotherapy. Chin J Integr Med. 2017;23(5):331–7.
164. Kim HS, Kim MK, Lee M, Kwon BS, Suh DH, Song YS. Effect of red ginseng on genotoxicity and health-related quality of life after adjuvant chemotherapy in patients with epithelial ovarian cancer: a randomized, double blind, placebo-controlled trial. Nutrients. 2017;9(7).
165. Choi MK, Song IS. Interactions of ginseng with therapeutic drugs. Arch Pharm Res. 2019;42(10):862–78.
166. Bilgi N, Bell K, Ananthakrishnan AN, Atallah E. Imatinib and Panax ginseng: a potential interaction resulting in liver toxicity. Ann Pharmacother. 2010;44(5):926–8.
167. Hwang S-W, Han H-S, Lim KY, Han J-Y. Drug interaction between complementary herbal medicines and Gefitinib. J Thorac Oncol. 2008;3(8):942–3.
168. Yennurajalingam S, Frisbee-Hume S, Palmer JL, Delgado-Guay MO, Bull J, Phan AT, et al. Reduction of cancer-related fatigue with dexamethasone: a double-blind, randomized, placebo-controlled trial in patients with advanced cancer. J Clin Oncol. 2013;31(25):3076–82.
169. Tomlinson D, Robinson PD, Oberoi S, Cataudella D, Culos-Reed N, Davis H, et al. Pharmacologic interventions for fatigue in cancer and transplantation: a meta-analysis. Curr Oncol. 2018;25(2):e152–e67.
170. Stockler MR, O'Connell R, Nowak AK, Goldstein D, Turner J, Wilcken NR, et al. Effect of sertraline on symptoms and survival in patients with advanced cancer, but without major depression: a placebo-controlled double-blind randomised trial. Lancet Oncol. 2007;8(7):603–12.
171. Palesh OG, Mustian KM, Peppone LJ, Janelsins M, Sprod LK, Kesler S, et al. Impact of paroxetine on sleep problems in 426 cancer patients receiving chemotherapy: a trial from the University of Rochester Cancer Center Community Clinical Oncology Program. Sleep Med. 2012;13(9):1184–90.
172. Minton O, Richardson A, Sharpe M, Hotopf M, Stone P. Drug therapy for the management of cancer-related fatigue. Cochrane Database Syst Rev. 2010;(7):Cd006704.

Sleep Issues and Insomnia

11

Ryan D. Davidson and Eric S. Zhou

Sleep Disturbances and Cancer

Sleep disturbances are common for patients across all types of cancer [1] with up to 60% of patients meeting criteria for a sleep disorder [2, 3]. Described as one of the most distressing symptoms associated with diagnosis and treatment of cancer, cancer patients report higher rates of sleep disturbances compared to the general adult population [4]. In addition to causing patient distress and compromising quality of life, sleep disturbances have significant health impacts. Some studies have indicated that poorer sleep also can impact tumor formation and cancer outcomes [5]. Chronically disrupted sleep has been associated with increased rates of colorectal cancer [6] and breast cancer in women [7] as well as prostate cancer in men [8]. Further, sleep disturbances are associated with more aggressive tumor characteristics for post-menopausal women with breast cancer [9].

There are differences in sleep disturbances based on the specific site of the cancer. Patients with breast or ovarian cancer are the most likely to have sleep disturbances while patients with prostate cancer are less likely to have sleep disturbances compared to other cancer diagnoses [10–12]. In addition to breast cancer being one of the most common types of cancer, particularly in women [13], the impact of the diagnosis itself, risk factors associated with breast cancer, and the treatment is associated with increased rates of sleep disturbances [14]. For patients with breast cancer, sleep disturbances are associated with worse quality of life compared to patients with other forms of cancer [15].

Differentiation Between Insufficient Sleep, Poor Sleep, and Sleep Disorders

It is important to recognize that the terms "insufficient sleep," "poor sleep quality," and/or a "sleep disorder" such as insomnia are often used interchangeably by patients and providers alike, but they are distinct problems. Insufficient sleep emphasizes the hours of sleep an individual gets on a nightly basis, whereas poor sleep quality focuses on how restful the night of sleep was

R. D. Davidson (✉)
Gastroenterology, Hepatology, and Nutrition, Boston Children's Hospital, Boston, MA, USA

Division of Psychiatry, Harvard Medical School, Boston, MA, USA
e-mail: ryan.davidson@childrens.harvard.edu

E. S. Zhou
Perini Family Survivor's Center, Dana-Farber Cancer Institute, Boston, MA, USA

Neurology, Boston Children's Hospital, Boston, MA, USA

Division of Sleep Medicine, Harvard Medical School, Boston, MA, USA
e-mail: eric_zhou@dcfi.harvard.edu

G. G. Kimmick et al. (eds.), *Common Issues in Breast Cancer Survivors*,
https://doi.org/10.1007/978-3-030-75377-1_11

based on subjective reports. Individuals who report poor sleep quality often report a sense of tossing and turning, having difficulty falling asleep, difficulty staying asleep, or feel like they were not in a deep sleep. Though individuals with insufficient sleep time may also report poor sleep quality, one study of breast cancer patients undergoing chemotherapy indicated that subjective reports of poor sleep quality and increased daytime dysfunction were associated with longer sleep duration [16]. Sleep disorders occur when symptoms of poor sleep duration, quality, or sleep behaviors reach a level which impairs daily functioning. It is important to note that neither insufficient sleep nor poor sleep quality is itself a sleep disorder. The most common sleep disorders in the general population include insomnia, obstructive sleep apnea (OSA), and sleep-related movement disorders (restless leg syndrome and periodic limb movement disorder) [17, 18]. For the purposes of this paper, we will use the term *sleep disturbances* as a broad term for insufficient sleep, poor sleep quality, and sleep disorders unless specified more narrowly.

Sleep Disturbances in Breast Cancer

There is limited research investigating relationships between sleep duration, specifically, and breast cancer. However, in one 20-year prospective study, short sleep duration was not associated with higher rates of breast cancer, but long-sleepers (over 9 h) were less at risk for developing breast cancer [19]. There is a greater breadth of research investigating the relationship of subjective sleep quality and cancer and related treatments. One limitation of the research within this field is the difficulty comparing rates of sleep disturbances across studies due to varying use of sleep disturbances, poor sleep quality, sleep problems, and insomnia as outcome measures with a wide range of definitions used. Women with breast cancer are more likely to experience insomnia than the general population [20, 21], but there is limited data about the rates of other sleep disorders such as OSA and restless leg syndrome in breast cancer populations.

Similar to patterns seen across all cancer types, women with breast cancer are more likely to experience insomnia and related symptoms compared to control groups of women without cancer [22, 23]. Some of the association between breast cancer and insomnia may be accounted for by overlapping risk factors. Two of these prominent risk factors for both include being female and having multiple health problems [12, 24, 25]. There are mixed findings regarding age and risk for insomnia for individuals with breast cancer, but some argue that women with breast cancer who are older are at greater risk, while in other studies age does not impact risk for insomnia [26]. Within breast cancer patients, there are several risk factors for vulnerability to developing insomnia or other sleep disturbances, including presence of hot flashes, menopausal symptoms, pain, fatigue, and depressive symptoms [27–29; see Table 11.1].

Insomnia is common in patients with breast cancer, regardless of stage. In an early seminal study of breast cancer patients (ranging from 2 to 357 months since diagnosis), 19% of non-metastatic patients had insomnia, and of these patients with insomnia, 95% of these patients had insomnia with symptoms lasting more than 6 months [21]. A third of the patients who reported insomnia, reported symptoms began

Table 11.1 Risk factors for insomnia for general population and breast cancer patients

Risk factors for insomnia in general population [24, 132]	Risk factors for insomnia in breast cancer patients [27–29]
History of insomnia	Hot flashes (slower onset and longer duration)
Family history of insomnia	Menopause
Female	Non-Caucasian
Older age	Younger age
Snoring	Pain
Poorer general health	Fatigue
Poorer mental health (depression, anxiety symptoms)	Depression symptoms
Pain	Decreased physical activity
Personality traits (lower extraversion, higher arousability)	Poorer reported general health

after diagnosis, and over half reported that the cancer diagnosis caused or exacerbated pre-existing sleep difficulties [21]. Even higher rates of sleep disturbances have been reported in women with metastatic breast cancer, with 63% reporting sleep disturbances and 35% reporting use of sleep medications within the previous month [30]. In a more recent study, these high rates of sleep disturbance persist, with more than half of female patients with breast cancer reporting poor sleep [29].

While early studies indicated that diagnosis of breast cancer was a key trigger for sleep disturbances and insomnia, other studies have highlighted the potential impact of chemotherapy on sleep. After chemotherapy, patients with breast cancer demonstrated lighter sleep with less deep sleep and REM sleep, as well as more time spent in bed awake [31]. Subjectively, women with breast cancer report a negative impact of chemotherapy on sleep quality [32]. Women in Egypt who underwent chemotherapy as a part of their treatment reported worse sleep quality than women who did not go through chemotherapy [3].

There are mixed findings about how chemotherapy impacts sleep disturbances over time for women with breast cancer. Some studies indicate there does not seem to be a change across chemotherapy cycles [32], while others indicate that as chemotherapy cycles continue, patients report worse subjective sleep [33]. An earlier study indicated that within the first 3 days of administration of chemotherapy, there were disruptions in the sleep-wake rhythm which worsened with each progressive administration of chemotherapy [34]. Whisenant and colleagues recently provided further insight regarding the trajectories of sleep disturbances reported by breast cancer patients across cycles of chemotherapy [35]. Within this study, there were two patterns of sleep disturbances noted; one group demonstrated mild improvements in sleep disturbances across the 2nd (89%) and 3rd (81%) cycle of chemotherapy, while the other group demonstrated a moderate worsening of sleep disturbances during the 2nd cycle of chemotherapy (11%) and a mild worsening of sleep disturbances in the 3rd cycle of chemotherapy (19%) [35]. Neither demographic nor treatment variables were predictive of sleep disturbance class.

Side effects of treatment, including the medical induction of menopause [36, 37] and increased hot flashes, also impact sleep disorders in women with breast cancer [38]. Breast cancer survivors were more likely to have hot flashes compared to a control group of matched healthy women [39]. In women with breast cancer, night-time hot flashes are associated with more time awake, less deep sleep, and more fragmented sleep [40]. There has been some research to identify the timing of symptoms and sleep disturbances. One study indicated that when prescribed tamoxifen, women experienced higher rates of depression than non-cancer mid-aged controls and that presence of hot flashes adversely impacted both depression and reported quality of life [41]. Though many women had also undergone chemotherapy and almost half had menopausal symptoms prior to starting tamoxifen, the frequency and burden of hot flashes were attributed to tamoxifen by the participants [41]. In this study, frequency of hot flashes was associated specifically with worse emotional functioning, higher levels of anxiety, and more sleep disturbances [41]. In another study, poor sleep was associated with increases in both pain and hot flashes, but these were preceded by dysfunctional sleep-related thoughts (worry about the consequences of insomnia) and sleep impairing behaviors (e.g., napping, staying in bed while awake, increasing time for sleep opportunities) [42].

Inflammatory cytokines, including interleukin-1 beta (IL-1β), interleukin-6 (IL-6), tumor necrosis factor-alpha (TNF-α), and interleukin-2 (IL-2), are thought to be one physiological link between cancer and sleep disturbances and may be produced as a response to tumor growth or chemotherapy. These cytokines can activate pathways which are also involved in sleep-wake cycles and pain responses [43, 44]. In addition, the stress associated with diagnosis and treatment can also exacerbate inflammatory cytokine response through activation of the hypothalamic-pituitary-adrenal axis [45]. Though the exact mechanism is still being understood, inflammatory cytokines may influence sleep through the impact on sleep-wake cycles, increased pain, fatigue, and production of corticosteroids associated with increased stress in adults with cancer [45, 46]. Other studies identified nausea, a common side effect of chemotherapy, as a potential mechanism for disturbed sleep in breast cancer patients. Nausea severity was found to impact both sleep disturbances and fatigue for women with breast cancer [47]. Many of the medications that are commonly used to improve treatment-related side effects such as opioids, anti-nausea medications, and corticosteroids can exacerbate sleep disturbances [48–50].

Differential Diagnoses and Importance of Assessment Within Cancer Populations

Sleep disturbances may begin or become exacerbated with cancer diagnosis, treatments, and/or side effects. For many patients with cancer generally, sleep disturbances (specifically insomnia symptoms) improve over time [23]. However, they do not necessarily resolve completely or along the same trajectory as other side effects of treatment such as pain and fatigue. Approximately 40% of individuals with a history of breast cancer without evidence of disease continue to report sleep disturbances 5 years posttreatment [51, 52]. With the high rates of sleep disturbances, it is important to address sleep disturbances specifically early, even before other side effects or symptoms associated with treatment have resolved.

Insomnia Disorder

Criteria for an insomnia disorder include difficulty initiating or maintaining sleep or experiencing nonrestorative sleep; difficulties must last for at least 1 month and sleep disturbances cause clinically significant distress or impairment in functioning [53]. These symptoms and experiences may be brief (transient), occur periodically (transient recurring), or can be chronic, and many people may experience a combination of symptoms. There are also side effects or consequences of insomnia, including tiredness, negative mood, inability to enjoy social activities, lack of concentration, impaired memory, decreased quality of life, exacerbated health conditions, as well as impacts on work such as higher rates of absenteeism and lower job performance [54]. Women with breast cancer may be twice as likely to experience insomnia compared to the general population [21]. As insomnia severity increases, postmenopausal women with breast cancer demonstrate worsening sequelae including cognitive impairments [55]. When assessing for insomnia, it is important to adequately assess mood symptoms as insomnia is often associated with increased rates of depression [30]. Furthermore, rates of anxiety, depression, and fatigue are higher in women after breast cancer diagnosis [56, 57].

Obstructive Sleep Apnea

Another common sleep disorder is obstructive sleep apnea (OSA) which involves frequent pauses in breathing overnight during sleep, associated with loud snoring and caused by obstruction of the airway, often associated with the tongue or airway dilator muscles [58]. Polysomnography is required to diagnose OSA as there are specific criteria associated with severity of desaturation, length of time of cessation of airflow, and the number of cessation events tallied throughout the night [59]. There are long-term health consequences associated with OSA, including cardiovascular, neurological, and endocrine implications [58]. There are mixed findings regarding whether OSA may be a contributing factor in the incidence or progression of cancer [60–62]. There are elevated rates of OSA in cancer populations, especially head and neck cancers [63, 64]. There is limited data about the frequency of OSA in patients with breast cancer specifically.

Periodic Limb Movement Disorder

Periodic Limb Movement Disorder (PLMD) is a neurological disorder that is associated with repeated limb movements, typically in lower limbs, which occurs in sleep [65]. Although impairment leading to the periodic limb movement disorder diagnosis is rare, the involuntary periodic limb movements during sleep are more common and may not reach the threshold to diagnose an individual with PLMD. Many individuals may experience restless leg syndrome which is associated with voluntary limb movements, but these occur while awake. As PLMD is a rare disorder, there is limited research regarding the relationship between periodic limb movements and cancer, and specifically patients with breast cancer. However, in one study of patients with breast cancer, women with cancer were more likely to experience periodic limb movements compared to women without cancer [31]. The increased rates of periodic limb movements may be a contributing factor to sleep disturbances in cancer patients as women with breast cancer with severe insomnia only differed from those with mild or moderate insomnia in number of periodic limb movements [66].

Interventions

Cognitive Behavioral Therapy for Insomnia

Given the significant distress regarding sleep disturbances and insomnia and its subsequent impact on quality of life, it is important for patients with sleep disturbances to receive treatment. Cognitive Behavioral Therapy for Insomnia (CBT-I) is considered the gold standard for insomnia treatment [67] and is typically administered within 4–8 sessions. It is associated with improvements in both subjective and objective measures of sleep [68]. CBT-I utilizes strategies from behavioral therapies and includes several components to create a brief, sleep-focused multimodal intervention [69, 70]. The components of CBT-I include sleep restriction, stimulus control, cognitive restructuring, sleep hygiene, and relaxation (see Table 11.2 for a more in-depth description of these components) [69–75]. It is hypothesized that in addition to the direct improvement on sleep measures resulting from both behavioral and cognitive methods, CBT-I is also associated with improvement in mood which then subsequently improves adherence and anxiety, further improving sleep quality [76].

Table 11.2 Description of components of CBT-I

Component of CBT-I	General description
Sleep restriction [72, 73]	Providers will "prescribe" a new window for sleep opportunity which typically would match the total amount of sleep the patient is currently receiving. Over time, the sleep opportunity window increases
Stimulus control [74]	Behavioral strategies for patients to begin to relearn associations between sleep and bed/bedroom. Strategies include going to bed when sleepy, only using the bed for sleep and sexual activities, and leaving the bed if unable to fall asleep within 20 min and not returning until one is sleepy again
Cognitive restructuring [71;75]	Patients are taught to identify unhelpful thoughts such as if one does not get enough sleep one night, they will be completely useless the next day. Over time, patients are taught to evaluate and modify their thoughts
Sleep hygiene [71]	Patients are encouraged to use behavioral strategies which improve sleep environment and routine, including going to bed and waking up at the same time every day, maintaining appropriate light and temperature in the bedroom, and minimization of caffeine, alcohol, and nicotine during the evening
Relaxation [71]	Providers work with patients to identify strategies which focus on decreasing physical tension as well as intrusive thoughts and worries at bedtime

[a]Note: Sleep disorders can be complex and often occur in the context of comorbid psychological and medical disorders. Specific interventions to address sleep should be provided by providers with specific training

CBT-I is effective for improving sleep using both subjective and objective outcome measures in breast cancer populations. Individuals with breast cancer who received CBT-I had decreased total wake time and improved sleep efficiency following treatment with sustained improvements at 3 and 6 months when using both sleep diaries and polysomnography [77–79]. Other studies showed that CBT-I was effective at improving reported insomnia [38, 80, 81]. However, one study indicated that there were no significant differences between CBT-I and a psychoeducation control group for women with breast cancer and insomnia for the following outcomes: wake after sleep onset, total sleep time, sleep efficiency, and sleep quality [82]. There was one difference between CBT-I and the psychoeducation control group as participants in the CBT-I group spent less time in bed at the end of treatment [82].

In addition to improving sleep, CBT-I relieves distress and improves quality of life [83]. For individuals with breast cancer specifically, there are reported improvements in depression and anxiety [84, 77] as well as fatigue and quality of life compared to control groups [80, 85]. Further, CBT targeting hot flashes was associated with reduction in menopausal symptoms using both physiological and subjective measures. Along with improvement in hot flashes, women also reported improved sleep quality and general quality of life [86]. Improvements in hot flashes and night sweats were maintained at 26-week follow-up [86]. CBT-I has also been shown to improve physical and cognitive functioning, lessen insomnia, improve attitudes towards sleep [81], and improve immune system functioning [84].

Despite proven benefits of CBT-I, there can be barriers to identifying sleep specialists to work with breast cancer patients. In order to address this potential barrier to accessing services and to address variations in adherence [87], investigators have explored a variety of alternate delivery options. Delivery methods evaluated in clinical trials include video-based intervention [88], self-help formats [89] some of which are delivered during chemotherapy [90], and web-based delivery [91]. Not only were these delivery methods effective in improving sleep quality, but, importantly, they were acceptable to patients, implying that the beneficial effects of CBT-I were credible to patients. Perceived credibility is important because it is associated with adherence to behavioral recommendations [92].

Stepped Care Interventions

A growing area of research within CBT-I is the idea of stepped care-interventions. With growing data to support alternative delivery options for CBT-I, there has been a growing need to identify appropriate methods to identify which form of delivery is most helpful for which patients. One potential mechanism by which to funnel patients to the appropriate care is through a stepped-care model. At the beginning all patients would enter into the treatment system through the "least restrictive therapy" [93]. If patients benefit from this level of intervention, they can leave the pathway, but if they need additional support they continue to move up the hierarchy of interventions until they reach the appropriate level of intervention and provider expertise. In the case of CBT-I, the first step or entry point could be a web-based delivery system or a single CBT-I-based workshop. If the patient's insomnia continues to be unremitting, they would eventually engage in a full course of in-person CBT-I with a behavioral sleep medicine expert.

Other Behavioral Interventions

In addition to CBT-I, there are other behavioral interventions which have been shown to be effective in treating insomnia for cancer patients [94]. A recent meta-analysis and systematic review of exercise interventions demonstrated that regular aerobic exercise can improve sleep quality for cancer patients [95, 96]. Mindfulness-based approaches also show promise [97, 98] with some recent feasibility and non-randomized studies indicating that mind-body interventions may be more acceptable and feasible for breast cancer survivors compared to CBT-I [99]. In addition to improvements in sleep outcomes, mind-body interventions like yoga can also impact daily cortisol rhythms and immune responses [100].

Pharmacotherapy

Up to 41% of cancer patients received a prescription for a sleep medication following diagnosis [101], and 28% of patients are prescribed sleep-related medications 9 years post cancer diagnosis [102]. Similar rates of medication use for sleep management were seen in breast cancer survivors [80, 103].

In the general population, CBT-I and pharmacotherapy are shown to be equally effective for short-term outcomes with CBT-I more effective in the long-term [104–106]. In one more recent randomized trial investigating the effect of a wake-promoting medication (armodafinil), study arms which included CBT-I (CBT-I plus placebo and CBT-I plus medication) demonstrated improvement in severity of insomnia and sleep quality compared to just medication study arms (armodafinil ad placebo) [107]. These improvements were maintained at follow-up 3-months post treatment [107]. The most common medications for the treatment of insomnia in the general population and for cancer patients include benzodiazepine, benzodiazepine receptor agonists, antidepressants, antihistamines, and melatonin receptor agonist [106]. The American Academy of Sleep Medicine has published a set of clinical practice guidelines for the use of pharmacologic treatment of insomnia for adults and should be referenced for more in-depth guidelines [108]. In one study, almost half of patients with breast cancer who use medication sleep aids were prescribed a hypnotic (benzodiazepine or benzodiazepine receptor agonist), but nearly a quarter used over-the-counter analgesics such as acetaminophen or ibuprofen as a sleep aid [103]. Meta-analyses reported within the European guidelines for the treatment of insomnia [106] indicate that benzodiazepines and benzodiazepine receptor agonists are effective when used for less than 4 weeks and are more effective than anti-depressants used in small doses to treat insomnia. There are limited meta-analyses assessing the effectiveness of antihistamines, antipsychotics, or other psychopharmacological options [106].

Though pharmacology is often utilized to treat sleep disturbances in general and cancer populations, many of these medications have not been tested in cancer populations and long-term effectiveness and efficacy are not understood [109]. There is even less data regarding the efficacy of these medications for breast cancer specifically. In addition, there are side effects as a consequence of many of these medications, and use of hypnotics has been associated with increased rates of cancer and mortality [110–112]. In older adult populations, specific antihistamines such as diphenhydramine, and doxylamine have been associated with liver and kidney complications, cognitive impairment, and increased rates of falls [113, 114]. Use of benzodiazepines at night for sleep is also associated with impairments in cognitive functioning, including memory, as well as both falls and motor vehicle accidents [115].

Intervention Recommendations

Although many patients receive sleep medication after diagnosis, a position statement from the American Academy of Sleep Medicine (AASM) notes that for the treatment of insomnia (not specific to cancer), there were no pharmacological agents that had stronger than "weak" supporting evidence [108]. Both the American College of Physicians (ACP) [116] and Canadian guidelines [117–119] indicate that CBT-I should be the first line of treatment for management of insomnia. Decisions about the addition of medication/pharmacotherapy to CBT-I should be made between providers and patients after discussions about the potential benefits and side effects. For patients who may have difficulty accessing CBT-I in person or administered by a sleep specialist, other modes of delivery of CBT-I (e.g., video-based, web-based) may be beneficial.

Algorithm for Assessment, Management, and Treatment for Sleep Disturbances and Insomnia in Breast Cancer Patients (See Fig. 11.1)

When working with patients with breast cancer, a comprehensive psychosocial assessment including questions about sleep can be helpful. Many patients with breast cancer experience depression, anxiety and/or worsening quality of life in addition to sleep disturbances. Providers should assess for mood disorders, sleep disorders, and side effects of medication in addition to sleep

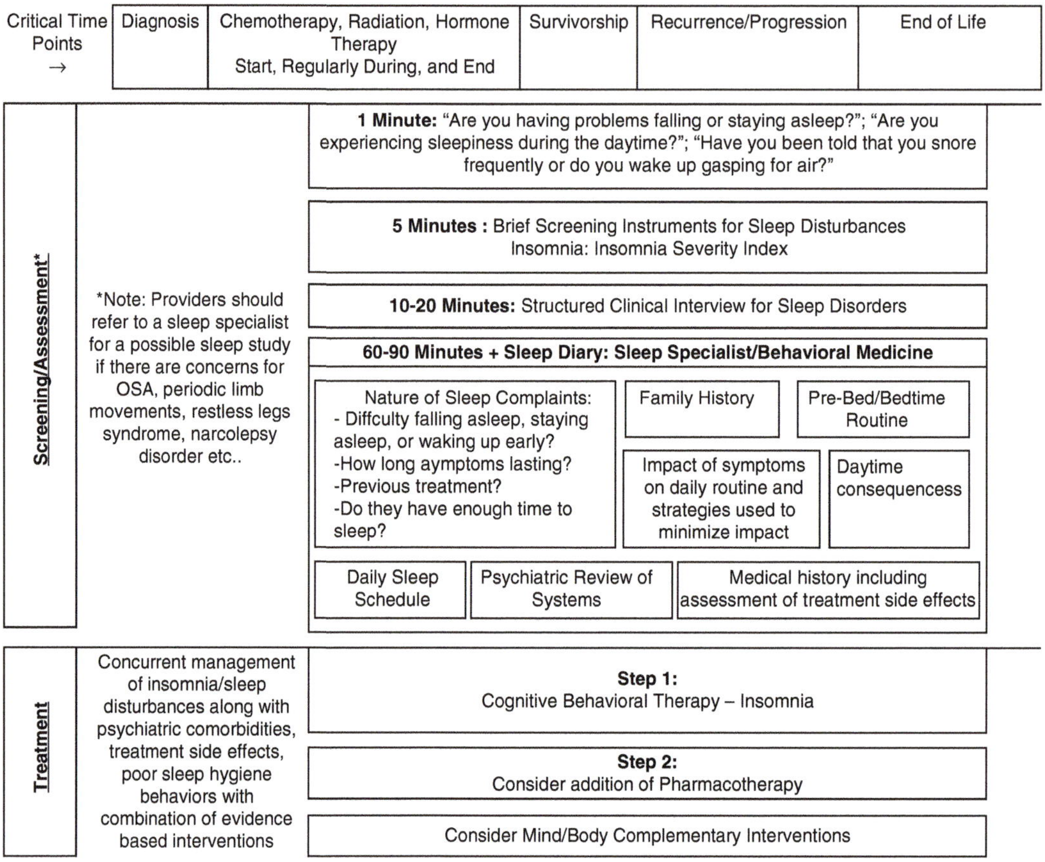

Fig. 11.1 Algorithm for assessment, management, and treatment for sleep disturbances and insomnia in breast cancer patients

problems, sleep schedule, and behaviors that augment sleep disturbances. A clinical interview is the gold standard for identification of insomnia within cancer populations [117, 118]. However, there are recent studies that indicate that extended interviews may not be feasible to administer to all patients within a busy clinic as extensive screening may require too much time [120]. The choice of method by which to screen for sleep disturbances will, therefore, depend on available time and resources.

Critical Time Points

Given the complex nature of cancer from diagnosis through treatment, and potential recurrence/progression, repeated screening for sleep disturbance is recommended. Screening is especially important at the following time points: at diagnosis, at start of treatment, after treatment completion, and at recurrence [117, 118]. Periodic screening for sleep disturbance should also occur during active treatment and during survivorship.

Screening

Providers can choose from many available tools to screen for insomnia, depending on time and resources (Fig. 11.1). Simple screening with several brief questions takes about 1 minute and determines whether additional screening is necessary. We suggest three key questions that briefly assess for perceived sleep quality, insufficient sleep, and OSA:

1. "Are you having problems falling or staying asleep?"
2. "Are you experiencing sleepiness during the daytime?"
3. "Have you been told that you snore frequently or do you wake up gasping for air?"

If a provider has 5 minutes, there are several brief screening instruments which providers can administer while a patient is in the office. To assess for insomnia, providers can use screening tools such as the Sleep Condition Indicator [121] or the Insomnia Severity Index (ISI) [122, 123]. The ISI has been widely used to assess not just insomnia symptoms but clinical improvement throughout treatment [123] and has been validated in cancer populations [124]. If the patient reports or the provider has concerns about potential OSA, the STOP-BANG [125] may be used. If the provider has 10–20 minutes to complete a screening/assessment for sleep disturbances and disorders, the Structured Clinical Interview for Sleep Disorders (SCISD) [126] can be administered (available at https://insomnia.arizona.edu/SCISD). The SCISD is an 8-page questionnaire which assesses for a variety of sleep disorders, including insomnia, hypersomnia, obstructive sleep apnea, periodic limb movements, and several other sleep disorders based on DSM-5 criteria [53].

Some cancer centers may have the benefit of social work, behavioral medicine, or sleep specialists available to conduct full-length assessments, which may take 60 to 90 minutes to complete. If this resource is available, medical providers may find it useful to complete an initial screen with standardized measures then refer to a social worker or other trained clinicians who can conduct an in-depth interview. The in-depth interview should include information about the nature of the sleep complaints, daily bedtime routines, impact of sleep symptoms on functioning, as well as a full psychiatric review of systems to assess for comorbid anxiety and or depression. In addition to the in-depth interview, a sleep diary may also be helpful to the assessment [127]. Sleep diaries are the gold standard for measuring subjective sleep and serves as a daily prospective self-monitoring tool. Patients use sleep diaries to report a wide range of information about their sleep including time they get in bed, time until they fall asleep, awakenings overnight, and when they wake up and get out of bed in the morning [127–129]. It may be helpful to provide patients with instructions on how to fill out the sleep diary prior to the patient's visit with a social worker or behavioral medicine/sleep specialist so that the provider conducting the in-depth assessment can collect and use as a part of their assessment. Polysomnography is considered the gold standard of objective sleep measurement; however, many providers will also use actigraphy (movement-based devices). It is important to note that actigraphy is different than many of the wearable devices publicly available. Wearable devices such as Fitbits, Apple watches, and other devices have been compared to these gold-standard measures of sleep, but with limited validation [130]. With the current state of the research, there is not enough evidence to support their use in clinical science, however, in the near future with more data, they may replace actigraphy.

Treatments

If sleep concerns are identified during the screening process, there are several treatment paths providers can take. Patients at risk for OSA or periodic limb movements based on initial screening measures should be referred to sleep centers for additional evaluation, and potential sleep study should be considered. Patients should be provided with information regarding the diagnoses under consideration. In addition to treating sleep disturbances, managing other conditions that interfere with sleep is necessary. These include pain, hot flashes, and side effects of cancer and its treatment. If sleep disturbance is identified and local resources do not include CBT-I, using a stepped care approach is recommended for patient education [93, 131]. One program targeted for cancer patients, the Sleep Training Education Program (STEP) model, demonstrated that providing psychoeducation, video, or self-help versions of CBT-I may be effective for many patients as the first step of intervention [131]. If there are persistent sleep issues after 4 or 8 weeks following the STEP intervention, CBT-I administered by an experienced professional should be considered. Providers should review the risks and benefits with patients regarding the addition of medication as an adjunct to CBT-I when warranted. Further, mind-body interventions may be available, such as yoga, that patients can engage in combination with CBT-I, but should be discussed with the sleep specialist or behavioral medicine provider to ensure that approach is not contraindicated, as some forms of yoga may exacerbate muscle soreness or joint pain.

Conclusion

Sleep disturbances, including poor sleep quality, insufficient sleep, and sleep disorders, are common among patients with breast cancer and often persist long after treatment and well into recovery. Sleep disturbances are associated with negative outcomes including poorer quality of life and higher risk for mortality. With the high prevalence rates, negative short- and long-term consequences, and complex nature of sleep disturbances, it is important to assess for them throughout cancer survivorship including diagnosis, treatment, recovery, and potential recurrence. This is particularly true for patients with breast cancer as they are at higher risk for sleep disturbances due to side effects of both cancer and treatment. Several treatments that have been found effective for treatment of sleep disorders have also been found to improve other variables associated with quality of life including pain, depression symptoms, and menopause symptoms. Unfortunately, access to trained providers is often a significant barrier to receiving the gold standard insomnia treatment, CBT-I. There is a growing body of research supporting a stepped care approach to the treatment of insomnia that start patients with the least restrictive interventions, such as a psychoeducation workshop or self-help intervention. If after several weeks, patients continue to report sleep disturbances, referral to sleep medicine specialist may be necessary.

References

1. Ancoli-Israel S. Sleep and fatigue in cancer patients. In: principles and practice of sleep medicine. Saunders; 2005.
2. Simeit R, Deck R, Conta-Marx B. Sleep management training for cancer patients with insomnia. Support Care Cancer. 2004;12(3):176–83.
3. Tag Eldin ES, Younis SG, Aziz LMAE, Eldin AT, Erfan ST. Evaluation of sleep pattern disorders in breast cancer patients receiving adjuvant treatment (chemotherapy and/or radiotherapy) using polysomnography. J BUON. 2019;24:529–34.
4. Ness S, Kokal J, Fee-Schroeder K, Novotny P, Satele D, Barton D. Concerns across the survivorship trajectory: results from a survey of cancer survivors. Oncol Nurs Forum. 2012;40(1):35–42.
5. Medic G, Wille M, Hemels MEH. Short- and long-term health consequences of sleep disruption. Nat Sci Sleep. 2017;9:151–61.
6. Schernhammer ES, Laden F, Speizer FE, Willett WC, Hunter DJ, Kawachi I, et al. Night-shift work and risk of colorectal cancer in the Nurses Health Study. J Natl Cancer Inst. 2003;95(11):825–8.
7. Schernhammer ES, Laden F, Speizer FE, Willett WC, Hunter DJ, Kawachi I, et al. Rotating night shifts and risk of breast cancer in women participating in the Nurses Health Study. J Natl Cancer Inst. 2001;93(20):1563–8.
8. Sigurdardottir LG, Valdimarsdottir UA, Mucci LA, Fall K, Rider JR, Schernhammer E, et al. Sleep disruption among older men and risk of prostate cancer. Cancer Epidemiol Biomark Prev. 2013;22(5):872–9.
9. Soucise A, Vaughn C, Thompson CL, Millen AE, Freudenheim JL, Wactawski-Wende J, Phipps AI, Hale L, Qi L, Ochs-Balcom HM. Sleep quality, duration, and breast cancer aggressiveness. Breast Cancer Res Treat. 2017;164(1):169–78. https://doi.org/10.1007/s10549-017-4245-1
10. Davidson JR, MacLean AW, Brundage MD. Sleep disturbance in cancer patients. Soc Sci Med. 2002;54:1309–21.
11. Portenoy RK, Thaler HT, Kornblith AB, Lepore JM, Friedlander-Klar H, Coyle N, et al. Symptom prevalence, characteristics and distress in a cancer population. Qual Life Res. 1994;3(3):183–9.
12. Zhou ES, Clark K, Recklitis CJ, Obenchain R, Loscalzo M. Sleepless from the get go: sleep problems prior to initiating cancer treatment. Int J Behav Med. 2018;25(5):502–16.
13. Ferlay J, Soerjomataram I, Dikshit R, Eser S, Mathers C, Rebelo M, Parkin DM, Forman D, Bray F. Cancer incidence and mortality worldwide: sources, meth-

ods and major patterns in GLOBOCAN 2012. Int J Cancer. 2015;136(5):E359–86.
14. Ancoli-Israel S. Sleep disturbances in cancer: a review. Sleep Med Res. 2015;6(2):45–9.
15. Fortner BV, Stepanksi EJ, Wang SC, Kasprowicz S, Durrence HH. Sleep and quality of life in breast cancer patients. J Pain Symptom Manage. 2002;24(5):471–80.
16. Ancoli-Israel S, Liu L, Marler MR, Parker BA, Jones V, Sadler GR, Dimsdale J, Cohen-Zion M, Fiorentino L. Fatigue, sleep, and circadian rhythms prior to chemotherapy for breast cancer. Support Care Cancer. 2006;14(3):201–9.
17. Ram S, Seirawan H, Kumar SK, Clark GT. Prevalence and impact of sleep disorders and sleep habits in the United States. Sleep Breath. 2010;14(1):63–70.
18. Wolkove N, Elkholy O, Baltzan M, Palayew M. Sleep and aging: 1. Sleep disorders commonly found in older people. CMAJ. 2007;176(9):1299–304.
19. Verkasalo PK, Lillberg K, Stevens RG, Hublin C, Partinen M, Koskenvuo M, Kaprio J. Sleep duration and breast cancer: a prospective cohort study. Cancer Res. 2005;65(20):9595–600.
20. Bower JE. Behavioral symptoms in breast cancer patients and survivors: fatigue, insomnia, depression, and cognitive disturbance. J Clin Oncol Off J Am Soc Clin Oncol. 2008;26(5):768.
21. Savard J, Simard S, Blanchet J, Ivers H, Morin CM. Prevalence, clinical characteristics, and risk factors for insomnia in the context of breast cancer. Sleep. 2001;24(5):583–90.
22. Savard J, Ivers H, Savard MH, Morin CM. Cancer treatments and their side effects are associated with aggravation of insomnia: results of a longitudinal study. Cancer. 2015;121(10):1703–11.
23. Palesh OG, Roscoe JA, Mustian KM, Roth T, Savard J, Ancoli-Israel S, Heckler C, Purnell JQ, Janelsins MC, Morrow GR. Prevalence, demographics, and psychological associations of sleep disruption in patients with cancer: University of Rochester Cancer Center–Community Clinical Oncology Program. J Clin Oncol. 2010;28(2):292.
24. Klink ME, Quan SF, Kaltenborn WT, Lebowitz MD. Risk factors associated with complaints of insomnia in a general adult population: influence of previous complaints of insomnia. Arch Intern Med. 1992;152(8):1634–7.
25. Savard J, Morin CM. Insomnia in the context of cancer: a review of a neglected problem. J Clin Oncol. 2001;19(3):895–908.
26. Bardwell WA, Profant J, Casden DR, Dimsdale JE, Ancoli-Israel S, Natarajan L, Rock CL, Pierce JP, Women's Healthy Eating & Living (WHEL) Study Group. The relative importance of specific risk factors for insomnia in women treated for early-stage breast cancer. Psycho-Oncology. 2008;17(1):9–18.
27. Leysen L, Lahousse A, Nijs J, Adriaenssens N, Mairesse O, Ivakhnov S, Bilterys T, Van Looveren E, Pas R, Beckwée D. Prevalence and risk factors of sleep disturbances in breast cancer survivors: systematic review and meta-analyses. Support Care Cancer. 2019;25:1–33.
28. Berger AM, Kupzyk KA, Djalilova DM, Cowan KH. Breast Cancer Collaborative Registry informs understanding of factors predicting sleep quality. Support Care Cancer. 2019;27(4):1365–73.
29. Savard MH, Savard J, Caplette-Gingras A, Ivers H, Bastien C. Relationship between objectively recorded hot flashes and sleep disturbances among breast cancer patients: investigating hot flash characteristics other than frequency. Menopause. 2013;20(10):997–1005.
30. Koopman C, Nouriani B, Erickson V, Anupindi R, Butler LD, Bachmann MH, Sephton SE, Spiegel D. Sleep disturbances in women with metastatic breast cancer. Breast J. 2002 Nov;8(6):362–70.
31. Fiorentino L, Mason W, Parker B, Johnson S, Amador X, Ancoli-Israel S. Sleep disruption in breast cancer patients post-chemotherapy. Sleep. 2005;28:A294.
32. Sanford SD, Wagner LI, Beaumont JL, Butt Z, Sweet JJ, Cella D. Longitudinal prospective assessment of sleep quality: before, during, and after adjuvant chemotherapy for breast cancer. Support Care Cancer. 2013;21(4):959–67.
33. Van Onselen C, Paul SM, Lee K, Dunn L, Aouizerat BE, West C, Dodd M, Cooper B, Miaskowski C. Trajectories of sleep disturbance and daytime sleepiness in women before and after surgery for breast cancer. J Pain Symptom Manag. 2013;45(2):244–60.
34. Savard J, Liu L, Natarajan L, Rissling MB, Neikrug AB, He F, Dimsdale JE, Mills PJ, Parker BA, Sadler GR, Ancoli-Israel S. Breast cancer patients have progressively impaired sleep-wake activity rhythms during chemotherapy. Sleep. 2009;32(9):1155–60.
35. Whisenant M, Wong B, Mitchell SA, Beck SL, Mooney K. Distinct trajectories of fatigue and sleep disturbance in women receiving chemotherapy for breast cancer. Oncol Nurs Forum. 2017;44(6):739.
36. Lower EE, Blau R, Gazder P, Tummala R. The risk of premature menopause induced by chemotherapy for early breast cancer. J Womens Health Gend Based Med. 1999;8(7):949–54.
37. Goodwin PJ, Ennis M, Pritchard KI, Trudeau M, Hood N. Risk of menopause during the first year after breast cancer diagnosis. J Clin Oncol. 1999;17(8):2365.
38. Fiorentino L, McQuaid JR, Liu L, Natarajan L, He F, Cornejo M, Lawton S, Parker BA, Sadler GR, Ancoli-Israel S. Individual cognitive behavioral therapy for insomnia in breast cancer survivors: a randomized controlled crossover pilot study. Nat Sci Sleep. 2010;2:1.
39. Carpenter JS, Elam JL, Ridner SH, Carney PH, Cherry GJ, Cucullu HL. Sleep, fatigue, and depressive symptoms in breast cancer survivors and matched healthy women experiencing hot flashes. Oncol Nurs Forum. 2004;31(3):591–8.

40. Savard J, Davidson JR, Ivers H, Quesnel C, Rioux D, Dupéré V, Lasnier M, Simard S, Morin CM. The association between nocturnal hot flashes and sleep in breast cancer survivors. J Pain Symptom Manage. 2004;27(6):513–22.
41. Hunter MS, Grunfeld EA, Mittal S, Sikka P, Ramirez AJ, Fentiman I, Hamed H. Menopausal symptoms in women with breast cancer: prevalence and treatment preferences. Psycho-Oncology. 2004;13(11):769–78.
42. Rumble ME, Keefe FJ, Edinger JD, Affleck G, Marcom PK, Shaw HS. Contribution of cancer symptoms, dysfunctional sleep related thoughts, and sleep inhibitory behaviors to the insomnia process in breast cancer survivors: a daily process analysis. Sleep. 2010;33(11):1501–9.
43. Miller AH, Ancoli-Israel S, Bower JE, Capuron L, Irwin MR. Neuroendocrine-immune mechanisms of behavioral comorbidities in patients with cancer. J Clin Oncol. 2008;28(6):971–82.
44. Wood LJ, Weymann K. Inflammation and neural signaling: etiologic mechanisms of the cancer treatment-related symptom cluster. Curr Opin Support Palliat Care. 2014;7(1):54–9.
45. Kwekkeboom KL, Tostrud L, Costanzo E, Coe CL, Serlin RC, Ward SE, Zhang Y. The role of inflammation in the pain, fatigue, and sleep disturbance symptom cluster in advanced cancer. J Pain Symptom Manag. 2018;55(5):1286–95.
46. Steel JL, Terhorst L, Collins KP, Geller DA, Vodovotz Y, Kim J, Krane A, Antoni M, Marsh JW, Burke LE, Butterfield LH. Prospective analyses of cytokine mediation of sleep and survival in the context of advanced cancer. Psychosom Med. 2018;80(5):483–91.
47. Peoples AR, Roscoe JA, Block RC, Heckler CE, Ryan JL, Mustian KM, Janelsins MC, Peppone LJ, Moore DF, Coles C, Hoelzer KL. Nausea and disturbed sleep as predictors of cancer-related fatigue in breast cancer patients: a multicenter NCORP study. Support Care Cancer. 2017;25(4):1271–8.
48. Cassileth PA, Lusk EJ, Torri S, DiNubile N, Gerson SL. Antiemetic efficacy of dexamethasone therapy in patients receiving cancer chemotherapy. Arch Intern Med. 1983;143(7):1347–9.
49. Ling MH, Perry PJ, Tsuang MT. Side effects of corticosteroid therapy: psychiatric aspects. Arch Gen Psychiatry. 1981;38(4):471–7.
50. Moore P, Dimsdale JE. Opioids, sleep, and cancer-related fatigue. Med Hypotheses. 2002;58(1):77–82.
51. Lowery-Allison AE, Passik SD, Cribbet MR, Reinsel RA, O'Sullivan B, Norton L, Kirsh KL, Kavey NB. Sleep problems in breast cancer survivors 1–10 years posttreatment. Palliat Support Care. 2018;16(3):325–34.
52. Schmidt ME, Wiskemann J, Steindorf K. Quality of life, problems, and needs of disease-free breast cancer survivors 5 years after diagnosis. Qual Life Res. 2018;27(8):2077–86.
53. American Psychiatric Association. Diagnostic and statistical manual of mental disorders (DSM-5®). American Psychiatric Pub; 2013.
54. Roth T, Ancoli-Israel S. Daytime consequences and correlates of insomnia in the United States: results of the 1991 National Sleep Foundation Survey. II. Sleep. 1999;22(Suppl 2):S354–8.
55. Liou KT, Ahles TA, Garland SN, Li QS, Bao T, Li Y, Root JC, Mao JJ. The relationship between insomnia and cognitive impairment in breast cancer survivors. JNCI Cancer Spectr. 2019;3(3):pkz041.
56. Kryger M. A woman's guide to sleep disorders. McGraw Hill Professional; 2004.
57. Reyes-Gibby CC, Aday LA, Anderson KO, Mendoza TR, Cleeland CS. Pain, depression, and fatigue in community-dwelling adults with and without a history of cancer. J Pain Symptom Manag. 2006;32(2):118–28.
58. Park JG, Ramar K, Olson EJ. Updates on definition, consequences, and management of obstructive sleep apnea. Mayo Clin Proc. 2011;86(6):549–55.
59. Iber C. The AASM manual for the scoring of sleep and associated events: rules. terminology and technical specification. American Academy of Sleep Medicine; 2007.
60. Christensen AS, Clark A, Salo P, Nymann P, Lange P, Prescott E, Rod NH. Symptoms of sleep disordered breathing and risk of cancer: a prospective cohort study. Sleep. 2013;36(10):1429–35.
61. Nieto FJ, Peppard PE, Young T, Finn L, Hla KM, Farré R. Sleep-disordered breathing and cancer mortality: results from the Wisconsin Sleep Cohort Study. Am J Respir Crit Care Med. 2012;186(2):190–4.
62. Kendzerska T, Leung RS, Hawker G, Tomlinson G, Gershon AS. Obstructive sleep apnea and the prevalence and incidence of cancer. CMAJ. 2014;186(13):985–92.
63. Nesse W, Hoekema A, Stegenga B, van der Hoeven JH, de Bont LG, Roodenburg JL. Prevalence of obstructive sleep apnea following head and neck cancer treatment: a cross-sectional study. Oral Oncol. 2006;42(1):107–13.
64. Payne RJ, Hier MP, Kost KM, Black MJ, Zeitouni AG, Frenkiel S, Naor N, Kimoff RJ. High prevalence of obstructive sleep apnea among patients with head and neck cancer. J Otolaryngol. 2005;34(5):304–11.
65. Aurora RN, Kristo DA, Bista SR, Rowley JA, Zak RS, Casey KR, Lamm CI, Tracy SL, Rosenberg RS. The treatment of restless legs syndrome and periodic limb movement disorder in adults—an update for 2012: practice parameters with an evidence-based systematic review and meta-analyses: an American Academy of Sleep Medicine Clinical Practice Guideline. Sleep. 2012;35(8):1039–62.
66. Reinsel RA, Starr TD, O'Sullivan B, Passik SD, Kavey NB. Polysomnographic study of sleep in survivors of breast cancer. Sleep Med. 2015;11(12):1361–70.
67. Morin CM, Benca R. Chronic insomnia. Lancet. 2012;379(9821):1129–41.

68. Cervena K, Dauvilliers Y, Espa F, Touchon J, Matousek M, Billiard M, Besset A. Effect of cognitive behavioural therapy for insomnia on sleep architecture and sleep EEG power spectra in psychophysiological insomnia. J Sleep Res. 2004;13(4):385–93.
69. Morin CM, Vallières A, Guay B, Ivers H, Savard J, Mérette C, Bastien C, Baillargeon L. Cognitive behavioral therapy, singly and combined with medication, for persistent insomnia: a randomized controlled trial. JAMA. 2009;301(19):2005–15.
70. Edinger JD, Carney CE. Overcoming insomnia: a cognitive-behavioral therapy approach, therapist guide. Oxford University Press; 2014.
71. Perlis ML, Smith MT, Jungquist C, et al. Cognitive-behavioral therapy for insomnia. In: Clinical handbook of insomnia. Humana Press; 2010. p. 281–96.
72. Miller CB, Espie CA, Epstein DR, et al. The evidence base of sleep restriction therapy for treating insomnia disorder. Sleep Med Rev. 2014;18(5):415–24.
73. Spielman AJ, Yang CM, Glovinsky PB. Sleep restriction therapy. In: Behavioral treatments for sleep disorders. Academic Press; 2011. p. 9–19.
74. Bootzin RR, Epstein D, Wood JM. Stimulus control instructions. In: Case studies in insomnia. Springer; 1991. p. 19–28.
75. Clark DA. Cognitive restructuring. In: The Wiley handbook of cognitive behavioral therapy. Wiley Blackwell; 2013. p. 1–22.
76. Aricò D, Raggi A, Ferri R. Cognitive behavioral therapy for insomnia in breast cancer survivors: a review of the literature. Front Psychol. 2016;7:1162.
77. Quesnel C, Savard J, Simard S, Ivers H, Morin CM. Efficacy of cognitive-behavioral therapy for insomnia in women treated for nonmetastic breast cancer. J Consult Clin Psychol. 2003;71(1):189.
78. Berger AM, VonEssen S, Kuhn BR, Piper BF, Farr L, Agrawal S, Lynch JC, Higgibotham P. Feasibility of a sleep intervention during adjuvant breast cancer chemotherapy. Oncol Nurs Forum. 2002;29(10):1431–41.
79. Berger AM, VonEssen S, Kuhn BR, Piper BF, Agrawal S, Lynch JC, Higginbotham P. Adherence, sleep, and fatigue outcomes after adjuvant breast cancer chemotherapy: results of a feasibility intervention study. Oncol Nurs Forum. 2003;30(3):513–22.
80. Savard J, Simard S, Ivers H, Morin CM. Randomized study on the efficacy of cognitive-behavioral therapy for insomnia secondary to breast cancer, part I: sleep and psychological effects. J Clin Oncol. 2005;23(25):6083–96.
81. Matthews EE, Berger AM, Schmiege SJ, Cook PF, McCarthy MS, Moore CM, Aloia MS. Cognitive behavioral therapy for insomnia outcomes in women after primary breast cancer treatment: a randomized, controlled trial. Oncol Nurs Forum. 2014;41(3):241–53.
82. Epstein DR, Dirksen SR. Randomized trial of a cognitive-behavioral intervention for insomnia in breast cancer survivors. Oncol Nurs Forum. 2007;34(5):E51–9.
83. Garland SN, Johnson JA, Savard J, Gehrman P, Perlis M, Carlson L, Campbell T. Sleeping well with cancer: a systematic review of cognitive behavioral therapy for insomnia in cancer patients. Neuropsychiatr Dis Treat. 2014;10:1113–24.
84. Savard J, Simard S, Ivers H, Morin CM. Randomized study on the efficacy of cognitive-behavioral therapy for insomnia secondary to breast cancer, part II: immunologic effects. J Clin Oncol. 2005;23(25):6097–106.
85. Dirksen SR, Epstein DR. Efficacy of an insomnia intervention on fatigue, mood and quality of life in breast cancer survivors. J Adv Nurs. 2008;61(6):664–75.
86. Mann E, Smith MJ, Hellier J, Balabanovic JA, Hamed H, Grunfeld EA, Hunter MS. Cognitive behavioural treatment for women who have menopausal symptoms after breast cancer treatment (MENOS 1): a randomised controlled trial. Lancet Oncol. 2012;13(3):309–18.
87. Matthews EE, Schmiege SJ, Cook PF, Berger AM, Aloia MS. Adherence to cognitive behavioral therapy for insomnia (CBTI) among women following primary breast cancer treatment: a pilot study. Behav Sleep Med. 2012;10(3):217–29.
88. Savard J, Ivers H, Savard MH, Morin CM. Is a video-based cognitive behavioral therapy for insomnia as efficacious as a professionally administered treatment in breast cancer? Results of a randomized controlled trial. Sleep. 2014;37(8):1305–14.
89. Savard J, Villa J, Simard S, Ivers H, Morin CM. Feasibility of a self-help treatment for insomnia comorbid with cancer. Psycho-Oncology. 2011;20(9):1013–9.
90. Marion LP, Ivers H, Savard J. Feasibility of a preventive intervention for insomnia in women with breast cancer receiving chemotherapy. Behav Sleep Med. 2019;26:1–3.
91. Dozeman E, Verdonck-de Leeuw IM, Savard J, van Straten A. Guided web-based intervention for insomnia targeting breast cancer patients: feasibility and effect. Internet Interv. 2017;9:1–6.
92. Tremblay V, Savard J, Ivers H. Predictors of the effect of cognitive behavioral therapy for chronic insomnia comorbid with breast cancer. J Consult Clin Psychol. 2009;77(4):742.
93. Espie CA. "Stepped care": a health technology solution for delivering cognitive behavioral therapy as a first line insomnia treatment. Sleep. 2009;32(12):1549–58.
94. Davidson JR, Waisberg JL, Brundage MD, MacLean AW. Nonpharmacologic group treatment of insomnia: a preliminary study with cancer survivors. Psycho-Oncology. 2001;10(5):389–97.
95. Fang YY, Hung CT, Chan JC, Huang SM, Lee YH. Meta-analysis: exercise intervention for sleep problems in cancer patients. Eur J Cancer Care. 2019;28(5):e13131.

96. Matthews EE, Janssen DW, Djalilova DM, Berger AM. Effects of exercise on sleep in women with breast cancer: a systematic review. Sleep Med Clin. 2018;13(3):395–417.
97. Carlson LE, Speca M, Patel KD, Goodey E. Mindfulness-based stress reduction in relation to quality of life, mood, symptoms of stress, and immune parameters in breast and prostate cancer outpatients. Psychosom Med. 2003;65(4):571–81.
98. Shapiro SL, Bootzin RR, Figueredo AJ, Lopez AM, Schwartz GE. The efficacy of mindfulness-based stress reduction in the treatment of sleep disturbance in women with breast cancer: an exploratory study. J Psychosom Res. 2003;54(1):85–91.
99. Arem H, Lewin D, Cifu G, Bires J, Goldberg E, Kaltman R, Power MC, Mauro LA, Kogan M. A feasibility study of group-delivered behavioral interventions for insomnia among breast cancer survivors: comparing cognitive behavioral therapy for insomnia and a mind–body intervention. J Altern Complement Med. 2019;25(8):840–4.
100. Rao RM, Vadiraja HS, Nagaratna R, Gopinath KS, Patil S, Diwakar RB, Shahsidhara HP, Ajaikumar BS, Nagendra HR. Effect of yoga on sleep quality and neuroendocrine immune response in metastatic breast cancer patients. Indian J Palliat Care. 2017;23(3):253.
101. Casault L, Savard J, Ivers H, Savard MH, Simard S. Utilization of hypnotic medication in the context of cancer: predictors and frequency of use. Support Care Cancer. 2012;20(6):1203–10.
102. Strollo SE, Fallon EA, Gapstur SM, Smith TG. Cancer-related problems, sleep quality, and sleep disturbance among long-term cancer survivors at 9-years post diagnosis. Sleep Med. 2020;65:177–85.
103. Moore TA, Berger AM, Dizona P. Sleep aid use during and following breast cancer adjuvant chemotherapy. Psycho-Oncology. 2011;20(3):321–5.
104. Smith MT, Perlis ML, Park A, Smith MS, Pennington J, Giles DE, Buysse DJ. Comparative meta-analysis of pharmacotherapy and behavior therapy for persistent insomnia. Am J Psychiatr. 2002;159(1):5–11.
105. Mitchell MD, Gehrman P, Perlis M, Umscheid CA. Comparative effectiveness of cognitive behavioral therapy for insomnia: a systematic review. BMC Fam Pract. 2012;13(1):40.
106. Riemann D, Baglioni C, Bassetti C, Bjorvatn B, Dolenc Groselj L, Ellis JG, Espie CA, Garcia-Borreguero D, Gjerstad M, Gonçalves M, Hertenstein E. European guideline for the diagnosis and treatment of insomnia. J Sleep Res. 2017;26(6):675–700.
107. Roscoe JA, Garland SN, Heckler CE, Perlis ML, Peoples AR, Shayne M, Savard J, Daniels NP, Morrow GR. Randomized placebo-controlled trial of cognitive behavioral therapy and armodafinil for insomnia after cancer treatment. J Clin Oncol. 2015;33(2):165.
108. Sateia MJ, Buysse DJ, Krystal AD, Neubauer DN, Heald JL. Clinical practice guideline for the pharmacologic treatment of chronic insomnia in adults: an American Academy of sleep medicine clinical practice guideline. J Clin Sleep Med. 2017;13(02):307–49.
109. Fiorentino L, Ancoli-Israel S. Insomnia and its treatment in women with breast cancer. Sleep Med Rev. 2006;10(6):419–29.
110. Kripke DF, Langer RD, Kline LE. Hypnotics' association with mortality or cancer: a matched cohort study. BMJ Open. 2012;2:e000850. https://doi.org/10.1136/bmjopen-2012-000850
111. Kripke DF. Mortality risk of hypnotics: strengths and limits of evidence. Drug Saf. 2016;39(2):93–107.
112. Lan TY, Zeng YF, Tang GJ, Kao HC, Chiu HJ, Lan TH, Ho HF. The use of hypnotics and mortality-a population-based retrospective cohort study. PLoS One. 2015;10(12):e0145271.
113. Zee PC, Turek FW. Sleep and health: everywhere and in both directions. Arch Intern Med. 2006;166(16):1686–8.
114. Johnson EO, Roehrs T, Roth T, Breslau N. Epidemiology of alcohol and medication as aids to sleep in early adulthood. Sleep. 1998;21(2):178–86.
115. Verster JC, Volkerts ER, Spence DW, Alford C, Pandi-Perumal SR. Effects of sleep medications on cognition, psychomotor skills, memory and driving performance in the elderly. Curr Psychiatr Rev. 2007;3(4):287–92.
116. Qaseem A, Kansagara D, Forciea MA, Cooke M, Denberg TD. Management of chronic insomnia disorder in adults: a clinical practice guideline from the American College of Physicians. Ann Intern Med. 2016;165(2):125–33.
117. Howell D, Keller-Olaman S, Oliver TK, Hack TF, Broadfield L, Biggs K, Chung J, Gravelle D, Green E, Hamel M, Harth T. A pan-Canadian practice guideline and algorithm: screening, assessment, and supportive care of adults with cancer-related fatigue. Curr Oncol. 2013;20(3):e233.
118. Howell D, Oliver TK, Keller-Olaman S, Davidson JR, Garland S, Samuels C, Savard J, Harris C, Aubin M, Olson K, Sussman J. Sleep disturbance in adults with cancer: a systematic review of evidence for best practices in assessment and management for clinical practice. Ann Oncol. 2014;25(4):791–800.
119. Matthews E, Carter P, Page M, Dean G, Berger A. Sleep-wake disturbance: a systematic review of evidence-based interventions for management in patients with cancer. Clin J Oncol Nurs. 2018;22(1):37–52.
120. Otte JL, Davis L, Carpenter JS, Krier C, Skaar TC, Rand KL, Weaver M, Landis C, Chernyak Y, Manchanda S. Sleep disorders in breast cancer survivors. Support Care Cancer. 2016;24(10):4197–205.
121. Espie CA, Kyle SD, Hames P, Gardani M, Fleming L, Cape J. The Sleep Condition Indicator: a clinical screening tool to evaluate insomnia disorder. BMJ Open. 2014;4(3):e004183.
122. Bastien CH, Vallières A, Morin CM. Validation of the insomnia severity index as an outcome measure for insomnia research. Sleep Med. 2001;2(4):297–307.

123. Morin CM, Belleville G, Bélanger L, Ivers H. The insomnia severity index: psychometric indicators to detect insomnia cases and evaluate treatment response. Sleep. 2011;34(5):601–8.
124. Savard MH, Savard J, Simard S, Ivers H. Empirical validation of the insomnia severity index in cancer patients. Psychooncology. 2005;14(6):429–41.
125. Chung F, Abdullah HR, Liao P. STOP-Bang questionnaire: a practical approach to screen for obstructive sleep apnea. Chest. 2016;149(3):631–8.
126. Taylor DJ, Wilkerson AK, Pruiksma KE, Williams JM, Ruggero CJ, Hale W, Mintz J, Organek KM, Nicholson KL, Litz BT, Young-McCaughan S. Reliability of the structured clinical interview for DSM-5 sleep disorders module. J Clin Sleep Med. 2018;14(3):459–64.
127. Carney CE, Buysse DJ, Ancoli-Israel S, Edinger JD, Krystal AD, Lichstein KL, Morin CM. The consensus sleep diary: standardizing prospective sleep self-monitoring. Sleep. 2012;35(2):287–302.
128. Bootzin RR, Engle-Friedman M. The assessment of insomnia. Behav Assess. 1981;3(2):107–26.
129. Buysse DJ, Ancoli-Israel S, Edinger JD, Lichstein KL, Morin CM. Recommendations for a standard research assessment of insomnia. Sleep. 2006;29(9):1155–73.
130. Depner CM, Cheng PC, Devine JK, Khosla S, de Zambotti M, Robillard R, Vakulin A, Drummond SPA. Wearable technologies for developing sleep and circadian biomarkers: a summary of workshop discussions. Sleep. 2020;43(2):1–13.
131. Zhou ES, Michaud AL, Recklitis CJ. Developing efficient and effective behavioral treatment for insomnia in cancer survivors: results of a stepped care trial. Cancer. 2020;126(1):165–73.
132. LeBlanc M, Merette C, Savard J, Ivers H, Baillargeon L, Morin CM. Incidence and risk factors of insomnia in a population-based sample. Sleep. 2009;32(8):1027–37.

Depressive and Anxiety Symptoms and Disorders

12

Caroline S. Dorfman, Nicole A. Arrato, Sarah S. Arthur, and Barbara L. Andersen

Introduction

Psychological distress—anxiety and/or depression—is prevalent for breast cancer patients throughout the survivorship trajectory, including diagnosis, during treatment, and in the initial recovery year [1–3]. For the majority, symptoms remit [4]; for others, especially those with a prior history of anxiety or mood disorders, symptoms may persist or may reemerge following an initial decline [5–7]. A small but significant portion of breast cancer survivors will meet Diagnostic and Statistical Manual of Mental Disorders 5 (DSM-5) diagnostic criteria for anxiety and depressive disorders. Screening for anxiety and depressive disorders is crucial, as these disorders have been shown to impact quality of life, treatment adherence (e.g., aromatase inhibitors), adherence to recommended follow-up care, subjective perception of physical symptoms, and survival [8–10].

In this chapter, recommendations for assessment of symptoms of anxiety and depression are discussed as is a review of the cardinal symptoms of anxiety and depressive disorders. Recommendations for appropriate triage, referral, and intervention are also provided.

C. S. Dorfman (✉)
Department of Psychiatry and Behavioral Sciences, Duke University Medical Center, Durham, NC, USA
e-mail: Caroline.dorfman@duke.edu

N. A. Arrato
Department of Psychology, The Ohio State University, Columbus, OH, USA
e-mail: Arrato.1@buckeyemail.osu.edu

S. S. Arthur
Department of Psychology and Neuroscience, Duke University, Durham, NC, USA
e-mail: Sarah.staley.arthur@duke.edu

B. L. Andersen
Department of Psychology, The Ohio State University, Columbus, OH, USA

Comprehensive Cancer Center and Solove Research Institute, The Ohio State University, Columbus, OH, USA
e-mail: Andersen.1@osu.edu

Screening for and Assessing Symptoms of Anxiety and Depression

The high prevalence of anxiety and depressive symptoms underscores the need for distress screening at diagnosis and throughout the survivorship trajectory and has been prescribed by accreditation bodies [e.g., American College of Surgeons Commission on Cancer (CoC)] and professional standards [11–14]. For example, CoC guidelines mandate routine screening using published, standardized, validated assessment measures with preference for ones with clinical cutoffs/symptom severity grading [11]. The American Society of Clinical Oncology (ASCO) provides specific guidelines (see Tables 12.1 and 12.2) including recommended assessment measures, patient characteristics that may co-occur

G. G. Kimmick et al. (eds.), *Common Issues in Breast Cancer Survivors*,
https://doi.org/10.1007/978-3-030-75377-1_12

Table 12.1 American Society of Clinical Oncology recommendations for the management of symptoms of depression

	Recommendations based on symptom severity		
Screening	None/mild (PHQ-9: 0–9) No or minimal symptoms of depression	Moderate (PHQ-9: 10–14) Subthreshold depressive symptoms; functional impairment from "mild" to "moderate"	Moderate-severe/severe (PHQ-9: 15–19) (PHQ-9: 20–27) Has most depressive symptoms; symptoms interfere moderately to markedly with functioning
Treatment recommendations	Offer referral to supportive care services; provide education and information about: • Stress management • Sources of informational support • Supportive care services (e.g., support groups) • Financial support • Symptom management • Non-pharmacological interventions (e.g., physical activity, nutrition)	Low intensity intervention options • Individually guided self-help (or computerized) based on CBT • Group-based CBT for depression • Psychosocial interventions (group) • Structured physical activity program	High intensity intervention options • Individual psychological interventions (e.g., CBT, ACT) • Pharmacotherapy (e.g., SSRIs)
Follow-up and ongoing reassessment		• Assess follow-through and adherence with individual or group psychological/psychosocial referrals and satisfaction with services • Assess adherence to pharmacologic treatment, concerns about side effects, and satisfaction with symptom relief • Create plan to improve adherence to treatment as necessary including plans to reduce barriers or offer alternative treatments • Make changes to medications/therapy recommendations if symptom reduction and satisfaction with treatment are poor after 8 weeks	

Note: *PHQ-9* Patient Health Questionnaire 9-symptom Depression scale [15]

with high symptom levels (e.g., history of depression or anxiety), and referral pathways for specific treatments [12].

ASCO recommends the Patient Health Questionnaire-9 (PHQ-9) [15] to assess depressive symptoms and the Generalized Anxiety Disorder 7-item scale (GAD-7) [16] to assess anxiety symptoms (see Box 12.1). Both the PHQ-9 and GAD-7 have data supporting acceptability by patients, ease of interpretation by staff, utility in medical settings (e.g., primary care), and confirmed reliability and validity in relationship to psychiatric diagnosis decisions [15–20]. The PHQ-9 asks patients to report on the frequency of nine symptoms (e.g., "feeling down, depressed, or hopeless"; "feeling tired or having little energy"; "poor appetite or overeating"; "trouble falling or staying asleep or sleeping too much") in the last 2 weeks using a Likert scale from 0 "Not at all" to 3 "Nearly Every Day." Symptoms assessed on the PHQ-9 map onto the nine Diagnostic and Statistical Manual of Mental Disorders IV (DSM-IV) [21] diagnostic criteria for Major Depressive Disorder (e.g., depressed mood, anhedonia, sleep problems, poor appetite, or overeating). The GAD-7 evaluates the presence and severity of seven symptoms (e.g., "feeling nervous, anxious, or on edge"; "not being able to stop or control worrying"; "trouble relaxing"; "feeling afraid as if something awful might happen") that map onto the DSM-IV criteria for Generalized Anxiety Disorder (e.g., feeling nervous, anxious or on edge, worrying too much about different things). Patients respond using a Likert scale

Table 12.2 American Society of Clinical Oncology recommendations for the management of symptoms of anxiety

	Recommendations based on symptom severity		
Screening	None/mild (GAD-7: 0–4, 5–9) No or mild symptoms of anxiety; no/minimal functional impairment	Moderate (GAD-7: 10–14) Functional impairment from mild to moderate	Moderate-severe/severe (GAD-7: 15–21) Symptoms interfere moderately to markedly with functioning
Treatment recommendations	Offer referral to supportive care services; provide education and information about: • Stress management • Sources of informational support • Supportive care services (e.g., support groups) • Financial support • Symptom management • Non-pharmacological interventions (e.g., physical activity, nutrition)	Low intensity intervention options • Education and active monitoring • Nonfacilitated or guided self-help (or computerized) based on CBT • Psychosocial interventions (groups)	High intensity intervention options • Individual psychological interventions (e.g., CBT, applied relaxation) • Pharmacotherapy (e.g., SSRIs)
Follow-up and ongoing reassessment		• Assess follow-through and adherence to individual or group psychological/psychosocial referrals and satisfaction with services • Assess adherence to pharmacologic treatment, concerns about side effects, and satisfaction with symptom relief • Create plan to improve adherence to treatment as necessary including plans to reduce barriers or offer alternative treatments • Make changes to medications/therapy recommendations if symptom reduction and satisfaction with treatment are poor after 8 weeks	

Note: *GAD-7* Generalized Anxiety Disorder 7-item Scale [16]

similar to the PHQ-9 with responses ranging from 0 "Not at all" to 3 "Nearly Every Day."

Both the PHQ-9 and GAD-7 have well-established cut-points (see Box 12.1). While the traditional cutoff for the PHQ-9 is ≥10 [15], ASCO has recommended a cutoff score of ≥8 based on research with cancer outpatients [12]. The established vs. recommended cutpoints for the PHQ-9 and GAD-7 will be referred to throughout this chapter. Adapted from the ASCO recommendations [12], Tables 12.1 and 12.2 provide guidance for further diagnostic assessment and referral for patients with scores on the PHQ-9 and GAD-7 in the moderate to severe range.

Other measures have been used, but collectively they are limited in their ability to detect symptomatology at the highest (moderately severe, severe) levels, which are more likely to be indicative of anxiety or depressive disorders [17, 22]. The Hospital Anxiety and Depression Scale (HADS) [23] and the National Comprehensive Cancer Network (NCCN) Distress Thermometer and Problem Checklist are two examples [13]. The NIH-Sponsored Patient Reported Outcomes Measurement Information System (PROMIS) Emotional Distress Short Forms [24] are labeled "emerging measures" by the American Psychiatric Association, but as of yet lack supporting validity data. Additional research is needed to understand their ability to identify patients with anxiety and depressive disorders. The PROMIS measures may reliably identify individuals with chronic illnesses screening positive for anxiety and depression on the PHQ-9 and GAD-7 [25, 26].

Box 12.1 PHQ-9 and GAD-7 Scores and Symptom Severity Classifications

Patient Health Questionnaire-9 (PHQ-9)	Generalized Anxiety Disorder-7 (GAD-7)
Score 0–4: Minimal Score 5–9: Mild Score 10–14: Moderate Score 15–19: Moderately Severe Score 20–27: Severe	Score 0–4: Minimal Score 5–9: Mild Score 10–14: Moderate Score 15–21: Severe

The full versions of the PHQ-9 and GAD-7, as well as administration and scoring instructions, can be accessed online at www.phqscreeners.com.

Diagnostic Criteria for Anxiety and Depressive Disorders

Prevalence rates of depression and anxiety differ based on time since diagnosis. In the first year after breast cancer diagnosis, it is estimated that 50% of women will meet diagnostic criteria for an anxiety or depressive disorder, with co-occurrence common [27, 28]. Prevalence estimates are 25% in the second, third, and fourth years since diagnosis, and 15% in the fifth year [29–32]. There is a low base rate (5%) of "late onset" anxiety and depressive disorders [33], excepting those with a pre-cancer psychiatric history. Long-term depression and anxiety are more common for those with previous psychological treatment, lack of an intimate confiding relationship, younger age, and severely stressful non-cancer life experiences [4, 30]. Maintenance of symptoms is also predicted by high initial subjective stress (i.e., self-reported perceived stress and emotional distress) or appraisals of one's life as stressful [34].

Depression

The most common depressive disorders are major depression, persistent depression, and adjustment disorder [9]. The cardinal symptoms of *major depressive disorder (MDD)* are depressed mood and a markedly diminished interest or pleasure in activities, i.e., anhedonia. In breast cancer survivors, these symptoms may co-occur with sexual dysfunction, infertility, and feelings of isolation [35]. Other symptoms of MDD are significant weight gain or loss, a slowing down of thought and physical movement, fatigue, feelings of worthlessness or guilt, cognitive difficulties, and recurrent thoughts of death. To be diagnosed with MDD, five or more of these symptoms must occur nearly all day, every day, for a 2-week period. Also, the individual must voice significant distress due to the symptoms or have impairment in social, occupational, or other major life areas. Further, the symptoms must not be a result of substance abuse or another medical condition (i.e., due to a disease-specific process) [36]. When examining psychiatric disorders in breast cancer survivors, one must differentiate between symptoms of depression/anxiety and those of cancer/treatment. Thus, it is important to either use diagnostic tools that allow for making this distinction, or to refer to qualified mental health specialists to do so [37].

Persistent depressive disorder (PDD) presents very similar symptoms as described above, but lasts for at least 2 years. During the 2-year period, the patient must not have been without the symptoms for more than 2 months at a time [36]. *Adjustment disorder* is defined as the development of emotional or behavioral symptoms in response to an identifiable stressor (such as cancer), evidenced by marked distress that is out of proportion to the stressor's intensity and/or causing significant impairment in functioning [36]. Adjustment disorder may be diagnosed when a patient does not meet criteria for another disorder such as MDD. Breast cancer survivors adjusting to a new set of stressors and living many years post-diagnosis may meet criteria for these disorders, but data for these more nuanced depressive disorders are scarce, and it is unknown whether they are a product of cancer-related phenomena or other stressors (e.g., other chronic illnesses of aging, partner loss, etc.) [9, 38].

Anxiety

After cancer treatment, anxiety often persists for a decade or more [39]. The most commonly diagnosed anxiety disorder is *generalized anxiety disorder (GAD)*, which is characterized by excessive anxiety or worry that is difficult to control and impairs function, along with at least three of the following present for 6 months: restlessness, fatigue, difficulty concentrating, irritability, muscle tension, and sleep disruptions [36]. Another anxiety disorder is *panic disorder (PD)*, involving sudden experiences of intense fear or discomfort, which include accelerated heart rate, sweating, shortness of breath, and even fear of death [36].

Two circumstances regarding survivors' anxieties merit mention. One is "fear of recurrence" defined as the "fear, worry, or concern relating to the possibility that cancer will come back or progress" [37, 40]. Another is the individual's feeling uncertain about the meaning and purpose of their life following cancer [39]. For both, the difference between realistic, normative worries about recurrence and life after cancer versus pathological worry is the degree to which the worry impacts the individual's daily functioning and leads to avoidance of normal activities or responsibilities.

Considering the fact that depressive and anxiety disorders are largely underrecognized and undertreated in this population [35], prevalence rates are likely higher than the literature suggests (depression, 16%; anxiety, 10%) [41]. Beyond formal diagnoses, an even greater number of breast cancer survivors experience subclinical symptoms of depression or anxiety [1–3].

Often, depressive and anxiety symptoms and disorders co-occur [42]. Two-thirds of patients with cancer who are diagnosed with a depressive disorder meet criteria for the mixed depression/anxiety phenotype [43], and a large portion of anxious patients experience depressive symptoms. While one disorder often contributes to the other, their diagnostic symptom overlap (i.e., fatigue, cognitive difficulties) must be considered. If comorbid diagnoses are detected, the recommendation is to treat the depression first [12].

Box 12.2 What to Look for: Cardinal Symptoms of MDD and GAD

MDD	GAD
Depressed mood	Excessive anxiety or worry (difficult to control and impairs function)
Markedly diminished interest or pleasure in activities (anhedonia)	Restlessness
Significant weight gain or loss	Fatigue
Slowing down of thought and physical movement	Difficulty concentrating
Fatigue	Irritability
Feelings of worthlessness or guilt	Muscle tension
Cognitive difficulties	Sleep disruptions
Recurrent thoughts of death	

Referral and Treatment in Clinical Settings

Triage and Referral

If moderate or severe symptomatology is detected based on patients' self-reports on the PHQ-9 or GAD-7 (see Box 12.1), further assessment is needed to determine the presence of an anxiety or depressive disorder [12]. Diagnosis with intention of providing referral for subsequent treatment will lead to optimal management of symptomatology. Failure to identify and treat anxiety and depression—particularly in the ranges discussed (see Tables 12.1 and 12.2)—will eventuate in survivors' increased morbidity and mortality [44–46]. Depression and greater depressive symptoms are associated with nonadherence to adjuvant endocrine therapy [10] and thus increased risk for recurrence and premature death [47, 48]. Studies have similarly shown breast cancer survivors with high levels of anxiety to have poor adherence to adjuvant endocrine therapy [49].

Implementation of psychological screening, referral for treatment, and continued follow-up is a multi-level process. As approaches for screening and the resources available for managing depression and anxiety may differ across practices and institutions, it is important to understand the screening and referral processes in your place of practice. If needed or not being conducted routinely, consider implementing screening in your own practice setting using assessment measures like those described previously (i.e., PHQ-9, GAD-7). Next, it is important to identify referral resources within your institution and/or in the community, including appropriately trained individuals who can conduct comprehensive diagnostic assessments and/or deliver empirically supported non-pharmacologic (e.g., cognitive behavior therapy, behavioral activation) treatments (e.g., psychologists, social workers) as well as providers who can manage pharmacologic treatments (e.g., psychiatrists, nurse practitioners). Referral pathways may or may not be established. National organizations, including the Association for Cognitive and Behavioral Therapy, American Psychological Association, and American Psychiatric Association as well as oncology-specific organizations (e.g., American Psychosocial Oncology Society, Cancer Support Community) may serve as resources for connecting with community clinicians. For example, the Cancer Support Community operates a helpline staffed by counselors and resource specialists who can provide information and referral to local, regional, and national resources [50]. Prior screening of the possible referral sources is important to find those familiar with cancer and its treatment and who provide empirically supported depression and/or anxiety treatment.

A practical implication of screening and referral is that strong patient-provider rapport and follow-up are key. This means collaborating with the patient as soon as possible for a plan for further mental health evaluation and eventual treatment that can also accommodate patients' prior experiences and current economic status. Many patients presenting with severe anxiety/depressive symptoms during survivorship will have had prior episodes of depression, with or without anxiety. These patients might return to a previous mental health provider if such services were satisfactory. If new to mental health treatment, patients will need information about the provider to whom she/he is referred. Continued support by the patients' medical team (e.g., oncology team if the patient is continued to be followed in this setting; patients' primary care provider) will be vital for reducing obstacles to treatment and ensuring patients' adherence and treatment success.

Even when a referral is made, it is common for persons with depressive symptoms to lack the motivation necessary to follow through on referrals and/or to adhere to treatment recommendations. Relatedly, cautiousness and a tendency to avoid are cardinal features of anxiety pathology. *Thus, it is critical to monitor patients' adherence to mental health referrals and services* [12]. Other factors which will impede an individual's adherence to treatment are not having a spouse or significant other, living alone or in a care facility, and/or limited financial means [51–54]. As oncology providers may be limited in their ability to follow survivors in the long-term, a multidisciplinary approach to follow up care may be beneficial. For example, involving social workers or patient navigators at your cancer center or the patients' primary care provider may help to promote follow-up and adherence to mental health treatment. If adherence is poor, these individuals may engage the patient in problem-solving barriers to care and creating a plan for participating in mental health treatment.

Box 12.3 Steps for Triage and Referral

Step 1: Identify and screen possible referral sources with knowledge of oncology and training in empirically supported treatments for anxiety and depression.
Step 2: Routinely assess patients' symptoms of anxiety and depression using the PHQ-9 and GAD-7.
Step 3: Refer patients whose scores fall in the moderate-severe or severe ranges for additional psychological assessment. If diagnoses are present, identify providers with expertise with cancer patients (ideal) and providing empirically supported treatments (essential).
Step 4: Monitor patients for referral adherence. Offer assistance and help patients problem-solve barriers to receiving treatment.

Interventions for Depression and Anxiety

Standard Care

As standard care, psychoeducation and physical exercise interventions are two important and universally applicable resources that have been found effective in the context of randomized clinical trials.

Psychoeducation

Providing relevant information can improve patients' quality of life, increase knowledge and feelings of preparedness, and reduce cancer-related stress and symptoms [55–57]. Readily available educational brochures and pamphlets, discussion of typical emotional and physiological symptoms common during treatment, and overview of available supportive care services are crucial. This information provides awareness of common problems and emotional and physiological symptoms and prompts engagement and coping. The National Institute of Mental Health (NIMH) has various psychoeducational resources available online that can be printed and provided to patients (e.g., Chronic Illness and Mental Health: Recognizing and Treating Depression [58]; Depression Basics [59]; 5 Things You Should Know about Stress [60]). Additionally, the American Cancer Society (ACS) has developed patient-directed brochures and pamphlets for coping with the psychosocial impact of cancer treatments (e.g., Getting Help for Distress [61]; When Cancer Comes Back [62]); these resources are available in both print and online formats.

Exercise Interventions

Physical exercise interventions can have beneficial effects on physical health (e.g., increases in muscle strength and endurance, improvements in blood pressure), symptoms (fatigue reduction), and mental health (mood improvement) [55]. A meta-analysis of 40 exercise interventions designed for cancer survivors found that increases in weekly aerobic exercise were associated with reductions in depressive symptoms [63]. Importantly, greater effects occurred when exercise sessions were conducted with trained professionals. Oncologists have a "teachable moment" that can improve survivors' health and well-being by discussing the safety and feasibility of an exercise plan and providing information on available programs in their community (e.g., Livestrong at the YMCA; the SilverSneakers program included with many Medicare Plans).

Psychotherapy

Treatment of patients' anxiety and depressive symptoms beyond standard care (e.g., informational and financial support, guidance regarding physical activity and nutrition) has immediate benefits and may improve long-term health and disease outcomes [64–66]. For breast cancer survivors coping with moderate to severe symptoms of anxiety and/or depression, psychotherapy (e.g., cognitive behavioral therapy, acceptance and commitment therapy) is indicated (see Tables 12.1 and 12.2). Depending on the extent of survivors' symptoms and needs, the intensity of intervention may differ. Although "low" and "high" intensity interventions often share content, they can be differentiated by factors such as the delivery setting, number of sessions, length of treatment, and format. Typically, low intensity interventions have fewer sessions and/or occur over a shorter period of time and may include several topics designed to enhance quality of life (e.g., stress reduction, problem-solving, social support). Intervention formats can vary from group-based therapies led by a licensed mental health practitioner to self-guided or online programs. High intensity treatments for anxiety or depressive disorders are manualized empirically supported treatments, typically delivered face-to-face, by a licensed mental health provider (e.g., a PhD-level clinical psychologist).

Cognitive Behavioral Therapy Among psychotherapies, the most successful and extensively studied treatment for anxiety and depressive disorders is cognitive behavioral therapy (CBT) [67–70]. Even among patients with severe depressive symptomology, several studies [71, 72] have found CBT to be effective during the acute phase of treatment, and, when compared to pharmacotherapy, patients who receive CBT have been found to be at lower risk for relapse than those treated with medication [73]. For some patients, the lower risk of relapse was sustained for as long as 2 years. For the treatment of generalized anxiety disorder (GAD), few randomized clinical trials (RCTs) have compared anxiolytic medications to CBT. Of those that have, CBT outperforms medications [74]. However, this conclusion is limited by the fact that benzodiazepines have been the primary drug with which CBT has been compared. Meta-analytic reviews demonstrate that CBT for GAD is superior to other treatments and conditions, such as wait-list conditions, no treatment control conditions, nondirective therapy, and pill placebo conditions [74].

Because breast cancer survivors can greatly benefit from CBT for anxiety and depressive disorders, it is important that providers are able to describe what is typically included in the treatment prior to making referrals.

- Components of CBT for depressive disorders: (i) behavioral activation to increase engagement in daily activities; (ii) change negative, automatic thoughts; (iii) identify and change core beliefs and schema that underlie persistent, negative attitudes.
- For cancer survivors with depressive symptoms, CBT targets distorted cognitions and feelings of helplessness and/or pessimism about the future.
- Components of CBT for GAD: (i) attend to internal and external cues that precede worry; (ii) use progressive muscle relaxation exercises to prevent and/or reduce symptom bother; (iii) change negative, automatic thoughts.
- For cancer survivors with GAD, CBT identifies and targets specific worries and addresses the common problem of overestimating the likelihood of negative events (e.g., the risk of recurrence/progression).

CBTs can be delivered in person, with printed materials, or remotely (e.g., via telephone, videoconferencing). A meta-analysis by Mayo-Wilson and Montgomery [75] of CBT for anxiety delivered via printed materials or other remote methods found support for improved symptoms of anxiety compared to no treatment/standard care. The findings were less compelling for reductions in depressive symptoms, as the short- and long-term effectiveness of these interventions need to be further studied in trials with larger samples. Overall, low intensity interventions can be a first-line treatment for breast cancer survivors with mild/moderate symptoms of depression or anxiety, whereas, at present, face-to-face CBT is recommended for individuals with moderate to severe symptomology.

Third-Wave Cognitive Behavioral Therapies Variants of CBT, known collectively as "third-wave" therapies, such as Acceptance and Commitment Therapy (ACT) and mindfulness-based therapies, have been used to treat anxiety and depressive symptoms, and there is early data suggesting utility for cancer survivors [76, 77].

- Components of ACT: (i) change the relationship individuals have with unwanted or feared thoughts, feelings, memories, and physical sensations; (ii) increase focus on the present moment; (iii) clarify goals and values and commit to behavioral change strategies.
- Components of mindfulness-based therapy protocols vary, but can include (i) attending to bodily sensations and emotional discomfort; (ii) using mindfulness practices such as walking meditation, body scan, or yoga exercises; and (iii) distancing from dysfunctional thought processes and recognizing that thoughts are not facts.
- Both ACT and mindfulness-based therapies address tendencies to avoid distressing thoughts and symptoms associated with cancer diagnosis and treatment through mindfulness and acceptance exercises and encourage the pursuit of valued goals.

Pharmacotherapy

Cancer survivors report medication use for symptoms of depression and/or anxiety at rates that are nearly two times those of adults without a cancer history [78]. Although pharmacologic treatments are commonly prescribed by oncologists, there are few studies supporting this general practice as effective. A 2018 meta-analysis of seven RCTs assessed the efficacy of using antidepressants for treating depression in cancer patients. The majority of trials compared antidepressants to placebo, while a few included head-to-head comparisons among several antidepressants. The authors found only minimal evidence for the effects of antidepressants compared to placebo [79]. Additionally, they concluded that more head-to-head trials are needed to inform the choice of which antidepressant (e.g., SSRI vs tricyclic antidepressant) to prescribe to patients. As for the treatment of anxiety symptoms, benzodiazepines and SSRIs are two of the most commonly prescribed treatments. A review by Traeger and colleagues (2012) of evidence-based treatments for anxiety in cancer patients identified three RCTs supporting the use of benzodiazepines for treating acute anxiety when compared to relaxation or standard care, while a fourth RCT found no evidence for the longer-term use of benzodiazepines when compared to placebo [69]. Additionally, the authors found that evidence from nine RCTs of antidepressants that included anxiety as an outcome provide mixed evidence for the use of antidepressants for longer-term anxiety treatment, while noting that many of the trials did not investigate doses that are considered therapeutic. More research is needed to demonstrate the efficacy of pharmacotherapy in cancer survivors and to inform best clinical practice. *Thus, health care providers should use caution when considering pharmacotherapy in this population.* Although pharmacotherapy is listed as both a low and high intensity treatment option in the ASCO guidelines for treatment of anxiety and depressive symptoms, this option should primarily be considered for survivors with high symptomatology on the PHQ-9 and/or GAD-7 (e.g., scores >15; see Tables 12.1 and 12.2) and meeting DSM-5 criteria for a depressive/anxiety disorder and after discussing all treatment options.

Because very little information is available to inform the use of pharmacologic treatment in this population, providers choosing this form of treatment must consider the following:

- Side effect profiles of the medications
- Tolerability of treatment, including the potential for interaction with other current medications (e.g., certain SSRIs, such as fluoxetine and paroxetine, may impact the metabolism of Tamoxifen, so caution is advised when coadministering these drugs) [80]
- Prior response to treatment
- Individual preference

It is common for individuals with symptoms of depression and/or anxiety to experience problems with adherence to mental health treatment recommendations and follow-up, as described previously; providers should monitor survivors regularly for adherence, concerns about adverse effects, and satisfaction with symptom relief [12]. Additionally, prior to being prescribed antidepressant or anxiolytic medication, survivors need information about other treatment options (e.g., psychological treatments) as some may be reluctant to take additional medications. Providers should also work with patients towards the goal of short-term use of certain medications, such as benzodiazepines in the treatment of anxiety, which are associated with an increased risk for dependence and/or abuse as well as certain adverse effects, such as cognitive impairment [81].

Conclusions

While ASCO outlines methods for screening for anxiety and depression symptoms [12], cancer patients with mood and anxiety disorders are infrequently identified. A 2016 study of more than 1200 adult cancer survivors found less than one-third reported having a detailed discussion with their provider about their emotional needs during survivorship care [82]. These results echo prior research suggesting that despite the high prevalence of symptoms of anxiety and depression among cancer survivors, discussions about emotional support are rare [83]. Even when identified, few patients receive appropriate treatment. This is highlighted by a recent study examining treatments received by cancer patients with major depressive disorder. At the time of the study, 73% were not receiving *any* psychological or pharmacologic treatment, with only 5% receiving psychotherapy of any kind [84]. The absence of treatment brings added sequelae including lower quality of life, greater symptom distress, maladaptive coping, and poor adherence to treatment and recommended follow-up care. Thus, it is imperative for oncology providers to routinely assess for symptoms of anxiety and depression and provide appropriate follow-up care for patients endorsing significant symptomatology.

The following summary points are provided:

1. Psychological distress is common for breast cancer survivors, and a significant number of women will meet diagnostic criteria for anxiety and mood disorders.
2. Prevalence rates of anxiety and depressive disorders differ based on time since diagnosis, with rates decreasing over time.
3. It is important to screen for and assess symptoms of anxiety and depression throughout the survivorship trajectory.
4. The PHQ-9 and GAD-7 are well-validated self-report measures that map onto the diagnostic criteria for major depressive disorder and generalized anxiety disorder, respectively. Scores in the moderate-severe range on these measures warrant further diagnostic assessment and referral for empirically supported treatments.
5. Psychoeducation about symptoms of anxiety and depression should be offered to patients as standard care.
6. Patients whose symptomatology warrant additional treatment should be referred for empirically supported treatments delivered by appropriately trained individuals with a background in cancer and its treatments.
7. Psychotherapy (e.g., cognitive behavioral therapy) is effective for reducing symptoms, and when compared to pharmacotherapy, may result in lower rates of relapse.
8. Although pharmacotherapies are commonly prescribed to address symptoms of anxiety and depression for patients with mild symptomatology, pharmacotherapies may be appropriate *only* for those with the greatest symptomatology (e.g., moderate-severe).
9. Adherence to psychotherapy and pharmacotherapy and follow-up care may be difficult for patients with high symptomatology; providers should regularly monitor patients for adherence, concerns about adverse effects, and satisfaction with symptom relief. Employing a multidisciplinary approach to follow-up care (e.g., involving the patients' primary care provider and/or social workers/patient navigators available through your institution) may help to promote adherence.

References

1. Zabora J, Britzenhofe-Szac K, Curbow B, Hooker C, Piantadosi S. The prevalence of psychological distress by cancer site. Psychooncology. 2001;10(1):19–28.
2. Carlson LE, Zelinski EL, Toivonen KI, Sundstrom L, Jobin CT, Damaskos P, et al. Prevalence of psychosocial distress in cancer patients across 55 North American cancer centers. J Psychosoc Oncol. 2019;37(1):5–21.
3. Mehnert A, Hartung TJ, Friedrich M, Vehling S, Brahler E, Harter M, et al. One in two cancer patients is significantly distressed: prevalence and indicators of distress. Psychooncology. 2018;27(1):75–82.
4. Andersen BL, Goyal NG, Westbrook TD, Bishop B, Carson WE 3rd. Trajectories of stress, depressive symptoms, and immunity in cancer survivors: diagnosis to 5 years. Clin Cancer Res. 2017;23(1):52–61.
5. Mitchell AJ, Ferguson DW, Gill J, Paul J, Symonds P. Depression and anxiety in long-term cancer survivors compared with spouses and healthy controls: a systematic review and meta-analysis. Lancet Oncol. 2013;14(8):721–32.
6. Park J-H, Chun M, Jung Y-S, Bae SH. Predictors of psychological distress trajectories in the first year after a breast cancer diagnosis. Asian Nurs Res. 2017;11(4):268–75.
7. Carreira H, Williams R, Müller M, Harewood R, Stanway S, Bhaskaran K. Associations between breast cancer survivorship and adverse mental health outcomes: a systematic review. J Natl Cancer Inst. 2018;110(12):1311–27.
8. Andersen BL, Yang HC, Farrar WB, Golden-Kreutz DM, Emery CF, Thornton LM, et al. Psychologic intervention improves survival for breast can-

cer patients: a randomized clinical trial. Cancer. 2008;113(12):3450–8.
9. Caruso R, GiuliaNanni M, Riba MB, Sabato S, Grassi L. Depressive spectrum disorders in cancer: diagnostic issues and intervention. A critical review. Curr Psychiatry Rep. 2017;19(6):33.
10. Mausbach BT, Schwab RB, Irwin SA. Depression as a predictor of adherence to adjuvant endocrine therapy (AET) in women with breast cancer: a systematic review and meta-analysis. Breast Cancer Res Treat. 2015;152(2):239–46.
11. American College of Surgeons Commission on Cancer. Cancer program standards: ensuring patient-centered care. American College of Surgeons; 2015.
12. Andersen BL, DeRubeis RJ, Berman BS, Gruman J, Champion V, Massie MJ, et al. Screening, assessment, and care of anxiety and depressive symptoms in adults with cancer: an American Society of Clinical Oncology guideline adaptation. J Clin Oncol. 2014;32(15):1605–19.
13. National Comprehensive Cancer Network. NCCN clinical practice guidelines in oncology (NCCN guidelines): distress management. Elsevier; 2020.
14. Hewitt M, Greenfield S, Stovall E, editors. Institute of medicine, national research council. From cancer patient to cancer survivor: lost in transition. The National Academies Press; 2006. 534 p.
15. Kroenke K, Spitzer RL, Williams JB. The PHQ-9: validity of a brief depression severity measure. J Gen Intern Med. 2001;16(9):606–13.
16. Spitzer RL, Kroenke K, Williams JB, Lowe B. A brief measure for assessing generalized anxiety disorder: the GAD-7. Arch Intern Med. 2006;166(10):1092–7.
17. Wagner LI, Pugh SL, Small W Jr, Kirshner J, Sidhu K, Bury MJ, et al. Screening for depression in cancer patients receiving radiotherapy: feasibility and identification of effective tools in the NRG Oncology RTOG 0841 trial. Cancer. 2017;123(3):485–93.
18. Lima MP, Longatto-Filho A, Osório FL. Predictor variables and screening protocol for depressive and anxiety disorders in cancer outpatients. PLoS One. 2016;11(3):e0149421.
19. Maurer DM. Screening for depression. Am Fam Physician. 2012;85(2):139–44.
20. Ebell MH. Diagnosis of anxiety disorders in primary care. Am Fam Physician. 2008;78(4):501–2.
21. American Psychiatric Association. Diagnostic and statistical manual of mental disorders (DSM-IV-TR). 4th ed. American Psychiatric Association; 2000.
22. Schellekens MPJ, van den Hurk DGM, Prins JB, Molema J, van der Drift MA, Speckens AEM. The suitability of the hospital anxiety and depression scale, distress thermometer and other instruments to screen for psychiatric disorders in both lung cancer patients and their partners. J Affect Disord. 2016;203:176–83.
23. Zigmond AS, Snaith RP. The hospital anxiety and depression scale. Acta Psychiatr Scand. 1983;67(6):361–70.
24. Cella D, Riley W, Stone A, Rothrock N, Reeve B, Yount S, et al. The Patient-Reported Outcomes Measurement Information System (PROMIS) developed and tested its first wave of adult self-reported health outcome item banks: 2005–2008. J Clin Epidemiol. 2010;63(11):1179–94.
25. Purvis TE, Neuman BJ, Riley LH, Skolasky RL. Comparison of PROMIS anxiety and depression, PHQ-8, and GAD-7 to screen for anxiety and depression among patients presenting for spine surgery. J Neurosurg Spine. 2019:1–8. https://doi.org/10.3171/2018.9.SPINE18521
26. Amtmann D, Kim J, Chung H, Bamer AM, Askew RL, Wu S, et al. Comparing CESD-10, PHQ-9, and PROMIS depression instruments in individuals with multiple sclerosis. Rehabil Psychol. 2014;59(2):220–9.
27. Stafford L, Komiti A, Bousman C, Judd F, Gibson P, Mann GB, et al. Predictors of depression and anxiety symptom trajectories in the 24 months following diagnosis of breast or gynaecologic cancer. Breast. 2016;26:100–5.
28. Weihs KL, McConnell MH, Wiley JF, Crespi CM, Sauer-Zavala S, Stanton AL. A preventive intervention to modify depression risk targets after breast cancer diagnosis: Design and single-arm pilot study. Psychooncology. 2019;28(4):880–7.
29. Avis NE, Levine BJ, Case LD, Naftalis EZ, Van Zee KJ. Trajectories of depressive symptoms following breast cancer diagnosis. Cancer Epidemiol Biomark Prev. 2015;24(11):1789–95.
30. Burgess C, Cornelius V, Love S, Graham J, Richards M, Ramirez A. Depression and anxiety in women with early breast cancer: five year observational cohort study. BMJ. 2005;330(7493):702.
31. Tsaras K, Papathanasiou IV, Mitsi D, Veneti A, Kelesi M, Zyga S, et al. Assessment of depression and anxiety in breast cancer patients: prevalence and associated factors. Asian Pac J Cancer Prev. 2018;19(6):1661–9.
32. Hubalek M, Sztankay M, Oberguggenberger A, Meraner V, Egle D, Mangweth-Matzek B, et al. Abstract P1-11-02: psychological morbidity in breast cancer survivors: prevalence rates and determinants. Cancer Res. 2016;76(4 Supplement):P1-11-02-P1-11-02.
33. Hoffman KE, McCarthy EP, Recklitis CJ, Ng AK. Psychological distress in long-term survivors of adult-onset cancer: results from a national survey. Arch Intern Med. 2009;169(14):1274–81.
34. Thornton LM, Andersen BL, Crespin TR, Carson WE. Individual trajectories in stress covary with immunity during recovery from cancer diagnosis and treatments. Brain Behav Immun. 2007;21(2):185–94.
35. Fann JR, Thomas-Rich AM, Katon WJ, Cowley D, Pepping M, McGregor BA, et al. Major depression after breast cancer: a review of epidemiology and treatment. Gen Hosp Psychiatry. 2008;30(2):112–26.
36. American Psychiatric Association. Diagnostic and statistical manual of mental disorders. 5th ed. American Psychiatric Association; 2013.

37. Yi JC, Syrjala KL. Anxiety and depression in cancer survivors. Med Clin North Am. 2017;101(6):1099–113.
38. Krok-Schoen JL, Naughton MJ, Bernardo BM, Young GS, Paskett ED. Fear of recurrence among older breast, ovarian, endometrial, and colorectal cancer survivors: findings from the WHI LILAC study. Psycho-Oncology. 2018;27(7):1810–5.
39. Arch JJ, Mitchell JL. An Acceptance and Commitment Therapy (ACT) group intervention for cancer survivors experiencing anxiety at re-entry. Psychooncology. 2016;25(5):610–5.
40. Lebel S, Ozakinci G, Humphris G, Mutsaers B, Thewes B, Prins J, et al. From normal response to clinical problem: definition and clinical features of fear of cancer recurrence. Support Care Cancer. 2016;24(8):3265–8.
41. Mehnert A, Koch U, Schulz H, Wegscheider K, Weis J, Faller H, et al. Prevalence of mental disorders, psychosocial distress and need for psychosocial support in cancer patients - study protocol of an epidemiological multi-center study. BMC Psychiatry. 2012;12:70.
42. Mehnert A, Brähler E, Faller H, Härter M, Keller M, Schulz H, et al. Four-week prevalence of mental disorders in patients with cancer across major tumor entities. J Clin Oncol. 2014;32(31):3540–6.
43. Brintzenhofe-Szoc KM, Levin TT, Li Y, Kissane DW, Zabora JR. Mixed anxiety/depression symptoms in a large cancer cohort: prevalence by cancer type. Psychosomatics. 2009;50(4):383–91.
44. Watson M, Haviland JS, Greer S, Davidson J, Bliss JM. Influence of psychological response on survival in breast cancer: a population-based cohort study. Lancet. 1999;354(9187):1331–6.
45. Pinquart M, Duberstein PR. Depression and cancer mortality: a meta-analysis. Psychol Med. 2010;40(11):1797–810.
46. Zhu J, Fang F, Sjölander A, Fall K, Adami HO, Valdimarsdóttir U. First-onset mental disorders after cancer diagnosis and cancer-specific mortality: a nationwide cohort study. Ann Oncol. 2017;28(8):1964–9.
47. Davies C, Pan H, Godwin J, Gray R, Arriagada R, Raina V, et al. Long-term effects of continuing adjuvant tamoxifen to 10 years versus stopping at 5 years after diagnosis of oestrogen receptor-positive breast cancer: ATLAS, a randomised trial. Lancet. 2013;381(9869):805–16.
48. Hershman DL, Shao T, Kushi LH, Buono D, Tsai WY, Fehrenbacher L, et al. Early discontinuation and nonadherence to adjuvant hormonal therapy are associated with increased mortality in women with breast cancer. Breast Cancer Res Treat. 2011;126(2):529–37.
49. Bender CM, Gentry AL, Brufsky AM, Casillo FE, Cohen SM, Dailey MM, et al. Influence of patient and treatment factors on adherence to adjuvant endocrine therapy in breast cancer. Oncol Nurs Forum. 2014;41(3):274–85.
50. Cancer Support Community. Cancer support helpline 2020. Available from: https://www.cancersupportcommunity.org/cancer-support-helpline
51. Jin J, Sklar GE, Min Sen Oh V, Chuen LS. Factors affecting therapeutic compliance: a review from the patient's perspective. Ther Clin Risk Manag. 2008;4(1):269–86.
52. Zivin K, Kales HC. Adherence to depression treatment in older adults. Drugs Aging. 2008;25(7):559–71.
53. Bull SA, Hu XH, Hunkeler EM, Lee JY, Ming EE, Markson LE, et al. Discontinuation of use and switching of antidepressants: influence of patient-physician communication. JAMA. 2002;288(11):1403–9.
54. Rivero-Santana A, Perestelo-Perez L, Pérez-Ramos J, Serrano-Aguilar P, De Las Cuevas C. Sociodemographic and clinical predictors of compliance with antidepressants for depressive disorders: systematic review of observational studies. Patient Prefer Adherence. 2013;7:151–69.
55. Duijts SF, Faber MM, Oldenburg HS, van Beurden M, Aaronson NK. Effectiveness of behavioral techniques and physical exercise on psychosocial functioning and health-related quality of life in breast cancer patients and survivors–a meta-analysis. Psychooncology. 2011;20(2):115–26.
56. Scheier MF, Helgeson VS, Schulz R, Colvin S, Berga S, Bridges MW, et al. Interventions to enhance physical and psychological functioning among younger women who are ending nonhormonal adjuvant treatment for early-stage breast cancer. J Clin Oncol. 2005;23(19):4298–311.
57. Jones JM, Cheng T, Jackman M, Walton T, Haines S, Rodin G, et al. Getting back on track: evaluation of a brief group psychoeducation intervention for women completing primary treatment for breast cancer. Psychooncology. 2013;22(1):117–24.
58. National Institute of Mental Health. Chronic illness and mental health: recognizing and treating depression. In: Health NIoM, editor. Bethesda: National Institutes of Health
59. National Institute of Mental Health. Depression basics. In: Health NIoM, editor. Bethesda: National Institutes of Health; 2016.
60. National Institute of Mental Health. 5 Things you should know about stress. In: Health NIoM, editor. Bethesda: National Institutes of Health.
61. American Cancer Society. Getting help for distress. In: American Cancer Society, editor. 2017.
62. American Cancer Society. When cancer comes back. In: American Cancer Society, editor. 2017.
63. Brown JC, Huedo-Medina TB, Pescatello LS, Ryan SM, Pescatello SM, Moker E, et al. The efficacy of exercise in reducing depressive symptoms among cancer survivors: a meta-analysis. PLoS One. 2012;7(1):e30955.
64. Antoni MH. Psychosocial intervention effects on adaptation, disease course and biobehavioral processes in cancer. Brain Behav Immun. 2013;30(Suppl):S88–98.

65. Lutgendorf SK, Andersen BL. Biobehavioral approaches to cancer progression and survival: mechanisms and interventions. Am Psychol. 2015;70(2):186–97.
66. Andersen BL, Thornton LM, Shapiro CL, Farrar WB, Mundy BL, Yang HC, et al. Biobehavioral, immune, and health benefits following recurrence for psychological intervention participants. Clin Cancer Res. 2010;16(12):3270–8.
67. Butler AC, Chapman JE, Forman EM, Beck AT. The empirical status of cognitive-behavioral therapy: a review of meta-analyses. Clin Psychol Rev. 2006;26(1):17–31.
68. Hollon SD, Stewart MO, Strunk D. Enduring effects for cognitive behavior therapy in the treatment of depression and anxiety. Annu Rev Psychol. 2006;57(1):285–315.
69. Traeger L, Greer JA, Fernandez-Robles C, Temel JS, Pirl WF. Evidence-based treatment of anxiety in patients with cancer. J Clin Oncol. 2012;30(11):1197–205.
70. Greer JA, Traeger L, Bemis H, Solis J, Hendriksen ES, Park ER, et al. A pilot randomized controlled trial of brief cognitive-behavioral therapy for anxiety in patients with terminal cancer. Oncologist. 2012;17(10):1337–45.
71. DeRubeis RJ, Hollon SD, Amsterdam JD, Shelton RC, Young PR, Salomon RM, et al. Cognitive therapy vs medications in the treatment of moderate to severe depression. Arch Gen Psychiatry. 2005;62(4):409–16.
72. Strunk DR, Adler AD, Hollon SD. Cognitive therapy of depression. The Oxford handbook of mood disorders. Oxford library of psychology. Oxford University Press; 2017. p. 411–22.
73. Hollon SD, DeRubeis RJ, Shelton RC, Amsterdam JD, Salomon RM, O'Reardon JP, et al. Prevention of relapse following cognitive therapy vs medications in moderate to severe depression. Annual Convention of the American Psychiatric Association 155th May 2002 Philadelphia PA US. 2005;62(4):417–22.
74. Mitte K. Meta-analysis of cognitive-behavioral treatments for generalized anxiety disorder: a comparison with pharmacotherapy. Psychol Bull. 2005;131(5):785–95.
75. Mayo-Wilson E, Montgomery P. Media-delivered cognitive behavioural therapy and behavioural therapy (self-help) for anxiety disorders in adults. Cochrane Database Syst Rev. 2013;(9):CD005330.
76. Piet J, Würtzen H, Zachariae R. The effect of mindfulness-based therapy on symptoms of anxiety and depression in adult cancer patients and survivors: a systematic review and meta-analysis. Annual Convention of the Association for Advancement of Behavior Therapy 37th Nov 2003 Boston MA US. 2012;80(6):1007–20.
77. Johns SA, Stutz PV, Talib TL, Cohee AA, Beck-Coon KA, Brown LF, et al. Acceptance and commitment therapy for breast cancer survivors with fear of cancer recurrence: a 3-arm pilot randomized controlled trial. Cancer. 2020;126(1):211–8.
78. Hawkins NA, Soman A, Buchanan Lunsford N, Leadbetter S, Rodriguez JL. Use of medications for treating anxiety and depression in cancer survivors in the United States. J Clin Oncol. 2017;35(1):78–85.
79. Ostuzzi G, Matcham F, Dauchy S, Barbui C, Hotopf M. Antidepressants for the treatment of depression in people with cancer. Cochrane Database Syst Rev. 2015;2015(6):CD011006.
80. National Comprehensive Cancer Network. NCCN clinical practice guidelines in oncology (NCCN guidelines): Breast Cancer, 2020.
81. Barker MJ, Greenwood KM, Jackson M, Crowe SF. Cognitive effects of long-term benzodiazepine use. CNS Drugs. 2004;18(1):37–48.
82. Chawla N, Blanch-Hartigan D, Virgo KS, Ekwueme DU, Han X, Forsythe L, et al. Quality of patient-provider communication among cancer survivors: findings from a nationally representative sample. J Oncol Pract. 2016;12(12):e964–e73.
83. Mello S, Tan ASL, Armstrong K, Sanford Schwartz J, Hornik RC. Anxiety and depression among cancer survivors: the role of engagement with sources of emotional support information. Health Commun. 2013;28(4):389–96.
84. Walker J, Hansen CH, Martin P, Symeonides S, Ramessur R, Murray G, et al. Prevalence, associations, and adequacy of treatment of major depression in patients with cancer: a cross-sectional analysis of routinely collected clinical data. Lancet Psychiatry. 2014;1(5):343–50.

Obesity, Weight Gain, and Weight Management

13

Kirsten A. Nyrop, Jordan T. Lee, Erin A. O'Hare, Chelsea Osterman, and Hyman B. Muss

Introduction

In their 2018 report, the World Cancer Research Fund (WCRF) and American Institute for Cancer Research (AICR) summarized the strength of evidence linking adult body composition and weight with risk for specific cancers [1]. The report states there is convincing evidence for increased risk of cancers of the esophagus, pancreas, liver, colorectal, breast (postmenopausal), endometrium, and kidney, as well as probable evidence for cancers of the mouth/pharynx/larynx, stomach (cardia), gallbladder, ovary, and prostate in obese persons [1]. Other reports have similarly identified these cancer sites as adiposity-related [2].

> *Clinical Cancer Advances 2015: Annual Report on Progress Against Cancer from the American Society of Clinical Oncology* (ASCO) [3]

> Obesity is quickly overtaking tobacco as the leading preventable cause of cancer. As many as 84,000 cancer diagnoses each year are attributed to obesity, and obesity or excess weight contributes up to one in five cancer-related deaths. If current obesity trends continue, it is estimated there could be an additional 500,000 cases of cancer by 2090.

The World Health Organization (WHO) defines overweight and obesity as abnormal or excessive fat accumulation that presents a risk to health [4]. Body Mass Index (BMI) is a measure that uses a person's height and weight to identify individuals with BMI 25–29.9 as overweight, and BMI 30 or higher as having obesity. In a review of cancer cases attributable to excess body weight in the USA [5], the relative risk for every 5-unit increase in BMI for cancers of the esophagus was

K. A. Nyrop (✉)
Department of Medicine, University of North Carolina at Chapel Hill School of Medicine, Chapel Hill, NC, USA
e-mail: kirsten_nyrop@med.unc.edu

J. T. Lee
Department of Exercise and Sport Science, University of North Carolina at Chapel Hill, Raleigh, NC, USA

E. A. O'Hare
Lineberger Comprehensive Cancer Center, University of North Carolina at Chapel Hill School of Medicine, Hillsborough, NC, USA

C. Osterman
Department of Medicine, Division of Oncology, University of North Carolina at Chapel Hill, Chapel Hill, NC, USA

H. B. Muss
Department of Medicine, University of North Carolina at Chapel Hill School of Medicine and Lineberger Comprehensive Cancer Center, Chapel Hill, NC, USA

G. G. Kimmick et al. (eds.), *Common Issues in Breast Cancer Survivors*,
https://doi.org/10.1007/978-3-030-75377-1_13

RR 1.48 (1.35–1.62) [6], stomach RR 1.31 (1.18–1.45) [6], gallbladder RR 1.29 (1.20–1.39) [6], kidney and renal pelvis RR 1.29 (1.20–1.39) [6], pancreas RR 1.14 (1.07–1.21) [7], breast (female, postmenopausal) RR 1.10 (1.08–1.12) [6], thyroid RR 1.09 (1.04–1.14) [8], multiple myeloma RR 1.09 (1.03–1.16) [9], and colorectal RR 1.04 (1.02–1.06) [10]. Illustrating the particular risk for adiposity-related cancers in women who are postmenopausal, a meta-analysis of prospective observational studies found that for every 5 kg (11 pounds) in adult weight gain, relative risks were breast cancer 1.11 (1.08–1.13) (no or low hormone replacement therapy/HRT users), endometrial cancer among HRT non-users 1.39 (1.29–1.49) and 1.09 (0.02–1.16) among HRT users, and ovarian cancer 1.13 (1.03–1.23) (no or low HRT users) [11].

In the USA, it has been estimated that overweight or obesity accounted for 40% of all cancers diagnosed in 2014 (630,000 persons) – 55% in women and 24% in men [12]. In women, rates (per 100,000 adjusted for age) for overweight/obesity-associated cancers also varied by race/ethnicity: black 226.3 (224.3–228.4), white 223.3 (221.5–223.1), and Hispanic 188.0 (1.86.0–189.9). In men, obesity-associated rates were black 134.2 (132.3–136.1), white 114.2 (113.6–114.8), and Hispanic 108.8 (107.1–110.6) [12].

Reflecting recent observations of rising obesity rates in younger people in the USA population [13, 14], a recent analysis of SEER data from 2000 to 2016 identified a shift towards younger age groups in obesity-associated cancer (OACs) [15]. It was noted that the percentage increase of incident OAC cases in this timeframe was highest in the 50–65 age group, which is consistent with previous studies showing rising incidence of cancers among younger adults [12, 16]. The report also noted concurrent decrease in the incidence of OACs among adults age 65 and older.

These data illustrate why the substantial evidence of an obesity-cancer link is of growing concern in cancer prevention and control, especially in countries where obesity rates are high and rising, as in the USA [17]. The evidence regarding risks, outcomes, and interventions is most developed in the literature pertaining to women with early breast cancer (Stage I–III). Primarily with the oncology clinician-patient relationship in mind [18], this chapter provides an overview of weight trajectories in women with early breast cancer, implications for prognosis and survival, nutrition and exercise for weight management, and the role of oncology clinicians. Lessons learned from the breast cancer population are illustrative for other types of cancers; however, it does not substitute for the need for further research specific to other patient populations.

Weight Trajectories After Breast Cancer Diagnosis

The earliest studies documenting weight gain in women with breast cancer date from the late 1970s [19], with chemotherapy emerging as a central risk factor for weight gain [20–24]. With the advent of newer chemotherapy regimens of shorter duration, weight gain has continued to be observed although at somewhat less dramatic levels [25, 26]. In addition to weight, studies have documented other treatment-related changes in body composition, such as fat mass [27–31].

Estimates of weight gain vary widely among studies, often depending on methodological factors such as patient recall versus objective measures of height and weight, time since breast cancer diagnosis if the study is cross-sectional, and duration of time when the data are longitudinal. Often, weight gain is reported as an average; however, it is important to note that many women with early breast cancer do not gain weight and even lose weight, which may be lost in reports of averages. In a recent chart review of US women seen at a university-affiliated hospital (29% non-white, 82% with hormone receptor positive tumors, 16% with HER-2 positive tumors), using nurse-assessed weight measures from breast cancer diagnosis to 2 years post primary treatment, it was found that one-third of study participants had relatively stable weight ±2 kilograms (kg), one-third lost more than 2 kg, and one-third gained more than 2 kg [32]. These findings reflect those of other studies reporting weight gain limited to about a third of patients [33–38], while other studies have reported higher proportions experiencing weight gain [31, 39, 40].

In addition to chemotherapy, endocrine treatment (ET) has been identified as a potential risk factor for weight gain, albeit with conflicting evidence [41]. Some studies have reported less weight gain among women on aromatase inhibitor (AI) therapy as compared to selective estrogen-receptor moderators (SERM) such as tamoxifen [42]. Other studies have reported that a majority of women on AI or tamoxifen do not experience weight gain during the first 2 years of ET [43, 44]. There has been similarly conflicting evidence regarding associations of menopausal status with weight trajectories, with some studies noting higher risk for weight gain in premenopausal women [22, 32, 34, 45] and others noting greater risk in postmenopausal women [23, 46].

Mostly, the focus has continued to be on chemotherapy as a risk factor [47], especially the longer-duration sequential regimens [31, 48] and anthracycline-based regimens [39, 49]. In a study of French women with early breast cancer, average weight gain was 5.1 kg at 18 months post-diagnosis [35]. Thirty-six percent of patients had greater than 5% weight gain, ranging from 7% of women on docetaxel plus cyclophosphamide to 60% of women on anthracycline plus paclitaxel or docetaxel. In a US sample of women with early breast cancer, the lowest proportion gaining 2+ kilograms at 2 years post primary treatment was observed in women who received no chemotherapy regardless of type of subsequent endocrine treatment (less than 30% of these patients gained weight), while the highest proportions of weight gain were observed in women who received no ET but had either anthracycline or non-anthracycline chemotherapy (42%) [32]. Of particular note in this study was that regardless of treatment plan (presence or absence of different chemotherapy regimens and plus/minus ET), premenopausal women gained far more weight than postmenopausal women. Although not statistically significant ($p > 0.05$), among women who received anthracycline-based chemotherapy but no ET, 45% of premenopausal compared to 38% of postmenopausal women gained 2 kg or more at 2 years post primary treatment. Significantly, in women who received anthracycline-based chemotherapy plus subsequent ET, these percentages were 50% and 26% for pre- and postmenopausal women, respectively ($p = 0.0005$).

These findings illustrate the impact that different treatment plans may have on the risk for weight gain. One hypothesis is that the differential impact may reflect substantial differences in fatigue levels and other toxicities associated with specific regimens [50, 51] that may affect the ability of patients to exercise during and after primary treatment. For example, to the extent extreme fatigue persists after chemotherapy completion, some patients may remain sedentary at the same time that they are regaining their appetite, thereby creating an energy imbalance. In fact, studies have shown that physical activity declines in breast cancer survivors, especially in black women [52, 53].

These findings underscore the need for further research into why premenopausal women are at greater risk for weight gain regardless of treatment plan. And, we need a better understanding of why some women considered "low risk" for weight gain (e.g., postmenopausal on a treatment plan that has the lowest proportion of patients experiencing weight gain) nevertheless gain substantial weight despite all efforts to avoid weight gain, while other women in "high risk for weight gain" treatment plans maintain their weight or even lose weight post primary treatment. In the interim, the specificity of current information can help clinicians address patient questions about whether their specific treatment plan and menopausal status may put them at high risk for weight gain. It also suggests that weight measurements should be routinely collected and monitored at follow-up visits, to identify patients at risk of gaining unhealthy amounts of weight and to permit timely interventions.

Excess Weight, Prognosis, and Survival

Many factors contribute to prognosis and survival in women with breast cancer, but here we focus only on the factor of excess weight.

Overall Mortality and Survival

Since 1975, the breast cancer mortality rate in the USA has declined by 40% largely due to a combination of treatment improvements and rising rates of early detection through mammography [54]. Five-year survival rates are especially promising for women with HR+ tumors – 92% for HR+/HER2- and 89% for HR+/HER2+ [55]. However, the impact of BMI is seen in a meta-analysis (21 studies) of HR+ breast cancer which reported a pooled hazard ratio for overall survival of 1.31 (1.17, 1.46) in women with obesity compared to no obesity [56]. The impact of post-diagnosis weight gain versus weight maintenance was assessed in a meta-analysis (12 studies) which reported an increased all-cause mortality hazard ratio of 1.12 (1.03, 1.22) for women experiencing >5% weight gain and 1.23 (1.09, 1.39) for >10% weight gain [57].

Overall survival rates represent a combination of breast cancer and non-breast cancer survival rates. Because most women diagnosed with breast cancer are above age 60, many have one or more comorbidities at diagnosis, and a majority die of non-breast cancer causes [58]. To the extent women with breast cancer have excess obesity, they are more likely to have obesity-related comorbidities, such as hypertension, diabetes mellitus, and cardiovascular disease [59, 60]. Competing comorbidities, rather than breast cancer diagnosis, are more likely to determine overall survival [61]. For example, in women age 65 or older diagnosed with Stage I breast cancer, the cumulative incidence of death due to non-cancer causes is 21.3% compared to 3.7% due to breast cancer at 100 months [62]. To the extent comorbidities can be managed through medications and/or lifestyles changes (weight management, diet, exercise), there are likely to be continued improvements in overall survival rates in women with breast cancer.

It is important to note that breast cancer death rates in white and black women were similar in the mid-1980s, but thereafter diverged dramatically to the point where the mortality rate is now 40% higher in black women [63]. This disparity is reflected in 5-year survival rates (2010–2015) for women with HR+/HER2- breast cancer, 93% for white and 86% for black women; similarly, for HR+/HER2+ breast cancer – 89% in white and 84% in black women [64]. This disparity reflects tumor, diagnostic, and treatment factors, but it also reflects differences in obesity rates and associated comorbidities [65]. Between 2007–2008 and 2015–2016, the prevalence of obesity in US women increased from 35% to 41% – from 36% to 43% in women age 40–59 and from 35% to 41% in women age 60 or older [66]. In women age 20 or older, the highest rates of obesity are seen in black women (55%) followed by Hispanic (51%) and white women (15%) [13]. This period of rising BMI coincides with rising breast cancer incidence rates, especially for HR+ disease and especially in black women with HR+ tumors [67].

In one of the earliest studies identifying comorbidities as a factor in survival disparities [68], it was found that among women with Stage I–IV breast cancer, black women had a higher proportion of 77 comorbidities that were associated with reduced survival. In that study, black women compared to white women had higher total number of comorbidities at baseline (2.26 versus 1.83, $p < 0.001$), diabetes without complications (23% versus 8%, $p < 0.001$), diabetes with complications (3% versus 1%, $p = 0.05$), and hypertension (63% versus 36%, $p < 0.001$). In that study, total comorbidities explained 49% of the overall survival difference between white and black women and 77% of competing cause of death disparity [68]. Hypertension alone has been estimated to account for 30% of the survival disparity between black and white women with breast cancer [69]. Other studies have shown differences between white and black women with breast cancer for cardiovascular disease and breast cancer mortality [70]. The management of obesity-related comorbidities is as important to overall survival as state-of-the-art breast cancer treatment; especially in black women, comorbidity management could greatly lessen the gap in disease mortality [61].

Breast Cancer-Specific Survival

Evidence regarding the impact of excess weight on breast cancer-specific survival is still evolving. In one meta-analysis (28 studies), increased risk for breast cancer mortality was observed for each 5 kg/m^2 increment of BMI – 18% if BMI was measured before diagnosis, 14% if measured within 12 months of diagnosis, and 29% if measured more than 12 months post diagnosis [71]. In another meta-analysis (13 studies), every 5 kg/m^2 increment of BMI was associated with increased risk for contralateral breast cancer RR 1.12 (1.06, 1.20) and breast second primary cancers RR 1.14 (1.07, 1.21) [72]. In a meta-analysis (21 studies) of women with HR+ breast cancer, the pooled hazard ratio was 1.36 (1.20, 1.54) for breast cancer-specific survival in women with obesity compared to no obesity [56]. In a study of women with estrogen receptor positive (ER+) tumors ($N = 6295$), the hazard ratio for late recurrence was 1.24 (1.00, 1.53) in women experiencing post-diagnosis weight gain of 10% or more; the analysis also found significantly increased risk for breast cancer-specific mortality in women with obesity [73]. Evidence is also emerging that wide fluctuations in weight from diagnosis – both loss and gain – can be problematic. In a recent analysis of a German cohort of 2216 women, greater than 10% weight loss since diagnosis doubled the risk for all-cause mortality and tripled the risk for breast cancer mortality [74].

In these studies, the focus is often on weight and BMI, but the underlying mechanism is likely to be body composition – total fat mass, muscle density, and fat infiltration of the muscle – as reflected by the exponentially growing interest in these metrics in cancer research [75–77]. A recent study of women with breast cancer found subcutaneous adipose tissue associated with increased risk for death HR 1.13 (1.02, 1.26) [78], and another study reported higher overall mortality HR 1.35 (1.08, 1.69) in women with the highest tertile of total adipose tissue (TAT) compared to the lowest tertile [79]. Other studies have reported an association between body composition metrics and treatment toxicities that may lead to dose delays and reductions and in turn impact survival [80].

Diet and Physical Activity for Weight Management

Maintaining energy balance through a physically active lifestyle and choosing healthy foods is the foundation of healthy weight maintenance for breast cancer survivors [6, 18]. For women with excess weight at breast cancer diagnosis, the challenge of avoiding weight gain is a common concern among same-age women without a cancer diagnosis who have a similar risk profile for weight gain [81–83]. A breast cancer diagnosis can provide a "teachable moment" for making important lifestyle changes [84–86]. However, for breast cancer survivors who all too often had a sedentary lifestyle prior to diagnosis [87], transitioning to a more physically active one and having the time, resources, and know-how to prepare diet-conscious meals are a great challenge. Increasing physical activity can be especially daunting for women struggling with fatigue, chemotherapy-induced peripheral neuropathy, and other lingering side effects of treatment.

The evidence supporting diet and exercise for weight management in women with breast cancer comes from decades of interventions studies. Among these studies, six have focused specifically on preventing or avoiding weight gain in women scheduled to receive chemotherapy [88, 89]. The decision to recruit women receiving chemotherapy reflects the evidence for chemotherapy as a risk factor for weight gain in early breast cancer. However, women often lose weight between diagnosis and start of endocrine treatment [43, 44], generally because they are experiencing chemotherapy side effects such as nausea, vomiting, and loss of appetite. For these women, the first 2 years after chemotherapy can then become a period of substantial weight gain that more than exceeds their weight loss [32]. In general, the period immediately following primary treatment is an especially important timeframe for initiating interventions to avoid weight gain.

At least 26 randomized controlled trials testing diet or diet/exercise interventions for weight loss have been published, with numerous additional studies still underway [90–92]. In these studies, most women were recruited within 6–12 months post primary treatment or an average of 3 or more years after treatment. Three studies were focused exclusively on black women with breast cancer [93–95]. In addition to weight loss and reduced BMI, several studies have included body composition outcomes such as fat mass/body fat, lean body mass, waist circumference, waist to hip ratio, or hip circumference [96–101]. Among the most recent RCTs that are still underway, there is a specific focus on measuring the potential impact of weight loss on cancer end points, such as breast cancer recurrence, disease-free survival, progression-free survival, and overall survival [92].

Among the studies that have been completed, multi-faceted approaches that include behavioral interventions in combination with diet and exercise have had the best results, achieving statistically significant as well as clinically significant outcomes (5–10% weight loss) in women with BMI of 25 or higher; intervention periods of 6–12 months have also had the most promising results [90, 91]. The downside of multi-faceted interventions is that they often entail intense contact with study participants and the investment of substantial resources (direct supervision by trained staff, facilities, equipment) to keep patients engaged and compliant/adherent with intervention regimens. Also, the evidence for maintenance of intervention effects (keeping the weight off, staying with the diet and exercise regimen) beyond 6 months post intervention is still limited [102]. It is important for intervention studies to include a focus on maintenance strategies for sustained compliance in addition to measuring immediate outcomes [103].

Interventions with promising results now need to be translated into practical advice that breast cancer survivors can follow on a self-directed basis at home. Weight management interventions should be designed for scalability and sustainability under "real-world" conditions. Interventions need to be "high reach" (relevant to most breast cancer survivors), but there is also a need for further research into interventions that are specifically tailored for diverse racial and ethnic perspectives on diet and exercise.

In the meantime, current evidence is strong that weight management interventions are feasible and safe for most women with early breast cancer. Women with unhealthy weight can be advised and encouraged to monitor their weight and waist circumference, and to discuss any weight-related concerns they may have with their oncology clinician and primary care provider. Breast cancer survivors need to understand that weight management, exercise, and diet can be as important to their health and wellness as completing their treatment.

Diet and Nutrition

For women aiming to avoid weight gain after primary treatment, the advice is that they should prioritize nutrient-dense foods over energy-dense foods, because they provide greater satiety while limiting caloric intake and providing high nutritional content [104, 105]. Within this broad guidance for energy balance, it is important to understand the nuances of healthy food choices. Breast cancer survivors should aim for a predominantly plant-based diet that includes plenty of colorful and nutrient-dense vegetables (4–5 servings/day) and fruits (2–3 servings/day) [106, 107]. The recommendation to "eat the rainbow" implies intake of a wide variety of vitamins and minerals [106, 108, 109].

Nutrient-dense vegetables	Kale, broccoli, spinach, sweet potato, brussel sprouts, cabbage, peas, chard, cauliflower, carrot, bell pepper, collard greens, kohlrabi, red cabbage
Nutrient-dense fruits	Grapefruit, blackberries, oranges, bananas, grapes, papaya, cherries, pineapple, avocado, apples, pomegranate, mango, strawberries, and cranberries

Increasing fruit and vegetables in the diet also satisfies the recommendation for adequate fiber intake (>25 g/day), which is an important factor in appetite regulation and may help prevent chronic diseases commonly associated with breast cancer, including cardiovascular disease and diabetes [107, 110]. Breast cancer survivors should choose foods with healthy fats such as nuts, seeds, avocados, and fatty fish to replace foods high in saturated fats such as fried food, savory snacks, baked sweets, and fast foods. Healthy fat from whole foods is crucial to a healthy diet, and patients should take care not to limit these in an effort to reduce overall calories [106, 111, 112]. Care should also be taken when choosing commercially produced condiments and salad dressings, as many contain added sugars and unhealthy fats [106].

While most Americans meet or exceed their protein needs, a disproportionate amount comes from red meat, much of which contains high levels of saturated fat [113]. Breast cancer survivors should focus on lean and plant-based proteins, limiting red meat intake to less than 11 oz. (2–3 servings) per week and consuming little, if any, cured or processed meats [6]. Carbohydrates should be chosen carefully to include nutrient- and fiber-rich options, including non-starchy vegetables, fruits, whole grains, and legumes [6, 18], and they should limit intake of refined carbohydrates such as baked goods and items containing sugar, other sweeteners, and white flour [6, 18]. While there is growing interest in studying the potential benefits of limiting total carbohydrates in women with breast cancer, the evidence is limited [114].

Calories from sweetened beverages are a common source of excess non-nutritive calories in the American diet and should be avoided, and instead focus on intake of water and non-sugar sweetened herbal or green tea [115, 116]. In addition to providing non-nutritive calories, alcoholic beverages are a risk factor for breast cancer and should be limited to one drink per day [6, 117]. Data suggest an increased risk of recurrence in breast cancer survivors who exceed 3–4 drinks/week [118].

Women should be advised to always consult with their oncology provider regarding administration of any herbal or nutrient supplement to avoid the risk of interactions with medications or other treatments [119]. The Memorial Sloan Kettering Cancer Center website includes a helpful web page pertaining to common herbal supplements and their effects – https://www.mskcc.org/cancer-care/patient-education/herbal-remedies-and-treatment. In the absence of a diagnosed nutrient deficiency, a "food first" policy is the best and safest way to ensure adequate nutrient intake.

Given the premium on clinic time with patients, having an in-depth discussion about dietary changes to support healthy weight maintenance may not be realistic for the oncologist. Registered Dietitians (RD) have specialized training in nutrition and cancer as well as the psychology of behavior change and are an excellent resource for the oncology provider and patient [17]. Referral to an RD for the newly diagnosed breast cancer patient is a cost-effective method to support healthy nutrition during and after cancer treatment. Weight loss and nutrition specialists may also provide guidance regarding the pros and cons of bariatric surgery, specific diet regimens (such as Atkins, ketogenic diets), prescription medications to treat overweight and obesity, and aids to behavior modification (e.g., hypnotherapy, cognitive behavior therapy).

Online resources pertaining to a healthy diet
American Institute for Cancer Research (AICR) – https://www.aicr.org/cancer-prevention/recommendations/eat-a-diet-rich-in-whole-grains-vegetables-fruits-and-beans/
American Cancer Society (ACS) – https://www.cancer.org/healthy/eat-healthy-get-active/eat-healthy.html
US Department of Agriculture (USDA) – https://www.choosemyplate.gov

Physical Activity

In a recent systematic review and meta-analysis, vigorous physical activity was associated with reduced risk for breast cancer in both premenopausal women (Relative Risk 0.79, 95% CI 0.69–0.91) and postmenopausal women (RR 0.90, 95% CI 10.85–0.95) [120]. The protective effects from physical activity, including recreational, occupational, and non-recreational activity, are greatest in women with physical activity exposure more than 1 year and less than 5 years (Overall Relative Risk 0.62, 95% CI 0.46–0.78) [121]. There is also emerging evidence of benefits from physical activity for reduced all-cause and breast cancer-specific mortality [122–125].

After breast cancer diagnosis, exercise can be an important tool for managing side effects from cancer and cancer treatment including adverse impacts on cardiorespiratory function, fatigue, depression, bone health, physical fitness, muscle strength, and body composition [126–134]. For women with breast cancer whose weight exceeds the healthy ideal, exercise may be an essential component to avoiding weight gain and even losing weight, when coupled with a healthy diet.

For both improved health-related outcomes and weight management, "exercise as medicine" has gained increased attention as a safe and potentially effective strategy to help women with breast cancer and other cancer survivors move through cancer and be as active and healthy as possible [135]. The American College of Sports Medicine (ACSM) has published guidelines for cancer survivors that include specific exercise prescriptions for targeting common side effects of cancer and cancer therapy [130, 136]. The general guideline is 150 minutes of moderate exercise per week (or 75 minutes of vigorous activity), coupled with 2–3 days of large muscle resistance training.

The 150 minutes of exercise need to be understood as specific time devoted to taking a walk, above and beyond the daily routine of work and chores, or other form of exercise. A pedometer or activity tracker can be helpful for monitoring the achievement of exercise goals. For example, at a moderate pace of 60 steps/minute, the achievement of 150 minutes of moderate aerobic exercise would be 9000 steps/week (60 steps × 150 minutes) [137], or about 1300 steps a day (22 minutes) above and beyond routine activities. This would be a minimum goal for the achievement ACSM aerobic exercise guidelines. With exercise approval from a clinician, breast cancer survivors can develop their own self-directed plan for raising their daily steps goal closer to 7000 steps/day, walking at a safe and sustainable pace [137].

Aerobic and resistance exercise have their own benefits individually, such as improved cardiorespiratory fitness and muscular strength, respectively; but a combination of modes provides variety and more multifaceted benefits [126, 136, 138–143]. For individuals with multiple comorbidities or side effects such as lymphedema, individualized or tailored exercise may be necessary and require referral to programs led by staff trained in exercise oncology [144–147]. Home- and community-based physical activity initiatives are also options for reversing physical decline and fatigue and maintaining quality of life, both during and after adjuvant treatment [148, 149], with the added benefits of flexibility in time and place and fewer requirements for equipment, facilities, or trained staff.

Exercise oncology is still an emerging area of research, with many areas requiring further investigation, such as the potential impact of exercise on peripheral neuropathy and cognitive functioning, treatment completion, and cancer recurrence and survival, and how these impacts may vary by cancer site and stage [136, 150]. However, there is enough evidence regarding safety, tolerability, and potential benefits in favor of moderate exercise for most women with breast cancer [151]. Exercise is not yet a part of standardized cancer care; but, the consistently demonstrated short- and long-term physical health benefits and increased quality of life warrant patient-provider conversations about the importance of safe and sustained physical activity [135, 152].

Online resources pertaining to exercise for adults with cancer
American Institute for Cancer Research (AICR) – https://www.aicr.org/cancer-prevention/recommendations/be-physically-active/
American Cancer Society (ACS) – https://www.cancer.org/treatment/survivorship-during-and-after-treatment/staying-active/physical-activity-and-the-cancer-patient.html

Role of Oncology Clinicians

Concern within the cancer community regarding the growing evidence of obesity-related cancers and their impact on cancer care is evidenced by guidelines and position statements from the American Society of Clinical Oncology (ASCO)

[17], American Cancer Society (ASC) [18, 107, 153], National Comprehensive Cancer Network (NCCN) [154], and international cancer entities [155, 156]. In 2012, the ACS updated their guidelines on nutrition and physical activity during and after cancer treatment [153], with the intention of presenting "health care providers with the best possible information with which to help cancer survivors and their families make informed choices related to nutrition and physical activity" during the continuum of cancer care [18]. The ASCO Obesity Initiative [157, 158] (https://www.asco.org/practice-policy/cancer-care-initiatives/prevention-survivorship/obesity-cancer) includes a website with tools and resources for clinicians [159] as well as for patients and families [160].

Talking with Patients About Weight

To avoid the weight stigma perceived by many patients in their clinician-patient relationships, it is important for clinicians to use person-centered or people-first language when discussing unhealthy weight [161, 162]. In general, preferred terms are weight, BMI, excess weight, weight problem, unhealthy body weight, or unhealthy BMI; least preferred terms are heaviness, excess fat, obesity, large size, and fatness [163, 164]. When in doubt, it is appropriate to use "person with" elevated BMI or excess weight [162].

Assessment and Screening

The NCCN guidelines for nutrition and weight management provide an algorithm for nutrition and weight management assessment and associated interventions [154]. The assessment includes (1) evaluating BMI, (2) conducting a clinical evaluation that includes asking the patient about their food intake and eating habits, physical activity, willingness to address weight, and barriers to nutrition and weight management, and (3) assessing treatment effects and medical issues that might affect nutrition and weight management including comorbidities, medications, dental health, and use of supplements. For patients identified as overweight or obese, the NCCN guidelines suggest (1) patient-provider discussions about nutrition, weight management, physical activity, and portion control, (2) referral to community resources for weight management, (3) referral to a dietician or weight management program for individualized help, and (4) consideration of evaluation for bariatric surgery or pharmacologic therapy [154].

The "5 A's Behavioral Change Model" provides levels of communication that an oncology clinician may decide to pursue with any given patient during any given clinic visit, ranging from "asking" if the patient would be interested in talking about weight management to "arranging" a referral to a nutritionist or weight counselor. It provides a range of options, rather than just one best approach. In the final analysis, there is also a need to address both real and perceived barriers to having weight-related conversations during a busy clinic visit [135, 165, 166].

Behavioral Change Model: Ask, Assess, Advise, Agree, Assist, Arrange – suggested conversations between oncology clinicians and their patients with obesity

Constructs	Illustrative examples
Ask (added to the model)	Clinician asks the patient if it is okay to discuss weight; OR clinician asks the patient about weight, nutrition, exercise
Assess	Clinician discusses the patient's current weight/BMI (electronic medical records data); OR clinician assesses patient's readiness to discuss healthy weight in breast cancer survivorship
Advise	Clinician makes a specific recommendation regarding weight (avoiding weight gain, losing weight), exercise, and energy balance; OR clinician explains the importance of weight management in breast cancer survivorship (risks and benefits)
Agree	Clinician seeks agreement with the patient to revisit their healthy weight discussion during subsequent clinic visits (this may include agreeing on specific realistic goals for no weight gain or weight loss)
Assist	Clinician provides brief counseling on how to pursue healthy weight and/or provides self-help materials
Arrange	Clinician refers the patient to a nutritionist or weight counseling program

Adapted from Vallis 2013 and Alexander 2011

Timing and Feasibility of Weight-Related Conversations

The ASCO Position Statement [17] notes: "Research shows that the time after a cancer diagnosis can serve as a teachable moment to motivate individuals to adopt risk-reducing behaviors. For this reason, the oncology care team – the providers with whom a patient has the closest relationships in the critical period after cancer diagnosis – is in a unique position to help patients lose weight and make other healthy lifestyle changes.... Knowing how and when to initiate a conversation about weight management is an important first step to helping patients lose weight and lead healthier lives after a cancer diagnosis" [17]. The statement notes that the teachable moment for behavioral change is not long and, hence, the urgency of oncologist and oncology care team engagement in messaging about weight management while the patient-provider contact is still fresh and frequent in the first few years post primary treatment, albeit not as intense as during active treatment.

To this point, the ASCO Cancer Prevention Committee recently conducted an "ASCO Obesity Survey" among its Health Equity Committee members, asking them "how and when they initiate conversations about weight management, as well as help their patients achieve and maintain healthy weight after a cancer diagnosis". Among the 971 respondents to the survey, awareness and interest in diet, physical activity, and weight management was high, and a majority agreed that addressing high BMI should be part of standard of care [166]. During clinic visits after active treatment, respondents reported they were more likely to ask patients about physical activity (43%) and advise increased physical activity (40.5%) than they were to ask patients about their diet (30%), advise weight loss to their overweight or obese patients (34%), or actively treat or refer patients for weight management (13%) [166].

In a study specific to women with early breast cancer, electronic medical records were reviewed for evidence of oncology clinicians conversations about weight with patients with a BMI of 30 or higher [167]. Charts were reviewed for 237 patients, mean age was 56.5 (range 25–86), and 37% were black women. Thirty-nine percent of these patients had evidence of weight-related interactions with at least one oncology clinician. A majority of these interactions were with medical oncologists (73%) and entailed mostly clinician notes describing weight-related interactions (67%) but also referrals to weight management programs (22%) and providing printed patient instructions about diet/exercise (12%) [167]. In a related study regarding physical activity communications between oncology providers and patients with early stage breast, colon, or prostate cancer, the proportion of medical oncologists having these interactions was 55% [168], again demonstrating greater willingness or ability to discuss exercise rather than weight management.

These and other studies [169, 170] suggest it is feasible for oncology clinicians to have nutrition, physical activity, and weight management communications with their patients, although the precise "when" and "how" deserves further research to ensure that these conversations are patient centered and culturally appropriate [171]. Patients often (but by no means universally) welcome guidance and encouragement from their treating clinician with regard to weight and diet [172–175], exercise [176], and healthy lifestyles [177–180]. But, great care and attention needs to surround these conversations so that they are not hurtful or harmful to women who may have a long history of trying to battle weight gain or may find themselves gaining perplexing amounts of weight despite good nutrition and exercise habits.

Conclusion

In this chapter, we have focused on issues and opportunities for addressing the cancer-obesity connection within the context of care provided by oncology clinicians. This is a timely focus, because there are increasing "calls to action" for oncology clinicians to become more actively involved with advising and encouraging their patients to achieve/maintain healthy weight and regular physical activity as essential strategies for their quality of life, prognosis, and survival [135, 181–186]. To greater and lesser extents, issues and intervention opportunities include surgical oncology and radiation oncology as well as medical oncology. We have also focused on actions that are likely to be the most feasible, such as letting the patient know that healthy weight is important to cancer outcomes and making referrals to specialists who can provide further guidance on exercise and nutrition.

Equally important, but not within the scope of this chapter, is the crucial urgency of lowering cancer risk and adverse outcomes through effective and widespread community-based obesity interventions [107]. To this point, the American Cancer Society has issued guidelines on nutrition and physical activity for cancer prevention, focusing on community action and messaging that is consistent with the American Heart Association and American Diabetes Association [107].

ACS guidelines on nutrition and physical activity for cancer survivors [18]
Achieve and maintain a healthy weight
If overweight or obese, limit consumption of high-calories foods and beverages and increase physical activity to promote weight loss
Engage in regular physical activity
Avoid inactivity and return to normal activity as soon as possible following diagnosis
Aim to exercise at moderate intensity at least 150 minutes per week
Include strength training at least 2 days per week
Achieve a dietary pattern that is high in vegetables, fruits, and whole grains
Follow the American Cancer Society Guidelines on Nutrition and Physical Activity for Cancer Prevention

Special Section: Excess Weight and Breast Cancer Risk

As with other cancers, breast cancer is largely a disease of aging, with 59% of new cases diagnosed in women age 60 or older [64]. As the US population continues to age [187], the USA has also experienced a rise in adult obesity, disproportionately affecting the black community and especially black women [188]. High BMI is an added risk factor for breast cancer, as explained in this section.

The most common tumor subtype is hormone receptor positive/human epidermal growth factor receptor 2 negative (HR+/HER2-), which accounts for 66% of new cases in US women – 69% in Non-Hispanic (NH) white, 55% in NH black, and 61% in Hispanic women [64]. Subtype HR-/HER2- is diagnosed in 10% of new cases (9% white, 19% black, 11% Hispanic); HR+/HER2+ in another 10% (9% white, 10% black, 11% Hispanic) and HR-HER2+ in 4% (4% white, 5% black, 5% Hispanic) [64]. Between 2004 and 2016, the annual increase in HR+ cases was 1.1% in white and Hispanic women; in black women, the rate of increase was 2.8% per year in 2004–2011 but leveled off thereafter [64]. These trends reflect the faster rise in obesity rates among black as compared to white women since the 1980s [188].

In a recent meta-analysis, adult weight gain and greater body adiposity increased the risk for HR+ breast cancer in postmenopausal women who were never users of postmenopausal hormones; this increased risk was not observed for HR- tumors or among current users of hormones [120].

In post-menopausal women, the risk for breast cancer increases for every … [120]	Relative risk (95% confidence interval)
5 kg/m^2 unit of higher BMI	RR 1.12 (1.10, 1.15)
5 kg unit of adult weight gain	RR 1.07 (1.05, 1.09)
Every 5 kg/m^2 gain in BMI	RR 1.17 (1.11, 1.23)
Every 10 cm unit of greater waist circumference	RR 1.11 (1.08, 1.14)
Every 10 cm unit of greater hip circumference	RR 1.06 (1.04, 1.09)
Every 0.1 unit greater waist-to-hip ratio	RR 1.10 (1.05, 1.16)

None of these associations were significant in premenopausal women. For all women (pre- as well as postmenopausal), every 5 kg unit of adult weight gain increased the risk for HR+ breast cancer RR 1.11 (1.06, 1.17) [120]. Other meta-analyses have reported similar associations between 5-unit increases in BMI and breast cancer risk [1, 189].

A recent analysis of women enrolled in the Women's Health Initiative (WHI) underscores the role of body fat, and not just BMI, in breast cancer risk. In a sample of 3460 postmenopausal women age 50–79 with "healthy" BMI of 18.5–24.9 [190], the hazard ratio for invasive breast cancer was 1.89 (1.21, 2.95) for women with the highest whole-body fat and 1.88 (1.18, 2.98) for women with the highest trunk fat mass [190]. This shows that weight and BMI are by no means the only metrics for assessing cancer risk. A combination of breast density and BMI greater than 25 increases the risk for any breast cancer, especially for ER- tumors in premenopausal women [191].

Potential Mechanisms

To understand the association of excess weight and breast cancer, it is important to understand how the combination of diet, nutrition, and physical activity – and hence body fat and weight gain – influence biological processes that in turn impact the development and progression of cancer [192]. High BMI due to an imbalance of high energy intake and low physical activity has been associated with a number of molecular changes that are also linked to cancer development, including altered cytokines/adipokines, chronic inflammation, hyperinsulinemia, and hypercholesterolemia [193]. Adiponectin and leptin have been identified as two of the most important adipokines mediating the link between obesity and breast cancer. While study findings have been mixed, adiponectin appears to be protective against carcinogenesis, and its decreased concentration in obese patients may negatively impact the prevention of tumor development [192]. Conversely, elevated leptin has a well-recognized role in increasing breast cancer risk and is an activator of tumor cell proliferation and progression in molecular pathways [192, 193]. Additionally, adipocytes undergo architectural changes as they grow and multiply, resulting in an unstable microenvironment due to hypoxia from reduced vascularization, which may directly enhance the ability for a cancer cell to grow and proliferate [192].

Obesity also contributes to a state of chronic low-grade inflammation, which can lead to increases in cyclooxygenase-2 (COX-2). COX-2 is overexpressed in invasive breast cancers [194] and can also promote cancer development and progression through increased prostaglandin signaling [195]. Similarly, insulin resistance and hyperinsulinemia are hallmarks of obesity that lead to increased insulin and insulin-like growth factor 1 (IGF-1) signaling, which increases cell survival and proliferation and decreases apoptosis [196]. Breast cancers are known to express both insulin and IGF-1 receptors, which do not appear to be down-regulated in the setting of hyperinsulinemia, and activation of these receptors may directly lead to tumor growth or progression [197]. Furthermore, metformin, an anti-diabetic medication, has shown some promise in mitigating the poorer prognosis of patients with breast cancer and diabetes [198, 199]. Finally, cholesterol is an essential component in cell membrane structure and a required precursor of sex hormones. Increased serum cholesterol levels have been directly linked with risk for hormone-dependent breast cancer [200, 201].

Factors beyond diet, nutrition, and physical activity that may independently contribute to both obesity and breast cancer, such as alcohol consumption [202], complicate the clarification of mechanisms by which obesity directly and indirectly impacts breast cancer risk and prognosis. The relative contributions of these myriad factors during the life course of a woman require further research for a deeper understanding of biological underpinnings of the obesity-breast cancer link.

References

1. World Cancer Research Fund/American Institute for Cancer Research. Continuous update project expert report 2018 – Body fatness and weight gain and the risk of cancer. 2018. dietandcancerreport.org. Accessed 30 Jan 2020.
2. Kyrgiou M, Kalliala I, Markozannes G, et al. Adiposity and cancer at major anatomical sites: umbrella review of the literature. BMJ. 2017;356:j477.

3. Masters GA, Krilov L, Bailey HH, et al. Clinical cancer advances 2015: annual report on progress against cancer from the American Society of Clinical Oncology. J Clin Oncol. 2015;33(7):786–809.
4. World Health Organization. BMI classification. 2016.
5. Islami F, Goding Sauer A, Gapstur SM, Jemal A. Proportion of cancer cases attributable to excess body weight by US State, 2011-2015. JAMA Oncol. 2019;5(3):384–92.
6. World Cancer Research Fund International/American Institute for Cancer Research. Diet, nutrition, physical activity and cancer: a global perspective. 2018. https://www.wcrf.org/dietandcancer/. Accessed 30 Jan 2020.
7. Genkinger JM, Spiegelman D, Anderson KE, et al. A pooled analysis of 14 cohort studies of anthropometric factors and pancreatic cancer risk. Int J Cancer. 2011;129(7):1708–17.
8. Kitahara CM, McCullough ML, Franceschi S, et al. Anthropometric factors and thyroid cancer risk by histological subtype: pooled analysis of 22 prospective studies. Thyroid. 2016;26(2):306–18.
9. Teras LR, Kitahara CM, Birmann BM, et al. Body size and multiple myeloma mortality: a pooled analysis of 20 prospective studies. Br J Haematol. 2014;166(5):667–76.
10. World Cancer Research Fund International/American Institute for Cancer Research. Continuous update project report: diet, nutrition, physical activity and colorectal cancer. 2017. http://www.aicr.org/continuous-update-project/reports/colorectal-cancer-2017-report.pdf. Accessed 30 Jan 2020.
11. Keum N, Greenwood DC, Lee DH, et al. Adult weight gain and adiposity-related cancers: a dose-response meta-analysis of prospective observational studies. J Natl Cancer Inst. 2015;107(2):djv088.
12. Steele CB, Thomas CC, Henley SJ, et al. Vital signs: trends in incidence of cancers associated with overweight and obesity - United States, 2005–2014. MMWR Morb Mortal Wkly Rep. 2017;66(39):1052–8.
13. Hales CM, Carroll MD, Fryar CD, Ogden CL. Prevalence of obesity among adults and youth: United States, 2015-2016. NCHS Data Brief. 2017;(288):1–8.
14. Fryar CD, Carroll MD, Ogden CL. Prevalence of overweight, obesity, and severe obesity among adults aged 20 and over: Unites States, 1960–1962 through 2015–2016: National Center for Health Statistics, 2018.
15. Koroukian SM, Dong W, Berger NA. Changes in age distribution of obesity-associated cancers. JAMA Netw Open. 2019;2(8):e199261.
16. Berger NA. Young adult cancer: influence of the obesity pandemic. Obesity (Silver Spring). 2018;26(4):641–50.
17. Ligibel JA, Alfano CM, Courneya KS, et al. American Society of Clinical Oncology position statement on obesity and cancer. J Clin Oncol. 2014;32(31):3568–74.
18. Rock CL, Doyle C, Demark-Wahnefried W, et al. Nutrition and physical activity guidelines for cancer survivors. CA Cancer J Clin. 2012;62(4):243–74.
19. Dixon JK, Moritz DA, Baker FL. Breast cancer and weight gain: an unexpected finding. Oncol Nurs Forum. 1978;5(3):5–7.
20. Levine EG, Raczynski JM, Carpenter JT. Weight gain with breast cancer adjuvant treatment. Cancer. 1991;67(7):1954–9.
21. Demark-Wahnefried W, Winer EP, Rimer BK. Why women gain weight with adjuvant chemotherapy for breast cancer. J Clin Oncol. 1993;11(7):1418–29.
22. Goodwin PJ, Ennis M, Pritchard KI, McCready D, Koo J, et al. Adjuvant treatment and onset of menopause predict weight gain after breast cancer diagnosis. J Clin Oncol. 1999;17(1):120–9.
23. Rock CL, Flatt SW, Newman V, Caan BJ, Haan MN, et al. Factors associated with weight gain in women after diagnosis of breast cancer. Women's Healthy Eating and Living Study Group. J Am Diet Assoc. 1999;99(10):1212–21.
24. Demark-Wahnefried W, Rimer BK, Winer EP. Weight gain in women diagnosed with breast cancer. J Am Diet Assoc. 1997;97(5):519–26, 29; quiz 27–8.
25. van den Berg MM, Winkels RM, de Kruif JT, et al. Weight change during chemotherapy in breast cancer patients: a meta-analysis. BMC Cancer. 2017;17(1):259.
26. Gross AL, May BJ, Axilbund JE, Armstrong DK, Roden RB, Visvanathan K. Weight change in breast cancer survivors compared to cancer-free women: a prospective study in women at familial risk of breast cancer. Cancer Epidemiol Biomarkers Prev. 2015;24(8):1262–9.
27. Campbell KL, Lane K, Martin AD, Gelmon KA, McKenzie DC. Resting energy expenditure and body mass changes in women during adjuvant chemotherapy for breast cancer. Cancer Nurs. 2007;30(2):95–100.
28. Freedman RJ, Aziz N, Albanes D, Hartman T, Danforth D, et al. Weight and body composition changes during and after adjuvant chemotherapy in women with breast cancer. J Clin Endocrinol Metab. 2004;89(5):2248–53.
29. Gordon AM, Hurwitz S, Shapiro CL, LeBoff MS. Premature ovarian failure and body composition changes with adjuvant chemotherapy for breast cancer. Menopause. 2011;18(11):1244–8.
30. Harvie M, Campbell IT, Baildam A, Howell A. Energy balance in early breast cancer patients receiving adjuvant chemotherapy. Breast Cancer Res Treat. 2004;83(3):201–10.
31. Vance V, Mourtzakis M, McCargar L, Hanning R. Weight gain in breast cancer survivors: prevalence, pattern and health consequences. Obes Rev. 2011;12(4):282–94.

32. Nyrop KA, Deal AM, Shachar SS, et al. Weight trajectories in women receiving systemic adjuvant therapy for breast cancer. Breast Cancer Res Treat. 2020;179(3):709–20.
33. Ingram C, Brown JK. Patterns of weight and body composition in premenopausal women with early stage breast cancer: has weight gain been overestimated? Cancer Nurs. 2004;27(6):483–90.
34. Raghavendra A, Sinha AK, Valle-Goffin J, Shen Y, Tripathy D, Barcenas CH. Determinants of weight gain during adjuvant endocrine therapy and association of such weight gain with recurrence in long-term breast cancer survivors. Clin Breast Cancer. 2018;18(1):e7–e13.
35. Reddy SM, Sadim M, Li J, et al. Clinical and genetic predictors of weight gain in patients diagnosed with breast cancer. Br J Cancer. 2013;109(4):872–81.
36. Kumar N, Allen KA, Riccardi D, et al. Fatigue, weight gain, lethargy and amenorrhea in breast cancer patients on chemotherapy: is subclinical hypothyroidism the culprit? Breast Cancer Res Treat. 2004;83(2):149–59.
37. Thivat E, Therondel S, Lapirot O, Abrial C, Gimbergues P, et al. Weight change during chemotherapy changes the prognosis in non-metastatic breast cancer for the worse. BMC Cancer. 2010;10(648):1–9.
38. Bradshaw PT, Ibrahim JG, Stevens J, Cleveland RJ, Abrahamson PE, et al. Postdiagnosis change in bodyweight and survival after breast cancer diagnosis. Epidemiology. 2012;23(2):320–7.
39. Tredan O, Bajard A, Meunier A, Roux P, Fiorletta I, et al. Body weight change in women receiving adjuvant chemotherapy for breast cancer: a French prospective study. Clin Nutr. 2010;29(2):187–91.
40. Makari-Judson G, Judson CH, Mertens WC. Longitudinal patterns of weight gain after breast cancer diagnosis: observations beyond the first year. Breast. 2007;13(3):258–65.
41. Nyrop KA, Williams GR, Muss HB, Shachar SS. Weight gain during adjuvant endocrine treatment for early-stage breast cancer: what is the evidence? Breast Cancer Res Treat. 2016;158(2):203–17.
42. Sedjo RL, Byers T, Ganz PA, et al. Weight gain prior to entry into a weight-loss intervention study among overweight and obese breast cancer survivors. J Cancer Surviv. 2014;8(3):410–8.
43. Nyrop KA, Deal AM, Lee JT, et al. Weight changes in postmenopausal breast cancer survivors over 2 years of endocrine therapy: a retrospective chart review. Breast Cancer Res Treat. 2017;162(2):375–88.
44. Nyrop KA, Deal AM, Lee JT, et al. Weight gain in hormone receptor-positive (HR+) early-stage breast cancer: is it menopause or something else. Breast Cancer Res Treat. 2018;167(1):235–48.
45. Befort CA, Austin H, Klemp JR. Weight control needs and experiences among rural breast cancer survivors. Psychooncology. 2011;20(10):1069–75.
46. Irwin ML, McTiernan A, Baumgartner RN, Bernstein L, Gilliland FD, Ballard-Barbash R. Changes in body fat and weight after a breast cancer diagnosis: influence of demographic, prognostic, and lifestyle factors. J Clin Oncol. 2005;23(4):774–82.
47. Saquib N, Flatt SW, Natarajan L, Thomson CA, Bardwell WA, et al. Weight gain and recovery of pre-cancer weight after breast cancer treatments: evidence from the Women's healthy Eating and Living (WHEL) study. Breast Cancer Res Treat. 2007;105(2):177–86.
48. Heideman WH, Russell NS, Gundy C, Rookus MA, Voskuil DW. The frequency, magnitude and timing of post-diagnosis body weight gain in Dutch breast cancer survivors. Eur J Cancer. 2009;45:119–26.
49. Sadim M, Xu Y, Selig K, et al. A prospective evaluation of clinical and genetic predictors of weight changes in breast cancer survivors. Cancer. 2017;123(13):2413–21. https://doi.org/10.1002/cncr.30628. Epub 2017 Feb 14. PMID: 28195643.
50. Nyrop KA, Deal AM, Shachar SS, et al. Patient-reported toxicities during chemotherapy regimens in current clinical practice for early breast cancer. Oncologist. 2019;24(6):762–71.
51. Schmidt ME, Chang-Claude J, Vrieling A, Heinz J, Flesch-Janys D, Steindorf K. Fatigue and quality of life in breast cancer survivors: temporal courses and long-term pattern. J Cancer Surviv. 2012;6(1):11–9.
52. Mason C, Alfano CM, Smith AW, et al. Long-term physical activity trends in breast cancer survivors. Cancer Epidemiol Biomarkers Prev. 2013;22(6):1153–61.
53. Hair BY, Hayes S, Tse CK, Bell MB, Olshan AF. Racial differences in physical activity among breast cancer survivors: implications for breast cancer care. Cancer. 2014;120(14):2174–82.
54. American Cancer Society. Breast cancer facts & figures 2017–2018. Atlanta: American Cancer Society Inc.; 2017.
55. DeSantis CE, Ma J, Gaudet MM, et al. Breast cancer statistics, 2019. Cancer. 2019;69(6):438–51.
56. Niraula S, Ocana A, Ennis M, Goodwin PJ. Body size and breast cancer prognosis in relation to hormone receptor and menopausal status: a meta-analysis. Breast Cancer Res Treat. 2012;134(2):769–81.
57. Playdon MC, Bracken MB, Sanft TB, Ligibel JA, Harrigan M, Irwin ML. Weight gain after breast cancer diagnosis and all-cause mortality: systematic review and meta-analysis. J Natl Cancer Inst. 2015;107(12):djv275.
58. Derks MGM, van de Velde CJH, Giardiello D, et al. Impact of comorbidities and age on cause-specific mortality in postmenopausal patients with breast cancer. Oncologist. 2019;24(7):e467–e74.
59. Patnaik J, Byers T, Diguiseppi C, Denberg T, Dabelea D. The influence of comorbidities on overall survival among older women diagnosed with breast cancer. J Natl Cancer Inst. 2011;103(14):1101–11.
60. Kim A, Scharf K, Senthil M, Solomon N, Garberoglio C, Lum SS. The prevalence of overweight and obesity in a breast clinic population:

consideration for weight loss as a therapeutic intervention. Surg Obes Relat Dis. 2014;10(2):348–53.
61. Hong CC, Ambrosone CB, Goodwin PJ. Comorbidities and their management: potential impact on breast cancer outcomes. Adv Exp Med Biol. 2015;862:155–75.
62. Wasif N, Neville M, Gray R, Cronin P, Pockaj BA. Competing risk of death in elderly patients with newly diagnosed stage I breast cancer. J Am Coll Surg. 2019;229(1):30–36.e1.
63. DeSantis CE, Miller KD, Goding Sauer A, Jemal A, Siegel RL. Cancer statistics for African Americans, 2019. Cancer. 2019;69(3):211–33.
64. DeSantis CE, Ma J. Breast cancer statistics, 2019. 2019.
65. Daly B, Olopade OI. A perfect storm: how tumor biology, genomics, and health care delivery patterns collide to create a racial survival disparity in breast cancer and proposed interventions for change. CA Cancer J Clin. 2015;65(3):221–38.
66. Hales CM, Fryar CD, Carroll MD, Freedman DS, Ogden CL. Trends in obesity and severe obesity prevalence in US youth and adults by sex and age, 2007-2008 to 2015-2016. JAMA. 2018;319(16):1723–5.
67. DeSantis CE, Fedewa SA, Goding Sauer A, Kramer JL, Smith RA, Jemal A. Breast cancer statistics, 2015: convergence of incidence rates between black and white women. CA Cancer J Clin. 2016;66(1):31–42.
68. Tammemagi CM, Nerenz D, Neslund-Dudas C, Feldkamp C, Nathanson D. Comorbidity and survival disparities among black and white patients with breast cancer. JAMA. 2005;2005:1765–72.
69. Braithwaite D, Tammemagi CM, Moore DH, et al. Hypertension is an independent predictor of survival disparity between African-American and white breast cancer patients. Int J Cancer. 2009;124(5):1213–9.
70. Troeschel AN, Liu Y, Collin LJ, et al. Race differences in cardiovascular disease and breast cancer mortality among US women diagnosed with invasive breast cancer. Int J Epidemiol. 2019;48(6):1897–905.
71. Chan DS, Vieira AR, Aune D, et al. Body mass index and survival in women with breast cancer-systematic literature review and meta-analysis of 82 follow-up studies. Ann Oncol. 2014;25(10):1901–14.
72. Druesne-Pecollo N, Touvier M, Barrandon E, et al. Excess body weight and second primary cancer risk after breast cancer: a systematic review and meta-analysis of prospective studies. Breast Cancer Res Treat. 2012;135(3):647–54.
73. Nechuta S, Chen WY, Cai H, et al. A pooled analysis of post-diagnosis lifestyle factors in association with late estrogen-receptor-positive breast cancer prognosis. Int J Cancer. 2016;138(9):2088–97.
74. Jung AY, Hüsing A, Behrens S, et al. Postdiagnosis weight change is associated with poorer survival in breast cancer survivors: a prospective population-based patient cohort study. Int J Cancer. 2021;148(1):18–27.
75. Aleixo GFP, Williams GR, Nyrop KA, Muss HB, Shachar SS. Muscle composition and outcomes in patients with breast cancer: meta-analysis and systematic review. Breast Cancer Res Treat. 2019;177(3):569–79.
76. Rossi F, Valdora F, Bignotti B, Torri L, Succio G, Tagliafico AS. Evaluation of body Computed Tomography-determined sarcopenia in breast cancer patients and clinical outcomes: a systematic review. Cancer Treat Res Commun. 2019;21:100154.
77. Shachar SS, Deal AM, Weinberg M, et al. Body composition as a predictor of toxicity in patients receiving anthracycline and taxane based chemotherapy for early stage breast cancer. Clin Cancer Res. 2017;23(14):3537–43.
78. Bradshaw PT, Cespedes Feliciano EM, Prado CM, et al. Adipose tissue distribution and survival among women with nonmetastatic breast cancer. Obesity (Silver Spring). 2019;27(6):997–1004.
79. Caan BJ, Cespedes Feliciano EM, Prado CM, et al. Association of muscle and adiposity measured by computed tomography with survival in patients with nonmetastatic breast cancer. JAMA Oncol. 2018;4(6):798–804.
80. Cespedes Feliciano EM, Chen WY, Lee V, et al. Body composition, adherence to anthracycline and taxane-based chemotherapy, and survival after nonmetastatic breast cancer. JAMA Oncol. 2020;6(2):264–70.
81. Sedjo RL, Hines LM, Byers T, et al. Long-term weight gain among Hispanic and non-Hispanic White women with and without breast cancer. Nutr Cancer. 2013;65(1):34–42.
82. Davis SR, Castelo-Branco C, Chedraui P, et al. Understanding weight gain at menopause. Climacteric. 2012;15(5):419–29.
83. Jung SY, Vitolins MZ, Fenton J, Frazier-Wood AC, Hursting SD, Chang S. Risk profiles for weight gain among postmenopausal women: a classification and regression tree analysis approach. PLoS One. 2015;10(3):e0121430.
84. Rabin C. Promoting lifestyle change among cancer survivors: when is the teachable moment? Am J Lifestyle Med. 2009;3:369.
85. Demark-Wahnefried W, Aziz NM, Rowland JH, Pinto BM. Riding the crest of the teachable moment: promoting long-term health after the diagnosis of cancer. J Clin Oncol. 2005;23(24):5814–30.
86. Anderson AS, Mackison D, Boath C, Steele R. Promoting changes in diet and physical activity in breast and colorectal cancer screening settings: an unexplored opportunity for endorsing healthy behaviors. Cancer Prev Res (Phila). 2013;6(3):165–72.
87. Cohen SS, Matthews CE, Bradshaw PT, et al. Sedentary behavior, physical activity, and likelihood of breast cancer among Black and White women: a report from the Southern Community Cohort Study. Cancer Prev Res (Phila). 2013;6(6):566–76.
88. Thomson ZO, Reeves MM. Can weight gain be prevented in women receiving treatment for breast cancer? A systematic review of intervention studies. Obes Rev. 2017;18(11):1364–73.

89. Chaudhry ZW, Brown RV, Fawole OA, et al. Comparative effectiveness of strategies to prevent weight gain among women with and at risk for breast cancer: a systematic review. Springerplus. 2013;2(1):277.
90. Playdon M, Thomas G, Sanft T, Harrigan M, Ligibel J, Irwin M. Weight loss intervention for breast cancer survivors: a systematic review. Curr Breast Cancer Rep. 2013;5(3):222–46.
91. Reeves MM, Terranova CO, Eakin EG, Demark-Wahnefried W. Weight loss intervention trials in women with breast cancer: a systematic review. Obes Rev. 2014;15(9):749–68.
92. Chlebowski RT, Reeves MM. Weight loss randomized intervention trials in female cancer survivors. J Clin Oncol. 2016;34(35):4238–48.
93. Djuric Z, Mirasolo J, Kimbrough L, et al. A pilot trial of spirituality counseling for weight loss maintenance in African American breast cancer survivors. J Natl Med Assoc. 2009;101(6):552–64.
94. Ferrante JM, Devine KA, Bator A, et al. Feasibility and potential efficacy of commercial mHealth/eHealth tools for weight loss in African American breast cancer survivors: pilot randomized controlled trial. Transl Behav Med. 2020;10(4):938–48.
95. Sheppard VB, Hicks J, Makambi K, Hurtado-de-Mendoza A, Demark-Wahnefried W, Adams-Campbell L. The feasibility and acceptability of a diet and exercise trial in overweight and obese black breast cancer survivors: the Stepping STONE study. Contemp Clin Trials. 2016;46:106–13.
96. Scott E, Daley AJ, Doll H, et al. Effects of an exercise and hypocaloric healthy eating program on biomarkers associated with long-term prognosis after early-stage breast cancer: a randomized controlled trial. Cancer Causes Control. 2013;24(1):181–91.
97. Harris MN, Swift DL, Myers VH, et al. Cancer survival through lifestyle change (CASTLE): a pilot study of weight loss. Int J Behav Med. 2013;20(3):403–12.
98. Greenlee HA, Crew KD, Mata JM, et al. A pilot randomized controlled trial of a commercial diet and exercise weight loss program in minority breast cancer survivors. Obesity (Silver Spring). 2013;21(1):65–76.
99. Thomson CA, Stopeck AT, Bea JW, et al. Changes in body weight and metabolic indexes in overweight breast cancer survivors enrolled in a randomized trial of low-fat vs. reduced carbohydrate diets. Nutr Cancer. 2010;62(8):1142–52.
100. Mefferd K, Nichols JF, Pakiz B, Rock CL. A cognitive behavioral therapy intervention to promote weight loss improves body composition and blood lipid profiles among overweight breast cancer survivors. Breast Cancer Res Treat. 2007;104(2):145–52.
101. Djuric Z, DiLaura NM, Jenkins I, et al. Combining weight-loss counseling with the weight watchers plan for obese breast cancer survivors. Obes Res. 2002;10(7):657–65.
102. Spark LC, Reeves MM, Fjeldsoe BS, Eakin EG. Physical activity and/or dietary interventions in breast cancer survivors: a systematic review of the maintenance of outcomes. J Cancer Surviv. 2013;7(1):74–82.
103. Befort CA, Klemp JR, Sullivan DK, et al. Weight loss maintenance strategies among rural breast cancer survivors: the rural women connecting for better health trial. Obesity (Silver Spring). 2016;24(10):2070–7.
104. Blatt AD, Roe LS, Rolls BJ. Hidden vegetables: an effective strategy to reduce energy intake and increase vegetable intake in adults. Am J Clin Nutr. 2011;93(4):756–63.
105. Rolls BJ, Drewnowski A, Ledikwe JH. Changing the energy density of the diet as a strategy for weight management. J Am Diet Assoc. 2005;105(5 Suppl 1):S98–103.
106. U.S. Department of Health and Human Services and U.S. Department of Agriculture. 2015–2020 Dietary Guidelines for Americans – 8th Edition. 2015. https://health.gov/our-work/food-nutrition/2015-2020-dietary-guidelines/guidelines/. Accessed 18 Feb 2020.
107. Kushi LH, Doyle C, McCullough M, et al. American Cancer Society guidelines on nutrition and physical activity for cancer prevention: reducing the risk of cancer with healthy food choices and physical activity. CA Cancer J Clin. 2012;62(1):30–67.
108. Jeurnink SM, Buchner FL, Bueno-de-Mesquita HB, et al. Variety in vegetable and fruit consumption and the risk of gastric and esophageal cancer in the European Prospective Investigation into Cancer and Nutrition. Int J Cancer. 2012;131(6):E963–73.
109. Liu RH. Potential synergy of phytochemicals in cancer prevention: mechanism of action. J Nutr. 2004;134(12 Suppl):3479s–85s.
110. Aune D, Chan DS, Greenwood DC, et al. Dietary fiber and breast cancer risk: a systematic review and meta-analysis of prospective studies. Ann Oncol. 2012;23(6):1394–402.
111. World Cancer Research Fund International. Continuous Update Project: diet, nutrition, physical activity and breast cancer survivors. 2014. http://www.wcrf.org/int/research-we-fund/continuous-update-project-findings-reports/breast-cancer-survivors. Accessed 28 Jun 2016.
112. Mozaffarian D, Hao T, Rimm EB, Willett WC, Hu FB. Changes in diet and lifestyle and long-term weight gain in women and men. N Engl J Med. 2011;364(25):2392–404.
113. Zeng L, Ruan M, Liu J, et al. Trends in processed meat, unprocessed red meat, poultry, and fish consumption in the United States, 1999–2016. J Acad Nutr Diet. 2019;119(7):1085–98.e12.
114. Champ CE, Volek JS, Siglin J, Jin L, Simone NL. Weight gain, metabolic syndrome, and breast cancer recurrence: are dietary recommendations supported by the data? Int J Breast Cancer. 2012;2012:506868.

115. Flood JE, Roe LS, Rolls BJ. The effect of increased beverage portion size on energy intake at a meal. J Am Diet Assoc. 2006;106(12):1984–90; discussion 90–1.
116. Pan A, Hu FB. Effects of carbohydrates on satiety: differences between liquid and solid food. Curr Opin Clin Nutr Metab Care. 2011;14(4):385–90.
117. Allen NE, Beral V, Casabonne D, et al. Moderate alcohol intake and cancer incidence in women. J Natl Cancer Inst. 2009;101(5):296–305.
118. Kwan ML, Kushi LH, Weltzien E, et al. Alcohol consumption and breast cancer recurrence and survival among women with early-stage breast cancer: the life after cancer epidemiology study. J Clin Oncol. 2010;28(29):4410–6.
119. Mayne ST, Ferrucci LM, Cartmel B. Lessons learned from randomized clinical trials of micronutrient supplementation for cancer prevention. Annu Rev Nutr. 2012;32:369–90.
120. Chan DSM, Abar L, Cariolou M, et al. World Cancer Research Fund International: Continuous Update Project-systematic literature review and meta-analysis of observational cohort studies on physical activity, sedentary behavior, adiposity, and weight change and breast cancer risk. Cancer Causes Control. 2019;30(11):1183–200.
121. Chen X, Wang Q, Zhang Y, Xie Q, Tan X. Physical activity and risk of breast cancer: a meta-analysis of 38 cohort studies in 45 study reports. Value Health. 2019;22(1):104–28.
122. Ballard-Barbash R, Friedenreich CM, Courneya KS, Siddiqi SM, McTiernan A, Alfano CM. Physical activity, biomarkers, and disease outcomes in cancer survivors: a systematic review. J Natl Cancer Inst. 2012;104:815–40.
123. Ibrahim EM, Al-Homaidh A. Physical activity and survival after breast cancer diagnosis: meta-analysis of published studies. Med Oncol. 2011;28(3):753–65.
124. Lahart IM, Metsios GS, Nevill AM, Carmichael AR. Physical activity, risk of death and recurrence in breast cancer survivors: a systematic review and meta-analysis of epidemiological studies. Acta Oncol. 2015;54(5):635–54.
125. Zhong S, Jiang T, Ma T, et al. Association between physical activity and mortality in breast cancer: a meta-analysis of cohort studies. Eur J Epidemiol. 2014;29(6):391–404.
126. Battaglini CL, Mills RC, Phillips BL, et al. Twenty-five years of research on the effects of exercise training in breast cancer survivors: a systematic review of the literature. World J Clin Oncol. 2014;5(2):177–90.
127. Casla S, Lopez-Tarruella S, Jerez Y, et al. Supervised physical exercise improves VO2max, quality of life, and health in early stage breast cancer patients: a randomized controlled trial. Breast Cancer Res Treat. 2015;153(2):371–82.
128. Kirkham AA, Bland KA, Sayyari S, Campbell KL, Davis MK. Clinically relevant physical benefits of exercise interventions in breast cancer survivors. Curr Oncol Rep. 2016;18(2):12.
129. Markes M, Brockow T, Resch KL. Exercise for women receiving adjuvant therapy for breast cancer. Cochrane Database Syst Rev. 2006;18(4):CD005001.
130. Schmitz KH, Courneya KS, Matthews C, Demark-Wahnefried W, Galvao DA, et al. American College of Sports Medicine roundtable on exercise guidelines for cancer survivors. Med Sci Sports Exerc. 2010;42(7):1409–26.
131. Godoy-Izquierdo D, Guevara NML, Toral MV, Galvan CT, Ballesteros AS, Garcia JFG. Improvements in health-related quality of life, cardio-metabolic health, and fitness in postmenopausal women after a supervised, multicomponent, adapted exercise program in a suited health promotion intervention: a multigroup study. Menopause. 2017;24(8):938–46.
132. Zhang X, Li Y, Liu D. Effects of exercise on the quality of life in breast cancer patients: a systematic review of randomized controlled trials. Support Care Cancer. 2019;27(1):9–21.
133. Furmaniak AC, Menig M, Markes MH. Exercise for women receiving adjuvant therapy for breast cancer. Cochrane Database Syst Rev. 2016;9:Cd005001.
134. Lee J. Effects of exercise interventions on breast cancer patients during adjuvant therapy: a systematic review and meta-analysis of randomized controlled trials. Cancer Nurs. 2018;43(2):115–25.
135. Schmitz KH, Campbell AM. Exercise is medicine in oncology: Engaging clinicians to help patients move through cancer. CA Cancer J Clin. 2019;69(6):468–84.
136. Campbell KL, Winters-Stone KM, Wiskemann J, et al. Exercise guidelines for cancer survivors: consensus statement from international multidisciplinary roundtable. Med Sci Sports Exerc. 2019;51(11):2375–90.
137. Nyrop KA, Deal AM, Choi SK, et al. Measuring and understanding adherence in a home-based exercise intervention during chemotherapy for early breast cancer. Breast Cancer Res Treat. 2018;168(1):43–55.
138. Hanson ED, Wagoner CW, Anderson T, Battaglini CL. The independent effects of strength training in cancer survivors: a systematic review. Curr Oncol Rep. 2016;18(5):31.
139. Courneya KS, Mackey JR, Bell GJ, Jones LW, Field CJ, Fairey AS. Randomized controlled trial of exercise training in postmenopausal breast cancer survivors: cardiopulmonary and quality of life outcomes. J Clin Oncol. 2003;21:1660–8.
140. Courneya KS, Segal RJ, Mackey JR, et al. Effects of aerobic and resistance exercise in breast cancer patients receiving adjuvant chemotherapy: a multicenter randomized controlled trial. J Clin Oncol. 2007;25(28):4396–404.
141. Courneya KS, McKenzie DC, Mackey JR, et al. Effects of exercise dose and type during breast cancer chemotherapy: multicenter randomized trial. J Natl Cancer Inst. 2013;105(23):1821–32.

142. McNeely ML, Campbell KL, Rowe BH, Klassen TP, Mackey JR, Courneya KS. Effects of exercise on breast cancer patients and survivors: a systematic review and meta-analysis. CMAJ. 2006;175(1):34–41.
143. van Waart H, Stuiver MM, van Harten WH, et al. Effect of low-intensity physical activity and moderate- to high-intensity physical exercise during adjuvant chemotherapy on physical fitness, fatigue, and chemotherapy completion rates: results of the PACES randomized clinical trial. J Clin Oncol. 2015;33(17):1918–27.
144. Kirkham AA, Bonsignore A, Bland KA, et al. Exercise prescription and adherence for breast cancer: one size does not FITT all. Med Sci Sports Exerc. 2018;50(2):177–86.
145. Lakoski SG, Eves ND, Douglas PS, Jones LW. Exercise rehabilitation in patients with cancer. Nat Rev Clin Oncol. 2012;9(5):288–96.
146. Sasso JP, Eves ND, Christensen JF, Koelwyn GJ, Scott J, Jones LW. A framework for prescription in exercise-oncology research. J Cachexia Sarcopenia Muscle. 2015;6(2):115–24.
147. Nelson NL. Breast cancer-related lymphedema and resistance exercise: a systematic review. J Strength Cond Res. 2016;30(9):2656–65.
148. Coughlin SS, Caplan LS, Williams V. Home-based physical activity interventions for breast cancer patients receiving primary therapy: a systematic review. Breast Cancer Res Treat. 2019;178(3):513–22.
149. Covington KR, Hidde MC, Pergolotti M, Leach HJ. Community-based exercise programs for cancer survivors: a scoping review of practice-based evidence. Support Care Cancer. 2019;27(12):4435–50.
150. Courneya KS, Rogers LQ, Campbell KL, Vallance JK, Friedenreich CM. Top 10 research questions related to physical activity and cancer survivorship. Res Q Exerc Sport. 2015;86(2):107–16.
151. van der Leeden M, Huijsmans RJ, Geleijn E, et al. Tailoring exercise interventions to comorbidities and treatment-induced adverse effects in patients with early stage breast cancer undergoing chemotherapy: a framework to support clinical decisions. Disabil Rehabil. 2018;40(4):486–96.
152. Burhenn PS, Bryant AL, Mustian KM. Exercise promotion in geriatric oncology. Curr Oncol Rep. 2016;18(9):58.
153. Doyle C, Kushi LH, Byers T, Courneya KS, et al. Nutrition and physical activity during and after cancer treatment: an American Cancer Society guide for informed choices. CA Cancer J Clin. 2006;56:323–53.
154. Denlinger CS, Ligibel JA, Are M, et al. Survivorship: nutrition and weight management, Version 2.2014. Clinical practice guidelines in oncology. J Natl Compr Cancer Netw. 2014;12(10):1396–406.
155. Anderson AS, Key TJ, Norat T, et al. European code against cancer 4th edition: obesity, body fatness and cancer. Cancer Epidemiol. 2015;39 Suppl 1:S34–45.
156. Lauby-Secretan B, Scoccianti C, Loomis D, Grosse Y, Bianchini F, Straif K. Body fatness and cancer – viewpoint of the IARC Working Group. N Engl J Med. 2016;375(8):794–8.
157. Ligibel JA, Wollins D. American Society of Clinical Oncology obesity initiative: rationale, progress, and future directions. J Clin Oncol. 2016;34(35):4256–60.
158. Ligibel JA, Alfano CM, Hershman D, et al. Recommendations for obesity clinical trials in cancer survivors: American Society of Clinical Oncology statement. J Clin Oncol. 2015;33(33):3961–7.
159. American Society for Clinical Oncology. Obesity and cancer: a guide for oncology providers. 2014. https://www.asco.org/sites/new-www.asco.org/files/content-files/blog-release/documents/obesity-provider-guide.pdf.
160. Managing your weight after a cancer diagnosis. Alexandria: American Society of Clinical Oncology; 2014.
161. Ferrante JM, Seaman K, Bator A, et al. Impact of perceived weight stigma among underserved women on doctor-patient relationships. Obes Sci Pract. 2016;2(2):128–35.
162. Pearl RL, Walton K, Allison KC, Tronieri JS, Wadden TA. Preference for people-first language among patients seeking bariatric surgery. JAMA Surg. 2018;153(12):1160–2.
163. Volger S, Vetter ML, Dougherty M, et al. Patients' preferred terms for describing their excess weight: discussing obesity in clinical practice. Obesity (Silver Spring). 2012;20(1):147–50.
164. Swift JA, Choi E, Puhl RM, Glazebrook C. Talking about obesity with clients: preferred terms and communication styles of U.K. pre-registration dieticians, doctors, and nurses. Patient Educ Couns. 2013;91(2):186–91.
165. Fong AJ, Faulkner G, Jones JM, Sabiston CM. A qualitative analysis of oncology clinicians' perceptions and barriers for physical activity counseling in breast cancer survivors. Support Care Cancer. 2018;26(9):3117–26.
166. Ligibel JA, Jones LW, Brewster AM, et al. Oncologists' attitudes and practice of addressing diet, physical activity, and weight management with patients with cancer: findings of an ASCO survey of the oncology workforce. J Oncol Pract. 2019;15(6):e520–8. Jop1900124.
167. Nyrop KA, Lee JT, Deal AM, Choi SK, Muss HB. Weight-related communications between oncology clinicians and women with obesity at early breast cancer diagnosis: findings from a review of the electronic health record. Nutr Cancer. 2020;72(4):576–83.
168. Nyrop KA, Deal AM, Williams GR, Guerard EJ, Pergolotti M, Muss HB. Physical activity communication between oncology providers and patients with early-stage breast, colon, or prostate cancer. Cancer. 2016;122(3):470–6.

169. Halilova KI, Pisu M. Healthy lifestyle discussions between healthcare providers and older cancer survivors: data from 12 cancer centers in the Southeastern United States. Cancer Med. 2019;8(16):7123–32.
170. Kirkham AA, Van Patten CL, Gelmon KA, et al. Effectiveness of oncologist-referred exercise and healthy eating programming as a part of supportive adjuvant care for early breast cancer. Oncologist. 2018;23(1):105–15.
171. Smith KC, Coa KI, Klassen AC. A qualitative study of dietary discussions as an emerging task for cancer clinicians. SAGE Open Med. 2016;4:2050312116665935.
172. Beeken RJ, Williams K, Wardle J, Croker H. "What about diet?" A qualitative study of cancer survivors' views on diet and cancer and their sources of information. Eur J Cancer Care. 2016;25(5):774–83.
173. Clark LH, Ko EM, Kernodle A, et al. Endometrial cancer survivors' perceptions of provider obesity counseling and attempted behavior change: are we seizing the moment? Int J Gynecol Cancer. 2016;26(2):318–24.
174. Tseng JH, Roche KL, Jernigan AM, Salani R, Bristow RE, Fader AN. Lifestyle and weight management counseling in uterine cancer survivors: a study of the uterine cancer action network. Int J Gynecol Cancer. 2015;25(7):1285–91.
175. Zhang FF, Meagher S, Koch-Weser S, et al. Weight management: perception, interest, and preferences in adult cancer survivors. Clin J Oncol Nurs. 2017;21(1):65–71.
176. Smith L, Croker H, Fisher A, Williams K, Wardle J, Beeken RJ. Cancer survivors' attitudes towards and knowledge of physical activity, sources of information, and barriers and facilitators of engagement: a qualitative study. Eur J Cancer Care. 2017;26(4).
177. Demark-Wahnefried W, Peterson B, McBride C, Lipkus I, Clipp E. Current health behaviors and readiness to pursue life-style changes among men and women diagnosed with early stage prostate and breast carcinomas. Cancer. 2000;88(3):674–84.
178. Fisher BA, Wilkinson L, Valencia A. Women's interest in a personal breast cancer risk assessment and lifestyle advice at NHS mammography screening. J Public Health (Oxf). 2017;39(1):113–21.
179. Sutton E, Hackshaw-McGeagh LE, Aning J, et al. The provision of dietary and physical activity advice for men diagnosed with prostate cancer: a qualitative study of the experiences and views of health care professionals, patients and partners. Cancer Causes Control. 2017;28(4):319–29.
180. Zaleta AK, Neff R, McCann GA, O'Malley DM, Carpenter KM. Perceptions of weight management counseling among gynecologic cancer survivors: opportunities for enhancing survivorship care. Support Care Cancer. 2017;25(5):1537–45.
181. Goodwin PJ. Obesity and breast cancer outcomes: how much evidence is needed to change practice? J Clin Oncol. 2016;34(7):646–8.
182. Massetti GM, Dietz WH, Richardson LC. Excessive weight gain, obesity, and cancer: opportunities for clinical intervention. JAMA. 2017;318(20):1975–6.
183. Frazelle ML, Friend PJ. Optimizing the teachable moment for health promotion for cancer survivors and their families. J Adv Pract Oncol. 2016;7(4):422–33.
184. Hardcastle SJ, Cohen PA. Effective physical activity promotion to survivors of cancer is likely to be home based and to require oncologist participation. J Clin Oncol. 2017;35(32):3635–7.
185. Brown JC, Ligibel JA. Putting exercise into oncology practice: state-of-the-science, innovation, and future directions. Cancer J. 2019;25(5):316–9.
186. Demark-Wahnefried W, Rogers LQ, Alfano CM, et al. Practical clinical interventions for diet, physical activity, and weight control in cancer survivors. CA Cancer J Clin. 2015;65(3):167–89.
187. United States Census Bureau. U.S. Census Bureau projections show a slower growing, older, more diverse nation a half century from now. 2012. http://www.census.gov/newsroom/releases/archives/population/cb12-243.html. Accessed 01/10/2014.
188. Jackson CL, Szklo M, Yeh HC, et al. Black-white disparities in overweight and obesity trends by educational attainment in the United States, 1997-2008. J Obes. 2013;2013:140743.
189. Liu K, Zhang W, Dai Z, et al. Association between body mass index and breast cancer risk: evidence based on a dose-response meta-analysis. Cancer Manag Res. 2018;10:143–51.
190. Iyengar NM, Arthur R, Manson JE, et al. Association of body fat and risk of breast cancer in postmenopausal women with normal body mass index: a secondary analysis of a randomized clinical trial and observational study. JAMA Oncol. 2019;5(2):155–63.
191. Shieh Y, Scott CG, Jensen MR, et al. Body mass index, mammographic density, and breast cancer risk by estrogen receptor subtype. Breast Cancer Res. 2019;21(1):48.
192. Ando S, Gelsomino L, Panza S, et al. Obesity, leptin and breast cancer: epidemiological evidence and proposed mechanisms. Cancers (Basel). 2019;11(1):62.
193. Niu J, Jiang L, Guo W, Shao L, Liu Y, Wang L. The association between leptin level and breast cancer: a meta-analysis. PLoS One. 2013;8(6):e67349.
194. Subbaramaiah K, Norton L, Gerald W, Dannenberg AJ. Cyclooxygenase-2 is overexpressed in HER-2/neu-positive breast cancer: evidence for involvement of AP-1 and PEA3. J Biol Chem. 2002;277(21):18649–57.
195. Subbaramaiah K, Morris PG, Zhou XK, et al. Increased levels of COX-2 and prostaglandin E2 contribute to elevated aromatase expression in inflamed breast tissue of obese women. Cancer Discov. 2012;2(4):356–65.
196. Lega IC, Lipscombe LL. Review: diabetes, obesity, and cancer – pathophysiology and clinical implications. Endocr Rev. 2020;41(1):1–20.

197. Hursting SD, Smith SM, Lashinger LM, Harvey AE, Perkins SN. Calories and carcinogenesis: lessons learned from 30 years of calorie restriction research. Carcinogenesis. 2010;31(1):83–9.
198. Allott EH, Hursting SD. Obesity and cancer: mechanistic insights from transdisciplinary studies. Endocr Relat Cancer. 2015;22(6):R365–86.
199. Sonnenblick A, Agbor-Rah D, Bradbury I, Di Cosima S, Azim HA. Impact of diabetes, insulin, and metformin use on the outcome of patients with human epidermal growth factor receptor-2 positive primary breast cancer: analysis from the ALTTO PHase III randomized trial. J Clin Oncol. 2017;35(13):1421–9.
200. Fagherazzi G, Fabre A, Boutron-Ruault MC, Clavel-Chapelon F. Serum cholesterol level, use of a cholesterol-lowering drug, and breast cancer: results from the prospective E3N cohort. Eur J Cancer Prev. 2010;19(2):120–5.
201. Kitahara CM, Berrington de Gonzalez A, Freedman ND, et al. Total cholesterol and cancer risk in a large prospective study in Korea. J Clin Oncol. 2011;29(12):1592–8.
202. Heng YJ, Hankinson SE, Wang J, Alexandrov LB, Ambrosone CB. The association of modifiable breast cancer risk factors and somatic genomic alterations in breast tumors: the cancer genome atlas network. Cancer Epidemiol Biomark Prev. 2020;29(3):599–605.

Breast Cancer-Related Lymphedema and Shoulder Impairments: Physical Therapy and Plastic Surgery

14

Carmen Kloer, Lisa Massa, Andrew Atia, and Sharon Clancy

Chapter Objectives

- Recognize and evaluate lymphedema and shoulder impairments early to improve outcomes and avoid secondary dysfunction.
- Prevent and reduce costly and unnecessary testing and treatment.
- Provide comprehensive knowledge for patients on their treatment options.

Section 1: Breast Cancer-Related Lymphedema (BCRL) – Arm Lymphedema

Example case:
Ms. J is a 48-year-old female with a past medical history of invasive ductal carcinoma for which she had bilateral mastectomy with axillary lymph node dissection and immediate breast reconstruction. One year ago, she started to complain of "heaviness" and swelling in her left arm. Two months ago, she started to notice that doing activities with her left arm was more difficult than it was with her right arm. She had been wearing compression garments on both arms for 3 hours per day since her surgery, but stopped doing so about 4 months ago. She does not exercise regularly, but walks occasionally. She reports decreased swelling with elevation of the arm. On examination, her blood pressure is 110/74, temperature is 98.6 °F (37 °C), and heart rate is 70 beats per minute. Her BMI is 32. Her left arm is grossly larger than her right, with a difference in circumference of 3 cm. Her left arm shows 1+ pitting edema without any signs of hardening or fibrosis within the arm.

- What's going on with Ms. J's left arm?
- Why is this happening to Ms. J?
- How can I help Ms. J?
- What are Ms. J's options?
- Will it get better?

C. Kloer · A. Atia
Department of Plastic Surgery, Duke University Hospital, Durham, NC, USA

L. Massa (✉)
Department of Physical and Occupational Therapy, Duke University Hospital, Durham, NC, USA
e-mail: lisa.massa@duke.edu

S. Clancy
Department of Plastic and Reconstructive Surgery, Duke University, Durham, NC, USA

An Introduction to Breast Cancer-Related Lymphedema (BCRL) of Upper Extremity

What's Going with Ms. J?

Ms. J's case is a classic example of a patient experiencing breast cancer-related lymphedema (BCRL), which typically arises after axillary

G. G. Kimmick et al. (eds.), *Common Issues in Breast Cancer Survivors*,
https://doi.org/10.1007/978-3-030-75377-1_14

lymph node dissection and/or radiotherapy to the axilla for breast cancer and, due to its progressive nature, can be a source of continuous distress, frustration, and reduced quality of life [1]. The reported incidence of BCRL ranges from 10% to 65%, depending on variability in reporting and diagnostic criteria used [1–5]. A recent meta-analysis notes the overall incidence likely to be 21.4% from 30 prospective cohort studies [7]. The incidence rate is higher in patients who have undergone axillary lymph node dissection (ALND) and regional lymph node radiation as part of their treatment plan [6].

In the United States, breast cancer treatment, especially procedures that manipulate the axillary lymph/lymph node system, is the most common cause of lymphedema [7]. Breast cancer treatments can disrupt the lymphatic system causing impairment of the lymphatic circulation of the remaining breast skin or tissue and/or ipsilateral arm. BCRL results from the dysfunctional lymph drainage, such that the arm becomes swollen, heavy, uncomfortable, and possibly painful.

Overview of the Lymphatic System

The lymphatic system is part of the circulatory system and has multiple functions. It collects and transports fluid from the interstitial space to the venous system. This lymphatic fluid also plays a critical role in immune response.

Lymphatic fluid, or lymph, is the fluid that is collected by superficial lymphoid capillaries from interstitial fluid surrounding vasculature and cells. The lymph flows from the lymphatic capillaries into collecting lymphatics, which carry it to lymph nodes. These collecting lymphatics have one-way valves to prevent back flow [8]. Lymph nodes house lymphocytes, T cells and B cells. In lymph nodes, protein-free fluid is extracted from lymph fluid and lymphocytes identify antigens in lymph [9]. The post-nodal lymphatic fluid then travels centrally to the thoracic duct or right lymph duct where it is returned to the venous system in the subclavian veins.

In summary, the lymphatic system is critical for the draining of interstitial fluid, transporting cells of the immune system and playing a role in the process of inflammation. Damage to this system results in stagnant fluid which increases arm swelling and subsequent deposition of excess adipose tissue and fibrosis, which are the hallmarks of lymphedema.

Classification of Lymphedema

There are two types of lymphedema, primary and secondary. Primary lymphedema is the result of a congenital malformation of the lymphatic system. Secondary lymphedema is the result of trauma to lymphatic system that causes disruption of its normal function. BCRL, the topic for this chapter, is due to trauma to the lymphatic system during breast cancer surgery and/or radiation, so is classified as a secondary lymphedema.

Histologically, lymphedema, whether primary or secondary, is defined by edema, fibroadipose tissue deposition, chronic inflammation, and hyperkeratosis [10]. Continuous stasis also leads to a state of chronic inflammation by activating inflammatory signals [11].

Why Is This Happening to Ms. J?

Many women undergo breast cancer treatment, similar to Ms. J. In fact, nearly all women with breast cancer undergo surgery, but only a minority of women develop clinically apparent lymphedema.

The pathophysiology of secondary lymphedema, however, is not fully understood. It appears that inciting factors, such as surgery or radiation, cause damage to the lymphatic channels and obstruct lymph flow, resulting in the clinical presentation of lymphedema. These inciting factors are necessary but not sufficient to guarantee the development of lymphedema [10]. It appears that the development of secondary lymphedema varies according to lymphatic vessel density and fluid flow patterns in the body region. Impairment of lymph flow causes persistent fluid stasis, lymphatic valvular incompetence, and dermal backflow of both the superficial and deep lymphatic systems.

The main risk factors that lead to BCRL are listed in Table 14.1 [12, 13].

Table 14.1 Risk factors for BCRL

Axillary lymph node dissection
≥ 8 axillary lymph nodes removed during axillary surgery
Radiation therapy to breast or axilla
History of postoperative complications (i.e., infections, seromas)
Ipsilateral venous compromise in the arm/axilla
Advanced or recurrent cancer
Subsequent, non-surgical, traumatic injury to the ipsilateral arm
History of having received taxane-based adjuvant chemotherapy
Extracapsular invasion by a tumor
Obesity and weight gain [14, 15]

Table 14.2 Risk-reducing behaviors (RRB)

Unproven but endorsed	Endorsed but proven unrelated
Avoiding BP checks in ipsilateral arm	Exercise
Avoiding phlebotomy in ipsilateral arm	Air travel
Avoiding IV placement in ipsilateral arm	House cleaning

Advances in surgical management of breast cancer have led to lower incidence of BCRL by using less extensive local procedures, such as sentinel lymph node (SLN) sampling instead of axillary lymph node dissection or lumpectomy instead of mastectomy [12]. Table 14.1 lists risk factors for acquiring BCRL. Some of the risk factors can be modified. In an attempt to modify the risk of developing lymphedema, experts in the field developed a list, most of which are anecdotal [16, 17]. The evidence supporting use of Risk Reducing Behaviors (RRB) are predominately anecdotal with a limited body of data that is controversial (Table 14.2). Specifically, air travel and exercise have been shown to be safe [16].

More data needs to be collected to verify the effects of these RRB behaviors in patients susceptible to BCRL. An important note: patients who had a sentinel lymph node sampling and did not have a complete ALND are at very low risk of BCRL and do not need to undergo RRB, even if they have received any type of mastectomy [18, 19].

Evaluation Process

How Can I Help Ms. J?

As care team members begin to understand more about lymphedema, there is a recognition of an increased need for proper evaluation and surveillance for patients who undergo breast cancer surgery and/or radiation. The methodology of evaluating BCRL continues to evolve, including improvements in lymphatic imaging such as outpatient MR lymphangiography and ICG lymphangiography, ease of monitoring in clinic with noninvasive volumetric measurements, and further research into potential treatments. To be able to help a patient such as Ms. J, the care team needs to be able to first recognize her symptoms in connection with her history. Once her symptoms are recognized as possibly related to BCRL, she can then be referred to the proper specialists to receive treatment. As we move through the case history, we are following the algorithm in Fig. 14.1, which outlines a systematic approach to this complex issue.

Symptoms and History

In the case vignette, the patient references a feeling of “heaviness” and “swelling” in her left arm – these and other symptoms in the arm, including paresthesia, fatigue, and general discomfort, can be the presenting complaints among patients with either subclinical or clinical BCRL [20]. These symptoms should prompt the provider to ask about any of the higher risk treatments (ALND or axillary radiation) or other BCRL risk factors. Also characterizing the lymphedema is important. Providers should ask if the swelling/lymphedema improves with elevation of the affected arm or not – this is an important distinguishing factor when considering surgical interventions since if there are reversible changes in the arm, they may be a candidate for surgery targeting increasing the fluid drainage from the arm. Taking a complete history will help direct the type of further management the patient could attempt or will need.

Lymphedema tends to have a delayed clinical presentation, appearing months to years after cancer treatments such as axillary lymph node surgery and/or radiation. On average, however,

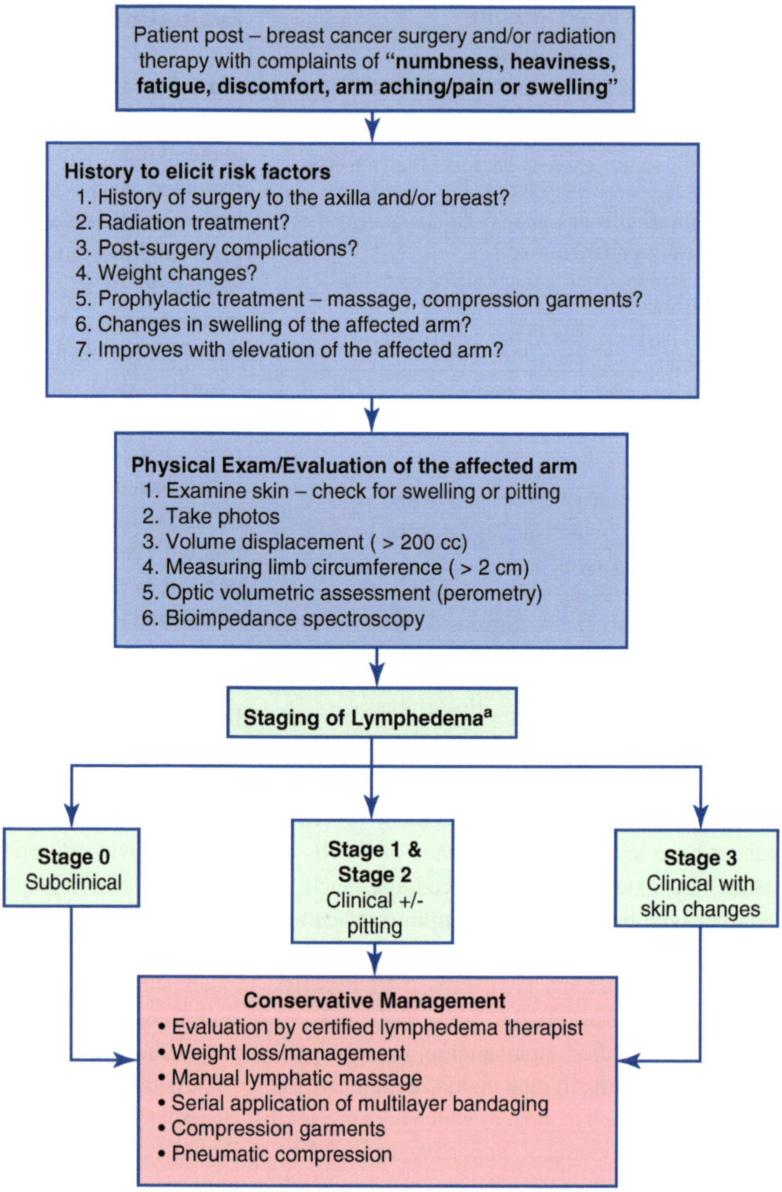

Fig. 14.1 Diagnostic approach: concern for BCRL. International Society of Lymphology [29]

BCRL appears about 8 months after interventions [20]. A thorough physical evaluation aids in diagnosis of lymphedema by eliminating other causes of arm swelling. Under some circumstances, CT or ultrasound is indicated to rule out cancer recurrence. In the absence of cancer, the differential for unilateral arm edema includes lipedema, myxedema, infection, or trauma. Lipedema is the abnormal accumulation of subcutaneous adipose and is more likely to be bilateral [21], while lymphedema typically presents unilaterally on the same side of the breast cancer and interventions [22]. Myxedema is usually associated with hypothyroidism, is also typically bilateral, and requires further history and laboratory testing, including thyroid function tests, for workup.

Physical Exam and Objective Assessment

In evaluating the severity of the lymphedema, we recommend starting with an examination of the skin. Evaluators need to notice if the skin is edematous and has pits or indentations when pressed and if the skin displays any changes in color, texture, or thickness. The presence or absence of skin changes is important in staging of the lymphedema. The care team should use photographs in their documentation process to aid in future evaluation for progression or response to treatments.

A simple physical exam is one method to evaluate arm swelling and/or volume by measuring the circumference of both arms. Lymphedema generally is limited to one arm; therefore, the less swollen or unaffected arm can be used for comparison. Measurements should be taken at standard locations, defined in relation to standard landmarks of the ulnar styloid process, olecranon, and shoulder. The number of measurements taken between these landmarks can vary based on a practice's preference, but, at a minimum, measurements about half way between the wrist to the elbow and elbow to shoulder should be collected [20, 23]. We recommend a minimum of 5 circumference measurements for each arm. The diagnosis of clinical lymphedema is made if the measurements between arms differ by greater than 2 cm [24]. A more accurate method to diagnose lymphedema is measuring volume with water displacement. This requires the patient to submerge their arms separately within a tank of water and the evaluator to measure the difference in volume between the two limbs. A diagnosis of clinical lymphedema is made if the volume is 200 cc greater in the affected than in the unaffected limb [24].

There are two evaluation methods, optoelectronic limb volumeter (perometry) and bioimpedance spectroscopy (BIS), that employ newer technology to evaluate lymphedema but are typically expensive and not easily accessible. Certified lymphedema therapists use these tools in their evaluation process. Perometry provides limb volume measurements through an infrared laser method [25]. The perometry machine itself is a large piece of equipment that features an adjustable arm to scan the limb. This method of measurement is quick with more accurate measurements of overall limb volume than tape circumference measurements [26, 27]. However, perometry does not provide information into the specific volume increase of extracellular fluid (ECF), while BIS does [25, 28]. BIS uses electrical currents to distinguish the amount of fluid collection in a lymphedematous limb versus the unaffected limb with a functional lymphatic system, specifically quantifying the ECF differential [12, 25]. Some researchers suggest the use of BIS as a method for screening for BCRL following the first year post-breast cancer treatment to evaluate for subclinical BCRL [12]. Using a combination of these measurement techniques allows for monitoring of lymphedema severity and may possibly curb the need for more expensive tests, imaging, or consultations.

Lymphedema Staging

There are many different methods for staging lymphedema. These include evaluating the degree of pitting and swelling (International Society of Lymphology staging system), using circumference measurements, utilizing ICG lymphangiography to distinguish level of lymphatic damage (NECST system), and classifying the level of dermal backflow using ICG lymphangiography (M.D. Anderson classification scheme) [10]. We recommend use of the International Society of Lymphology staging metric because it relies predominately on clinical assessment (Table 14.3) [29].

Conservative, Non-surgical, Management

Conservative therapies are the first-line approach to management of lymphedema. These options include complex decongestive therapy, weight management, compression garments, and intermittent pneumatic compression. Complex Decongestive Therapy (CDT) is a combination of manual lymph drainage, compression therapy, therapeutic exercise, and skin care.

(a) *Manual Lymph Drainage (MLD)*:

This is a gentle manual technique that gently stretches the subcutaneous tissues to facilitate lymphatic flow in the affected region. The stretch pressure is gently released which allows the lymphatic vessels to pull additional fluid out of the interstitial space. The effects of MLD include reversing lym-

Table 14.3 Staging of lymphedema – International Society of Lymphology

Stage		
0 Subclinical swelling not apparent on clinical exam despite impaired lymph flow	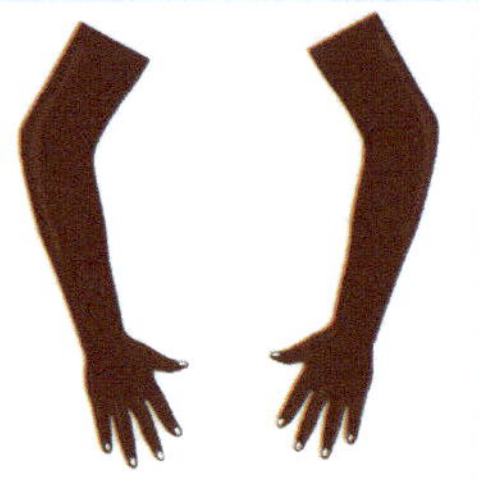	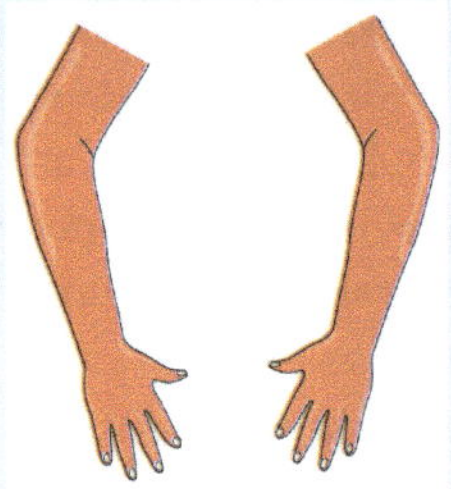
1 Soft edema that pits with no dermal fibrosis and subsides with limb elevation within 24 hours	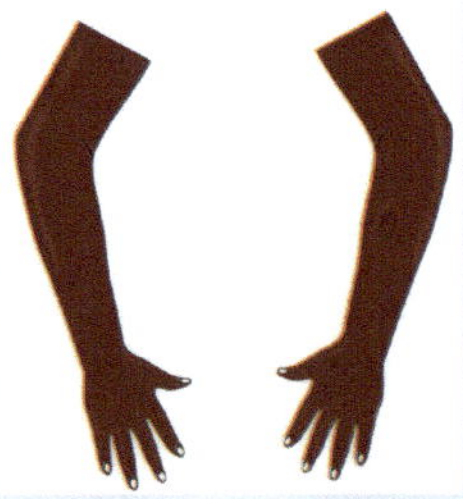	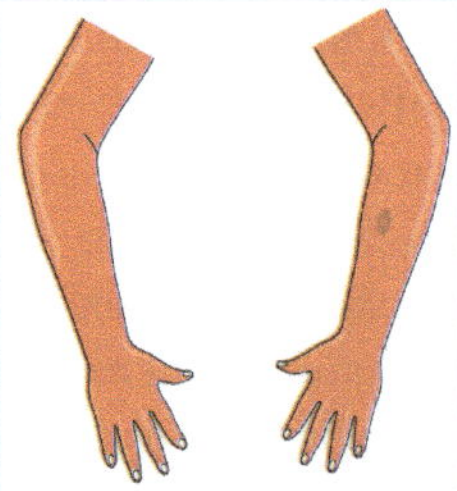
2 Nonpitting lymphedema that does not resolve with limb elevation, reflecting evolution of dermal fibrosis	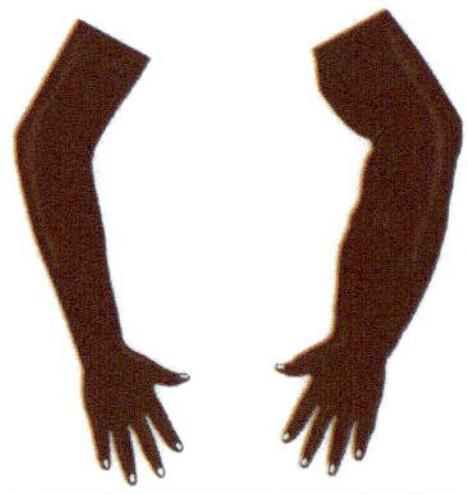	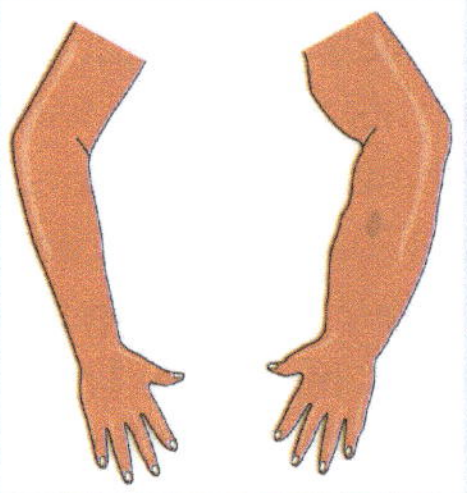
3 Lymphostatic elephantiasis with nonpitting edema with skin changes of acanthosis and warty overgrowths	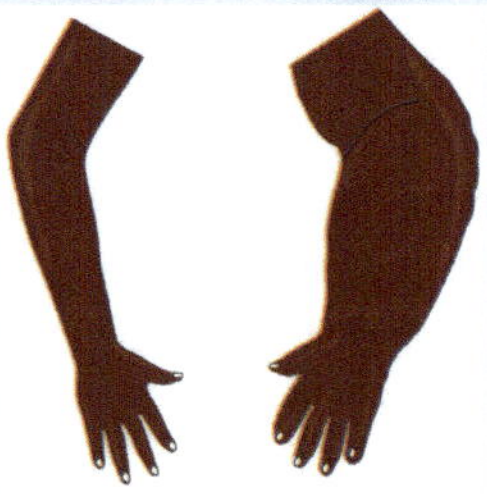	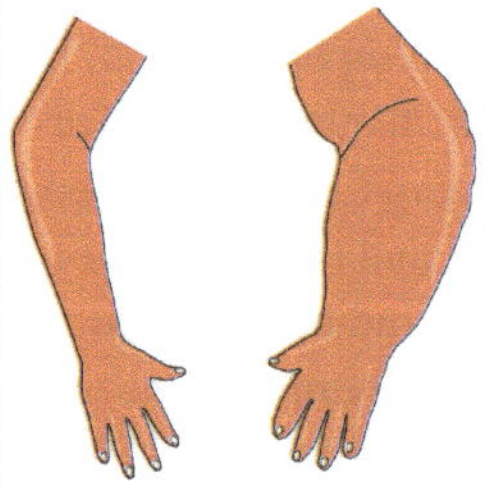

Graphic art created by Amelia Kloer
Refer to Table 14.2. in International Society of Lymphology [29]

phatic flow, increasing contractile rate of lymph vessels, increasing venous flow, and decreasing pain.

(b) *Compression Therapy*

Once lymphedema is present, the elastic fibers of cutaneous tissues are altered and will require some form of external compression. This is necessary to prevent re-accumulation of fluid in the affected area. This can be in the form of bandages or a garment. Some of the other benefits of compression therapy include improving venous return, improving the effectiveness of the muscles to pump and propel the lymphatic fluid centrally, soften fibrosis, and increase flexibility of scar tissue.

(c) *Exercise*

Exercise is an integral part of lymphedema management. During the intensive phase of lymphedema treatment, exercises help facilitate lymphatic flow. These exercises should be done when compression bandages are on the affected limb. Aerobic, resistive, and breathing exercises can all be included. Two systematic reviews have supported resistance exercise as safe and effective for individuals with BCRL [30, 31]. It is important to provide supervision and a gradual exercise progression for these programs to achieve maximal success.

(d) *Skin Care*

Patients should be instructed in skin and nail care. This includes proper cleaning and moisturizing of skin. Cleansers and moisturizers should be hypoallergenic and pH balanced. Patients should also be taught how to inspect their skin/nails for infection and inflammation. Encouraging our patients to maintain a general first aid kit in both their home and car is important, as this can be a helpful tool if they acquire a cut, scrape, or minor burn. The first aid kit should include an OTC antibiotic ointment and clean dry bandages to cover open areas.

(e) *Weight Management*

As previously mentioned, obesity is a risk factor for BCRL. When reviewing the Body Mass Index (BMI) of your patient, make a note if their BMI is between 25 and 29.9 (overweight) or over 30 (obese). There is evidence to suggest that a higher BMI correlates with a greater likelihood that patients will develop lymphedema [32]. It is important that we advocate that our breast cancer survivors to develop an active lifestyle. Mitigating lymphedema risk is certainly not the only benefit of routine exercise for breast cancer survivors. Exercise has also been identified as one of the most important modifiable risk factors regarding recurrence of disease [14, 33]. Please see also Chap. 13, Obesity, Weight Gain and Weight Managementin Women with Early Stage Breast Cancer.

(f) *Compression Garments*

Compression garments are used to prevent the recurrence of lymphedema once the affected area is decongested and these should become part of our survivor's lifelong routine. There are a range of sleeves and gloves made from a variety of materials. Compression garment fitting should be done by trained professionals, as an ill-fitting garment can actually exacerbate lymphedema.

(g) *Intermittent Pneumatic Compression (ICP)*

An Intermittent Compression Pump (IPC) is comprised of an inflatable garment and electrical pneumatic pump [34]. The inflatable garment has multiple chambers which are placed around the affected area. The chambers can have varying amounts of pressure to facilitate lymphatic flow. IPCs should not be used as a stand-alone treatment for lymphedema, always used as an adjunct only. It can be used along with other treatment interventions previously mentioned.

What Are Ms. J's Options?

As we review Ms. J's case history, it would appear that she could potentially benefit from all components of the conservative management described above. There are many factors a lymphedema specialist will need to consider when developing Ms. J's plan of care. Some of those factors would include transportation concerns, financial concerns, presence of supportive caregivers/family members, and any pre-morbid cognitive issues. Another consideration is that the plan of care needs to not only reduce the lymphedema but also empower the patient to independently use all. Unfortunately, there are occasions where these measures are ineffectual, despite patient best efforts and compliance using appropriate tools to manage this lifetime condition. In these cases, a referral for surgical management of lymphedema may be appropriate.

Surgical Management of Lymphedema

Once a patient begins to consider surgical interventions for lymphedema, it is important to have a thorough workup from a lymphatic specialist. Patients should be referred to a plastic surgeon to evaluate for surgical candidacy. Surgical interventions are chosen based on the level of physiologic availability that the patient's lymphatic system offers. Figure 14.2 shows the care pathway for patients interested in surgical interventions for BCRL. We utilize the Barcelona Lymphedema Algorithm for Surgical Treatment

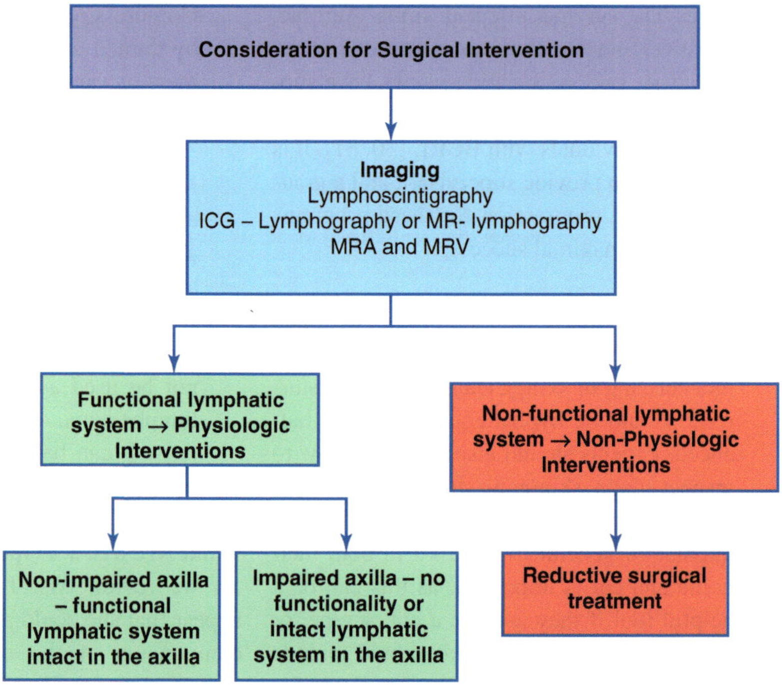

Fig. 14.2 Diagnostic approach after trial of Conservation Management: using the Barcelona Lymphedema Algorithm for Surgical Treatment (BLAST) [35]. ICG indocyanine green (ICG) lymphangiography, MR magnetic resonance, MRA magnetic resonance angiography, MRV magnetic resonance venography

(BLAST) to determine appropriate surgical interventions for patients [35].

Imaging

Imaging provides critical information along with history, physical exam, and response to conservative management into the health and viability of the patient's lymphatic system. Table 14.4 introduces the various imaging modalities used for surgical treatment planning of BCRL along with their benefits and limitations. We recommend starting with lymphoscintigraphy (LS) to determine if the axilla has functional lymphatic uptake. To determine the optimal surgical procedure, the initial step is establishing if the lymphatics within the arm and/or axilla have any functional capacity. Without any functionality of the lymphatic system, the only intervention options become non-physiologic interventions.

If there is any functionality in the axilla or arm, we investigate the level of functionality and the location of blockage or dysfunction. ICG lymphangiography and MR-lymphography map the lymphatic vessels and the sites of dysfunction. In practice, ICG lymphangiography is more readily accessible than MR-lymphography, and thus, is more often used for the surgical planning. However, MR-lymphography provides more information than ICG lymphangiography via its visualization of deeper lymphatic channels and yields useful information in some cases.

There are exciting advances and research being done regarding imaging of lymphatics. For example, researchers have found that LS offers visualization of lymphangiogenesis post-ALNT [38]. Of note, ultrasound and CT have low sensitivity and should not be used for diagnosis or evaluation of lymphedema, except to rule out presence of cancer mass as cause of arm swelling.

Surgical Treatment

What Are Ms. J's Options?

Many reconstructive techniques have been developed with improvements in imaging technology and the advancement in the field of microsurgery and supermicrosurgery from both a technical skill aspect and improvements with instrumentation [39]. In thinking of Ms. J's case, it is important to

Table 14.4 Imaging options for surgical evaluation

Imaging modality	Description	Benefit/reason for acquiring	Limitations
Lymphoscintigraphy	Nuclear medicine imaging with radiolabeled colloid injected. The rate of uptake determines the amount of lymph drainage	No prep necessary Identifies blockage in lymphatic vessels Helpful for evaluating if a patient is a candidate for ALNT	Less sensitive than ICG and MRI
ICG lymphangiography	An infrared camera visualizes ICG dye as it passes through the functioning lymphatic vessels	High sensitivity [36] Can visualize lymphatic drainage pathways and determine salvageable lymphatic structures Can measure the velocity of lymphatic transport Helpful for determining if a patient is a candidate for LVA surgery	Only see superficial lymphatic channels <2 cm from skin surface Lymphatic mapping is not an FDA-approved usage of ICG yet, and only approved for intravenous injections
MR-lymphography	Magnetic resonance imaging with contrast injected which shows the anatomical structures in space and time with high resolution for both lymphatic vessels and nodes [37]	High sensitivity [36] Can visualize lymphatic channels deeper than 2 cm from skin surface Helpful for determining if a patient is a candidate for LVA surgery	Requires a radiologist to optimize the technique Not widely accessible because of cost of equipment and training
MRA	Magnetic resonance imaging that focuses on the arterial vasculature	Helpful in evaluation for ALNT surgery	An additional study
MRV	Magnetic resonance imaging that focuses on the venous vasculature	Helpful in evaluation for LVA surgery	An additional study

ICG indocyanine green (ICG) lymphangiography, *MR* magnetic resonance, *MRA* magnetic resonance angiography, *MRI* magnetic resonance Imaging, *MRV* magnetic resonance venography, *LVA* lymph-venous anastomosis, *ALNT* axillary lymph node transfer

consider all aspects of her story – decreased swelling with limb elevation, minimal exercise, and pitting edema. Her physical exam and response to conservative treatment can provide great detail into how she will respond to surgical intervention since with response to conservative treatment and reversibility of some of her physical issues with lymphedema correlate with success of surgical intervention. Surgical procedures are classified as non-physiologic interventions and physiologic interventions. Given the description of Ms. J's lymphedema physical findings, she most likely is Stage 1 BCRL. The different recommendations for physiologic versus non-physiologic interventions depends on the functionality of her lymphatic system. Table 14.5 provides a summary for the most common procedures offered.

- Non-physiologic interventions are indicated when there are no working lymphatics or very minimal function of lymphatics; surgical interventions are aimed only at managing symptoms such as increased limb circumference.
- Physiologic interventions are considered when there are functioning lymphatics; surgical intervention can make use of intact lymphatic channels to help relieve BCRL.

As Ms. J undergoes conservative management with a certified lymphedema therapist, tracking her response to therapy will help in her surgical evaluation. If she responds well to treatment and shows decreased swelling with therapy, this furthers the likelihood that she is a good candidate for physiologic surgical interventions. Plastic surgeons who are trained in lymphatic microsur-

Table 14.5 Surgical procedure options [40–44, 46–48]

	Non-physiologic intervention		Physiologic interventions	
Procedure	Liposuction	Direct excisional debulking	VLNT	LVA
Potential patient	Stage 2–3 lymphedema No/limited response to conservative management Cannot undergo a longer surgical procedure	Stage 3 lymphedema No/limited response to conservative management Able to tolerate a longer surgical procedure	Stage 0–2 lymphedema Response to conservative management	Stage 0–2 lymphedema Response to conservative management
Imaging	LS ➔ significant blockage in lymphatics system	LS ➔ significant blockage in lymphatics system	LS ➔ signs of functionality with limited or no axilla uptake ICG lymphangiography or MR-lymphography Consider MRA and MRV	LS ➔ signs of functionality with functional axillary nodes ICG lymphangiography or MR-lymphography MRV
Procedure synopsis	Extract hypertrophied fat from the affected limb	Direct removal of skin and subcutaneous tissue above the muscle with skin grafting	Transplant a flap containing three to six lymph nodes with a vascularized pedicle from a low-risk donor site, such as the superficial inferior epigastric area, into the damaged axilla region	Harvest the functional lymphatic vessels until blockages to be anastomosed with a superficial vein
Benefits	Minimal scarring and damage to the skin Reduction in limb volume Less morbid than Charles procedure Improvement in blood flow	Significant decrease in limb circumference	Reduction in symptomatic limb volume and other symptoms of pain and heaviness	Reduction in symptomatic limb volume and other symptoms of pain and heaviness
Potential risks/ complications	Skin numbness 3–6 months following surgery	Recurrence of lymphedema Skin graft loss Poor cosmetic result Prolonged numbness	Donor site seroma Iatrogenic lymphedema of donor site Lymphocele	Skin ulceration
Barriers to care	Lifelong need to wear compression garment post-operatively	Requires significant wound care for proper healing	Continue conservative treatments in conjunction with surgical intervention ➔ need multiple appointments	Continue conservative treatments in conjunction with surgical intervention ➔ need multiple appointments
Volume reduction (%)	80–100	16–52	25–50	14–50
Post-operative treatment	Compression garment	Compression garment Complete decongestive therapy	Compression garment Suction drain in place Manual lymphatic drainage Start rehabilitation program	Compression garment Consider physiotherapy Lymphatic pumping Start rehabilitation program

See Table 14.3 for lymphedema staging

VLNT vascular lymph node transplant, *LVA* lymphatic-venous anastomosis, *LS* lymphoscintigraphy, *ICG* indocyanine green, *MR* magnetic resonance, *MRA* magnetic resonance angiography, *MRI* magnetic resonance imaging

gery and supermicrosurgery provide these interventions.

It is important to remind patients of overall guidelines to surgical success when considering surgical intervention, as healing relies on the patient's health. This implies that good surgical candidates do not smoke, have controlled diabetes, eat a healthy diet, maintain a reasonable BMI (ideally <30 kg/m^2), and are able to comply with post-operative instructions as well as ongoing MDT. Every patient needs to be evaluated to develop an individualized treatment care plan.

Some unique requirements for physiologic interventions include the need to continue wearing compression garments and working with a lymphedema therapist. These therapies will be prescribed to patients based on their procedure and will be re-evaluated during their recovery process. The rigorous post-operative care required may be overwhelming to many patients but has been shown to improve quality of life [40–44]. It is also important to be mindful of the financial burden that these patients experience. Because of the Breast and Cervical Cancer Prevention and Treatment Act approved by Congress in 2000, women can be covered with Medicaid for their breast cancer treatments, and this should include BCRL interventions [45].

The main physiologic surgical interventions consist of the Vascularized Lymph Node Transplant (VLNT) and Lymphatic-Venous Anastomosis (LVA). Both of these procedures require some form of lymphatic system function in the patient's arm and/or axilla. These procedures are helpful and more effective for patients with earlier stages of BCRL.

Non-physiologic interventions are an important option for patients with advanced disease who no longer have functionality in their lymphatic structures and have primarily fibroadipose tissue deposition. Non-physiologic procedures focus on volume reduction to improve symptoms and quality of life. The main non-physiologic interventions are liposuction and direct excision.

Will It Get Better?

Most research indicates that lymphedema interventions have high rates of success and improve the quality of life for many patients [42]. Patients find that their symptoms are relieved or reduced. There is an opportunity for further innovation in this field.

There is a rare disease associated with long-standing lymphedema called Stewart-Treves syndrome (STS), a cutaneous angiosarcoma with poor prognosis. This pathology develops from 4 to up to 50 years following axillary trauma due to breast cancer interventions followed by lymphedema. It features extensive skin changes with nodules and mauve coloring [49]. The treatment for STS is limited mostly to amputation or extensive cutaneous excision [50]. Following surgical interventions, patients with STS have an average of 20-month survival [51]. The incidence of STS continues to decrease with improvements in breast cancer treatment and management, but it is important to be aware of this rare but dangerous complication of lymphedema.

Section 2: BCRL – Breast Lymphedema

Case Study #2

Ms. L is a 45-year-old female with Stage IB right breast cancer. She underwent a lumpectomy, sentinel lymph node (SLN) dissection, low axillary node dissection (ALND), and radiation to her breast. At her first follow-up appointment after she completed her radiation treatment, she complained of pain and tenderness in her right breast. She also has observed that her right breast seems to be "too large for her bra." She has noticed that when she takes her bra off at night, there are indentions in her skin under her breast where her bra rests against her skin. You observe a mild erythema in the two lower quadrants of her breast.

- What is the most likely explanation for Ms. L's presentation?
- What are the key points we need to consider in addressing this issue?

BCRL: Breast Lymphedema (BLE)

Overview

Breast lymphedema is characterized by diffuse skin edema and erythema and symptoms such as

Table 14.6 Risk factors for breast lymphedema [55, 56]

1. History of axillary node dissection
2. Higher body mass index (BMI)
3. Location of surgical incision in the UOQ, LIQ, and central breast
4. Adjuvant chemotherapy
5. Ongoing breast pain
6. History of breast radiation therapy/radiation therapy boost
7. Large tumor size (>17 mm at time of surgery)

UOQ upper outer quadrant, *LIQ* lower inner quadrant

breast heaviness, redness, and swelling [52]. It is a well-recognized complication of breast and axillary surgery, yet it has not garnered as much attention as BCRL of the upper extremity. It is important that this condition is detected, evaluated, and treated as early as possible to decrease risk of infection, impaired wound healing, and chronic cellulitis associated with chronically lymphedematous tissues [53, 54]. In addition, the differentiation between cellulitis and BLE can avoid unnecessary use of antibiotics. Table 14.6 has a list of risk factors that have been associated with increased incidence of BLE.

In these studies, axillary node dissection increased the risk of BLE but the number of nodes dissected did not increase risk. The mean BMI of the individuals with BLE was 31. Surgical incisions in the upper outer quadrant, lower internal quadrant, and central (areolar) region had an increased risk for BLE compared to tumors located in the upper inner and lower outer quadrants. BLE was more often present in the two lower quadrants of the breast. Erythema was equally distributed throughout all four quadrants and the central region in patients with BLE. Tumors >17 mm were associated with BLE as compared to tumors <13 mm.

Table 14.7 Possible signs and symptoms of BLE

1. Redness in breast and adjacent trunk
2. Hypomobility of breast scar tissue
3. Asymmetrical bra fit
4. Pain in breast
5. Asymmetrical truncal skin folds
6. Report of heaviness in the breast
7. Skin irritation in lateral aspect of breast/axilla

Table 14.8 Typical cellulitis presentation [48]

1. Chills, followed by a high fever
2. Severe malaise
3. Nausea
4. Headache
5. Local pain in the breast or area of the breast
6. Warm/hot skin of the breast
7. Map-like borders to the skin erythema
8. Rapid course progression

Clinical Presentation

The clinical presentation of BLE can be somewhat variable. A thorough examination of the integument of the breast and truncal region is imperative. An important point to consider that the presence of erythema with edema in the breast does not necessarily indicate the presence of cellulitis. A checklist of signs and symptoms to consider in the diagnosis of BLE is listed in Table 14.7.

It is important to discern between BLE and cellulitis. Common cellulitis symptoms are listed in Table 14.8.

Consider the following algorithm when assessing the patient.

Algorithm for Breast Lymphedema (BLE)

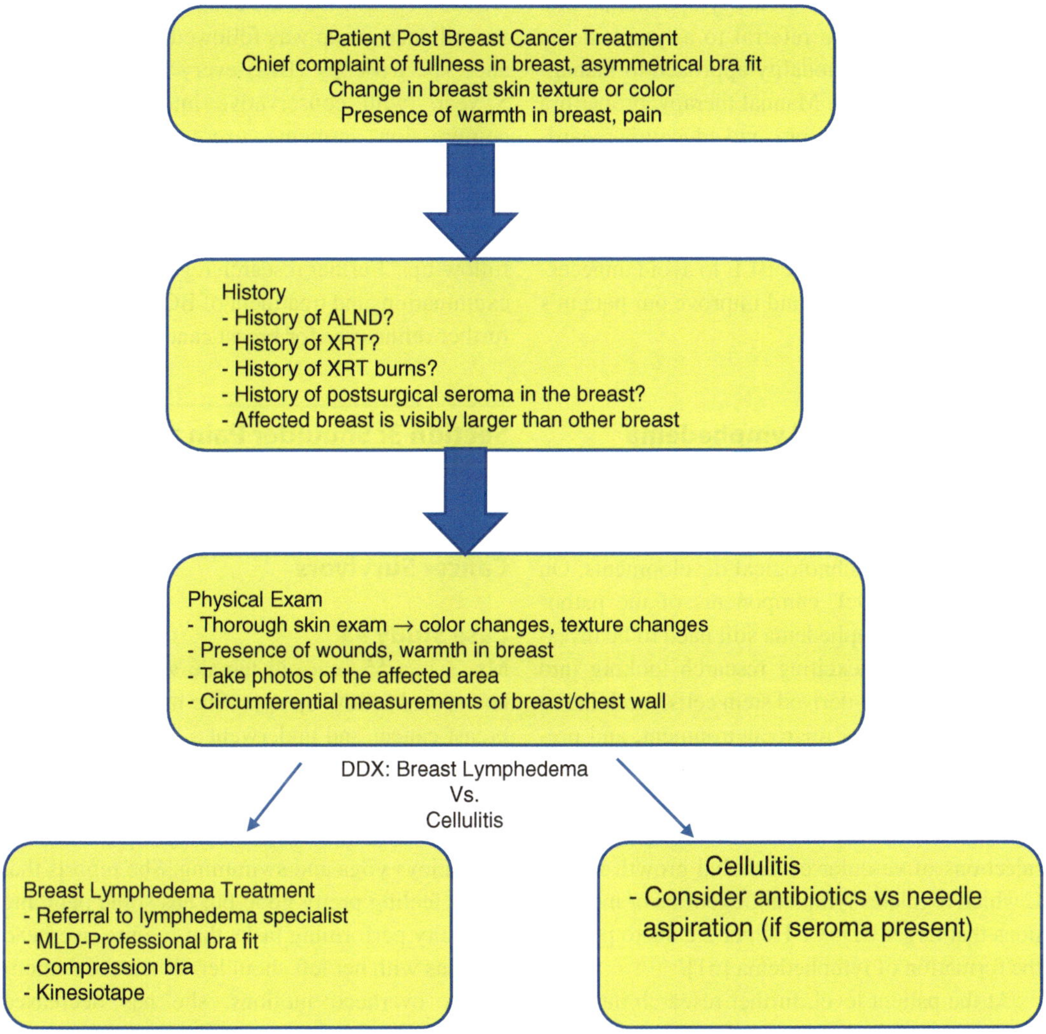

Treatment Options

Research for BLE is presently lacking. The most common management strategies for BLE include manual lymph drainage, kinesiotape to facilitate truncal/breast drainage, use of compression bra, skin/nail care education, and professional fitting for a daily bra. Many women have never been professionally fitted for a bra and often wear bras that are too small with regard to cup size and band width. Poor bra fit can restrict lymphatic flow in the breast and adjacent truncal region and lead to congestion of lymphatic fluid in the breast. Kinesiotape has been shown to improve tissue texture in BLE [57]. A recent pilot study demonstrated that a compression bra can reduce both pain and edema in breast cancer survivors [58]. Manual Lymph Drainage (MLD) has been shown to help with breast lymphedema with varying degrees of success. Compression bandaging of the torso is another anecdotal, unproven management technique, though it causes restriction around the rib cage and may be difficult to tolerate.

What are Ms. L's options?
Ms. L appears to have breast lymphedema. She would benefit from a referral to a lymphedema specialist. A multi-modality approach to managing BLE is preferred. Manual therapy, proper bra fit, use of compression bra, and education regarding skin care can all be an integral part of Ms. L's care plan. BLE has been associated with lower QOL and body image [56]. It is important to be able to correctly diagnose BLE to avoid unnecessary medical treatment and improve our patient's quality of life.

Future of BCRL and Lymphedema Interventions

The field of lymphedema management continues to advance with technological developments. On the molecular level, components of the pathophysiology of lymphedema still need to be investigated. There is exciting research looking into the use of adipose-derived stem cells, modulation of the lymphedema microenvironment, and preemptive treatment for BCRL through primary lymphatic anastomosis with breast reconstruction [59, 60]. The future of BCRL might include injections of vascular endothelial growth factor-C which regulates lymphangiogenesis or medications that target $CD4^{+}$ T Helper 2 cells to prevent the formation of lymphedema [61].

At the patient level, further research into best diagnostic practices, preventative techniques, and surveillance methods would be helpful in treating patients with BCRL. While there is some disagreement among experts regarding specific clinical practice guidelines for BCRL, it is generally agreed that a multidisciplinary approach is optimal for managing this condition. For now, we can focus on diagnosing these patients early and preventing the progression of BCRL. Among researchers in the field of BCRL, there are movements for providers to engage in "surveillance practices" – monitoring patients preemptively for subclinical or clinical signs of lymphedema through physical exam and imaging methods [62]. In a prospective study of 186 patients treated for breast cancer, Soran, et al. (2014) found that the surveillance group experienced clinical BCRL 30% less than the control group [62]. The surveillance group was followed with bioimpedance spectroscopy (BIS) every 3–6 months for 5 years with conservative interventions (i.e., compression garments, exercises, etc.) started with signs of subclinical lymphedema. The control group had an initial preoperative BIS measurement and were limited to only clinical follow-ups. Further research regarding diagnosis, examination, and treatment of BCRL is needed to further refine care for breast cancer survivors.

Section 3: Shoulder Pain and Joint Dysfunction

Shoulder Impairment in Breast Cancer Survivors

Case Study #3

Ms. Z is a 55-year-old female who presents for her annual follow-up appt. She had Stage IIC left breast cancer and underwent a mastectomy with an axillary lymph node dissection, chemotherapy, and radiation treatment 2 years ago. She returned to her job as elementary school teacher. She enjoys yoga and swimming. She reports that she is feeling pretty good but has some pain and difficulty performing tasks that require overhead motions with her left shoulder. When she demonstrates overhead motions, she has decreased range on the left side compared to the right side. She reports she cannot hold her arm in an overhead position for more than 30–60 seconds. She points to her anterior shoulder as the area that is most painful.

Is this presentation related to her previous treatment or worrisome for new onset of disease?

Is her primary complaint something that can be addressed, or does the patient need to be instructed on adaptive techniques because there is no likelihood of improvement?

Overview

Pain and joint dysfunction of the shoulder are frequent side effects experienced by breast cancer

Table 14.9 Shoulder pain categories after breast cancer surgery [65, 66]

1. Musculoskeletal nociceptive
2. Neuropathic pain
A. Cancer-related
B. Drug-induced
3. Radiotherapy-induced pain
4. Chronic persistent pain

survivors [63]. The prevalence rate for pain ranges from 12% to 51%. The prevalence rate for joint dysfunction ranges from 1.5% to 50% [64]. Categories of shoulder pain are listed in Table 14.9.

Musculoskeletal nociceptive pain can result from any intervention that impacts the neuromusculoskeletal tissues of the shoulder region, including surgery and radiation for breast cancer. This results in pain, limitation of joint range of motion, and hypoesthesia [67]. Pain that results from breast surgery may result in individuals using a variety of motor strategies to avoid pain, resulting in reduced shoulder range of motion, subacromial impingement, and pain. Shortening of the pectoral muscle often occurs secondary to protective splinting, scar formation, and poor posture. This can lead to depression and protraction of the adjacent shoulder joint.

Neuropathic pain can occur because of the cancer lesion or secondary to the hormonal therapy that includes aromatase inhibitors required to manage the disease [68]. Post mastectomy pain syndrome is an example of a neuropathic pain syndrome. Postmastectomy pain syndrome (PMPS) remains poorly defined, although it is applied to chronic neuropathic pain following surgical procedures of the breast, including mastectomy and breast-conserving surgery. It is characterized by persistent pain affecting the anterior thorax, axilla, and/or medial upper arm following mastectomy or lumpectomy. Though the onset of pain is most likely after surgery, there may also be onset following adjuvant therapy, including chemotherapy or radiation therapy [69]. (Also see Chaps. 7 and 8, Persistent Breast Pain (PBP) and Common Issues in Breast Cancer Survivors: A Practical Guide to Evaluation and Management of Neuropathy.)

Radiotherapy-induced shoulder pain is often present, due to skin changes/burns, pain, and scarring of the chest wall/pectoral muscles. Radiation to skeletal muscles can cause fibrosis, atrophy, and pain.

Chronic persistent pain is present in as many as 50% of breast cancer patients 6 months after surgery [68]. These individuals often have higher depression and anxiety scores as well. Even when the pain is not directly in the shoulder, it can affect the willingness and confidence of the patient to use the shoulder with their activities of daily living, job-related tasks, and recreational activities.

Referral/Interventions

Any time a survivor presents to your clinic with complaints of shoulder pain or decreased shoulder function, it is recommended to place a referral to physical therapy. Multimodal physical therapy has been shown to be an effective intervention after breast cancer surgery. These interventions include manual therapy, flexibility, and resistance exercises. Education regarding pain pathophysiology and assessment for lymphedema are also important components for patient care. Exercise not only improves the motion and movement patterns of the shoulder but can also help reduce the anxiety a patient may be experiencing regarding their condition [70]. Cognitive behavioral techniques and education on proper sleep hygiene in conjunction with a supervised exercise program can further enhance patient outcomes. A multidisciplinary team approach that includes expertise of both medical and rehabilitation professionals provides the best care.

References

1. Merchant SJ, Chen SL. Prevention and management of lymphedema after breast cancer treatment. Breast J. 2015;21(3):276–84. https://doi.org/10.1111/tbj.12391. Epub 2015 Mar 13. Review. PubMed PMID: 25772311.
2. Shah C, Vicini FA. Breast cancer-related arm lymphedema: incidence rates, diagnostic techniques, optimal management and risk reduction strategies. Int J Radiat Oncol Biol Phys. 2011;81:907–14.

3. Ganju RG, Savvides G, Korentager S, Ward MJ, TenNapel M, Amin A, Wagner J, Mitchell M. Incidence of breast lymphedema and predictors of its development in patients receiving whole breast radiation therapy after breast-conservation surgery. Lymphology. 2019;52(3):126–33. PubMed PMID: 31874124.
4. Ribeiro Pereira ACP, Koifman RJ, Bergmann A. Incidence and risk factors of lymphedema after breast cancer treatment: 10 years of follow-up. Breast. 2017;36:67–73. https://doi.org/10.1016/j.breast.2017.09.006. Epub 2017 Oct 6. PubMed PMID: 28992556.
5. Rebegea L, Firescu D, Dumitru M, Anghel R. The incidence and risk factors for occurrence of arm lymphedema after treatment of breast cancer. Chirurgia (Bucur). 2015;110(1):33–7. PubMed PMID: 25800313.
6. McDuff SGR, Mina AI, Brunelle CL, Salama L, Warren LEG, Abouegylah M, Swaroop M, Skolny MN, Asdourian M, Gillespie T, Daniell K, Sayegh HE, Naoum GE, Zheng H, Taghian AG. Timing of lymphedema after treatment for breast cancer: when are patients most at risk? Int J Radiat Oncol Biol Phys. 2019;103(1):62–70. https://doi.org/10.1016/j.ijrobp.2018.08.036. Epub 2018 Aug 28. PubMed PMID: 30165125; PubMed Central PMCID: PMC6524147.
7. DiSipio T, Rye S, Newman B, Hayes S. Incidence of unilateral arm lymphoedema after breast cancer: a systematic review and meta-analysis. Lancet Oncol. 2013;14(6):500–15. https://doi.org/10.1016/S1470-2045(13)70076-7. Epub 2013 Mar 27. Review. PubMed PMID: 23540561.
8. Baluk P, Fuxe J, Hashizume H, Romano T, Lashnits E, Butz S, Vestweber D, Corada M, Molendini C, Dejana E, McDonald DM. Functionally specialized junctions between endothelial cells of lymphatic vessels. J Exp Med. 2007;204(10):2349–62. https://doi.org/10.1084/jem.20062596. Epub 2007 Sep 10. PMID: 17846148; PMCID: PMC2118470.
9. Breslin JW, Yang Y, Scallan JP, Sweat RS, Adderley SP, Murfee WL. Lymphatic vessel network structure and physiology. Compr Physiol. 2018;9(1):207–99. https://doi.org/10.1002/cphy.c180015. Review. PubMed PMID: 30549020; PubMed Central PMCID: PMC6459625.
10. Rubin JP, Neligan PC. Plastic Surgery. 4th rev. ed. Elsevier; 2018. 832 p.
11. Ly CL, Kataru RP, Mehrara BJ. Inflammatory manifestations of lymphedema. Int J Mol Sci. 2017;18(1):171. https://doi.org/10.3390/ijms18010171. PMID: 28106728; PMCID: PMC5297803.
12. Rockson SG. Lymphedema after breast cancer treatment. N Engl J Med. 2018;379(20):1937–44. https://doi.org/10.1056/NEJMcp1803290. Review. PubMed PMID: 30428297.
13. Keeley V. Advances in understanding and management of lymphoedema (cancer, primary). Curr Opin Support Palliat Care. 2017;11(4):355–60. https://doi.org/10.1097/SPC.0000000000000311. Review. PubMed PMID: 28984676.
14. Armer JM, Ballman KV, McCall L, Ostby PL, Zagar E, Kuerer HM, Hunt KK, Boughey JC. Factors associated with lymphedema in women with node-positive breast cancer treated with neoadjuvant chemotherapy and axillary dissection. JAMA Surg. 2019;154(9):800–9. https://doi.org/10.1001/jamasurg.2019.1742. PMID: 31314062; PMCID: PMC6647005.
15. Eyigör S, Cinar E, Caramat I, Unlu BK. Factors influencing response to lymphedema treatment in patients with breast cancer-related lymphedema. Support Care Cancer. 2015;23:2705.
16. McLaughlin SA, DeSnyder SM, Klimberg S, et al. Considerations for clinicians in the diagnosis, prevention, and treatment of breast cancer-related lymphedema: recommendations from an expert panel — Part 2: preventive and therapeutic options. Ann Surg Oncol. 2017;24:2827–35.
17. Larocque G, McDiarmid S. The legacy of lymphedema: Impact on nursing practice and vascular access. Can Oncol Nurs J. 2019;29(3):194–203. eCollection 2019 Summer. PubMed PMID: 31966004; PubMed Central PMCID: PMC6970461.
18. Penn IW, Chang YC, Chuang E, Chen CM, Chung CF, Kuo CY, Chuang TY. Risk factors and prediction model for persistent breast-cancer-related lymphedema: a 5-year cohort study. Support Care Cancer. 2019;27(3):991–1000. https://doi.org/10.1007/s00520-018-4388-6. Epub 2018 Aug 14. PMID: 30105666; PMCID: PMC6373263.
19. Purushotham AD, Upponi S, Klevesath MB, et al. Morbidity after sentinel lymph node biopsy in primary breast cancer: results from a randomized controlled trial. J Clin Oncol. 2005;23:4312.
20. Rausky J, Robert N, Binder JP, Revol M. In search of the ideal surgical treatment for lymphedema. Report of 2nd European Conference on supermicrosurgery (Barcelona – March 2012). Ann Chir Plast Esthet. 2012;57(6):594–9. https://doi.org/10.1016/j.anplas.2012.08.003. Epub 2012 Oct 11. PubMed PMID: 23063020.
21. Buck DW 2nd, Herbst KL. Lipedema: a relatively common disease with extremely common misconceptions. Plast Reconstr Surg Glob Open. 2016;4(9):e1043. https://doi.org/10.1097/GOX.0000000000001043. PMID: 27757353; PMCID: PMC5055019.
22. Norman SA, Localio AR, Potashnik SL, et al. Lymphedema in breast cancer survivors: incidence, degree, time course, treatment, and symptoms. J Clin Oncol. 2009;27:390–7.
23. Taylor R, Jayasinghe UW, Koelmeyer L, Ung O, Boyages J. Reliability and validity of arm volume measurements for assessment of lymphedema. Phys Ther. 2006;86(2):205–14. PubMed PMID: 16445334.
24. Levenhagen K, Davies C, Perdomo M, Ryans K, Gilchrist L. Diagnosis of upper quadrant lymphedema secondary to cancer: clinical practice guideline from the Oncology Section of the American Physical Therapy Association. Phys Ther. 2017;97(7):729–45. https://doi.org/10.1093/ptj/pzx050.
25. Dylke ES, Ward LC, Kilbreath SL. Standardized approach to lymphedema screening. Oncologist.

2013;18(11):1242. https://doi.org/10.1634/theoncologist.2013-0238. PMID: 24218003; PMCID: PMC3825313.
26. Sharkey AR, King SW, Kuo RY, Bickerton SB, Ramsden AJ, Furniss D. Measuring limb volume: accuracy and reliability of tape measurement versus perometer measurement. Lymphat Res Biol. 2018;16(2):182–6. https://doi.org/10.1089/lrb.2017.0039. Epub 2017 Sep 28. PubMed PMID: 28956715.
27. Sun F, Hall A, Tighe MP, Brunelle CL, Sayegh HE, Gillespie TC, Daniell KM, Taghian AG. Perometry versus simulated circumferential tape measurement for the detection of breast cancer-related lymphedema. Breast Cancer Res Treat. 2018;172(1):83–91. https://doi.org/10.1007/s10549-018-4902-z. Epub 2018 Jul 30. PMID: 30062571; PMCID: PMC6191334.
28. Czerniec SA, Ward LC, Lee M, et al. Segmental measurement of breast cancer-related arm lymphoedema using perometry and bioimpedance spectroscopy. Support Care Cancer. 2011;19:703–10. https://doi.org/10.1007/s00520-010-0896-8.
29. International Society of Lymphology. The diagnosis and treatment of peripheral lymphedema: 2013 consensus document of the International Society of Lymphology. Lymphology. 2013;46:1–11.
30. Keilani M, Haenorhl T, Neubauer M, Crevenna R. Resistance exercise and secondary lymphedema in breast cancer survivors a systematic review. Support Care Cancer. 2016;24(4):1907–16.
31. Nelson NL. Breast cancer related lymphedema and resistance exercise- a systematic review. J Strength Cond Res. 2016;30(9):2656–65.
32. Wu R, Huang X, Dong X, Zhang H, Zhnag L. Obese Patients have a higher incidence of lymphedema after breast cancer than overweight ones- a meta-analysis. Ann Transl Med. 2019;7(8):172. https://doi.org/10.21037/atm.2019.03.44.
33. Dieli-Conwright CM, Orozco BZ. Exercise after breast cancer treatment- current perspectives. Breast Cancer (Dove Med Press). 2015;7:353–62.
34. Zuther JE, Norton S. Lymphedema management. Thieme Publishers; 2018.
35. Masià J, Pons G, Rodríguez-Bauzà E. Barcelona lymphedema algorithm for surgical treatment in breast cancer-related lymphedema. J Reconstr Microsurg. 2016;32:329–35.
36. Mihara M, Hara H, Araki J, Kikuchi K, Narushima M, Yamamoto T, Iida T, Yoshimatsu H, Murai N, Mitsui K, Okitsu T, Koshima I. Indocyanine green (ICG) lymphography is superior to lymphoscintigraphy for diagnostic imaging of early lymphedema of the upper limbs. PLoS One. 2012;7(6):e38182. https://doi.org/10.1371/journal.pone.0038182. Epub 2012 Jun 4. PMID: 22675520; PMCID: PMC3366958.
37. Mazzei FG, Gentili F, Guerrini S, Cioffi Squitieri N, Guerrieri D, Gennaro P, Scialpi M, Volterrani L, Mazzei MA. MR lymphangiography: a practical guide to perform it and a brief review of the literature from a technical point of view. Biomed Res Int. 2017;2017:2598358. https://doi.org/10.1155/2017/2598358. Epub 2017 Mar 7. PubMed PMID: 28367439; PubMed Central PMCID: PMC5359436.
38. Forte AJ, Boczar D, Huayllani MT, Lu X, Ciudad P. Lymphoscintigraphy for evaluation of lymphedema treatment: a systematic review. Cureus. 2019;11(12):e6363. https://doi.org/10.7759/cureus.6363. Review. PubMed PMID: 31886094; PubMed Central PMCID: PMC6907718.
39. Badash I, Gould DJ, Patel KM. Supermicrosurgery: history, applications, training and the future. Front Surg. 2018;5:23. https://doi.org/10.3389/fsurg.2018.00023. PMID: 29740586; PMCID: PMC5931174.
40. Sapountzis S, Ciudad P, Lim SY, Chilgar RM, Kiranantawat K, Nicoli F, Constantinides J, Wei MY, Sönmez TT, Singhal D, Chen HC. Modified Charles procedure and lymph node flap transfer for advanced lower extremity lymphedema. Microsurgery. 2014;34(6):439–47. https://doi.org/10.1002/micr.22235. Epub 2014 Feb 14. PubMed PMID: 24677042.
41. Garza R 3rd, Skoracki R, Hock K, Povoski SP. A comprehensive overview on the surgical management of secondary lymphedema of the upper and lower extremities related to prior oncologic therapies. BMC Cancer. 2017;17(1):468. https://doi.org/10.1186/s12885-017-3444-9. PMID: 28679373; PMCID: PMC5497342.
42. Brorson H. Liposuction in lymphedema treatment. J Reconstr Microsurg. 2016;32(01):56–65.
43. Schaverien MV, Coroneos CJ. Surgical treatment of lymphedema. Plast Reconstr Surg. 2019;144(3):738–58. https://doi.org/10.1097/PRS.0000000000005993. Review. PubMed PMID: 31461041.
44. Carl HM, Walia G, Bello R, Clarke-Pearson E, Hassanein AH, Cho B, Pedreira R, Sacks JM. Systematic review of the surgical treatment of extremity lymphedema. J Reconstr Microsurg. 2017;33(6):412–25. https://doi.org/10.1055/s--0037-1599100. Epub 2017 Feb 24. Review. PubMed PMID: 28235214.
45. 106th Congress. PUBLIC LAW 106–354—OCT. 24, 2000.
46. Scaglioni MF, Fontein DBY, Arvanitakis M, Giovanoli P. Systematic review of lymphovenous anastomosis (LVA) for the treatment of lymphedema. Microsurgery. 2017;37(8):947–53. https://doi.org/10.1002/micr.30246. Epub 2017 Oct 3. Review. PubMed PMID: 28972280.
47. Cornelissen AJM, Kool M, Lopez Penha TR, Keuter XHA, Piatkowski AA, Heuts E, van der Hulst RRWJ, Qiu SS. Lymphatico-venous anastomosis as treatment for breast cancer-related lymphedema: a prospective study on quality of life. Breast Cancer Res Treat. 2017;163(2):281–6. https://doi.org/10.1007/s10549-017-4180-1. Epub 2017 Mar 7. PubMed PMID: 28265793; PubMed Central PMCID: PMC5410204.
48. Schaverien MV, Badash I, Patel KM, Selber JC, Cheng MH. Vascularized lymph node transfer for lymphedema. Semin Plast Surg. 2018;32(1):28–35.

https://doi.org/10.1055/s-0038-1632401. Epub 2018 Apr 9. Review. PubMed PMID: 29636651; PubMed Central PMCID: PMC5891655.
49. Mesli SN, Ghouali AK, Benamara F, Taleb FA, Tahraoui H, Abi-Ayad C. Stewart-Treves syndrome involving chronic lymphedema after mastectomy of breast cancer. Case Rep Surg. 2017;2017:4056459. https://doi.org/10.1155/2017/4056459. Epub 2017 Feb 9. PMID: 28280645; PMCID: PMC5322458.
50. Sharma A, Schwartz RA. Stewart-Treves syndrome: pathogenesis and management. J Am Acad Dermatol. 2012;67(6):1342–8. https://doi.org/10.1016/j.jaad.2012.04.028. Epub 2012 Jun 8. PMID: 22682884.
51. Cui L, Zhang J, Zhang X, Chang H, Qu C, Zhang J, Zhong D. Angiosarcoma (Stewart-Treves syndrome) in postmastectomy patients: report of 10 cases and review of literature. Int J Clin Exp Pathol. 2015;8(9):11108–15. PMID: 26617830; PMCID: PMC4637645.
52. Denigrim AC, Miller J, Hoskin TL, et al. A prospective study of breast lymphedema-frequency, symptoms and quality of life. Breast Cancer Res Treat. 2012;134(3):915–22.
53. Staren ED, Klepec S, Smith AP, Hartsell WF, Segretti J, Witt TR, Griem KL, Bines SD. The dilemma of delayed cellulitis after breast conservation therapy. Arch Surgery. 1996;131(6):651–4. Pub Med: 8645074.
54. Baddour LM. Breast Cellulitis complicating breast conservation therapy. J Intern Med. 1999;245(1):5–9. Pub Med: 10095811.
55. Boughey JC, Hoskin TL, Cheville AL, Miller J, Loprinzi MD, Thomsen KM, Maloney S, Baddour LM, Degnim MD. Risk factors associated with breast lymphedema following breast surgery. Ann Surg Oncologia. 2014;21(4):1202–8. https://doi.org/10.1245/s10434-013-3408-5.
56. Young-Afat DA, Gregorowitsch ML, van den Bongard DH, Burgmans I, van der Pol CC, Witkamp AJ, Biljsma RM, Koelemij R, Schoemakers EJ, Jonasse Y, van Gils CH, Varkooijen HM. Breast edema following breast conserving surgery and radiotherapy: patient-reported prevalence, determinants and effect on health-related quality of life. JNCI Cancer Spectrum. 2019;3(2):pkz011. https://doi.org/10.1093/jncics/pkz011.
57. Finnerty S, Thomason S, Woods M. Audit the use of kinesiotape for breast oedema. J lymphoedema. 2010;5:38–44.
58. Gregorwitsch ML, Van den Bongard DH, Batenburg MC, Van de Grootevheen MJ, Fuhler N, Van het Westeinde T, Van der Pol CC, Young-Afat DA, Verkijooen HM. Compression vest treatment for symptomatic breast edema in women treated for breast cancer: a pilot study. Lymph Res Bio. 2020; https://doi.org/10.1089/lrb.2018.0067.
59. Nguyen AT, Chang EI, Suami H, Chang DW. An algorithmic approach to simultaneous vascularized lymph node transfer with microvascular breast reconstruction. Ann Surg Oncol. 2015;22(9):2919–24. https://doi.org/10.1245/s10434-015-4408-4. Epub 2015 Jan 27. PubMed PMID: 25623599.
60. Ahmadzadeh N, Robering JW, Kengelbach-Weigand A, Al-Abboodi M, Beier JP, Horch RE, Boos AM. Human adipose-derived stem cells support lymphangiogenesis in vitro by secretion of lymphangiogenic factors. Exp Cell Res. 2020:111816. https://doi.org/10.1016/j.yexcr.2020.111816. [Epub ahead of print] PubMed PMID: 31923426.
61. Schaverien MV, Aldrich MB. New and emerging treatments for lymphedema. Semin Plast Surg. 2018;32(1):48–52. https://doi.org/10.1055/s--0038-1632403. Epub 2018 Apr 9. PMID: 29636654; PMCID: PMC5891649.
62. Soran A, Ozmen T, McGuire KP, et al. The importance of detection of subclinical lymphedema for the prevention of breast cancer-related clinical lymphedema after axillary lymph node dissection; a prospective observational study. Lymphat Res Biol. 2014;12:289–94.
63. Rietman JS, Dijlkstra PU, Hoekstra HJ, Eisma WH, Szabo BG, Groothoff JW, JHB G. Late morbidity after treatment of breast cancer in relation to daily activities and quality of life: a system. Eur J Surg Oncol. 2003;29(3):229–38. https://doi.org/10.1053/ejso.20021403.
64. Van Kampen DGA, Dieltjens M, E. Christiaens MR. Neven P. Geraerts I. Devoogdt N. Effectiveness of post-operative physical therapy for upper limb impairments after breast cancer treatment: a systematic review. Arch Phys Med Rehab. 2015;6:2015–23. https://doi.org/10.1111/j.1365-2354.2009.01141x.
65. Niljs J, Torres-Cueco R, van Wilgen CP, et al. Applying modern pain neuroscience in clinical practice: criteria for classification of central sensitization pain. Pain Physician. 2014;17:447–57.
66. Nijs J, Leysen L, Pas R, et al. Treatment of pain following cancer: applying neuroimmunology in rehabilitation practice. Disabil Rehabil. 2018;40:714–21. https://doi.org/10.1080/09638288.2016.1261418.
67. Brookham RL, Cudlip AC, Dickerson CR. Examining upper limb kinetics and dysfunction of breast cancer survivors in functional dynamic tasks. Clin Biomech. 2018;55:86–93. https://doi.org/10.1016/clinbiomech.2018.126418.
68. Giacolone A, Alessandria P, Ruberti E. The physiotherapy intervention for shoulder pin in patients with breast cancer: systematic review. Cureus. 11(12):e6416. https://doi.org/10.7759/cureus.6416.
69. Capuco A, Urits I, Orhurhu V, Chun R, Shukla B, Burke M, Kaye AD, Viswanath O. A comprehensive review of diagnosis, treatment and management of postmastectomy pain syndrome. Curr Pan Headache Rep. 2020;24:41.
70. Olsson MU, Beck I, Ryden L, Malmstrom M. A comprehensive approach to rehabilitation interventions following breast cancer treatment a systematic review of systematic reviews. BMC Cancer. 2019;19:472. https://doi.org/10.1186/s12885-019-5648-7.

Bone Loss

15

Patrick B. Cacchio, Jennie Petruney, and Kenneth W. Lyles

Introduction

Due to continuous improvements in early detection and treatment, the number of breast cancer survivors has grown steadily over the past three decades. Five-year survival rates now eclipse 90%, though significant regional and ethnic disparities exist [1]. Estimates suggest that there are over three million breast cancer survivors in the USA with over 70% of these aged 60 and older [2]. While historically most of these patients have been followed closely by oncology teams, given the growing number of survivors, much of their health care will now ultimately be delivered through primary care [3]. The majority of breast cancer survivors will have received a combination of surgical, radiation, and chemotherapy treatments for their cancer, many with long-term effects as discussed elsewhere in this text. The net effects of these treatments often result in a significant loss of bone mass, such as that from local radiation effects, premature menopause from oophorectomy or chemotherapy, and increased resorption due to adjuvant endocrine therapies.

Therefore, it is not a surprising finding that breast cancer survivors have a significantly increased risk of clinical fractures [4]. Studies have shown fragility fracture rates as high as 13.6% over a 5-year period [5]. In particular, breast cancer survivors may have as high as a 20-fold increased risk of vertebral fracture, even among those without skeletal metastases [6]. Fractures are significant clinical events that incur high morbidity, resulting in chronic pain, deformity, and loss of function. It has been shown that after hip fracture, only 50% of patients will regain their pre-fracture level of activity and independence; in addition, 10–20% of patients will become institutionalized after hip fracture [7]. Most importantly, numerous studies have shown mortality rates of as high as 25% in the first year after hip fracture [7]. Breast cancer survivors with history of a pre-existing fragility fracture have also been shown to have decreased survival [8].

Despite the established association between breast cancer, bone loss, fractures, and survival, several gaps in screening and treatment exist. Joint ACS and ASCO guidelines recommend a baseline dual-energy X-ray absorptiometry (DXA) screening for all postmenopausal breast cancer survivors, as well as baseline screening for premenopausal women treated with selective estrogen receptor modulators (SERMs) [9]. Follow-up DXA is recommended every 2 years

P. B. Cacchio (✉)
Duke University Department of Medicine, Durham, NC, USA
e-mail: patrick.cacchio@duke.edu

J. Petruney
Duke University Cancer Center, Durham, NC, USA

K. W. Lyles
Duke University School of Medicine, Durham VA Medical Center, Durham, NC, USA

G. G. Kimmick et al. (eds.), *Common Issues in Breast Cancer Survivors*,
https://doi.org/10.1007/978-3-030-75377-1_15

in these populations. Unfortunately, recent studies suggest that less than half of these highest-risk patients are appropriately screened with DXA, and treatment rates are similarly low [10]. Therefore, opportunity exists for clinicians to improve screening and treatment practices to further improve clinical outcomes for breast cancer survivors.

Pathophysiology

Estrogen plays an important role in the growth of bone and maintenance of skeletal strength. The net actions of estrogen cause essentially a decrease in bone resorption, primarily by causing a decrease in osteoclast precursors and an increase in osteoclast apoptosis [11]. These actions occur predominantly through signaling at the estrogen receptors, alpha and beta. In contrast, estrogen deficiency, such as in the post-menopausal state, causes a net increase in bone resorption. Therefore, breast cancer survivors who undergo premature menopause induced by surgery or chemotherapy are at risk for significant bone loss. In premenopausal women treated with gonadotropin-releasing hormone (GnRH) agonists, pituitary gonadotropins are reduced, and the resulting hypogonadism induces bone loss [12]. Similarly, use of aromatase inhibitors, which block conversion of androgens to estrogen and result in estrogen deprivation, also results in net bone loss. This has been confirmed in clinical trials, where results have shown not only a decrease in bone density in patients treated with aromatase inhibitors but also an increase in fracture risk [13–15]. Similar rates of bone loss and fracture have been shown with both steroidal and nonsteroidal aromatase inhibitors [16].

Limited data also suggests an association between chemotherapy regimens and bone loss [17]. The etiology of bone loss during chemotherapy remains unclear, but is likely due to a combination of ovarian dysfunction, effects of the chemotherapy itself on slowing bone turnover, renal dysfunction, as well as increased bone resorption and decreased bone formation from supportive therapies such as glucocorticoids [12].

Radiation therapy is also associated with bone injury, with predominantly local effects occurring within the irradiated field. This occurs secondary to changes in the bone microenvironment, resulting in fibrosis and osteoblast and osteoclast imbalances [12]. Therefore, it is not surprising that in breast cancer survivors receiving radiation, an increase in low-trauma rib fractures has been reported [5].

Some data also suggests that patients with hormone receptor-positive breast cancer may have occult disseminated tumor cells within bone. While the process of metastatic spread is complex, there is evidence that the presence of tumor cells in bone likely correlates with relapse [18]. Therefore, it might be expected that adjuvant bone-directed therapies could have beneficial effects on both skeletal-related events and disease-free survival for breast cancer survivors.

Clinical Evaluation

To accurately assess an individual's bone health and fracture risk as they transition from active treatment to surveillance and survivorship, a carefully updated medical history is essential. While net bone loss is expected to occur during adult life, it can also occur as a result of secondary processes such as diseases and medications. Peak bone mass is achieved by the third decade of life [19]. Therefore, poor nutrition, concomitant disease, or prolonged amenorrhea in females may negatively affect peak bone mass accrual. In addition, as many as one fourth of adults with osteoporosis may have secondary processes influencing their skeletal status and fracture risk. A list of secondary causes of bone loss are listed in Table 15.1. Surgical history, particularly as it may pertain to previous fractures or bony abnormalities, may also be revealing, as well as a history of bariatric procedures, which can lead to bone loss and secondary hyperparathyroidism from malabsorption.

Table 15.1 Secondary causes of osteoporosis including pertinent testing

	Condition	Pertinent testing
Endocrine disorders	Hypercalciuria Hypercortisolism Hyperparathyroidism Hyperthyroidism Hypogonadism Panhypopituitarism Type 1 and type 2 diabetes mellitus	24-hour urine studies for calcium, cortisol, and creatinine Dexamethasone suppression testing Midnight salivary cortisol Intact parathyroid hormone and ionized calcium Thyroid stimulating hormone (TSH) and free thyroxine (T4) Follicle stimulating hormone, luteinizing hormone, estradiol Morning fasting total testosterone Prolactin Hemoglobin A1c, fasting blood glucose
Gastrointestinal disorders	Celiac disease Cirrhosis Gastric bypass Inflammatory bowel disease Primary biliary cirrhosis	TTG-IgA testing Hepatic function panel Gamma-glutamyl transferase Esophagogastroduodenoscopy Colonoscopy
Genetic and connective tissue disorders	Ankylosing spondylitis Ehlers-Danlos syndrome Gaucher disease Marfan syndrome Osteogenesis imperfecta Pompe disease Rheumatoid arthritis	Genetic testing as clinically indicated
Hematologic disorders	Hemochromatosis Mastocytosis Multiple myeloma Sickle cell disease Thalassemia	Complete blood count Iron studies Serum tryptase Serum and urine protein electrophoresis
Nutritional deficiencies	Anorexia nervosa, bulimia Calcium Magnesium Vitamin D	Serum calcium and albumin Serum magnesium 25-OH vitamin D
Medications	Antiepileptics Depot medroxyprogesterone acetate Glucocorticoids Gonadotropin-releasing hormone agonists Heparin Immunosuppressants: Cyclosporine, tacrolimus Methotrexate Proton pump inhibitors Selective serotonin reuptake inhibitors	Pharmacy records
Other	Alcohol Tobacco Heart failure Cystic fibrosis End stage renal disease Immobilization Multiple sclerosis Amyloidosis Sarcoidosis Pregnancy-associated osteoporosis Transient osteoporosis	Ethanol Nicotine Brain natriuretic peptide Creatinine Bone biopsy Magnetic resonance imaging 1,25-dihyroxyvitamin D Angiotensin converting enzyme Chest x-ray

Family history is an important determinant of one's fracture risk, as current estimates indicate as much as two-thirds of peak bone mass is genetically determined [19]. Therefore, a family history of osteoporosis is predictive of an individual's bone density. In addition, a history of hip fracture in either parent has been shown to be a strong independent risk factor for osteoporotic fracture [20].

Similarly, a personal history of low-trauma fracture has been shown to be a powerful predictor of subsequent fracture [21]. Low-trauma fractures are defined as fractures involving the force from a standing height fall or less. These most commonly affect the vertebrae, proximal femur, distal forearm, and proximal humerus. In addition, data would suggest that the ribs, proximal tibia, and pelvis are also prone to fragility fractures. Recent studies have shown that the risk for subsequent fracture is highest within the first 2 years following a low-trauma fracture [22].

Physical examination is helpful to indicate the presence of osteoporotic fracture but also may potentially identify secondary processes influencing bone health. Height loss, best measured with a calibrated device such as stadiometer, of greater than 4 cm from maximum reported adult height is predictive of vertebral fracture [23]. In addition, the rib-to-pelvis distance and wall-to-occiput measurements have also been well-correlated with the presence of existing vertebral compression fractures [24]. Lateral x-rays of the thoracic and lumbar spine can confirm the presence of vertebral compression fractures. Other examples of physical exam findings pertinent to fracture risk would include such observations such as bony tenderness associated with osteomalacia, blue sclerae seen with osteogenesis imperfecta, facial plethora and striae of Cushing syndrome, and goiter or proptosis from hyperthyroidism. In addition, functional testing such as sit-to-stand and gait analysis can be helpful to identify patients at high risk for falls and fracture, or those who might benefit most from formal physical therapy assessment.

Laboratory studies are useful as an adjunct to the evaluation of the bone health of breast cancer survivors. Standard chemistries to evaluate renal and liver function, as well as serum calcium and 25-OH vitamin D levels, are recommended as part of the initial evaluation. Many clinics also screen for hypercalciuria and hypocalciuira with 24-hour urine calcium studies, as these conditions can negatively impact bone health. As clinically indicated, we recommend measuring intact parathyroid hormone levels to screen for primary or secondary hyperparathyroidism, thyroid function testing for hyperthyroidism, serum phosphorus levels for hypophosphatemic disorders, alkaline phosphatase levels for hypophosphatasia, urinary 24-hour cortisol levels for Cushing syndrome, and serum/urine protein electrophoresis for multiple myeloma. Recent guidelines suggest potential utility of serum and urinary bone turnover markers, including bone-specific alkaline phosphatase, procollagen type 1 N-terminal propeptide, C-terminal telopeptide, and N-terminal telopeptide, in the assessment of osteoporosis treatment response or adherence, though optimal parameters for monitoring remain unclear due to diurnal variability, effects of food, and interassay differences [25].

Dual-energy X-ray absorptiometry (DXA) remains the gold standard imaging modality for the diagnosis of osteoporosis. This is primarily due to its ability to predict fractures, wide availability, low cost, low radiation dose, and the presence of robust normative databases [26]. Commonly measured sites include the lumbar spine and proximal femur, since these sites appear to correlate best with fracture risk [27]. Conditions such as hyperparathyroidism and malabsorption may induce more cortical bone loss, and therefore if clinically indicated, the distal forearm may also be included in a DXA study [28]. For postmenopausal women, the T-score, which is a comparison to the young adult mean, is used for diagnosis. A T-score at the spine, femoral neck, total hip, or distal third of the radius of less than or equal to −2.5 is diagnostic of osteoporosis. T-score values at any of the same sites between −1.0 and −2.5

are classified as osteopenia or low bone mass. The lowest T-score is utilized for diagnosis. For premenopausal women, a Z-score is utilized for diagnosis, which represents a comparison to a healthy age, gender, and ethnic-matched mean. A Z-score at any site less than −2.0 is considered to be low bone density for age. Advances in imaging technology such as trabecular bone scores (TBS), vertebral fracture assessment (VFA), and quantitative computed tomography (QcT) can be additive to DXA measurements in certain populations, though are currently limited by cost, availability, and radiation exposure in the case of QcT. While DXA remains the gold standard for assessment of bone density, it is important to note that errors are not uncommon due to a combination of technical aspects as well as inconsistencies in analysis [29]. Therefore, it is paramount that clinicians have an understanding of the high-quality DXA standards as set forth by the International Society for Clinical Densitometry (ISCD). It is recommended that clinicians review actual DXA scan images to differentiate technical problems such as artifacts or positioning errors, from clinically significant biological changes in bone density.

In addition to DXA assessment, several fracture risk prediction models exist, with the most widely utilized being FRAX. FRAX is a computer-based algorithm made publicly available through the World Health Organization (https://www.sheffield.ac.uk/FRAX/). It utilizes easily obtained clinical risk factors such as fracture history, parenteral history of hip fracture, and glucocorticoid use, along with femoral neck BMD, to provide individualized 10-year risk of osteoporotic fracture. The algorithm is able to adjust for observed differences among fracture rates between countries and in the USA, among ethnicities. In the USA, guidance exists to institute pharmacologic treatment based on specific thresholds, which are currently 20% for major osteoporotic fracture or 3% for hip fracture. The predictive value of FRAX has been replicated in breast cancer survivors, including those receiving aromatase inhibitor therapy [30].

Management of Bone Loss and Fracture Risk

Lifestyle Modification

In many regards, the first step in addressing the bone health of breast cancer survivors is to ensure appropriate lifestyle modifications to reduce further bone loss and fracture risk. While some debate exists regarding the utility of various supplements, most clinicians support the recommendation for adequate intake of calcium and vitamin D as important for bone health. Current guidelines recommend daily calcium intake of 1200 mg for women, which can be obtained from any combination of dietary sources and/or supplements [31]. Available data does not demonstrate increased cardiovascular risk at this level of daily calcium intake [32], though there is a concern for risk of nephrolithiasis with calcium supplements in certain individuals, and therefore dietary calcium is preferred for those with a history of nephrolithiasis [33]. Adequate vitamin D intake is necessary for calcium absorption, as well as bone and muscle health; the Institute of Medicine advocates for serum 25OH-D levels of at least 20 ng/mL, while other guidelines would recommend maintenance of levels >30 ng/mL in those with osteoporosis [31]. For most patients, daily intake of 800–1000 units of vitamin D should be sufficient, though for those with lower baseline levels, doses as high as 4000 units daily may be required and are considered safe. Available data suggests a potential reduction in fractures with vitamin D and calcium [34], though this has not been demonstrated in breast cancer survivors [35].

As a majority of osteoporotic fractures occur from falls, a comprehensive falls risk assessment is essential for the management of breast cancer survivors at increased risk for fracture. This may consist of any combination of functional testing by the clinician, formal physical therapy assessment, home-based occupational therapy evaluation, as well as vision and hearing studies. A combination of regular weight-bearing and muscle-strengthening exercise is recommended and has demonstrated beneficial effects in breast cancer survivors [36].

Weight-bearing exercise may include modalities such as walking, jogging, elliptical machines, tennis, dance, step aerobics, and Tai Chi. Common resistance exercises include utilization of light weights, resistance bands, yoga, and Pilates. For patients with osteoporosis and especially those with a history of vertebral fractures, formal physical therapy guidance for instruction on proper spine mechanics can be particularly helpful prior to initiating an exercise program.

Additional lifestyle modifications for fracture risk reduction include appropriate counseling and referrals for smoking and alcohol cessation, as both have been shown to be independent predictors of fracture and are incorporated into the FRAX assessment. The negative health effects of smoking are well-described, and alcohol intake of greater than 2 drinks per day has also demonstrated negative skeletal effects.

Pharmacologic Treatment

The decision to initiate pharmacologic treatment for bone protection remains individualized, though an extensive literature exists to support the efficacy of various medications to prevent bone loss and fracture and to potentially improve survival for breast cancer survivors. A list of available pharmacologic treatments is included in Table 15.2, with a proposed algorithm for breast cancer survivors on adjuvant aromatase inhibitor therapy provided in Fig. 15.1.

Table 15.2 Available bone-directed medications studied in breast cancer survivors

Class	Agents	Advantages	Disadvantages
Selective estrogen receptor modulators (SERMs)	Tamoxifen Raloxifene	Reduction in breast cancer recurrence (tamoxifen only) Prevention of breast cancer in high-risk patients Prevention of bone loss in postmenopausal patients Fracture prevention in breast cancer survivors (tamoxifen only)	Bone loss in premenopausal women Risk of thromboembolism Bone loss with discontinuation
Oral bisphosphonates	Alendronate Risedronate Ibandronate	Prevention of bone loss Well-tolerated Cost-effective Potential survival benefits in postmenopausal patients Potential persistent bone protection with discontinuation	Lack of fracture prevention data in breast cancer survivors Poor compliance
Parenteral bisphosphonates	Zoledronic acid	Prevention of bone loss in breast cancer survivors Fracture prevention in breast cancer survivors Demonstrated survival benefit Well-tolerated Good compliance Cost-effective Potential persistent bone protection with discontinuation	Potential acute phase reaction Risk of osteonecrosis of the jaw and atypical femur fractures Contraindicated in renal insufficiency (CrCl <35 mL/min)
RANKL inhibitor	Denosumab	Prevention of bone loss in breast cancer survivors Fracture prevention in breast cancer survivors Potential disease-free survival benefit Well-tolerated Good-compliance Generally safe in patients with renal insufficiency	Rebound bone loss and vertebral fracture with discontinuation Potential immunosuppression Risk of osteonecrosis of the jaw and atypical femur fracture Cost

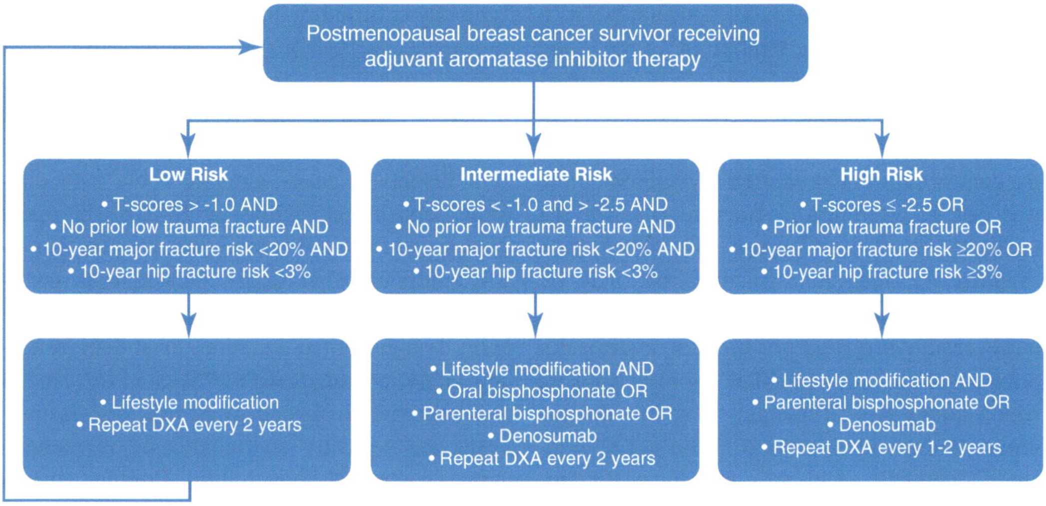

Fig. 15.1 Potential algorithm for treatment of postmenopausal breast cancer survivors receiving aromatase inhibitor treatment

Selective Estrogen Receptor Modulators (SERMs)

Selective estrogen receptor modulators (SERMs) have long been shown to prevent osteoporosis in postmenopausal women. With respect to breast cancer prevention and treatment, tamoxifen, a first-generation SERM is primarily used to reduce breast cancer recurrence in women with a history of hormone positive breast cancer. It has also been shown to be effective as chemoprevention in women at high risk of developing breast cancer [37]. Raloxifene, a second-generation SERM is used as chemoprevention in high-risk women but has not been shown to reduce recurrence risk in women with a history of breast cancer [38].

Tamoxifen has estrogenic effects in some tissue, such as the endometrium, bone, and cardiovascular system, while antiestrogenic in others, such as breast cells. For this reason, tamoxifen is regarded to be relatively bone protective while also reducing breast cancer recurrence risk. There is evidence to support improvements in bone mineral density (BMD) for postmenopausal women receiving tamoxifen as a treatment for breast cancer. A prospective study of 140 women randomized to tamoxifen vs placebo and found the mean bone mineral density in the lumbar spine increased by 0.61 percent compared to a decrease of 1.0 percent per year in the placebo group [39]. Even more striking, data from the NASBP Breast Cancer Prevention Trial including 13,388 women found a 32% reduction in osteoporotic fractures in postmenopausal women taking tamoxifen vs placebo at 7-year follow-up [37].

Unfortunately, the bone effect of tamoxifen differs in premenopausal women. Although tamoxifen acts like estrogen in the bones of postmenopausal women, it may antagonize the more potent activity of endogenous estrogen in premenopausal women. Tamoxifen, compared to placebo, decreases bone density in the hip and spine of premenopausal women [40]. For young women with a history of breast cancer receiving the LHRH agonist goserelin, BMD decreased significantly compared to the control arm. For women on combined LHRH agonist and tamoxifen and for women receiving tamoxifen alone, BMD still was shown to be significantly decreased compared to the control group; however the decrease was less than with ovarian suppression alone [41].

Additional evidence of a differential effect for tamoxifen in premenopausal women comes from a large statistical analysis involving greater than 11,000 women. The study evaluating 5520 women between the ages of 18 and 90 with breast cancer receiving tamoxifen vs 5520 age matched healthy controls reveals that the cumulative incidence of fractures was 6.5% for premenopausal women on tamoxifen vs 3.6% in the control group. For women ages 55–90, there was not a difference in fracture risk for the tamoxifen vs control groups [42]. This study supports the idea that fracture risk may be higher for premenopausal women on tamoxifen; however the investigators did not control for prior chemotherapy or LHRH agonist exposure which could also accelerate bone loss in this group. Unfortunately, this trial did not demonstrate a decrease in fracture risk for postmenopausal women with tamoxifen use. Nonetheless others have found a potential fracture risk reduction related to tamoxifen use [37].

Raloxifene has been shown to have antiestrogenic effects on breast and endometrial tissue and estrogenic effects on bone, lipid metabolism, and blood clotting. Raloxifene is approved for the prevention of osteoporosis in postmenopausal women and has been found to reduce the risk of invasive breast cancer in high-risk women [38, 43]. Raloxifene however is not indicated as adjuvant therapy in women with a history of breast cancer.

Oral Bisphosphonates

The oral bisphosphonates alendronate, risedronate, and ibandronate have been studied and used for the treatment of postmenopausal osteoporosis for the past three decades. They are widely available, cost-effective, and available for daily, weekly, or monthly dosing. Due to potential for esophagitis and generally poor drug absorption, these medications must be administered on an empty stomach with water, and patients are advised to remain upright for at least 30 minutes after each dose. In general, they are well-tolerated, though upper gastrointestinal and musculoskeletal adverse effects are not uncommon. With long-term use, there is increased risk for osteonecrosis of the jaw and atypical femur fracture, though these risks remain low and are typically eclipsed by the benefit of reducing the high risk of osteoporotic fracture for most patients undergoing treatment. However, due to concerns regarding these rare adverse effects, as well as inconvenient dosing, compliance with oral bisphosphonates remains poor, with one-year persistence as low as 20–30% in many instances [44]. Oral bisphosphonates are generally contraindicated for patients with renal insufficiency and creatinine clearance (CrCl) <35 mL/min, though limited data does exist demonstrating safety in patients with GFR <35 [45]. Due to the potential for esophagitis, oral bisphosphonates are typically contraindicated in patients with esophageal dysmotility, stricture, or an inability to remain upright after dosing. In the postmenopausal population, alendronate and risedronate have demonstrated efficacy in reducing both vertebral and nonvertebral fractures, while ibandronate has shown a significant reduction in vertebral fracture risk. All three oral bisphosphonates have been well-studied in breast cancer survivors, and in particular patients undergoing adjuvant aromatase inhibitor therapy. Alendronate has been shown to prevent aromatase-inhibitor associated bone loss [46], as has risedronate [47, 48] and ibandronate [49, 50]. It is notable that most studies of oral bisphosphonates were not powered to demonstrate fracture risk reduction in breast cancer survivors, though risedronate has demonstrated improvements in quality of life outcomes [51]. Most importantly, however, cohort studies and pooled analyses suggest a potential survival benefit for breast cancer survivors treated with oral bisphosphonates [52, 53]; this effect is most pronounced in postmenopausal patients [54]. In the postmenopausal osteoporosis setting, a treatment holiday is often considered for lower-risk patients after 5 years of treatment with an oral bisphosphonate based on available data [55], though continued treatment may be considered for higher-risk patients. Data is currently lacking regarding the value of a bisphosphonate treatment holiday for breast cancer survivors, though intuitively these patients would remain at high risk of bone loss as long as they remain on an aromatase inhibitor.

Parenteral Bisphosphonates

While ibandronate and pamidronate are available in parenteral formulations, zoledronic acid remains the predominant parenteral bisphosphonate used in the clinical setting, and this use is supported by substantial clinical trial data within the breast cancer survivor population. In these patients, typical protocols advocate for use of 4 mg of zoledronic acid dosed either every 6, 12, or 18 months. However, due to institutional, population, and protocol differences, the optimal dosing of zoledronic acid in breast cancer survivors remains somewhat unclear. Multiple large trials have consistently demonstrated efficacy for zoledronic acid at prevention of aromatase-inhibitor associated bone loss in post- [56–59] and pre-menopausal women [60]. More recently, randomized clinical trial data has demonstrated a significant reduction in fracture rate in breast cancer survivors treated with zoledronic acid [61]. As with oral bisphosphonates, pooled clinical trial data is suggestive of potential disease-free and overall survival benefits for zoledronic acid within postmenopausal breast cancer survivors [53, 54, 62]. These benefits appear to be independent of ER status, tumor grade, and level of bone density, but have not been demonstrated within a premenopausal breast cancer survivor population [54]. It is also particularly noteworthy that within patients who have recently suffered a hip fracture, zoledronic acid has demonstrated a substantial mortality benefit [63], perhaps making it a preferred treatment in that specific clinical setting. Zoledronic acid is typically contraindicated in patients with CrCl <35 mL/min, though reduced dosing can be considered in certain situations; it also should not be utilized in patients with hypocalcemia. The most common adverse effect to zoledronic acid is an acute phase reaction consisting of fever, myalgias, and fatigue, which occurs within 3 days of administration and typically resolves within 14 days; it has been reported in as many as 25% of patients. Recent data has demonstrated that prior oral bisphosphonate use, vitamin D sufficiency, and slower infusion rates may all be protective against the acute phase reaction, which is also less frequent with subsequent treatments [64]. As with oral bisphosphonates, there are rare incidences of osteonecrosis of the jaw and atypical femur fractures reported with zoledronic acid, with higher risk likely seen due to the more potent nature of the drug. Also as with oral bisphosphonates, treatment holidays are often considered for low-risk non-cancer patients after 5 years of therapy [55], though again, definitive data is lacking to guide this decision-making regarding frequency and duration of bisphosphonate in the breast cancer survivor population.

Denosumab

Denosumab is a monoclonal antibody to receptor activator of nuclear factor kappa-beta ligand (RANKL) administered by subcutaneous injection. In the osteoporosis and breast cancer survivor populations, denosumab is dosed every 6 months. The efficacy of denosumab in the breast cancer survivor population is supported primarily by two clinical trials, HALT-BC and ABCSG-18. The HALT-BC trial was the first to demonstrate a BMD benefit for breast cancer survivors treated with denosumab and adjuvant aromatase inhibitors [65]. More recently, the ABCSG-18 study has demonstrated a clear fracture benefit, as well as potential disease-free survival benefits in those with ER+/PR+ cancer with use of denosumab [66, 67]. Denosumab is typically well-tolerated, though can cause significant hypocalcemia, and those with renal insufficiency are at highest risk of this complication. As RANKL is expressed in lymphocytes, inhibition with denosumab can lead to immunosuppression, and an increase in infections has been seen in clinical trials of immunosuppressed patients with denosumab [68]. As with other antiresorptive therapies, both osteonecrosis of the jaw and atypical femur fractures have also been reported with denosumab. Perhaps of greatest clinical significance is the observation of rapid bone loss and the risk of multiple vertebral fractures with abrupt discontinuation of denosumab [69, 70]. For this reason, a holiday from denosumab is not recommended [71]. Current data has demonstrated safety and efficacy for up to 10 years of continuous use of denosumab in the postmenopausal osteoporosis population [72]. The optimal strategy for discontinuation of denosumab is yet to be determined, though dosing of a parenteral bisphosphonate, such as zoledronic acid, at the end of therapy has been studied with limited success [73].

Hormone Replacement Therapy

Estradiol has long been shown to improve bone health and reduce fracture risk for aging women. After the results of the Women's Health Initiative (WHI) revealed the risks of hormone replacement therapy may outweigh the benefits, oral estradiol became less commonly prescribed for postmenopausal women [74]. More recently there is some thought that using estradiol at low doses or transdermally may be a safe and cost-effective strategy to prevent or treat osteoporosis [75]. This approach has not been shown to be safe in women with a history of breast cancer or who are at high risk of developing breast cancer in their lifetime. In fact, a recent meta-analysis suggests that the use of estradiol in breast cancer survivors who are older than age 50 years at diagnosis may increase the risk of recurrence [76]. As there are several other options that have been established for safe and effective use in breast cancer survivors, estradiol is not generally recommended for bone protection.

Recombinant Parathyroid Hormone

Teriparatide and abaloparatide are recombinant analogs of parathyroid hormone approved for treatment of postmenopausal osteoporosis in the USA. They must be self-administered subcutaneously on a daily basis. Clinical trials demonstrate that these agents improve bone density and reduce vertebral and nonvertebral fractures [77, 78]. However, these treatments were both associated with osteosarcoma in preclinical studies and carry a black box warning as a result. There is currently no published clinical trial data demonstrating safety or efficacy for these agents in breast cancer survivors. They are contraindicated in patients with skeletal metastases, prior radiation therapy involving the skeleton, Paget disease, and hypercalcemia. Given the potential risks, cost of treatment, and lack of available safety data, most clinicians choose to avoid these agents in breast cancer survivors.

Romosozumab

Romosozumab is a monoclonal antibody that inhibits sclerostin, resulting in a net increase in bone formation and decrease in bone resorption. It is administered via monthly subcutaneous injections and has been shown to improve bone density as well as reduce vertebral and nonvertebral fractures [79]. Romosozumab is currently indicated for postmenopausal women with osteoporosis at high risk of fracture defined as those women with a history of osteoporotic fracture, multiple risk factors for fracture, or with failure/intolerance of other available osteoporotic therapies. Based on clinical trial data, it carries a black box warning for myocardial infarction and stroke risk, and is contraindicated in patients who have had an ischemic event within the past year. Romosozumab is typically well-tolerated, but its use is limited to 12 monthly doses and can also induce hypocalcemia and cause headache, rash, and arthralgias. In clinical trials, it was also associated with potential osteonecrosis of the jaw and atypical femur fractures. As there is currently no available data demonstrating safety or efficacy in breast cancer survivors, its use cannot be routinely recommended at this time.

Summary

Given the continued improvements in detection and treatment of breast cancer, the age and number of survivors continues to increase. Bone loss and fractures are among the most common long-term adverse treatment effects in this population. An appropriate clinical evaluation including

DXA allows for appropriate risk stratification in order to reduce the morbidity and mortality associated with fragility fractures. Data exists to support the use of SERMs, bisphosphonates, and denosumab in breast cancer survivors, with potential beneficial effects with respect to reductions in bone loss and fracture rates and improvements in disease-free and overall survival rates. Treatment decisions remain individualized based on patient preferences, comorbidities, and clinical experience.

References

1. DeSantis CE, et al. Breast cancer statistics, 2017, racial disparity in mortality by state. CA Cancer J Clin. 2017;67(6):439–48.
2. DeSantis CE, et al. Cancer treatment and survivorship statistics, 2014. CA Cancer J Clin. 2014;64(4):252–71.
3. Ganz PA. Survivorship: adult cancer survivors. Prim Care. 2009;36(4):721–41.
4. Chen Z, et al. Fracture risk among breast cancer survivors: results from the Women's Health Initiative Observational Study. Arch Intern Med. 2005;165(5):552–8.
5. Robinson PJ, et al. Minimal-trauma fracture in women with breast cancer surviving for at least 5 years from diagnosis. Osteoporos Int. 2015;26(2):795–800.
6. Kanis JA, et al. A high incidence of vertebral fracture in women with breast cancer. Br J Cancer. 1999;79(7–8):1179–81.
7. Dyer SM, et al. A critical review of the long-term disability outcomes following hip fracture. BMC Geriatr. 2016;16:158.
8. Newcomb PA, et al. Postmenopausal fracture history and survival after reproductive cancer diagnosis. JNCI Cancer Spectr. 2018;2(1):pky001.
9. Runowicz CD, et al. American Cancer Society/American Society of Clinical Oncology breast cancer survivorship care guideline. J Clin Oncol. 2016;34(6):611–35.
10. Gyori DJ, et al. Evaluation of appropriate use of bisphosphonates and denosumab in patients with cancer. J Oncol Pharm Pract. 2020;26(2):286–92.
11. Boyce BF. Advances in osteoclast biology reveal potential new drug targets and new roles for osteoclasts. J Bone Miner Res. 2013;28(4):711–22.
12. D'Oronzo S, et al. Cancer treatment-induced bone loss (CTIBL): pathogenesis and clinical implications. Cancer Treat Rev. 2015;41(9):798–808.
13. Coleman RE, et al. Skeletal effects of exemestane on bone-mineral density, bone biomarkers, and fracture incidence in postmenopausal women with early breast cancer participating in the Intergroup Exemestane Study (IES): a randomised controlled study. Lancet Oncol. 2007;8(2):119–27.
14. Eastell R, et al. Long-term effects of anastrozole on bone mineral density: 7-year results from the ATAC trial. Ann Oncol. 2011;22(4):857–62.
15. Rabaglio M, et al. Bone fractures among postmenopausal patients with endocrine-responsive early breast cancer treated with 5 years of letrozole or tamoxifen in the BIG 1-98 trial. Ann Oncol. 2009;20(9):1489–98.
16. Goss PE, et al. Exemestane versus anastrozole in postmenopausal women with early breast cancer: NCIC CTG MA.27–a randomized controlled phase III trial. J Clin Oncol. 2013;31(11):1398–404.
17. Greep NC, et al. The effects of adjuvant chemotherapy on bone density in postmenopausal women with early breast cancer. Am J Med. 2003;114(8):653–9.
18. Kennecke H, et al. Metastatic behavior of breast cancer subtypes. J Clin Oncol. 2010;28(20):3271–7.
19. Weaver CM, et al. The National Osteoporosis Foundation's position statement on peak bone mass development and lifestyle factors: a systematic review and implementation recommendations. Osteoporos Int. 2016;27(4):1281–386.
20. Yang S, et al. Objectively verified parental hip fracture is an independent risk factor for fracture: a linkage analysis of 478,792 parents and 261,705 offspring. J Bone Miner Res. 2016;31(9):1753–9.
21. Johansson H, et al. Imminent risk of fracture after fracture. Osteoporos Int. 2017;28(3):775–80.
22. van Geel TA, et al. Timing of subsequent fractures after an initial fracture. Curr Osteoporos Rep. 2010;8(3):118–22.
23. Leslie WD, et al. Measured height loss predicts incident clinical fractures independently from FRAX: a registry-based cohort study. Osteoporos Int. 2020;31(6):1079–87.
24. Siminoski K, et al. Accuracy of physical examination using the rib-pelvis distance for detection of lumbar vertebral fractures. Am J Med. 2003;115(3):233–6.
25. Eastell R, et al. Pharmacological management of osteoporosis in postmenopausal women: an Endocrine Society* Clinical Practice Guideline. J Clin Endocrinol Metab. 2019;104(5):1595–622.
26. Johnell O, et al. Predictive value of BMD for hip and other fractures. J Bone Miner Res. 2005;20(7):1185–94.
27. Leslie WD, Lix LM. Absolute fracture risk assessment using lumbar spine and femoral neck bone density measurements: derivation and validation of a hybrid system. J Bone Miner Res. 2011;26(3):460–7.
28. Wood K, et al. What is the utility of distal forearm DXA in primary hyperparathyroidism? Oncologist. 2012;17(3):322–5.
29. Licata AA, et al. Consensus statement by the American association of clinical endocrinologists and American college of endocrinology on the quality of DXA scans and reports. Endocr Pract. 2018;24(2):220–9.
30. Leslie WD, et al. Performance of FRAX in women with breast cancer initiating aromatase inhibitor therapy: a registry-based cohort study. J Bone Miner Res. 2019;34(8):1428–35.

31. Cosman F, et al. Clinician's guide to prevention and treatment of osteoporosis. Osteoporos Int. 2014;25(10):2359–81.
32. Kopecky SL, et al. Lack of evidence linking calcium with or without vitamin D supplementation to cardiovascular disease in generally healthy adults: a clinical guideline from the National Osteoporosis Foundation and the American Society for Preventive Cardiology. Ann Intern Med. 2016;165(12):867–8.
33. Curhan GC, et al. Comparison of dietary calcium with supplemental calcium and other nutrients as factors affecting the risk for kidney stones in women. Ann Intern Med. 1997;126(7):497–504.
34. Yao P, et al. Vitamin D and calcium for the prevention of fracture: a systematic review and meta-analysis. JAMA Netw Open. 2019;2(12):e1917789.
35. Datta M, Schwartz GG. Calcium and vitamin D supplementation and loss of bone mineral density in women undergoing breast cancer therapy. Crit Rev Oncol Hematol. 2013;88(3):613–24.
36. Lahart IM, et al. Physical activity for women with breast cancer after adjuvant therapy. Cochrane Database Syst Rev. 2018;1(1):Cd011292.
37. Fisher B, et al. Tamoxifen for the prevention of breast cancer: current status of the National Surgical Adjuvant Breast and Bowel Project P-1 study. J Natl Cancer Inst. 2005;97(22):1652–62.
38. Vogel VG, et al. Effects of tamoxifen vs raloxifene on the risk of developing invasive breast cancer and other disease outcomes: the NSABP Study of Tamoxifen and Raloxifene (STAR) P-2 trial. JAMA. 2006;295(23):2727–41.
39. Love RR, et al. Effects of tamoxifen on bone mineral density in postmenopausal women with breast cancer. N Engl J Med. 1992;326(13):852–6.
40. Powles TJ, et al. Effect of tamoxifen on bone mineral density measured by dual-energy x-ray absorptiometry in healthy premenopausal and postmenopausal women. J Clin Oncol. 1996;14(1):78–84.
41. Sverrisdottir A, et al. Bone mineral density among premenopausal women with early breast cancer in a randomized trial of adjuvant endocrine therapy. J Clin Oncol. 2004;22(18):3694–9.
42. Kyvernitakis I, Kostev K, Hadji P. The tamoxifen paradox-influence of adjuvant tamoxifen on fracture risk in pre- and postmenopausal women with breast cancer. Osteoporos Int. 2018;29(11):2557–64.
43. Cummings SR, et al. The effect of raloxifene on risk of breast cancer in postmenopausal women: results from the MORE randomized trial. Multiple Outcomes of Raloxifene Evaluation. JAMA. 1999;281(23):2189–97.
44. Silverman SL, Gold DT. Compliance and persistence with osteoporosis therapies. Curr Rheumatol Rep. 2008;10(2):118–22.
45. Miller PD, et al. Renal safety in patients treated with bisphosphonates for osteoporosis: a review. J Bone Miner Res. 2013;28(10):2049–59.
46. Lomax AJ, et al. Prevention of aromatase inhibitor-induced bone loss with alendronate in postmenopausal women: the BATMAN Trial. J Bone Oncol. 2013;2(4):145–53.
47. Greenspan SL, et al. Prevention of bone loss with risedronate in breast cancer survivors: a randomized, controlled clinical trial. Osteoporos Int. 2015;26(6):1857–64.
48. Van Poznak C, et al. Prevention of aromatase inhibitor-induced bone loss using risedronate: the SABRE trial. J Clin Oncol. 2010;28(6):967–75.
49. Livi L, et al. Phase 2 placebo-controlled, single-blind trial to evaluate the impact of oral ibandronate on bone mineral density in osteopenic breast cancer patients receiving adjuvant aromatase inhibitors: 5-year results of the single-centre BONADIUV trial. Eur J Cancer. 2019;108:100–10.
50. Lester JE, et al. Prevention of anastrozole induced bone loss with monthly oral ibandronate: final 5 year results from the ARIBON trial. J Bone Oncol. 2012;1(2):57–62.
51. Monda V, et al. Improvement of Bone physiology and life quality due to association of risedronate and anastrozole. Front Pharmacol. 2017;8:632.
52. Rennert G, et al. Oral bisphosphonates and improved survival of breast cancer. Clin Cancer Res. 2017;23(7):1684–9.
53. Hadji P, et al. Effect of adjuvant bisphosphonates on disease-free survival in early breast cancer: retrospective analysis results in an unselected single-center cohort. J Bone Oncol. 2013;2(1):2–10.
54. Early Breast Cancer Trialists' Collaborative, G. Adjuvant bisphosphonate treatment in early breast cancer: meta-analyses of individual patient data from randomised trials. Lancet. 2015;386(10001):1353–61.
55. Adler RA, et al. Managing osteoporosis in patients on long-term bisphosphonate treatment: report of a task force of the American Society for Bone and Mineral Research. J Bone Miner Res. 2016;31(1):16–35.
56. Coleman R, et al. Zoledronic acid (zoledronate) for postmenopausal women with early breast cancer receiving adjuvant letrozole (ZO-FAST study): final 60-month results. Ann Oncol. 2013;24(2):398–405.
57. Gnant M, et al. Zoledronic acid combined with adjuvant endocrine therapy of tamoxifen versus anastrozol plus ovarian function suppression in premenopausal early breast cancer: final analysis of the Austrian Breast and Colorectal Cancer Study Group Trial 12. Ann Oncol. 2015;26(2):313–20.
58. Nuzzo F, et al. Bone effect of adjuvant tamoxifen, letrozole or letrozole plus zoledronic acid in early-stage breast cancer: the randomized phase 3 HOBOE study. Ann Oncol. 2012;23(8):2027–33.
59. Brufsky AM, et al. Final 5-year results of Z-FAST trial: adjuvant zoledronic acid maintains bone mass in postmenopausal breast cancer patients receiving letrozole. Cancer. 2012;118(5):1192–201.
60. Gnant M, et al. Endocrine therapy plus zoledronic acid in premenopausal breast cancer. N Engl J Med. 2009;360(7):679–91.
61. Wilson C, et al. Adjuvant zoledronic acid reduces fractures in breast cancer patients; an AZURE (BIG 01/04) study. Eur J Cancer. 2018;94:70–8.

62. Coleman RE, et al. Benefits and risks of adjuvant treatment with zoledronic acid in stage II/III breast cancer. 10 years follow-up of the AZURE randomized clinical trial (BIG 01/04). J Bone Oncol. 2018;13:123–35.
63. Lyles KW, et al. Zoledronic acid and clinical fractures and mortality after hip fracture. N Engl J Med. 2007;357(18):1799–809.
64. Crotti C, et al. Acute phase reactions after Zoledronic acid infusion: protective role of 25-Hydroxyvitamin d and previous oral bisphosphonate therapy. Endocr Pract. 2018;24(5):405–10.
65. Ellis GK, et al. Randomized trial of denosumab in patients receiving adjuvant aromatase inhibitors for nonmetastatic breast cancer. J Clin Oncol. 2008;26(30):4875–82.
66. Gnant M, et al. Adjuvant denosumab in breast cancer (ABCSG-18): a multicentre, randomised, double-blind, placebo-controlled trial. Lancet. 2015;386(9992):433–43.
67. Gnant M, et al. Adjuvant denosumab in postmenopausal patients with hormone receptor-positive breast cancer (ABCSG-18): disease-free survival results from a randomised, double-blind, placebo-controlled, phase 3 trial. Lancet Oncol. 2019;20(3):339–51.
68. Bonani M, et al. Infections in De novo kidney transplant recipients treated with the RANKL inhibitor denosumab. Transplantation. 2017;101(9):2139–45.
69. Bone HG, et al. Effects of denosumab treatment and discontinuation on bone mineral density and bone turnover markers in postmenopausal women with low bone mass. J Clin Endocrinol Metab. 2011;96(4):972–80.
70. Cummings SR, et al. Vertebral fractures after discontinuation of denosumab: a post hoc analysis of the randomized placebo-controlled FREEDOM trial and its extension. J Bone Miner Res. 2018;33(2):190–8.
71. Tsourdi E, et al. Discontinuation of denosumab therapy for osteoporosis: a systematic review and position statement by ECTS. Bone. 2017;105:11–7.
72. Bone HG, et al. 10 years of denosumab treatment in postmenopausal women with osteoporosis: results from the phase 3 randomised FREEDOM trial and open-label extension. Lancet Diabetes Endocrinol. 2017;5(7):513–23.
73. Reid IR, et al. Bone loss after denosumab: only partial protection with zoledronate. Calcif Tissue Int. 2017;101(4):371–4.
74. Crawford SL, et al. Menopausal hormone therapy trends before versus after 2002: impact of the Women's Health Initiative Study Results. Menopause. 2018;26(6):588–97.
75. Levin VA, Jiang X, Kagan R. Estrogen therapy for osteoporosis in the modern era. Osteoporos Int. 2018;29(5):1049–55.
76. Mudhune GH, Armour M, McBride KA. Safety of menopausal hormone therapy in breast cancer survivors older than fifty at diagnosis: a systematic review and meta-analysis. Breast. 2019;47:43–55.
77. Neer RM, et al. Effect of parathyroid hormone (1–34) on fractures and bone mineral density in postmenopausal women with osteoporosis. N Engl J Med. 2001;344(19):1434–41.
78. Miller PD, et al. Effect of abaloparatide vs placebo on new vertebral fractures in postmenopausal women with osteoporosis: a randomized clinical trial. JAMA. 2016;316(7):722–33.
79. Cosman F, et al. Romosozumab treatment in postmenopausal women with osteoporosis. N Engl J Med. 2016;375(16):1532–43.

16 Cardiovascular Health

Susan F. Dent, Robin Kikuchi, Susan C. Gilchrist, and Chiara Melloni

Introduction

Breast cancer (BC) affects 1 in 8 women in the USA, making it the most common cancer diagnosis in women [1]. Advances in cancer treatments have led to increased numbers of survivors, with the average 5-year survival rate for women with invasive BC exceeding 90% [2, 3]. As long-term survival continues to improve, a better understanding of the long-term impact of cancer treatments is essential, particularly with regard to cardiovascular (CV) complications. There is a greater risk of hospitalization due to cardiovascular disease (CVD) among BC survivors compared to the general population [4]. Additionally, several years after cancer diagnosis, post-menopausal BC patients are at a greater risk of CV mortality than BC-related mortality [5]. This is especially concerning for older patients who often have comorbid risk factors for CVD [4, 6]. Cardio-oncology is a new sub-specialty of medicine that focuses on the identification and management of CV complications that can arise during and following completion of anticancer therapy. In this chapter, we review BC treatments associated with CV morbidity and mortality and discuss potential strategies, including a multidisciplinary approach, to mitigate the impact of these treatments in BC survivors.

Impact of Cancer Treatments on Cardiovascular Health

Several cancer treatment modalities (e.g., chemotherapy, targeted therapies, radiation, and endocrine therapies) have led to improvement in survival rates among BC patients but are associated with a detrimental impact on CV health [7]. Anthracycline-containing chemotherapies have led to significant improvements in disease-free and overall survival, especially among patients with aggressive cancers [8]. In addition, human epidermal growth factor receptor positive (HER2+) targeted therapies such as trastuzumab, previously administered in conjunction with anthracycline-containing regimens, have also improved outcomes for patients with HER2+ BC [9]. However, these treatment modalities are associated with an increased risk of heart failure, arrhythmias (e.g., premature ventricular contractions, ventricular tachycardia, bradycardia, atrio-

S. F. Dent (✉)
Duke Cancer Institute, Durham, NC, USA
e-mail: susan.dent@duke.edu

R. Kikuchi
Duke University, Durham, NC, USA
e-mail: robin.kikuchi@duke.edu

S. C. Gilchrist
Clinical Cancer Prevention and Cardiology, the University of Texas MD Anderson Cancer Center, Houston, TX, USA
e-mail: sgilchrist@mdanderson.org

C. Melloni
Duke University, Durham, NC, USA

IQVIA, Durham, NC, USA
e-mail: chiara.melloni@duke.edu

G. G. Kimmick et al. (eds.), *Common Issues in Breast Cancer Survivors*,
https://doi.org/10.1007/978-3-030-75377-1_16

ventricular block, bundle-branch block, QT prolongation), CV hospitalization, and death, which can manifest years after completion of treatment [10–16]. Radiation therapy is associated with an increased risk of developing ischemic heart disease, in particular for those individuals exposed to left-sided breast and chest wall radiation [17]. These CV consequences (e.g., coronary disease, valvular disease, and vasculopathy) can appear years to decades after radiation therapy [17, 18]. Early menopause and adjuvant endocrine therapy with aromatase inhibitors may place women at an increased risk for developing CVD. There is mixed data regarding use of aromatase inhibitors on CVD events among women with BC. Although the absolute increase in CVD risk is likely to be low, there have been some studies associating aromatase inhibitors and hyperlipidemia [19, 20]. In addition, adjuvant endocrine therapy with selective estrogen receptor modulators (i.e., tamoxifen) increases the risk of venous thromboembolism and other thromboembolic issues [21]. Some anticancer therapies have been associated with arrhythmias (e.g., anthracyclines, trastuzumab, cyclophosphamide, paclitaxel) and QTc prolongations (e.g., cyclophosphamide, 5-fluorouracil, paclitaxel) which may continue into survivorship; [16] however, data on the long-term CV impact of many anticancer therapies is limited in BC survivors.

Many cancer treatments indirectly increase CVD risk by accelerating weight gain and interrupting normal physical activity (PA) [22]. BC treatment can result in physical deconditioning, weight gain, and metabolic dysregulation, which contribute to an increased risk of CVD among BC patients [23]. Approximately 36% of BC patients are sedentary [24], and 50–96% experience weight gain during treatment [25, 26]. The Health, Eating, Activity, and Lifestyle (HEAL) study noted that, from pre- to post- diagnosis, PA among BC patients decreased approximately 2 hours/week with the greatest decrease in PA (60%) noted among women with the most aggressive treatment regimens [27]. This may be in part due to the most commonly reported side effect reported by women during BC treatment, fatigue. Up to 70% of women report fatigue during BC treatment, and 30% continue to report problems with fatigue into survivorship [28]. Although the specific cause of fatigue is not known, it is theorized to be due to the combined physiologic, psychologic, and social effects of cancer treatment [28]. Indeed, Bower et al. conducted a large-scale study (n = 1957) of BC survivors to explore the epidemiology of fatigue in this population [29]. Approximately a third of the study population reported severe fatigue. Reports of severe fatigue were associated with receiving chemotherapy and with higher levels of depression, pain, sleep disturbance, and menopausal symptoms [29]. These findings corroborated the earlier findings of Broeckel et al. who found severe fatigue to be associated with receiving chemotherapy, a comorbid psychiatric disorder, and/or those individuals who are post-menopausal [30]. Fatigue adversely effects survivors' quality of life (QOL), as they are often unable to perform at the same levels of fitness or complete the same functions of daily life they were able to prior to treatment, resulting in a decrease in physical functional status [31].

Furthermore, comorbid risk factors, such as diabetes, hyperlipidemia, hypertension, and smoking, at the time of BC diagnosis, can further increase the risk of CVD [32]. Thus, screening and managing these risk factors before, during, and after anticancer therapy is recommended to mitigate this increased risk [7, 33]. Taken together, the combination of treatment-related exposures, change in lifestyle behaviors following a BC diagnosis, and comorbid conditions, often described as the multi-hit hypothesis, leads to an increased risk of CVD among BC survivors [34] (Fig. 16.1).

It has been shown these "multiple-hits" to the CV system often manifest with a decline in cardiorespiratory fitness, even prior to a measurable decline in left ventricular ejection fraction (LVEF) among BC patients [35, 36]. Cardiorespiratory fitness is defined as the highest rate at which oxygen is transported and utilized by the body during maximal exercise (VO_{2peak}) [35, 36]. Among 248 BC patients with normal cardiac function (LVEF >50%), Jones et al. found

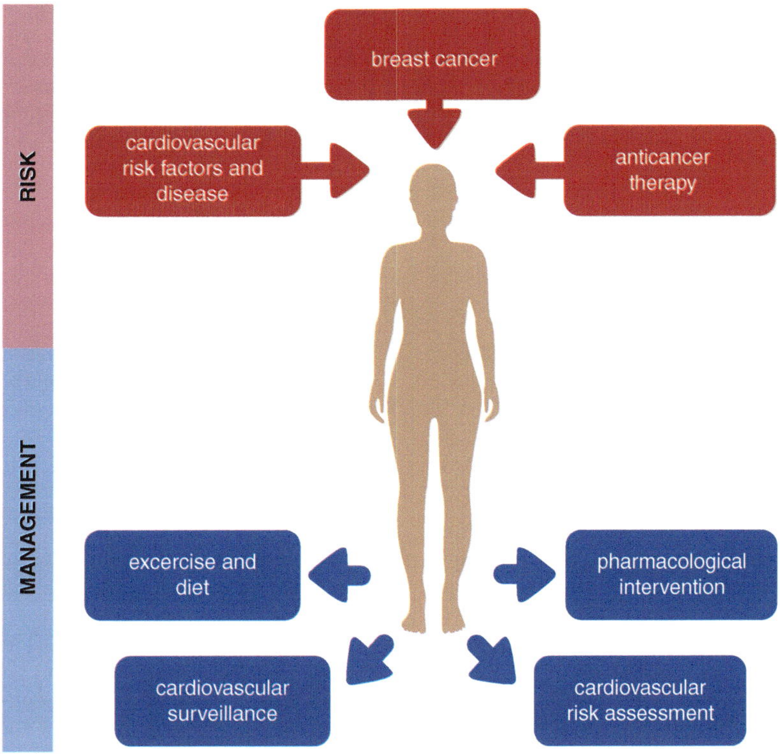

Fig. 16.1 Modifying cardiovascular risk factors in breast cancer

the average VO_{2peak} in the population to be 27% less than that of age-matched sedentary but otherwise healthy women without a history of BC [37]. In both patients with advanced BC and other cancer types, low VO_{2peak} has been shown to be a prognostic marker of survival in these populations [38, 39]. Additionally, this decrease in fitness can compound other issues seen in BC patients such as exercise intolerance, lower functional status, and fatigue, further elevating a patient's risk for CV complications [28–30].

CV Survivorship Imaging Guidelines

Several organizations, including the European Society of Medical Oncology (ESMO), the American Society of Clinical Oncology (ASCO), the American Heart Association (AHA), the European Society of Cardiology (ESC), the American Society of Echocardiography (ASE), and the European Association of Cardiovascular Imaging (EACVI), have put forth guidelines for monitoring and managing the CV health of cancer patients and survivors [7, 22, 40–42]. ESMO, ASCO, ESC, and NCCN guidelines are summarized in Table 16.1. All of the guidelines agree that monitoring of BC patients' cardiac function and CV comorbidities throughout treatment and into survivorship is critical to the early detection and prevention of CVD. Problems with cardiac function and CVD can appear from treatment onset to years after completion of anthracycline therapy [22, 43] and from years to decades after completion of radiation therapy [17, 18]. The standard measure of CV dysfunction among BC patients exposed to potentially cardiotoxic treatments, such as anthracyclines and/or trastuzumab, is a decrease in LVEF [22]. 3D echocardiogram (echo) and cardiac magnetic resonance (CMR) are the preferred methods of cardiac monitoring; however, CMR is not widely used do to availability, cost, and required expertise [40, 41]. Although still sometimes used in oncology practice, multigated acquisition (MUGA) imaging is no longer recommended as the primary modality, due to the associated radiation exposure [40]. The evidence for cardiac

Table 16.1 Recommendations for cardiovascular surveillance in cancer patients

	ESMO [40]	ASCO [7]	ESC [42]	NCCN [47]
Type of screening	Cardiac imaging (3D Echo, CMR) with cardiac biomarkers (BNP, troponin)	Echocardiogram (+biomarkers if symptomatic)	Cardiac imaging and biomarkers (such as BNP)	Echocardiogram + Doppler flow studies
Timeframe	*6–12 months, at 2 years* post-treatment and possibly periodically thereafter (patients treated with cardiotoxic agents)	*6–12 months* after the completion of treatment (asymptomatic) *Immediate* full diagnostic workup (symptomatic)	*Periodic* screening	*Within 12 months* post-treatment for patients treated with anthracyclines with 1 or more risk factors
Action if findings arise	Cardiology consultation Consider pharmacological treatment	Referral to cardio-oncologist or cardiologist	Any suggestive findings should be investigated immediately	Referral to a cardiologist

ASCO American Society of Clinical Oncology, *ESC* European Society of Cardiology, *ESMO* European Society for Medical Oncology, *NCCN* National Comprehensive Cancer Network

serum biomarkers, specifically troponin I and brain natriuretic peptides (BNP), to detect or predict CV toxicities such as heart failure and cardiomyopathy continues to evolve [40, 44, 45]. Biomarkers are now recommended by ASCO and ESMO for monitoring those patients most at risk of developing CV dysfunction due to high anthracycline doses, preexisting CVD, or CV risk factors during treatment [7, 40]. Patients with significant elevation of these serum biomarker levels beyond alarm levels (0.08 ng/mL for troponin I; 0.1 ng/mL for BNP) or baseline readings should be referred to a cardiologist [44, 46]. However, there is a lack of data regarding the efficacy of these biomarkers in survivorship.

The frequency of cardiac monitoring in survivorship differs between guidelines due to lack of long-term data on the CV consequences of cancer therapy in survivors of adult onset cancers. It is for this reason that many recommendations in survivorship are based on expert opinion. The 2020 ESMO consensus recommendation suggests that in asymptomatic patients who have received potentially cardiotoxic therapy, monitoring, including measurement of biomarkers (BNP and/or troponin) and cardiac imaging, should be performed at 6–12 months, after completion of cancer therapy, 2 years, and periodically throughout survivorship [40]. Survivors should be referred to a cardiologist for management if asymptomatic cardiac dysfunction (LVEF <50%) is identified during routine surveillance. In symptomatic patients, monitoring should be conducted regularly, and CV care should be continued indefinitely [7, 40]. These recommendations remain in line with previous recommendations by ASCO and ESC [7, 42]. NCCN guidelines are based on studies of the prevalence of late onset cardiotoxicity [47]. They recommend patients treated with anthracyclines and with one or more additional risk factors be imaged once within 12 months of anticancer therapy completion [47]. These recommendations are based on patients treated with anthracyclines with or without the addition of trastuzumab. These guidelines are relevant to BC patients but do not take into account the CV consequences of other BC treatments (Table 16.1).

Interventions

Managing CV Risk Factors

Among BC survivors, there is a greater risk of hospitalization due to CVD compared to the general population [4]. Therefore, one of the most important interventions for managing CVD risk in BC survivors is regular monitoring and management of CV risk factors throughout survivorship. Risk factors, such as smoking, hypertension, dyslipidemia, diabetes, and obesity, left unmanaged significantly increase the risk of developing CVD, especially in conjunction with a history of cardiotoxic therapy [7, 40]. In the Kaiser Permanente Southern California-SEER (Surveillance, Epidemiology, and End Results) cancer registry, hypertension was more prevalent in patients with cancer and was also an independent risk factor for CV events [48]. In the Dietary Approaches to Stop Hypertension (DASH) study, participants following a diet with fruits, vegetables, legumes, whole grains, and low saturated fats were more successful in reducing blood pressure [49]. In addition to lifestyle changes, appropriate pharmacological management of hypertension should be considered [40]. Hyperlipidemia has been implicated in promoting cardiac inflammation and contributing to atherosclerosis [32, 50]. Cancer patients should receive standard risk assessment based on the 2019 ACC/AHA primary prevention guidelines to see if they would benefit from lipid lowering therapy [32, 40]. Diabetes has been shown to increase the risk of cancer treatment-related cardiovascular dysfunction (CTRCD) in several studies; thus, it is critical to manage this risk factor throughout survivorship [40, 51, 52].

Exercise:
Exercise has several well-known positive CV effects, such as improving CV efficiency, increasing stroke volume and cardiac output, decreasing resting heart rate, and enhancing ventilation and oxygen transport [53]. Several reports have underscored the importance of CV health for women with BC and suggest that physicians should recommend BC survivors engage in an exercise training program to improve cardiorespiratory fitness [54]. For example, Jones et al., in a large cohort of 2973 women with nonmetastatic BC, demonstrated the positive impact of exercise on the incidence of CVD-specific mortality and morbidity. Based on surveys, they found that women who exercised after cancer diagnosis had a substantial reduction in newly diagnosed CV events or CV death. The observed positive effect was consistent across different groups of patients based on baseline CV risk factors and type of anticancer therapy received [55]. Despite the evidence for the positive impact of exercise to address the acute, short-, and long-term effects of cancer treatments, data for the optimal exercise prescription in this population remain unclear. The basis for many exercise recommendations and study paradigms for cancer patients at risk of CTRCD are extrapolated based on preexisting guidelines regarding CVD risk and heart failure [32, 56]. Approximately 150 minutes of moderate-intensity exercise is recommended by the AHA, for all people regardless of health status, to reduce the risk of CVD [32]. Additionally, those asymptomatic patients with preexisting risk factors and treated with cardiotoxic anticancer therapies are considered stage A heart failure patients [47, 57]. The AHA guidelines for patients with stable early stage heart failure (stage A) recommend encouraging patients to exercise regularly to improve physical conditioning and, therefore, CV health [56]. A recent study by Scott et al. in 174 postmenopausal BC survivors randomized patients to receive either a supervised fixed dose intensity per exercise session intervention, a supervised variable dose intensity per exercise session intervention, or stretching sessions. No difference in the improvement of cardiorespiratory fitness between the dosing schedules was seen [58].

Although dosing schedule remains unclear, several recent studies have explored variable-intensity supervised exercise recommendations for improving cardiorespiratory fitness in BC patients, which has positive implications for improving CV fitness and mitigating CTRCD risk. Giallauria et al., in a study of 51 women with BC following an exercise training program of moderate intensity (3 session/week on a bicycle at 60–70% VO_{2peak} for 3 months, followed by one session/week until 1-year follow-up), demonstrated an improvement in both cardiopulmonary functional capacity and vascular endothelial function after 12 months when compared to a control group of women not performing a formal exercise program [36]. The peak oxygen consumption (VO_{2peak}) significantly increased in the exercise group (from 12.4 ± 2.9 to 14.3 ± 3.3 mL/kg/min, $p < 0.001$) compared to the control group (from 12.8 ± 2.5 to 12.6 ± 2.8 mL/kg/min, $p = 0.55$; $p < 0.001$ between groups) [36]. A more recent pilot study by Hornsby et al., evaluating the safety and efficacy of aerobic training in 21 BC patients receiving neoadjuvant chemotherapy, demonstrated that a supervised aerobic training program incorporating high-intensity (60–100% of VO_{2peak}) aerobic interval training three times per week is a safe and well-tolerated adjunct therapy in women undergoing anthracycline-containing chemotherapy for operable BC. This study also demonstrated that while anthracycline-containing chemotherapy alone is associated with marked reductions in cardiopulmonary function [VO_{2peak} decreased by 1.5 ± 2.2 ml/kg/min (−8.6%)], aerobic training not only negates the unfavorable impact of chemotherapy but causes significant improvements in cardiopulmonary function (VO_{2peak} increased by 2.6 ± 3.5 ml/kg/min (+ 13.3%) during concurrent neoadjuvant therapy) [59].

Some studies have investigated at-home interventions to improve cardiorespiratory fitness in BC patients. A study by Segal et al. compared both self-directed and supervised exercise to usual care among 123 women with stage I and II BC undergoing anticancer therapy [60]. A standardized series of warm-up and cool-down exercises and a progressive walking program at an exercise intensity of 50% to 60% of the predicted maximal oxygen uptake was provided to all participants. Those in the self-directed exercise group received a home exercise prescription and were asked to exercise five times per week for a 26-week period. Supervised exercise group participants received a supervised exercise program three times per week for 26 weeks in the rehabilitation area of the Ottawa Regional Cancer Centre. Compared with usual care, a self-directed exercise led to a moderately large and clinically significant 9.8-point improvement in subjective physical functioning, as measured by the physical functioning scale of the SF-36, while supervised exercise led to a moderate difference (6.3-point improvement). The authors concluded that physical exercise can blunt some of the negative side effects of BC treatment, including reduced physical functioning [60]. Lahart et al. conducted a similar randomized controlled trial evaluating the effect of a six-month home-based PA intervention, with face-to-face and telephone counselling versus usual care, on cardiorespiratory fitness in 80 BC survivors [35]. They found a small beneficial effect (effect sizes ≥0.20) on absolute and relative VO_2 max (d = 0.44 and 0.40, respectively) and total and moderate PA (d = 0.73 and 0.59, respectively) in the intervention arm [35].

Although the literature tends to focus on exercise interventions and the direct effect on fitness and exercise tolerance, some trials have investigated the effect of exercise on the more subjective measures of QOL and fatigue. These parameters, especially fatigue, can impact survivors' lifestyles leading to more sedentary behavior and further exacerbating the physical deconditioning associated with anticancer therapy. For example, a study led by Courneya et al. showed that postmenopausal women with BC undergoing supervised exercise program using recumbent or upright cycle ergometers (at approximately 70% to 75% of maximal oxygen consumption) had benefits not only on changes in peak oxygen consumption (peak oxygen consumption increased by 0.24 L/min in the exercise group), but also in happiness, self-esteem, fatigue, and several subcomponents of overall QOL [61]. Moreover, a meta-analysis of 20 exercise intervention groups, comprised of 748 BC patients receiving adjuvant chemotherapy, examined the outcomes of fatigue and QOL measures and found that exercise led to significant decreases in fatigue and depression and that lower doses of exercise (<12 MET-h/week) were more effective in improving fatigue and QOL outcomes than higher doses of exercise [62]. Therefore, moderate to high intensity aerobic interventions, such as those studied in cardiorespiratory fitness, may not be suitable in a population severely impacted by fatigue. A multicenter study in 119 sedentary women with Stage 0–III BC focused on the effect of exercise on fatigue, one of the most prevalent and debilitating symptoms experienced by BC patients receiving adjuvant chemotherapy or radiation therapy [63]. Participants were instructed to walk 5–6 times/week at 50–70% of maximum heart rate as tolerated. There were no differences between the home-based exercise and usual care in the intention to treat analysis, mostly due to significant crossover between arms. There was a clinically important and statistically significant ($p = 0.03$) effect of exercise on pretest-to-posttest change in fatigue levels demonstrated when exercise participation was considered using the data analysis method of *instrumental variables* with *principal stratification*. This study reinforces that adherence to a home-based moderate-intensity walking exercise program may effectively mitigate high levels of fatigue experienced during cancer treatment and improve functional capacity [63]. Additionally, in a study of 27 women with stage I-IV BC, participants were instructed to follow an 8-week at home exercise program and to keep a daily fatigue diary. Women who exercised regularly during this time recorded fewer days of high fatigue levels and more days of low fatigue levels in comparison to women who did not exercise [64].

Yoga has become a novel area of inquiry in recent years for improving QOL in cancer patients; however, there are large knowledge gaps and further research is needed. This is especially important for women whose fitness may not be suited for aerobic interventions. Yoga and stretching interventions may offer PA suitable to their functional level although there is no evidence that it is a more effective intervention than other exercise modalities [65]. A study by Vadiraja et al. evaluated the effects of yoga on cancer-related fatigue in 91 metastatic BC patients randomized to receive 3 months of either yoga or education and supportive therapy. In this population, they found that yoga reduced fatigue frequency ($p < 0.001$) and severity ($p < 0.001$) [66]. Dong et al., in a meta-analysis of 17 studies comprising 2183 BC patients, demonstrated a large effect of yoga on fatigue. They found that yoga interventions had a significant benefit in mitigating physical fatigue [Standardized Mean Difference = −0.63, 95% CI (−0.90, −0.35), $p = 0.09$)] with supervised classes offering the most benefit [Standardized Mean Difference = −0.92, 95% CI (−1.53, −0.32), $p = 0.003$)] [67]. Although further inquiry is needed, yoga may offer BC patients and survivors a PA suitable for various physical functional abilities.

The American College of Sports Medicine (ACSM) convened an expert panel to review the extent of literature on exercise interventions among cancer survivors and update relevant exercise recommendations. The ACSM statement recommended 90 to 150 minutes of moderate-intensity aerobic PA weekly in addition to 2–3 days of resistance exercises to reduce fatigue, improve QOL, and physical functioning [68]. While there was not enough evidence to provide an exercise dose recommendation to prevent CVD among cancer survivors, a recent meta-analysis suggests that exercise training at the recommended dose (~150 minutes/week) in BC survivors improves cardiorespiratory fitness, a key subclinical CVD endpoint as discussed in this review [69]. It is clear there is a high level of variability in prescription and response among patient populations with these exercise interventions; thus, it is important to consider that individualized exercise plans that take into account a patient's previously existing risk factors, history of anti-cancer therapy, and functional status may be more appropriate than one-size-fits-all interventions [70]. Additionally, although many studies have investigated exercise interventions in BC patient populations, cardiorespiratory fitness, rather than CVD outcomes, are often the outcomes measured. Nevertheless, exercise, especially aerobic exercise, offers a lifestyle intervention that has been shown to improve BC patients' exercise tolerance, cardiopulmonary fitness, QOL, fatigue, CV health, and CV outcomes. It is recommended for all cancer survivors regardless of risk [40].

Integration into Clinical Practice

Although the literature clearly supports exercise for all BC patients, a study by Coletta et al. has previously shown that, in the outpatient setting, <20% of BC survivors obtain the recommended levels of activity [71]. Being overweight or obese and having prior exposure to chemotherapy were key predictors of non-adherence in this study. A novel meta-analysis by Berkman and Gilchrist concluded that the best adherence to lifestyle changes occurs through use of social cognitive theory and motivational interviewing [72]. Social cognitive theory holds that the influence of an individual's experiences, their interactions with others, and their environmental factors impact their health behaviors; exploring these perceptions can influence behavioral change. Motivational interviewing is a patient-based counseling technique that guides patients through exploring and resolving their own ambivalence to elicit behavioral change. These strategies should be considered by clinicians when working with patients to determine a practical survivorship plan for exercise and other lifestyle changes. In addition to these strategies, it is critical to create the infrastructure needed to address poor PA adherence in this population. An oncologist's recommendation is an important step to increase uptake of PA [24]. Oncology clinics should work towards providing all BC survivors with education regarding the PA guidelines. Moreover, alliances between oncology clinics, the community (e.g., Lifestrong YMCA, Active after Cancer), and institutional partners (e.g., physical therapy) are important to address barriers to exercise and to provide opportunities for patients to engage in PA.

In the MD Anderson system, Gilchrist et al. have developed an approach at the beginning of cancer treatment to measure and mitigate existing CV risk factors (e.g., smoking, blood pressure, cholesterol, diabetes) and determine whether prior exposures in combination with existing 10-year CVD risk warrants preventative CVD therapies, such as statins for BC survivors at heightened risk (Fig. 16.2) [7, 73, 74]. In all patients, healthy lifestyle behaviors are recommended, a referral to a dietician is made (when appropriate), and a discussion regarding exercise goals and reducing sedentary behavior is performed [7, 40, 74]. A 6-minute walk or cardiopulmonary exercise test is completed to determine baseline functional capacity and readiness for moderate-intensity exercise. Both aerobic and resistance training is prescribed along with modifications for patients with lymphedema or bone metastases. Remote feedback is provided by an exercise physiologist over an initial 12-week period to help BC survivors make modifications or overcome barriers to reaching guideline-based PA levels with the goal to transition patients to community-based programs to maintain PA. Follow-up in clinic with the cardiologist is based on need to monitor and/or treat uncontrolled risk factors, symptoms, or exercise intolerance [74]. While this approach is interesting, objective measures such as improvements in cardiorespiratory fitness and fatigue and reduction in CVD risk are needed prior to widespread adoption of this approach into clinical practice.

Given limited resources, it is difficult to provide personalized exercise prescriptions and preventative cardiology visits for all BC survivors at risk of CVD within the existing cardio-oncology infrastructure. In addition, a majority of community-based programs have no access to specialized clinics to address this need. Gilchrist's American Heart Association Scientific Statement, describing MD Anderson's approach to CV risk management program, further outlines how to leverage existing cardiac rehabilitation (CR) infrastructure to scale preventative cardiology and exercise training among BC survivors [74]. CR is widely available in both academic and community settings. It has been shown that exercise training within the CR setting improves physical functioning, reduces fatigue, and improves QOL [74]. The biggest barrier currently is a lack of third party reimbursement for CR among cancer patients. In those situations, a partnership between oncology and cardiology is needed to negotiate time and space within CR to address the needs of BC survivors. Partnering with aligned private foundations to support the ACSM cancer trainers to oversee training is important. Lastly, streamlining processes and creating automated referrals (e.g., following last chemotherapy infusion or clinic survivorship visit) to ensure BC survivors are provided the opportunity to engage in PA is critical [74]. By leveraging these existing resources, cardiologists and oncologists can take steps to improve the overall health and wellness of their patients in survivorship.

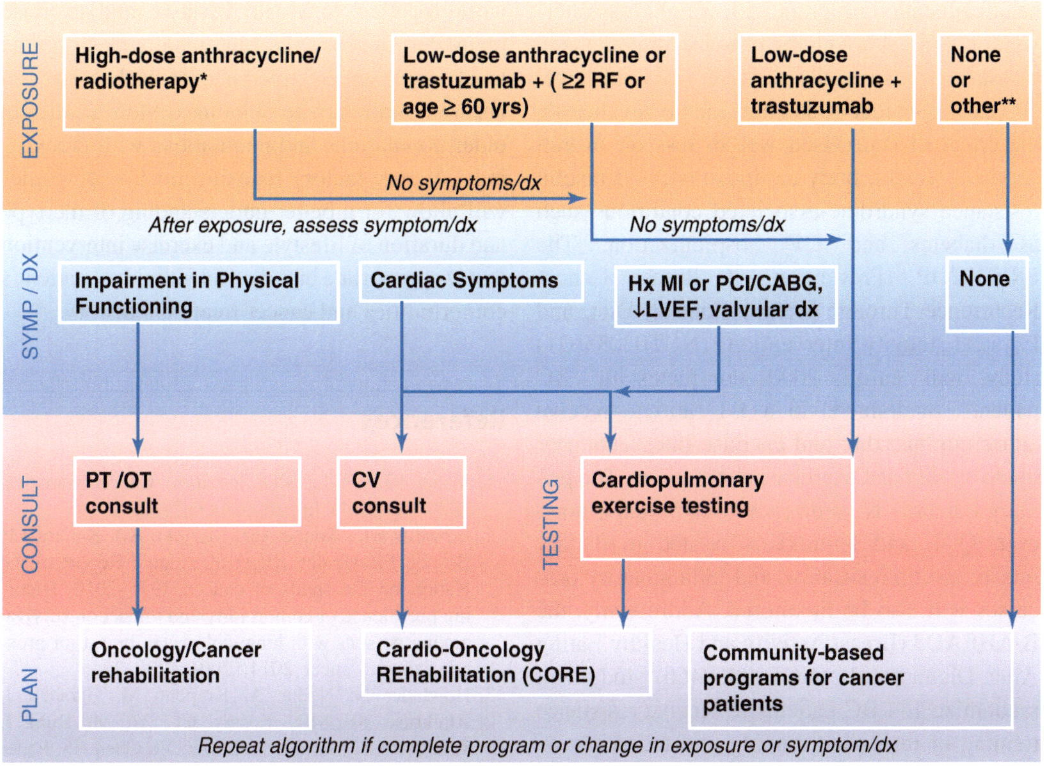

Fig. 16.2 Cardio-oncology rehabilitation (CORE) algorithm for patients treated with cancer therapy [74]. Risk factors (RFs) include hypertension, dyslipidemia, diabetes mellitus, smoking, and obesity. CABG coronary artery bypass graft, CV cardiovascular, dx diagnosis, Hx history, LVEF left ventricular ejection fraction, MI myocardial infarction, OT occupational therapy, PCI percutaneous coronary intervention, and PT physical therapy. High-dose anthracycline (e.g., doxorubicin ≥250 mg/m^2); high-dose radiotherapy (RT; ≥30 Gy) where the heart is in the treatment field; or lower-dose anthracycline + lower-dose RT (<30 Gy). Other therapies should be reviewed by treating healthcare provider to determine appropriateness for community-based program vs need for consultation or other testing. (Copyright American Heart Association 2019. This table has been modified from its original form)

Future Directions

We have made significant gains in the clinical outcomes of individuals diagnosed with BC; however, the long-term consequences, including cardiovascular complications, of these cancer treatments in adult cancer survivors have not been fully explored. UPBEAT (Understanding and Predicting Breast Cancer Events After Treatment) (NCT02791581) is a multicenter prospective cohort study of 840 early stage BC patients scheduled to receive chemotherapy and 160 healthy volunteers who will be followed for 9 years to determine the long-term impact of anticancer therapy on the heart, the ability to exercise, and fatigue. The results of this study will provide valuable information on the CV consequences of breast cancer therapy and identify those individuals at greatest risk to enable more focused research on primary prevention strategies.

In addition, exercise is now widely recommended among cancer patients and survivors [40, 74]; however, questions remain on the optimal exercise prescriptions for individual patients. Several trials are exploring the impact of exercise and lifestyle interventions on the cardiovascular health and well-being of BC survivors. The BWEL (Breast Cancer Weight Loss) (NCT02750826) study will enroll approximately 3200 early BC patients, randomized in a 1:1 ratio to the health education program arm alone or the health education program with weight loss intervention arm. Although the primary outcome is to measure invasive disease-free survival over 10 years, secondary outcomes include evaluating the effect of supervised weight loss on overall survival, weight, body composition, and insulin resistance syndrome-associated conditions such as diabetes and CV hospitalization. The PREDICOP (Prevention of Breast Cancer Recurrence Through Weight Control, Diet, and Physical Activity Intervention) (NCT02035631) study will enroll 2000 non-metastatic BC patients, randomized in a 1:1 ratio to receive either minimal diet and exercise intervention or intensive diet and exercise interventions. The primary outcome is recurrence over 5 years; however, QOL and biomarkers related to dietary intake, insulin resistance, and inflammatory processes will also be monitored. Additionally, the B-AHEAD3 (Breast Activity and Healthy Eating After Diagnosis 3) (NCT00869466) study will randomize 134 BC patients to receive resistance training or resistance training and tailored low-calorie diet counseling. Patients' time to disease progression, chemotherapy toxicity, QOL, fatigue, change in weight, waist circumference, and fat and muscle mass will be evaluated.

The results of these studies, consisting of large cohorts and long follow-up periods, may yield promising data on the practical application of lifestyle interventions in survivorship specifically in BC patients. While these studies will provide important data on the impact of lifestyle interventions in BC survivors, further studies focusing on older BC patients with concomitant CV comorbidities evaluating CV outcomes are needed if we are to improve the CV health of BC survivors.

Conclusion

It is critical that BC survivors maintain healthy and active lifestyles after completion of cancer therapy and throughout survivorship to buoy their CV health against the impact of anticancer therapy, CV risk factors, and lifestyle disruptions. Cardiologists, oncologists, primary care providers, and other allied health professionals must work together to create lifestyle and exercise plans that improve the functional status, fatigue level, and exercise tolerance of each patient to ensure optimal health outcomes. More studies in older populations and populations with preexisting CV risk factors focusing on CV outcomes will allow for a better understanding of the type and duration of lifestyle and exercise intervention that is appropriate based on an individual patient's comorbidities and cancer treatment history.

References

1. Siegel RL, Miller KD, Jemal A. Cancer statistics, 2020. CA Ca J Clin. 2020;70(1):7–30.
2. Edwards BK, Noone AM, Mariotto AB, Simard EP, Boscoe FP, Henley SJ, et al. Annual Report to the Nation on the status of cancer, 1975–2010, featuring prevalence of comorbidity and impact on survival among persons with lung, colorectal, breast, or prostate cancer. Cancer. 2014;120(9):1290–314.
3. Howlader N, Noone A, Krapcho M, Garshell J, Altekruse SF MD, Kosary CL, Yu M, Ruhl J, Tatalovich Z, Mariotto A, Lewis DR, Chen HS, Feuer EJ, Cronin KA, editors. SEER Cancer Statistics Review, 1975–2012. Bethesda, MD: National Cancer Institute; 2015.
4. Buddeke J, Gernaat SA, Bots ML, van den Bongard DH, Grobbee DE, Vaartjes I, et al. Trends in the risk of cardiovascular disease in women with breast cancer in a Dutch nationwide cohort study. BMJ Open. 2019;9(5):e022664.
5. Hooning MJ, Botma A, Aleman BM, Baaijens MH, Bartelink H, Klijn JG, et al. Long-term risk of cardiovascular disease in 10-year survivors of breast cancer. J Natl Cancer Inst. 2007;99(5):365–75.
6. Accordino MK, Neugut AI, Hershman DL. Cardiac effects of anticancer therapy in the elderly. J Clin Oncol. 2014;32(24):2654.
7. Armenian SH, Lacchetti C, Barac A, Carver J, Constine LS, Denduluri N, et al. Prevention and monitoring of cardiac dysfunction in survivors of adult cancers: American Society of Clinical Oncology Clinical Practice Guideline. J Clin Oncol. 2016;
8. Turner N, Biganzoli L, Di Leo A. Continued value of adjuvant anthracyclines as treatment for early breast cancer. Lancet Oncol. 2015;16(7):e362–e9.
9. Romond EH, Perez EA, Bryant J, Suman VJ, Geyer CE Jr, Davidson NE, et al. Trastuzumab plus adjuvant chemotherapy for operable HER2-positive breast cancer. N Engl J Med. 2005;353(16):1673–84.
10. Pinder MC, Duan Z, Goodwin JS, Hortobagyi GN, Giordano SH. Congestive heart failure in older women treated with adjuvant anthracycline chemotherapy for breast cancer. J Clin Oncol. 2007;25(25):3808–15.

11. Doyle JJ, Neugut AI, Jacobson JS, Grann VR, Hershman DL. Chemotherapy and cardiotoxicity in older breast cancer patients: a population-based study. J Clin Oncol. 2005;23(34):8597–605.
12. Seidman A, Hudis C, Pierri MK, Shak S, Paton V, Ashby M, et al. Cardiac dysfunction in the trastuzumab clinical trials experience. J Clin Oncol. 2002;20(5):1215–21.
13. Doxorubicin Hydrochloride for Injection, U SP [package insert]. Phramacia & Upjohn Company, Division of Pfizer Inc, NY, NY 10017. 2010.
14. Murbraech K, Wethal T, Smeland KB, Holte H, Loge JH, Holte E, et al. Valvular dysfunction in lymphoma survivors treated with autologous stem cell transplantation: a national cross-sectional study. JACC Cardiovasc Imaging. 2016;9(3):230–9.
15. Epirubicin Hydrochloride for Injection [package insert]. Mayne Pharma Limited Mulgrave, VIC 3170, Australia. 2006.
16. Buza V, Rajagopalan B, Curtis AB. Cancer treatment–induced arrhythmias: focus on chemotherapy and targeted therapies. Circ Arrhythm Electrophysiol. 2017;10(8):e005443.
17. Darby SC, Ewertz M, Hall P. Ischemic heart disease after breast cancer radiotherapy. N Engl J Med. 2013;368(26):2527.
18. Desai MY, Jellis CL, Kotecha R, Johnston DR, Griffin BP. Radiation-associated cardiac disease: a practical approach to diagnosis and management. JACC Cardiovasc Imaging. 2018;11(8):1132–49.
19. Cuppone F, Bria E, Verma S, Pritchard KI, Gandhi S, Carlini P, et al. Do adjuvant aromatase inhibitors increase the cardiovascular risk in postmenopausal women with early breast cancer: meta-analysis of randomized trials. Cancer. 2008;112(2):260–7.
20. Dent SF, Gaspo R, Kissner M, Pritchard KI. Aromatase inhibitor therapy: toxicities and management strategies in the treatment of postmenopausal women with hormone-sensitive early breast cancer. Breast Cancer Res Treat. 2011;126(2):295–310.
21. Xu X, Chlebowski RT, Shi J, Barac A, Haque R. Aromatase inhibitor and tamoxifen use and the risk of venous thromboembolism in breast cancer survivors. Breast Cancer Res Treat. 2019;174(3):785–94.
22. Mehta LS, Watson KE, Barac A, Beckie TM, Bittner V, Cruz-Flores S, et al. Cardiovascular disease and breast cancer: where these entities intersect: a scientific statement from the American Heart Association. Circulation. 2018;137(8):e30–66.
23. Koelwyn GJ, Khouri M, Mackey JR, Douglas PS, Jones LW. Running on empty: cardiovascular reserve capacity and late effects of therapy in cancer survivorship. J Clin Oncol. 2012;30(36):4458.
24. Jones LW, Courneya KS, Fairey AS, Mackey JR. Effects of an oncologist's recommendation to exercise on self-reported exercise behavior in newly diagnosed breast cancer survivors: a single-blind, randomized controlled trial. Ann Behav Med. 2004;28(2):105–13.
25. Vance V, Mourtzakis M, McCargar L, Hanning R. Weight gain in breast cancer survivors: prevalence, pattern and health consequences. Obes Rev. 2011;12(4):282–94.
26. Demark-Wahnefried W, Campbell KL, Hayes SC. Weight management and its role in breast cancer rehabilitation. Cancer. 2012;118(S8):2277–87.
27. Irwin ML, Crumley D, McTiernan A, Bernstein L, Baumgartner R, Gilliland FD, et al. Physical activity levels before and after a diagnosis of breast carcinoma: the Health, Eating, Activity, and Lifestyle (HEAL) study. Cancer. 2003;97(7):1746–57.
28. Dimeo FC, Stieglitz RD, Novelli-Fischer U, Fetscher S, Keul J. Effects of physical activity on the fatigue and psychologic status of cancer patients during chemotherapy. Cancer. 1999;85(10):2273–7.
29. Bower JE, Ganz PA, Desmond KA, Rowland JH, Meyerowitz BE, Belin TR. Fatigue in breast cancer survivors: occurrence, correlates, and impact on quality of life. J Clin Oncol. 2000;18(4):743.
30. Broeckel JA, Jacobsen PB, Horton J, Balducci L, Lyman GH. Characteristics and correlates of fatigue after adjuvant chemotherapy for breast cancer. J Clin Oncol. 1998;16(5):1689–96.
31. De Ligt K, Heins M, Verloop J, Ezendam N, Smorenburg C, Korevaar J, et al. The impact of health symptoms on health-related quality of life in early-stage breast cancer survivors. Breast Cancer Res Treat. 2019;178(3):703–11.
32. Arnett DK, Blumenthal RS, Albert MA, Buroker AB, Goldberger ZD, Hahn EJ, et al. 2019 ACC/AHA guideline on the primary prevention of cardiovascular disease: executive summary: a report of the American College of Cardiology/American Heart Association Task Force on Clinical Practice Guidelines. J Am Coll Cardiol. 2019;74(10):1376–414.
33. Curigliano G, Cardinale D, Suter T, Plataniotis G, De Azambuja E, Sandri MT, et al. Cardiovascular toxicity induced by chemotherapy, targeted agents and radiotherapy: ESMO Clinical Practice Guidelines. Ann Oncol. 2012;23(suppl_7):vii155–vii66.
34. Jones LW, Haykowsky MJ, Swartz JJ, Douglas PS, Mackey JR. Early breast cancer therapy and cardiovascular injury. J Am Coll Cardiol. 2007;50(15):1435–41.
35. Lahart IM, Carmichael AR, Nevill AM, Kitas GD, Metsios GS. The effects of a home-based physical activity intervention on cardiorespiratory fitness in breast cancer survivors; a randomised controlled trial. J Sports Sci. 2018;36(10):1077–86.
36. Giallauria F, Vitelli A, Maresca L, De Magistris MS, Chiodini P, Mattiello A, et al. Exercise training improves cardiopulmonary and endothelial function in women with breast cancer: findings from the Diana-5 dietary intervention study. Intern Emerg Med. 2016;11(2):183–9.
37. Jones LW, Courneya KS, Mackey JR, Muss HB, Pituskin EN, Scott JM, et al. Cardiopulmonary function and age-related decline across the breast cancer survivorship continuum. J Clin Oncol. 2012;30(20):2530.

38. Lakoski SG, Eves ND, Douglas PS, Jones LW. Exercise rehabilitation in patients with cancer. Nat Rev Clin Oncol. 2012;9(5):288.
39. Jones LW, Watson D, Herndon JE, Eves ND, Haithcock BE, Loewen G, et al. Peak oxygen consumption and long-term all-cause mortality in nonsmall cell lung cancer. Cancer. 2010;116(20):4825–32.
40. Curigliano G, Lenihan D, Fradley M, Ganatra S, Barac A, Blaes A, et al. Management of cardiac disease in cancer patients throughout oncological treatment: ESMO consensus recommendations. Ann Oncol. 2020;31(2):171–90.
41. Plana JC, Galderisi M, Barac A, Ewer MS, Ky B, Scherrer-Crosbie M, et al. Expert consensus for multimodality imaging evaluation of adult patients during and after cancer therapy: a report from the American Society of Echocardiography and the European Association of Cardiovascular Imaging. Eur Heart J Cardiovasc Imag. 2014;15(10):1063–93.
42. Zamorano J, Lancellotti P, Rodriguez Muñoz D, Aboyans V, Asteggiano R, Galderisi M, et al. ESC Scientific Document Group. 2016 ESC Position Paper on cancer treatments and cardiovascular toxicity developed under the auspices of the ESC Committee for Practice Guidelines: The Task Force for cancer treatments and cardiovascular toxicity of the European Society of Cardiology (ESC). Eur Heart J. 2016;37(36):2768–801.
43. Seferina SC, de Boer M, Derksen MW, van den Berkmortel F, van Kampen RJ, van de Wouw AJ, et al. Cardiotoxicity and cardiac monitoring during adjuvant trastuzumab in daily Dutch practice: a study of the Southeast Netherlands Breast Cancer Consortium. Oncologist. 2016;21(5):555–62.
44. Cardinale D, Colombo A, Torrisi R, Sandri MT, Civelli M, Salvatici M, et al. Trastuzumab-induced cardiotoxicity: clinical and prognostic implications of troponin I evaluation. J Clin Oncol. 2010;28(25):3910–6.
45. Sandri MT, Salvatici M, Cardinale D, Zorzino L, Passerini R, Lentati P, et al. N-terminal pro-B-type natriuretic peptide after high-dose chemotherapy: a marker predictive of cardiac dysfunction? Clin Chem. 2005;51(8):1405–10.
46. Doust J, Lehman R, Glasziou P. The role of BNP testing in heart failure. Am Fam Physician. 2006;74(11):1893–8.
47. Denlinger CS, Sanft T, Baker KS, Broderick G, Demark-Wahnefried W, Friedman DL, et al. Survivorship, version 2.2018, NCCN clinical practice guidelines in oncology. J Natl Compr Cancer Netw. 2018;16(10):1216–47.
48. Armenian SH, Xu L, Ky B, Sun C, Farol LT, Pal SK, et al. Cardiovascular disease among survivors of adult-onset cancer: a community-based retrospective cohort study. J Clin Oncol. 2016;34(10):1122–30.
49. Arps K, Pallazola VA, Cardoso R, Meyer J, Jones R II, Latina J, et al. Clinician's guide to the updated ABCs of cardiovascular disease prevention: a review part 1. Am J Med. 2019;
50. O'Keefe JH, Bell DS. Postprandial hyperglycemia/hyperlipidemia (postprandial dysmetabolism) is a cardiovascular risk factor. Am J Cardiol. 2007;100(5):899–904.
51. Wolf I, Sadetzki S, Catane R, Karasik A, Kaufman B. Diabetes mellitus and breast cancer. Lancet Oncol. 2005;6(2):103–11.
52. Jawa Z, Perez RM, Garlie L, Singh M, Qamar R, Khandheria BK, et al. Risk factors of trastuzumab-induced cardiotoxicity in breast cancer: a meta-analysis. Medicine. 2016;95(44)
53. Schneider CM, Dennehy CA, Carter SD. Exercise and cancer recovery: human kinetics 1; 2003.
54. Xie Y, Collins WJ, Audeh MW, Shiao SL, Gottlieb RA, Goodman MT, et al. Breast cancer survivorship and cardiovascular disease: emerging approaches in cardio-oncology. Curr Treat Options Cardiovasc Med. 2015;17(12):60.
55. Jones LW, Habel LA, Weltzien E, Castillo A, Gupta D, Kroenke CH, et al. Exercise and risk of cardiovascular events in women with nonmetastatic breast cancer. J Clin Oncol. 2016;34(23):2743.
56. MEMBERS WC, Hunt SA, Abraham WT, Chin MH, Feldman AM, Francis GS, et al. 2009 focused update incorporated into the ACC/AHA 2005 Guidelines for the Diagnosis and Management of Heart Failure in Adults: a report of the American College of Cardiology Foundation/American Heart Association Task Force on Practice Guidelines: developed in collaboration with the International Society for Heart and Lung Transplantation. Circulation. 2009;119(14):e391–479.
57. Finet JE, Tang WW. Protecting the heart in cancer therapy. F1000Research. 2018;7
58. Scott JM, Thomas SM, Peppercorn JM, Herndon JE, Douglas PS, Khouri MG, et al. Effects of exercise therapy dosing schedule on impaired cardiorespiratory fitness in patients with primary breast cancer: a randomized controlled trial. Circulation. 2020;141(7):560–70.
59. Hornsby WE, Douglas PS, West MJ, Kenjale AA, Lane AR, Schwitzer ER, et al. Safety and efficacy of aerobic training in operable breast cancer patients receiving neoadjuvant chemotherapy: a phase II randomized trial. Acta Oncol. 2014;53(1):65–74.
60. Segal R, Evans W, Johnson D, Smith J, Colletta S, Gayton J, et al. Structured exercise improves physical functioning in women with stages I and II breast cancer: results of a randomized controlled trial. J Clin Oncol. 2001;19(3):657–65.
61. Courneya KS, Mackey JR, Bell GJ, Jones LW, Field CJ, Fairey AS. Randomized controlled trial of exercise training in postmenopausal breast cancer survivors: cardiopulmonary and quality of life outcomes. J Clin Oncol. 2003;21(9):1660–8.
62. Carayol M, Bernard P, Boiche J, Riou F, Mercier B, Cousson-Gélie F, et al. Psychological effect of exercise in women with breast cancer receiving adjuvant therapy: what is the optimal dose needed? Ann Oncol. 2013;24(2):291–300.

63. Mock V, Frangakis C, Davidson NE, Ropka ME, Pickett M, Poniatowski B, et al. Exercise manages fatigue during breast cancer treatment: a randomized controlled trial. Psycho Oncol. 2005;14(6):464–77.
64. Schwartz AL. Daily fatigue patterns and effect of exercise in women with breast cancer. Cancer Pract. 2000;8(1):16–24.
65. El-Hashimi D, Gorey KM. Yoga-specific enhancement of quality of life among women with breast cancer: systematic review and exploratory meta-analysis of randomized controlled trials. J Evid Based Integr Med. 2019;24:2515690X19828325.
66. Vadiraja H, Rao RM, Nagarathna R, Nagendra H, Patil S, Diwakar RB, et al. Effects of yoga in managing fatigue in breast cancer patients: a randomized controlled trial. Indian J Palliat Care. 2017;23(3):247.
67. Dong B, Xie C, Jing X, Lin L, Tian L. Yoga has a solid effect on cancer-related fatigue in patients with breast cancer: a meta-analysis. Breast Cancer Res Treat. 2019:1–12.
68. Schmitz KH, Courneya KS, Matthews C, Demark-Wahnefried W, Galvão DA, Pinto BM, et al. American College of Sports Medicine roundtable on exercise guidelines for cancer survivors. Med Sci Sports Exerc. 2010;42(7):1409–26.
69. Grimmett C, Corbett T, Brunet J, Shepherd J, Pinto BM, May CR, et al. Systematic review and meta-analysis of maintenance of physical activity behaviour change in cancer survivors. Int J Behav Nutr Phys Act. 2019;16(1):37.
70. Scott JM, Zabor EC, Schwitzer E, Koelwyn GJ, Adams SC, Nilsen TS, et al. Efficacy of exercise therapy on cardiorespiratory fitness in patients with cancer: a systematic review and meta-analysis. Am Soc Clin Oncol. 2018;
71. Coletta AM, Marquez G, Thomas P, Thoman W, Bevers T, Brewster AM, et al. Clinical factors associated with adherence to aerobic and resistance physical activity guidelines among cancer prevention patients and survivors. PloS one. 2019;14(8)
72. Berkman AM, Gilchrist SC. Behavioral change strategies to improve physical activity after cancer treatment. Rehabil Oncol. 2018;36(3):152–60.
73. Yin AB, Brewster AM, Barac A, Thoman W, Oeffinger KC, Gilchrist SC. Cardiovascular prevention strategies in breast cancer. JACC. 2019;1(2):322–5.
74. Gilchrist SC, Barac A, Ades PA, Alfano CM, Franklin BA, Jones LW, et al. Cardio-oncology rehabilitation to manage cardiovascular outcomes in cancer patients and survivors: a scientific statement from the American Heart Association. Circulation. 2019;139(21):e997–e1012.

17 Diabetes and Breast Cancer

Leonor Corsino and Jasmine Mcneill

Introduction

Women with diabetes are more likely to develop breast cancer [1], are less likely to be screened for breast cancer [2], and have greater mortality once diagnosed with breast cancer as compared to women without diabetes [3]. Women who have been diagnosed with both breast cancer and diabetes are therefore particularly vulnerable to poor health outcomes that could potentially be preventable through early diagnosis and treatment of diabetes to support their breast cancer care.

Previous studies have shown the prevalence of diabetes among patients with breast cancer to be much higher than in the general population. A 2011 meta-analysis of women with breast cancer reported diabetes prevalence ranging from 8% to 31%, which was significantly higher than the US national prevalence of diabetes of 8.3% at the time [4, 5].

Although the exact mechanism explaining the observed association between breast cancer and diabetes is not elucidated, several potential pathophysiologic mechanics have been proposed. The most studied potential mechanism involves the role of hyperinsulinemia. Hyperinsulinemia, common in patients with type 2 diabetes, is thought to be a contributing factor in breast cancer and other obesity-related cancers. This is due to insulin inhibition of the sex hormone-binding globulin increasing free steroid hormones, including estrogen [6]. Additionally, hyperinsulinemia leads to higher levels of IGF-1 and inflammatory cytokines that may promote carcinogenesis by promoting cell proliferation and inhibiting apoptosis [7]. Other potential mediators include hyperglycemia, adipokines, dyslipidemia, and changes in the gut microbiome [8].

Concurrent diagnosis of diabetes in a breast cancer survivor has implications not only for the management of each of these diseases and for their mortality but also for the patient's quality of life [9]. Improving a breast cancer survivor's quality of life is not only important in and of itself but also is associated with reduced cancer recurrence and improved mortality rates [10]. These results support the mutli-faceted importance of diabetes management in breast cancer survivors.

In this chapter, we will summarize the existing evidence about the impact of diabetes on breast cancer outcomes, including diagnosis, treatment, treatment response, mortality, and cancer recurrence, and we will outline an approach to diabetes management in a patient with breast cancer.

L. Corsino (✉)
Department of Medicine, Division of Endocrinology, Metabolism, and Nutrition, Duke University School of Medicine, Durham, NC, USA
e-mail: Corsi002@mc.duke.edu

J. Mcneill
Keck School of Medicine of University of Southern California, Los Angeles, CA, USA
e-mail: Jasmine.McNeill@med.usc.edu

G. G. Kimmick et al. (eds.), *Common Issues in Breast Cancer Survivors*,
https://doi.org/10.1007/978-3-030-75377-1_17

Diagnosis, Treatment, and Treatment Response

Breast Cancer Screening and Diagnosis

Despite the existing evidence supporting the association between breast cancer and diabetes, in general, preventive care underutilization in patients with diabetes has been reported [11]. The underutilization of preventive care and screening can be explained in part by the burden diabetes imposes on patients and their health-care providers, making services that are less directly related to diabetes rendered less often [12]. Two epidemiologic studies examined use of screening mammograms in women with diabetes compared to women without diabetes. The first was a case-control study looking at whether women with diabetes received recommended screening mammograms compared with women without diabetes that included a total of 424 women with diabetes between the ages of 50 and 75 years treated at primary care in the mid-western United States and a comparison group of 845 women without diabetes. Findings showed that women with diabetes had significantly lower rates of screening mammograms than women without diabetes. This lower rate persisted after adjusting for insurance status and race [12]. In contrast, the Southern Community Cohort Study (*N* = 45,511; age 40–79), a cohort study conducted primarily among low-income persons in the southeastern United States, found no differences in rates of having a screening mammogram in the past 12 months among white women with diabetes and those without diabetes [13]. There was also no association of diabetes and having received a screening mammogram with the past 12 months among black women.

Diabetes has been shown to predict use of screening mammogram in large cohort studies. A study looking at patient and provider characteristics as predictors of screening mammograms in a cohort of 44,318 Israeli women aged 56–74 showed that having diabetes was associated with lower adherence with screening mammogram recommendations [14]. Further, a study conducted with a total of 841 eastern Caribbean women showed that having diabetes and hypertension was associated with not receiving timely screening mammograms [15]. Similarly, a study using a large cohort (*N* = 2056) of women in France showed that adherence to breast cancer screening was lower in women with obesity and diabetes, and this persisted after adjusting for the complete range of screening determinants [16]. A population-based retrospective cohort study conducted in Canada with a total of 188,759 with diabetes and 315,529 with no diabetes showed that, after adjusting for socioeconomic status, women with diabetes were less likely to have a mammogram [2]. All of this confirms the underutilization of screening mammograms in patients with diabetes. A more recently published meta-analysis looking at cancer screening in patients with diabetes confirmed that having diabetes is associated with a significantly lower likelihood of breast cancer screening [17].

Current recommendations emphasize the importance of screening patients with diabetes for breast cancer with the recommended age-appropriate cancer screening. Further, it is highly recommended that cancer screening be part of the routine diabetes assessment [11, 18].

Screening for Diabetes

In 2019, it was estimated that a total of 232 million people around the world met the criteria for a diagnosis of diabetes and yet had not been formally diagnosed. This alarming rate of underdiagnosis prompts questions regarding the potential role of diabetes screening in patients diagnosed with breast cancer. Currently, the American Diabetes Association (ADA) standard of care guidelines does not specifically recommend routine screening for diabetes in asymptomatic patients with breast cancer. However, providers should keep in mind that diabetes and cancer share many risk factors, such as aging, obesity, and physical inactivity. Patients not previously or not recently screened for diabetes who meet the current ADA recommendation for screening (Table 17.1) [19] and who are diagnosed with breast cancer should be tested.

Table 17.1 Indications for testing for diabetes in adults. Adapted from the ADA 2020 standard of care [54]

Overweight or obese adult (BMI >/= 25 kg/m^2 or >/= 23 kg/m^2 in Asian-American) that has one or more risk factors including: First-degree relative with diabetes High-risk race/ethnicity (e.g., African-American, Latino, Native American, Asian-American, and Pacific Islander) History of cardiovascular disease Hypertension (>/= 140/90 mm hg or on therapy for hypertension) HDL cholesterol <35 mg/dL (0.90 mmol/L) and/or a triglyceride level >250 mg/dL (2.82 mmol/L) Women with polycystic ovary syndrome Physical inactivity Other conditions associated with insulin resistance (e.g., severe obesity, acanthosis nigricans)
Patients with prediabetes (A1C >/= 5.7% [39 mmol/Mol], impaired glucose tolerance (IGT), or impaired fasting glucose (IFG) should be tested yearly
Women who were diagnosed with gestational diabetes mellitus (GDM) should have a lifelong testing at least every 3 years
For all other patients, testing should begin at the age of 45 years
If results are normal, testing should be repeated at minimum every 3 years with consideration of more frequency testing depending on initial results and risk status

Treatment and Treatment Response

In this section, we will summarize the available evidence exploring the role of diabetes medications in the prevention of breast cancer, the role of diabetes in breast cancer regimen choices, and the impact of diabetes in breast cancer treatment response.

Diabetes Medications and Breast Cancer

Metformin is an oral antidiabetic medication recommended as the first-line agent for the management of patients with type 2 diabetes. Metformin has been the most studied diabetes medication in cancer for its potential effect on cancer prevention and cancer cell proliferation. Metformin works by reducing hepatic glucose production and insulin resistance. The exact mechanism of action of metformin is complex and not clearly understood. However, recent studies showed several potential mechanisms by which metformin produces a reduction in hepatic glucose production. A recently identified mechanism includes the inhibition of mitochondrial glycerol-3-phosphate dehydrogenase (GPD2), which increases the cellular redox state and results in the inhibition of the conversion of some substrates (such as lactate and glycerol) to glucose in vitro. The additional mechanism includes metformin action on the liver via AMP-activated protein kinase (AMPK) activation, inhibits mTOR activity by activating ataxia-telangiectasia mutated (ATM) and liver kinase B1 (LKB1), and thus prevents protein synthesis and cell growth [20, 21]. Laboratory studies provided the initial signals towards a potential role of metformin in the prevention and treatment of cancers, including breast cancer [22, 23].

Studies in humans, including observational and randomized controlled trials, have been conducted exploring these potential uses of metformin in breast cancer. In recent years, an array of publications has emerged showing inconclusive results when it comes to the role of metformin in the prevention and treatment of patients with breast cancer [24]. A 2018 review of 12 observational studies on the role of metformin in breast cancer incidence concluded that there was insufficient evidence to support the role of metformin as a preventive drug for breast cancer, although authors acknowledged the limitations of their conclusion, primarily because the review was based on observational studies [25].

In a 2017 Surveillance, Epidemiology, and End Results (SEER) study, authors looked at diabetes medications including metformin and the risk of adverse outcomes in early-stage breast cancer patients [26]. In this study, a total of 14,766 women aged 66–80 were included. Of those, 4544 (30.8%) women had a diagnosis of diabetes, and 2558 (17.3%) reported ever using metformin after a breast cancer diagnosis. The study showed that women with a prior diagnosis of diabetes were more likely to have tumors that were stage II, node positive, and of higher grade and larger size. These characteristics were similar in women with diabetes independent of the use of metformin. Among those with diabetes, after multivariable-adjusted analyses, women ever reporting the use of metformin had a 28% lower risk of a second breast cancer event, 31% lower breast cancer recurrence, and 49% lower breast cancer death compared with nonusers of metformin. Among all patients with diabetes treated with medications ($N = 3189$), the use of sulfonylurea or insulin was associated with higher risks of breast cancer death, but not with secondary breast cancer events or recurrence risk. Further analysis looking at patients on multiple medications for diabetes showed no meaningful changes in risk estimates. Similar results were observed when the analysis was conducted to reduce confounding. The use of metformin was associated with 38%, 42%, and 66% lower risks of secondary breast cancer events, recurrence, and breast cancer death, respectively, whereas the use of insulin was associated with a 2.42-fold higher risk of breast cancer death. When looking at the patients using one medication at a time, the use of sulfonylurea or insulin remained associated with a higher risk of all adverse breast cancer outcomes when compared to the use of metformin alone [26].

The use of metformin and insulin and the effect on breast cancer outcomes were analyzed in data from the Adjuvant Lapatinib and/or Trastuzumab Treatment Optimization (ALTTO) trial, a phase III randomized trial in women with human epidermal growth factor receptor 2 (HER2)-positive primary breast cancer in which patients were randomized to one of four arms: (1) trastuzumab, (2) lapatinib, (3) their sequence, and (4) combination of both. Of the 8381 patients included in the study, 446 (5.3%) had diabetes. Two hundred and sixty (3.1%) were on metformin and 186 (2.2%) were not. The median follow-up time was 4.5 years. Patients with diabetes who had not been treated with metformin experienced worse disease-free survival, distant disease-free survival, and overall survival. Similar to the SEER study, insulin use was associated with worse outcomes [27].

A prospective phase II trial was conducted to compare metformin plus chemotherapy versus chemotherapy alone in the first-line treatment of HER2-negative metastatic breast cancer. The MYME trial, a phase II clinical trial of metformin plus chemotherapy versus chemotherapy alone in the first-line treatment of HER2-negative metastatic breast cancer, enrolled patients without diabetes. A total of 126 participants between the ages of 18 and 75 years were enrolled from 16 centers in Italy. Participants were randomized to chemotherapy (non-pegylated liposomal doxorubicin (NPLD) 60 mg/m2 + cyclophosphamide (C) 600 mg/m2 × 8 cycles Q21 days) with or without metformin (2000 mg/day). The study's primary outcome was progression-free survival (PFS; calculated from the date of randomization to the date of disease progression). At a median follow-up of 39.6 months, with 112 PFS events, median progression-free survival was not statistically different between arms (HR 1.09, 95% CI 0.75–1.58, $p = 0.653$); median PFS was 9.4 months (95% CI 7.8–10.4) with chemotherapy + metformin and 9.9 months (95% CI 7.4–11.5) with chemotherapy alone. Median overall survival was, likewise, no different. In this study, the addition of metformin to chemotherapy did not improve outcome among patients with HER2-negative metastatic breast cancer [28].

The association of diabetes, diabetes treatment, and breast cancer gene expression profile (GEP) was analyzed in a retrospective single-center cohort study. The GEP, Oncotype DX® (ODX) test, is a prognosticator of breast cancer recurrence and a predictor of the benefit of chemotherapy for patients with node-negative, hormone receptor-positive, HER2-negative breast cancer. A study assessing the impact of diabetes and metformin use in the ODX score showed that neither a diagnosis of diabetes/prediabetes nor the use of metformin is associated with GEP score. The study included a cohort of 514 early-stage, hormone-positive breast cancer patients. Of those, 67 (13%) had diabetes or prediabetes [29]. Given the known poor outcomes for breast cancer patients with diabetes, further research studying the association between diabetes and breast cancer GEP is warranted.

In sum, the above data demonstrate the need for additional research to determine the role of metformin in the prevention or treatment of patients with breast cancer.

Key Points

- Metformin has been the most studied diabetes medication in cancer including the prevention and potential treatment of breast cancer.
- Observational and randomized controlled trials have been reported with conflicting results.
- Currently, metformin is not recommended for breast cancer prevention or treatment.
- Additional research is needed to further determine the role of metformin in breast cancer prevention and treatment.

Mortality and Recurrence

In addition to the higher-than-average diabetes prevalence among patients with breast cancer, many studies have explored the prognostic implications of diabetes as comorbidity on women with breast cancer. Due to the multifactorial contributions of both breast cancer and diabetes to a patient's health, prognostication is equally as complex and variable based on the factors examined. This segment will review the all-cause mortality of breast cancer survivors with diabetes and will further explore cancer-specific mortality and mortality associated with other causes. Other related considerations will also be reviewed, including the timing of the diagnosis and duration of diabetes, the observed effect of obesity on mortality, and how high sugar states (hyperglycemia, high fructosamine levels) may be used as prognostic factors among women with breast cancer.

Overall Survival and Disease-Free Survival

In 2016, Zhao et al. performed a systematic review and meta-analysis of pertinent evidence over the past 15 years with a focus on studying how diabetes as a comorbidity was associated with overall survival, disease-free survival, and relapse-free period among women with breast cancer [30]. In this study, overall survival was defined as the time from diagnosis or surgery to death due to any cause or last follow-up visit and is analogous with "all-cause mortality" within the same time parameters. There was great heterogeneity of evidence on the overall survival of breast cancer patients with diabetes as compared to those without diabetes with hazard ratios (HR) ranging from 0.85 (95% CI 0.55–1.33) [31] to 2.35 (95% CI 1.56–3.54) [32]. The authors attributed this heterogeneity, in part, to variability in age of populations and type of anti-hyperglycemic used (if any). On meta-analysis, the pooled adjusted HR for those with versus without diabetes was 1.51 (95% CI 1.34–1.70) for overall survival and 1.28 (95% CI, 1.09–1.50) for disease-free survival. There was, however, no significant difference in the relapse-free period between patients with and without diabetes (HR 1.42, 95% CI 0.90–2.23). More recent studies have shown similar findings of higher rates of all-cause mortality in breast cancer patients with diabetes, as discussed below [33–45].

Although most studies on mortality have focused on women with early-stage breast cancer, a similar pattern was seen in a study of women with brain metastases from breast cancer in which women with either diabetes or obesity had worse overall survival and progression-free survival than women without diabetes or obesity [33].

In a study of 190 women with HER2+ breast cancer who were treated with surgical resection and trastuzumab, women with diabetes had worse overall and disease-free survival than women without diabetes [34].

Specific Causes of Mortality

The risk of death from all-causes, cancer specifically, and other causes has been shown to be greater among breast cancer patients with diabetes compared to those without diabetes. In order to explore these associations, several studies have examined sociodemographic, patient, and tumor characteristics to find confounders. In addition, studies have explored diabetes treatment and outcomes.

One study, published in 2020, reported causes of death among Medicaid-insured women aged <64 years with breast cancer that was reported to the New York State Cancer Registry between 2014 and 2016, by presence or absence of a diagnosis of diabetes [35]. Of the included 9221 women with breast cancer in the study, 1477 had a diagnosis of type 2 diabetes *before* their diagnosis of breast cancer. After adjusting for confounding factors, women with preexisting type 2 diabetes were not only at greater risk of all-cause mortality (HR 1.40, 95% CI 1.21–1.63), consistent with the above studies, but also for cancer-specific mortality (HR 1.24, 95% CI 1.04–1.47) and cardiovascular-specific mortality (HR 2.46, 95% CI 1.54–3.90). Interestingly, in this group of Medicaid-insured women, the higher risk of all-cause mortality among women with type 2 diabetes compared to those without diabetes was most marked among non-Hispanic white (HR 1.78, 95% CI 1.38–2.30), those with localized SEER Summary Stage (HR 1.62, 95% CI 1.23–2.14), postmenopausal (HR 1.47, 95% CI 1.23–1.77), and nonobese (HR 1.49, 95% CI 1.22–1.82) women. Analyses also explored risk factors for all-cause mortality among patients with diabetes. Among women with coexistent diabetes and breast cancer, higher risk of all-cause mortality was noted among postmenopausal (versus premenopausal; HR 1.60, 95% CI 1.02–2.50) and those with triple-negative breast cancer (versus hormone receptor positive; HR 1.76, 95% CI 1.11–2.80) and lower risk of all-cause mortality among obese (versus nonobese; HR 0.65, 95% CI 0.52–0.83). In addition, compared to those treated with metformin for type 2 diabetes, higher all-cause mortality was seen among and those treated with sulfonylurea (HR 1.44, 95% CI 1.06–1.94) or insulin (HR 1.54, 95% CI 1.12–2.11).

The association of breast cancer-specific mortality with diabetes has been inconsistent in the literature, which may be due to modification by receipt of chemotherapy and antihyperglycemic use. A 2009 SEER-Medicare analysis including over 70,000 patients found that, although patients with diabetes had higher all-cause mortality (HR 1.35, 95% CI 1.31–1.39), only patients with diabetes who received chemotherapy had higher breast cancer-specific mortality (HR 1.20, 95% CI 1.07–1.35) than patients without diabetes who also received chemotherapy [36]. There was no difference in breast cancer-specific mortality among patients with or without diabetes if they did not receive chemotherapy (HR 0.95, 95% CI 0.88–1.03).

A 2015 study of 1763 patients with both breast cancer and type 2 diabetes reported that a decreased breast cancer-specific mortality was associated with each year of metformin use, especially with at least 2 years of use (adjusted HR 0.47, 95% CI 0.26–0.82) [37]. This same study found a large increase (adjusted HR 3.64, 95% CI 2.16–6.16) in breast cancer-specific mortality associated with sulfonylurea derivative use; however, the authors cautioned that this association may be due to selective prescribing among patients with more advanced cancer.

As part of the Long Island Breast Cancer Study Project, Parada et al. examined the risk of breast cancer incidence and all-cause and breast cancer-specific mortality based on single nucleotide polymorphisms (SNPs) found to be associated with diabetes [38]. Among these diabetes-associated SNPs, three SNPs were found to be associated with all-cause mortality in additive models ($\alpha = 0.05$) but were not significant at Bonferroni corrected α of 0.0003. Three SNPs were associated with breast cancer-specific mortality, two of which were associated with reduced mortality and one with greater mortality. Continued research into how these diseases interact at a genetic level may provide a further understanding of factors modifying breast cancer-specific mortality and how mortality is impacted by cancer or diabetes treatments.

Timing of Diagnosis and Duration of Diabetes

A large retrospective study of women in the United States Military Health System examined the significance of the timing of diagnosis of diabetes with respect to mortality among 9398 women with breast cancer [39]. Women who were diagnosed with type 2 diabetes before their diagnosis of breast cancer had a modestly increased risk of mortality compared to women without diabetes (HR 1.17, 95% CI 0.95–1.44). Women who had diabetes diagnosed at or after their breast cancer diagnosis was made had an even higher risk of mortality compared to women without diabetes (HR 1.39, 95% CI 1.16–1.66). These results suggest a moderately increased mortality for women with diabetes, which may be modified by the timing of this diagnosis compared to their diagnosis with breast cancer.

The timing of the diagnosis of diabetes may also be associated with other aspects of patient care, including receipt of differential treatment. The above study also found that women who were diagnosed with diabetes before their diagnosis with breast cancer were less likely to receive radiation or chemotherapy. Although there is a reasonable concern for the interaction between diabetes, diabetes treatment, and breast cancer treatment, in this population, there was not a mortality difference among women with diabetes between women diagnosed *before* and *at/after* a breast cancer diagnosis. There was greater mortality among women with diabetes regardless of timing of diagnosis compared to women without diabetes. These findings suggest that the difference of mortality is multifactorial beyond (but including) severity of diabetes and receipt of differential breast cancer treatment.

The final point about timing from this study is the finding that women with diabetes diagnosed before breast cancer were less likely to have a recurrence of the disease as compared to women diagnosed at/after breast cancer or women without diabetes (15.9% before, 21.5% at/after, 20% no diabetes, $p = 0.01$). It is unclear if this finding is due to better control of diabetes with an earlier diagnosis of diabetes and if this better glycemic control is associated with lower likelihood of breast cancer recurrence or if there are other variables (such as genetics or lifestyle) that may confound this association.

In a retrospective cohort study of almost 5000 women, Lega et al. found, overall, that among women with breast cancer, women with diabetes had greater all-cause mortality (adjusted HR 1.16, 95% CI 1.06–1.27) but that this was not true of women who had a duration of diabetes which was less than 5 years (adjusted HR 1.02, 95% CI 0.86–1.21) [3]. Further, although, among all women with diabetes, breast cancer-specific mortality was not significantly increased as compared to the breast cancer-specific mortality of women without diabetes, women with a duration of diabetes greater than 5 years did have an increased breast cancer-specific mortality (adjusted HR 1.25, 95% CI 1.02–154). These findings show that a longer duration of diabetes is associated with greater all-cause and cancer-specific mortality.

Key Points

- Women with breast cancer and diabetes might have a higher risk of death.
- These findings might be influenced by many factors including time of diabetes diagnosis and use of chemotherapy and medications to treat diabetes.
- Additional research is needed to determine the factors that influence mortality in women with breast cancer and diabetes.

Obesity

A study associated with Long Island Breast Cancer Study Project reported that among women with breast cancer, women with diabetes had greater all-cause mortality but that this finding was even stronger among women who were obese at the time of their diagnosis with breast cancer [40]. However, this has not been a finding in every study.

When women with breast cancer and type 2 diabetes are further stratified into groups by obesity status, Lawrence et al. found that women who were obese had lower all-cause mortality than their nonobese counterparts (HR 0.65, 95% CI 0.52–0.83) [36]. Possible explanations for this "obesity paradox" include differences in body composition, lower weight of patients who are more chronically ill or with more aggressive cancers, or the greater nutritional reserves associated with being obese [41, 42].

A recent prospective observational study of 841 patients with early breast cancer performed analyses of overall survival and disease-free survival comparing women with and without diabetes, with and without obesity, and with both/either obesity and/or diabetes or none [43]. Buono et al. found that women with either or both diabetes and/or obesity were more likely to relapse and die from breast cancer than women without either. Consistent with prior findings, this study found that patients with diabetes had worse overall survival and worse disease-free-survival. In multivariate analyses, comorbid diabetes with obesity was found to be an independent prognostic factor for disease-free survival (HR 2.62, 95% CI 1.23–5.60, $p = 0.001$), but not overall survival (HR 2.52, 95% CI 0.97–6.58, $p = 0.058$).

Hyperglycemia

Even relatively small differences in chronic hyperglycemia may dramatically increase mortality as shown among a sample of women with clinically defined diabetes. Women with early-stage breast cancer with a hemoglobin A1c of ≥7% have more than twice the risk of all-cause mortality as compared to women with hemoglobin A1c <6.5% [32].

To further understand this process, Connor et al. evaluated the fructosamine levels of a subgroup of women who participated in the prospective case-cohort New Mexico HEAL study [44]. Fructosamine is a glycoprotein that has previously been used as an indicator of hyperglycemia that reflects a glycemic history of weeks rather than minutes in blood glucose levels or months in hemoglobin A1c levels [45]. Although Connor et al. found only minimal positive associations between fructosamine and mortality as a *continuous measure*, women with clinically high fructosamine levels had a much greater risk of mortality as compared to women with normal levels of fructosamine (all-cause HR 2.32, 95% CI 1.30–4.14; breast cancer-specific HR 4.25, 95% CI 1.67–10.80). This finding suggests that fructosamine may have prognostic value for patients with breast cancer in addition to or as an alternative to hemoglobin A1c.

Managing Diabetes in Patients with Breast Cancer

The management of diabetes in patients with breast cancer is important [46]. Patients with a diagnosis of diabetes and those that develop hyperglycemia while undergoing treatment for malignancies should have rigorous and multifactorial approaches for the control of their diabetes [47]. Currently, limited published studies are testing different approaches to managing diabetes and hyperglycemia in patients while being treated for cancer. However, there are existing recommendations from major professional organizations that provide detailed instructions on how to manage diabetes in inpatient and outpatient settings [48–51]. Below, we will provide some practical suggestions based on current recommendations that will ease the management of diabetes and hyperglycemia in breast cancer survivors.

While treating these patients, it is important to consider the patient's short- and long-term health goals. Further, treatment goals should be revisited regularly as the patient's cancer progresses or improves. Treatment decisions should be personalized and patient centered [52].

Many factors of cancer treatment might contribute to the worsening glycemic control in patients undergoing cancer treatment. Those factors are chemotherapeutic agents and their side effects, glucocorticoid use, lack of physical activity, dietary changes including enteral feeding, comorbidities, and psychosocial factors.

Patients newly diagnosed with diabetes, while undergoing cancer treatment, should receive diabetes education and nutrition. Mental health provider referral should be considered in patients with impairment of self-care, depression, diabetes distress syndrome, anxiety, declining ability to perform diabetes self-care, and symptoms suspicious of eating disorders [46, 52]. Medication choices should be driven by patient preference, overall health, comorbidities, life expectancy, nutrition status, degree of hyperglycemia, risk of hypoglycemia, cost, and complexity of the regimen.

Below is the proposed approach to diabetes screening and management in patients with a history of breast cancer [53]:

> All patients not previously diagnosed with diabetes who meet ADA recommendations should be screened using one of the methods recommended by the ADA including a fasting glucose test, a 2-hour oral glucose tolerance test, a hemoglobin A1c test, and a random blood glucose test in patients with classic symptoms of hyperglycemia or hyperglycemic crisis (Table 17.2).
>
> Unless the patient presents with a clear hyperglycemia crisis and random blood glucose of equal or more than 200 mg/dl (11.1 mmol/L), the diagnosis of diabetes requires two abnormal test results from the same sample or in two separate test samples [55]. Health-care providers should become familiarized with some of the caveats of each test. For example, in patients with anemia, the hemoglobin A1c might not be reliable as it might be lower than expected. Providers will need to utilize other methods like fructosamine to assess level of control.

1. Patients with a previous diagnosis of diabetes and no hemoglobin A1c within the last 3–6 months should get an A1c to determine the degree of glycemic control before the cancer diagnosis and treatment.
2. Review, in detail, the patient's current diabetes management regimen including medication names and doses to determine the need for adjustments on medication doses and/or regimen.
3. Determine the need for mental health referral as mentioned above.
4. Refer patients to diabetes education and nutritionist.
5. Obtain a detailed dietary and activity record.
6. Patients managed by an endocrinologist should continue working with their providers. Communication between the oncology team and other providers should remain open and frequent to allow appropriate transition of care and regimen adjustments.
7. Referral to endocrinology should be considered in all patients not able to control their diabetes on current regimen or those with difficulty controlling diabetes.
8. Medication(s) should be carefully chosen based on the medication mechanism of action, side effects, additional benefits, cost, route of administration, and frequency of administration [54]. Regimens should focus on simplifying the patient's already complex medical management while getting cancer treatment.
9. Considering the constantly changing drugs to manage type 2 diabetes, providers should become aware of the available and emerging drugs and their benefits and side effects (Table 17.3).
10. The patient requiring insulin (Table 17.4) should receive appropriate teaching on how to take their insulin and how to monitor their blood glucose. For example, patients on the basal/bolus regimen should check their blood glucose three to four times per day or use continuous glucose monitoring (sensor). Patients on basal insulin only can check fasting and when symptomatic or with concern of hypoglycemia.
11. The use of insulin pens is encouraged as it will facilitate adherence to the regimen and will minimize the complexity of insulin administration.
12. During hospitalizations, patients' medications should be revised. The use of metfor-

Table 17.2 American Diabetes Association diagnosis criteria for diabetes. From the ADA 2020 standard of care [54]

Fasting plasma glucose of > or = to 126 mg/dl (7.0 mmol/L) - fasting refers to no intake for at least 8 hours
2-hour plasma glucose of > or = to 200 mg/dl (11.1 mmol/L) during 75 gr OGTT
Hemoglobin A1c > or = to 6.5% (48 mmol/Mol) test completed using a method that is NGSP certified and standardized to the Diabetes Control and Complications Trial (DCCT) assay
Random blood glucose of > or = to 200 mg/dl (11.1 mmol/L) in patients with classic symptoms of diabetes

Table 17.3 Commonly used and approved drugs to the management of adults with type 2 diabetes and their side effects [54, 55]

	Special considerations and side effects*	Route of administration
Metformin	Oral medication, low cost, no risk of hypoglycemia, recommended with food, gastrointestinal side effects (diarrhea and nausea), contraindicated in patients with GFR <30 ml/min/1.73 m^2, potential for B12 deficiency. Avoid if expecting to use IV contrast	Oral
SGLT-2 inhibitors	Oral medication, high cost, renal dose adjustment required, risk of volume depletion and hypotension, risk of amputation and bone fracture (canagliflozin), genitourinary infection, increased LDL, Fournier gangrene	Oral
DDP-4 inhibitors	Oral medication, high cost, risk of acute pancreatitis and joint pain, renal dose adjustment required except for linagliptin	Oral
GLP 1- receptor agonist	Injectable and oral (semaglutide), renal dose adjustment required (exenatide, lixisenatide), potential for acute kidney injury, risk of C-cell tumor of the thyroid (liraglutide, albiglutide, dulaglutide, exenatide extended release), gastrointestinal side effects (nausea, vomiting, diarrhea), injection site reaction, and questionable risk of acute pancreatitis	Oral (only one in this class recently approved - semaglutide) Injections
Thiazolidinediones	Oral, less commonly used, side effects include weight gain and fluid retention, risk of congestive heart failure, risk of bone fracture, risk of bladder cancer (pioglitazone), increased LDL	Oral
Sulfonylureas	Oral, less commonly used, risk of hypoglycemia, glyburide not recommended, potential risk of cardiovascular mortality with older generations of sulfonureas	Oral

*Providers should constantly review changes to indications and side effects

Table 17.4 Type of insulin and duration of action [56, 57]

Insulin type	Onset	Peak	Duration
Rapid acting Aspart Glulisine Lispro	15 minutes	1 hour	2–4 hours
Short acting Regular	30 minutes	2–3 hours	3–6 hours
Intermediate acting NPH	2–4 hours	4–12 hours	12–18 hours
Long acting Detemir Glargine Basaglar	Several hours	No peak	Up to 24 hours
Ultra-long acting Degludec Glargine u-300	6 hours	No peak	36 hours or longer
Combinations NPH/regular 70/30 Rapid acting 70/30 Rapid acting 75/25 Rapid acting 50/50 NPH/regular 50/50	30 min–1 hour 5–20 minutes 5–20 minutes 5–20 minutes 30 min–1 hour	2–12 hours 1–2 hours 1–2 hours 1–2 hours 2–12 hours	10–16 hours 10–16 hours 10–16 hours 10–16 hours 10–16 hours

min should be revisited if there is an anticipated need to receive contrast material for imaging. Further, oral medications are not ideal in patients with nausea, vomiting, or at risk of dehydration.

13. Patients with type 1 diabetes should always take their basal insulin, and the dose can be adjusted as needed in patients with significant weight loss and risk of hypoglycemia.
14. Patients with significant elevation of postprandial glucose might require short- or rapid-acting insulin.
15. Rapid-acting insulin should be considered in patients on steroids. The insulin dose for patients on preexisting insulin therapy might need to be increased two to three times the original dose. These patients will need close follow-up to titrate the insulin as needed based on the steroid dose, duration of steroids, and associated symptoms.
16. The management of patients on enteral nutrition is complex, and an endocrinologist or diabetes specialist should be included as soon as possible in the management of these patients.

References

1. Boyle P, Boniol M, Koechlin A, Robertson C, Valentini F, Coppens K, et al. Diabetes and breast cancer risk: a meta-analysis. Br J Cancer. 2012;107(9):1608–17.
2. Chan W, Yun L, Austin PC, Jaakkimainen RL, Booth GL, Hux J, et al. Impact of socioeconomic status on breast cancer screening in women with diabetes: a population-based study. Diabet Med. 2014;31(7):806–12.
3. Lega IC, Austin PC, Fischer HD, Fung K, Krzyzanowska MK, Amir E, et al. The impact of diabetes on breast Cancer treatments and outcomes: a population-based study. Diabetes Care. 2018;41(4):755–61.
4. Peairs KS, Barone BB, Snyder CF, Yeh H-C, Stein KB, Derr RL, et al. Diabetes mellitus and breast Cancer outcomes: a systematic review and meta-analysis. J Clin Oncol. 2011;29(1):40–6.
5. Centers for Disease Control and Prevention. National Diabetes Statistics Report. Atlanta, GA: centers for disease control and prevention. US Department of Health and Human Services. 2011;2011
6. Kaaks R. Nutrition, hormones, and breast cancer: is insulin the missing link? Cancer Causes Control. 1996;7(6):605–25.
7. Cohen DH, LeRoith D. Obesity, type 2 diabetes, and cancer: the insulin and IGF connection. Endocr Relat Cancer. 2012;19(5):F27–45.
8. Kang C, LeRoith D, Gallagher EJ. Diabetes, obesity, and breast Cancer. Endocrinology. 2018;159(11):3801–12.
9. Tang Z, Wang J, Zhang H, Sun L, Tang F, Deng Q, et al. Associations between diabetes and quality of life among breast cancer survivors. Chu P-Y, editor. PLOS ONE. 2016;11(6):e0157791.
10. Epplein M, Zheng Y, Zheng W, Chen Z, Gu K, Penson D, et al. Quality of life after breast Cancer diagnosis and survival. J Clin Oncol. 2011;29(4):406–12.
11. Suh S, Kim K-W. Diabetes and Cancer: Cancer should be screened in routine diabetes assessment. Diabetes Metab J. 2019;43(6):733.
12. Beckman TJ, Cuddihy RM, Scheitel SM, Naessens JM, Killian JM, Pankratz VS. Screening mammogram utilization in women with diabetes. Diabetes Care. 2001;24(12):2049–53.
13. Sanderson M, Lipworth L, Han X, Beeghly-Fadiel A, Shen-Miller D, Patel K, et al. Mammography use among women with and without diabetes: results from the southern community cohort study. J Epidemiol Glob Health. 2014;4(3):223.
14. Katz D, Tengekyon AJ, Kahan NR, Calderon-Margalit R. Patient and physician characteristics affect adherence to screening mammography: A population-based cohort study. Miller AB, editor. PLOS ONE. 2018;13(3):e0194409.
15. Wang KH, Galusha D, Friedman H, Nazario CM, Nunez M, Maharaj RG, et al. Non-communicable chronic diseases and timely breast cancer screening among women of the eastern Caribbean health outcomes research network (ECHORN) cohort study. Cancer Causes Control. 2018;29(3):315–24.
16. Constantinou P, Dray-Spira R, Menvielle G. Cervical and breast cancer screening participation for women with chronic conditions in France: results from a national health survey. BMC Cancer. 2016;16(1):255.
17. Bhatia D, Lega IC, Wu W, Lipscombe LL. Breast, cervical and colorectal cancer screening in adults with diabetes: a systematic review and meta-analysis. Diabetologia. 2020;63(1):34–48.
18. American Diabetes Association. 4. Comprehensive medical evaluation and assessment of comorbidities: standards of medical care in diabetes—2020. Diabetes Care. 2020;43(Supplement 1):S37–47.
19. Giovannucci E, Harlan DM, Archer MC, Bergenstal RM, Gapstur SM, Habel LA, et al. Diabetes and cancer: a consensus report. Diabetes Care. 2010;33(7):1674–85.
20. Rena G, Hardie DG, Pearson ER. The mechanisms of action of metformin. Diabetologia. 2017;60(9):1577–85.
21. Saraei P, Asadi I, Kakar MA, Moradi-Kor N. The beneficial effects of metformin on cancer prevention and

therapy: a comprehensive review of recent advances. Cancer Manag Res. 2019;11:3295–313.
22. Heckman-Stoddard BM, DeCensi A, Sahasrabuddhe VV, Ford LG. Repurposing metformin for the prevention of cancer and cancer recurrence. Diabetologia. 2017;60(9):1639–47.
23. Zhuang Y, Ly RC, Frazier CV, Yu J, Qin S, Fan X-Y, et al. The novel function of tumor protein D54 in regulating pyruvate dehydrogenase and metformin cytotoxicity in breast cancer. Cancer Metab. 2019;7(1):1.
24. Mallik R, Chowdhury TA. Metformin in cancer. Diabetes Res Clin Pract. 2018;143:409–19.
25. Tang GH, Satkunam M, Pond GR, Steinberg GR, Blandino G, Schünemann HJ, et al. Association of Metformin with breast Cancer incidence and mortality in patients with type II diabetes: a GRADE-assessed systematic review and meta-analysis. Cancer Epidemiol Biomark Prev. 2018;27(6):627–35.
26. Chen L, Chubak J, Boudreau DM, Barlow WE, Weiss NS, Li CI. Diabetes treatments and risks of adverse breast Cancer outcomes among early-stage breast Cancer patients: a SEER-Medicare analysis. Cancer Res. 2017;77(21):6033–41.
27. Sonnenblick A, Agbor-Tarh D, Bradbury I, Di Cosimo S, Azim HA, Fumagalli D, et al. Impact of diabetes, insulin, and metformin use on the outcome of patients with human epidermal growth factor receptor 2–positive primary breast Cancer: analysis from the ALTTO phase III randomized trial. J Clin Oncol. 2017;35(13):1421–9.
28. MYME investigators, Nanni O, Amadori D, De Censi A, Rocca A, Freschi A, et al. Metformin plus chemotherapy versus chemotherapy alone in the first-line treatment of HER2-negative metastatic breast cancer. The MYME randomized, phase 2 clinical trial. Breast Cancer Res Treat. 2019;174(2):433–42.
29. Tharakan S, Zimmerman B, Ru M, Blanter J, Cascetta K, Tiersten A. Diabetes and metformin association with recurrence score in a large Oncotype database of breast Cancer patients. Oncology. 2020;17:1–4.
30. Zhao X-B, Ren G-S. Diabetes mellitus and prognosis in women with breast cancer: a systematic review and meta-analysis. Medicine (Baltimore). 2016;95(49):e5602.
31. Kiderlen M, de Glas NA, Bastiaannet E, Engels CC, van de Water W, de Craen AJM, et al. Diabetes in relation to breast cancer relapse and all-cause mortality in elderly breast cancer patients: a FOCUS study analysis. Ann Oncol. 2013;24(12):3011–6.
32. Erickson K, Patterson RE, Flatt SW, Natarajan L, Parker BA, Heath DD, et al. Clinically defined type 2 diabetes mellitus and prognosis in early-stage breast Cancer. J Clin Oncol. 2011;29(1):54–60.
33. McCall NS, Simone BA, Mehta M, Zhan T, Ko K, Nowak-Choi K, et al. Onco-metabolism: defining the prognostic significance of obesity and diabetes in women with brain metastases from breast cancer. Breast Cancer Res Treat. 2018;172(1):221–30.
34. Lee A, Jo S, Lee C, Shin H-H, Kim TH, Ahn KJ, et al. Diabetes as a prognostic factor in HER-2 positive breast cancer patients treated with targeted therapy. Breast Cancer. 2019;26(5):672–80.
35. Lawrence WR, Hosler AS, Gates Kuliszewski M, Leinung MC, Zhang X, Schymura MJ, et al. Impact of preexisting type 2 diabetes mellitus and antidiabetic drugs on all-cause and cause-specific mortality among Medicaid-insured women diagnosed with breast cancer. Cancer Epidemiol. 2020;66:101710.
36. Srokowski TP, Fang S, Hortobagyi GN, Giordano SH. Impact of diabetes mellitus on complications and outcomes of adjuvant chemotherapy in older patients with breast cancer. J Clin Oncol Off J Am Soc Clin Oncol. 2009;27(13):2170–6.
37. Vissers PAJ, Cardwell CR, van de Poll-Franse LV, Young IS, Pouwer F, Murray LJ. The association between glucose-lowering drug use and mortality among breast cancer patients with type 2 diabetes. Breast Cancer Res Treat. 2015;150(2):427–37.
38. Parada H, Cleveland RJ, North KE, Stevens J, Teitelbaum SL, Neugut AI, et al. Genetic polymorphisms of diabetes-related genes, their interaction with diabetes status, and breast cancer incidence and mortality: The Long Island Breast Cancer Study Project. Mol Carcinog. 2018;mc.22940.
39. Shao S, Gill AA, Zahm SH, Jatoi I, Shriver CD, McGlynn KA, et al. Diabetes and overall survival among breast cancer patients in the U.S. military health system. Cancer Epidemiol Biomark Prev. 2018;27(1):50–7.
40. Cleveland RJ, North KE, Stevens J, Teitelbaum SL, Neugut AI, Gammon MD. The association of diabetes with breast cancer incidence and mortality in the Long Island breast cancer study project. Cancer Causes Control. 2012;23(7):1193–203.
41. Strulov Shachar S, Williams GR. The obesity paradox in cancer—moving beyond BMI. Cancer Epidemiol Biomark Prev. 2017;26(1):13–6.
42. Han SJ, Boyko EJ. The evidence for an obesity paradox in type 2 diabetes mellitus. Diabetes Metab J. 2018;42(3):179.
43. Buono G, Crispo A, Giuliano M, De Angelis C, Schettini F, Forestieri V, et al. Combined effect of obesity and diabetes on early breast cancer outcome: a prospective observational study. Oncotarget. 2017 [cited 2020 Apr 28];8(70).
44. Connor AE, Visvanathan K, Boone SD, Rifai N, Baumgartner KB, Baumgartner RN. Fructosamine and diabetes as predictors of mortality among Hispanic and non-Hispanic white breast cancer survivors. NPJ Breast Cancer. 2019;5(1):3.
45. Malmström H, Walldius G, Grill V, Jungner I, Gudbjörnsdottir S, Hammar N. Fructosamine is a useful indicator of hyperglycaemia and glucose control in clinical and epidemiological studies – cross-sectional and longitudinal experience from the AMORIS Cohort. Hribal ML, editor. PLoS ONE. 2014;9(10):e111463.
46. Shelby RA, Dorfman CS, Arthur SS, Bosworth HB, Corsino L, Sutton L, et al. Improving health

engagement and lifestyle management for breast cancer survivors with diabetes. Contemp Clin Trials. 2020;92:105998.

47. Handelsman Y, Leroith D, Bloomgarden ZT, Dagogo-Jack S, Einhorn D, Garber AJ, et al. Diabetes and cancer--an AACE/ACE consensus statement. Endocr Pract Off J Am Coll Endocrinol Am Assoc Clin Endocrinol. 2013;19(4):675–93.
48. Corsino L, Dhatariya K, Umpierrez G. Management of Diabetes and Hyperglycemia in hospitalized patients. In: Feingold KR, Anawalt B, Boyce A, Chrousos G, Dungan K, Grossman A, et al., editors. Endotext. South Dartmouth (MA): MDText.com, Inc.; 2000.
49. Mabrey ME, Barton AB, Corsino L, Freeman SB, Davis ED, Bell EL, et al. Managing hyperglycemia and diabetes in patients receiving enteral feedings: a health system approach. Hosp Pract. 2015;43(2):74–8.
50. American Diabetes Association. introduction: standards of medical care in diabetes—2020. Diabetes Care. 2020;43(Supplement 1):S1–2.
51. Garber AJ, Handelsman Y, Grunberger G, Einhorn D, Abrahamson MJ, Barzilay JI, et al. Consensus statement by the American Association of Clinical Endocriniologists and American College of endocrinology on the comprehensive type 2 diabetes management algorithm - 2020 executive summary. Endocr Pract. 2020;26(1):107–39.
52. American Diabetes Association. 5. Facilitating behavior change and well-being to improve health outcomes: standards of medical care in diabetes—2020. Diabetes Care. 2020;43(Supplement 1):S48–65.
53. American Diabetes Association. 9. Pharmacologic approaches to glycemic treatment: standards of medical care in diabetes—2020. Diabetes Care. 2020;43(Supplement 1):S98–110.
54. American Diabetes Association. 2. Classification and diagnosis of diabetes: standards of medical care in diabetes—2020. Diabetes Care. 2020;43(Supplement 1):S14–31.
55. American Diabetes Association. 9. Pharmacologic approaches to glycemic treatment: standards of medical care in diabetes—2020. Diabetes Care. 2020;43(Supplement 1):S98–110.
56. American Diabetes Association. Insulin Basics [Internet]. [cited 2020 Apr 29]. Available from: https://www.diabetes.org/diabetes/medication-management/insulin-other-injectables/insulin-basics
57. Cleveland Clinic. Injectable Insulin Medications [Internet]. [cited 2020 Apr 29]. Available from: https://my.clevelandclinic.org/health/drugs/13902-injectable-insulin-medications

Hair Loss

18

Elise A. Olsen

Introduction

One in every eight women in the United States will get breast cancer in her lifetime [1], and there are 250,000 new cases of invasive breast cancer per year in women in the USA with an incidence of 125 per 100,000 persons [2]. Survival in breast cancer has increased over the past 20 years due to both new chemotherapeutic agents and the use of endocrine therapy (ET). The overall 5-year relative survival rate in the USA is now 99% for localized disease, 85% for regional disease, and 27% for distant-stage disease [3]. Survival within each stage varies by tumor size with the 5-year relative survival of patients with regional disease now 95% for tumors less than or equal to 2.0 cm, 85% for tumors 2.1–5.0 cm, and 72% for tumors greater than 5.0 cm [4]. Breast cancer survivors now represent more than 3.5 million US women [5].

The initial concerns of the patient upon diagnosis of breast cancer usually are regarding prognosis and the acute side effects of therapy. Hair loss or alopecia, a disorder characterized by a decrease in the density of scalp hair compared to normal for a given individual at a given age, is identified by 58% of women as the most disturbing anticipated adverse event of chemotherapy [6] and the second most troublesome side effect after the effect on family or partner [7]. With the knowledge that a long life after initial treatment is possible, or even probable, focus should be on preventing or ameliorating the long-term treatment sequelae that adversely affect the quality of life in survivors.

Hair loss in breast cancer survivors is common and variable in degree but may be related not only to former chemotherapy but also to ET, sudden menopause, underlying hair disorders present prior to the diagnosis of breast cancer, or new hair disorders not uncommon in women. Each of these types of hair loss has its own clinical characteristics, pathological findings, potential for progression or regrowth, and effective treatments, which may or may not be safe to use in this population. This chapter will focus on how to recognize the types and potential treatments of hair loss in breast cancer survivors.

The Hair Loss Cycle

To understand hair loss, it is important to understand the basic components of the hair growth cycle (Fig. 18.1). Each mature follicle consists of a germinative bulb of matrix cells with high mitotic activity and melanocytes that surround a dermal collection of cells with inductive properties (the dermal papilla). The matrix cells produce a fused bundle of keratin fibers (hair shaft)

E. A. Olsen (✉)
Hair Disorders Research and Treatment Center, Duke University Medical Center, Durham, NC, USA
e-mail: Elise.olsen@dm.duke.edu

G. G. Kimmick et al. (eds.), *Common Issues in Breast Cancer Survivors*,
https://doi.org/10.1007/978-3-030-75377-1_18

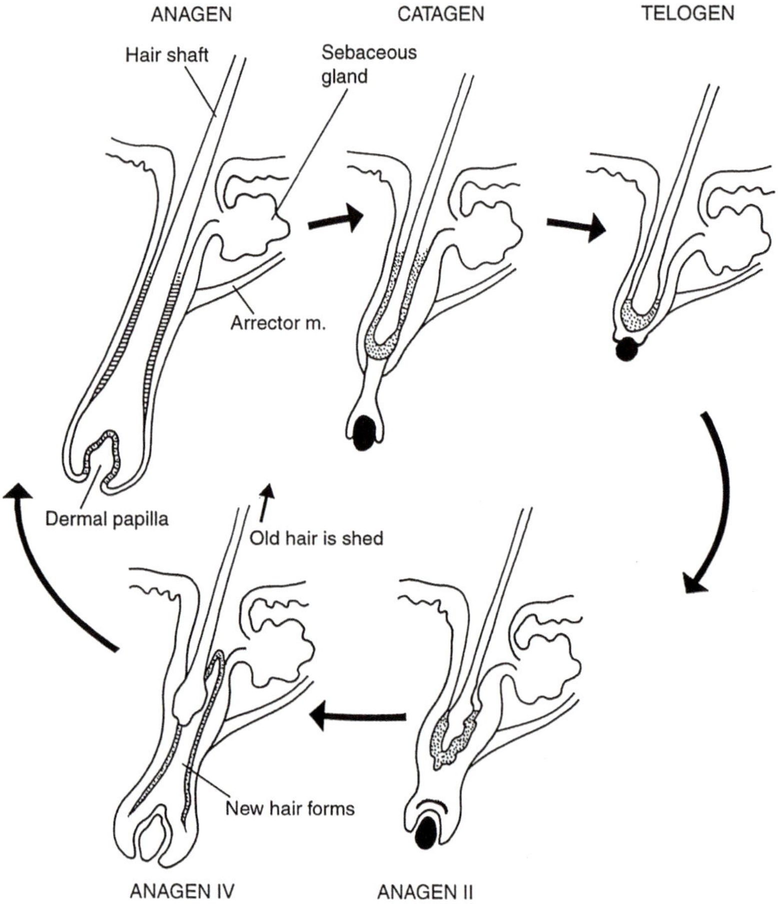

Fig. 18.1 Hair loss cycle (Messenger A, The Control of Hair Growth and Pigmentation in Olsen. EA (editor). *Hair Disorders: Diagnosis and Treatment*, McGraw Hill, NY, 2004, page 50

that are surrounded by inner and outer root sheaths that provide a protective coating, anchor the growing hair, and provide a reservoir of pluripotential cells. Attached to the follicle are a sebaceous gland and an arrector pili muscle that inserts close to the sebaceous gland. A specialized collection of hair stem cells is tucked into the area known as the "bulge" close to the insertion of the arrector pili muscle [8]. All hairs, regardless of body location, go through a cycle that includes, in order, growth (anagen), involution (catagen), rest (telogen), and regrowth/creation of a new growing hair. Anagen lasts for a variable period of time depending on body area, presence or absence of underlying pattern hair loss (also referred to as androgenetic alopecia), and prior exposure to treatments that may have permanently altered the matrix cells. At the conclusion of anagen, catagen ensues during which the bulb matrix and lower root sheaths undergo apoptosis causing cessation of cellular proliferation and melanocytes discontinue melanin production. The inferior follicle and dermal papilla then separate and move up into the dermis from the subcutaneous tissue, albeit at different rates, coming to rest near the insertion of the arrector pili muscle [8]. For all hair-bearing areas of the body, catagen lasts about 2–4 weeks and telogen normally 2–4 months [9]. Hairs in telogen, which are poorly anchored due to changes in the surrounding root sheath, are often dislodged with traction from shampooing, combing, and styling during this time period. At the end of telogen, the follicular cells move inferiorly to their former position, envelop the dermal papilla once again, and begin proliferation; if still present, the remaining telogen hair is ejected. It is during the proliferative phase of anagen that the hair follicle matrix cells are most vulnerable, whereas the stem cells, due to slow cycling, are better protected from damage due to chemotherapy or radiation therapy.

In the normal scalp, 85–90% of hair is in anagen. The duration of anagen will determine the length of hair and is relatively fixed per body site [9]. The perception of scalp "coverage" with hair is due to a number of factors including the number of viable follicular units, the number of hairs per follicular unit (typically more than one), the diameter of the hairs projecting from the scalp, and the ratio of anagen to telogen hairs. Typical hair growth is 1 cm/month. Two common hair loss conditions in women, chronic telogen effluvium (CTE) and female-pattern hair loss (FPHL), cause potentially reversible hair loss and may contribute to the hair loss seen in breast cancer survivors.

Psychological Effect of Scalp Hair Loss

Hair loss is a problem that may create significant anxiety and depression in patients of all ages. In cancer survivors, alopecia has been associated with depression, anxiety, low self-esteem, negative body image, and a decrease in health-related quality of life (HRQOL) [6, 10]. The lack of ability to camouflage the hair loss, the lack of stability in social relationships or job, and the degree to which the individual's positive self-image is related to her scalp hair all potentially relate to the negative feelings of self-worth. It is important to note that the degree of distress may not correlate with the severity of hair loss [11, 12] and that there may be more concern about hair loss with early disease when survival is more assured than with metastatic disease when survival is threatened [12].

Persistent Chemotherapy-Induced Alopecia

Most agents used in multiagent chemotherapy for breast cancer will cause some decrease in hair density/shedding during treatment, but certain agents will cause complete alopecia. The agents used to treat breast cancer that may induce increased shedding or mild hair loss include methotrexate, cisplatin, and 5-fluorouracil; these agents are unlikely to cause long-term hair loss after the agents are discontinued [10, 13]. The regimens used for breast cancer therapy that are most likely to cause severe or complete hair loss are those that include cyclophosphamide, anthracyclines and taxanes [13]. These latter agents cause immediate cell death of the matrix keratinocytes and melanocytes [14, 15], leading to anagen arrest with constriction, thinning, and potential fracture of affected hairs [16]. Scalp cooling, by decreasing the blood flow and thereby exposure of hair follicles to chemotherapy, may prevent chemotherapy-induced alopecia (CIA) in up to 59% of patients on a taxane-based regimen but only 16% of those on an anthracycline-based regimen [17]. Hair loss with those agents, which likely leads to total or near-total hair loss, usually begins with profound shedding within 1–3 weeks after initiation of therapy [(18 days ± 12.6 (SD) in one study] [18] and is usually most prominent by 6 weeks [19]. This may be accompanied by transient folliculitis of the scalp. Hair regrowth usually begins within 2–4 months after discontinuation of therapy with the maximum recovery at about 1 year [18]. The new hair may be different in color, texture (straight/curly), or thickness compared to pre-chemotherapy. Topical minoxidil may accelerate the initiation of hair regrowth; although reported with 2% topical minoxidil [20], most hair experts would recommend 5% topical minoxidil foam or solution twice a day as safe and more effective than 2% topical minoxidil solution twice a day (personal communication, E Olsen) based on data in male and female-pattern hair loss [21, 22].

Persistent chemotherapy-induced alopecia (pCIA) is a term used to describe patients treated with chemotherapy who experience incomplete hair regrowth >6 months following completion of chemotherapy (Fig. 18.2) [23]. The incidence of pCIA at 6 and 36 months post-chemotherapy in one prospective cohort study in Korea of breast cancer patients who received either doxorubicin plus cyclophosphamide (AC), fluorouracil plus cyclophosphamide and doxorubicin (FAC), or AC plus docetaxel as adjuvant therapy was 39.5% and 42.3%, respectively. Although in this study, pCIA was defined as absent or incomplete hair

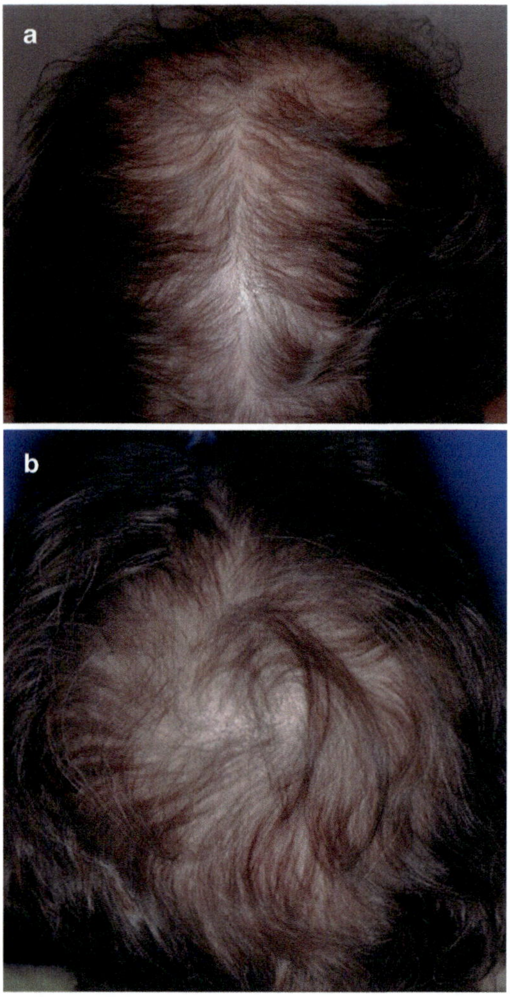

Fig. 18.2 Patient with pCIA following docetaxel/carboplatin/trastuzumab and tamoxifen. (**a**) Midline part (**b**) Back of scalp

growth based on two standard deviations below the values pre-chemotherapy for either a decrease of hair density or thickness (diameter), the major long-term change was related to a decrease in hair thickness [24]. The primary complaints of patients were thinning hair (75%) and reduced hair volume (54%). A second Korean study at a different site of 265 breast cancer patients treated with an anthracycline plus cyclophosphamide (AC) or anthracycline-based therapy plus taxane (with or without trastuzumab or ET) found similar results of alopecia in 43.2% of patients at 3–5 years post-chemotherapy [25]. In a single-center study in France, patients with early breast cancer treated with fluorouracil/epirubicin/cyclophosphamide (FEC-100) and docetaxel, with pre-chemotherapy scalp cooling, had a 5-year incidence of alopecia of 32.9% based on photographic review of their scalp hair [26]. The degree of hair loss may be related to the particular chemotherapeutic agent, the combination of agents, the drug half-life, dose, dosing frequency, and duration of treatment. Severe hair loss (Common Terminology Criteria for Adverse Events (CTCAE) Grade 2 or >50% hair loss) has been reported to be higher with taxane- and anthracycline-based chemotherapy (10.5%) than doxorubicin and cyclophosphamide (2.7%) [25]. In these cases of severe pCIA, there may have been permanent damage to the hair follicle stem cells during therapy [27, 28], so there is actual loss of follicular units. Patients treated with taxane-based treatment regimens are more likely to experience pCIA than those with other treatments [24, 29–31].

Clinical Evaluation

Before immediately ascribing all scalp hair loss to the preceding chemotherapy, one has to consider other concomitant factors or conditions. *Early-onset FPHL* (presentation teens to third decade) is a progressive lifelong hair loss related to follicular androgen sensitivity [32]. *Late-onset FPHL* may first appear at the time of perimenopause or menopause and phenotypically overlaps with early-onset FPHL and the onset of senescent alopecia. Both early- and late-onset FPHL are related to a progressive miniaturization of affected hair follicles (thinner, shorter hairs) in the involved section of the central scalp. Other features of FPHL include a shorter anagen duration, prolongation of a latent phase of the cycle after the telogen hair has been shed (termed kenogen) [33], and a lower anagen/telogen ratio [34]. Chemotherapy or ET may exacerbate either early- or late-onset FPHL.

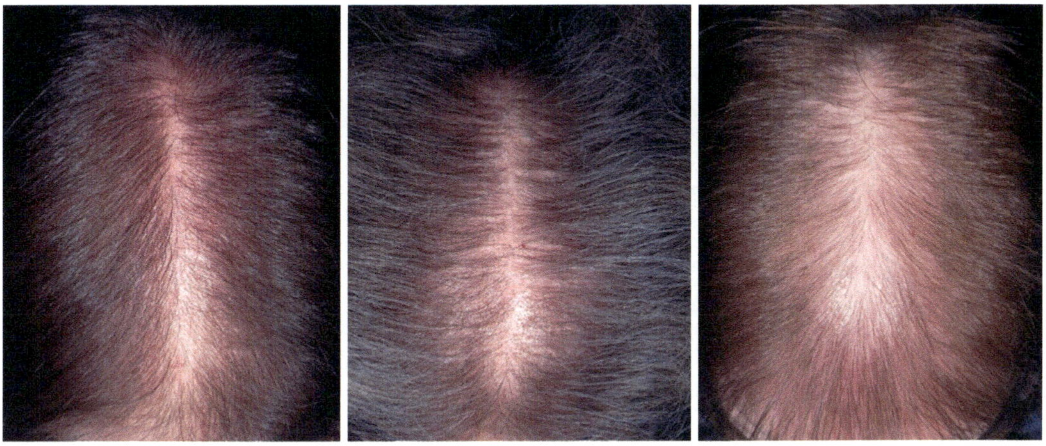

Fig. 18.3 Female-pattern hair loss (FPHL). Presentation of FPHL in three different women as shown by midline part of hair in central scalp. Frontal accentuation may be subtle but is an important clue to distinguishing FPHL vs chronic telogen effluvium. With extensive hair loss, part will widen markedly across central scalp

FPHL is characterized clinically by a decrease in hair density in the central scalp with usually one of two patterns of hair loss: central thinning (Ludwig pattern) or frontal accentuation/Christmas tree pattern (Olsen pattern, Fig. 18.3a–c) [32, 35]. Preservation of follicular ostia (visible pores) in areas of hair loss ensures that the follicular apparatus is still present and, hence, the condition potentially reversible. A midline central part width compared to a similar parting of hair in the occiput is a simple way of documenting the relative decrease in hair density in FPHL in the central scalp since the occipital hair is not under androgen control and thus not subject to the balding process.

Chronic telogen effluvium (CTE) is characterized by an increase in the percentage of hairs in telogen all over the scalp that leads to a marked increase in hair shedding and a global decrease in hair density that persists for greater than 6 months [34]. This is a potentially reversible process with intact ostia but one without an obvious etiology. In CTE, a hair pull, which involves grasping several groups of 50–60 hairs at the base and pulling gently towards the ends [9], will usually produce >2 telogen hairs per pull in multiple areas of the scalp [36]. A hair pull is an easy test to do at the bedside to corroborate the history of an increase in shedding. Telogen hairs can be recognized clinically by their rounded-up proximal end. The degree of shedding may be graded according to the Hair Shedding Visual Scale based on the amount of shed hairs collected on a daily basis [37]. There is a potential for overlap between FPHL and CTE.

Text Box

Differential diagnosis of hair loss in breast cancer survivors:

- Female-pattern hair loss (FPHL)
- Chronic telogen effluvium (CTE)
- Frontal fibrosing alopecia (FFA)
- Central centrifugal cicatricial alopecia (CCCA) (primarily in African-American women)

Another type of scalp hair loss that commonly occurs in postmenopausal women who are over the age of 50 years, similar to the peak age of onset of breast cancer, is frontal fibrosing alopecia (FFA) (Fig. 18.4). This is a condition of primarily postmenopausal Caucasian women characterized by frontal/parietal hairline recession and eyebrow loss accompanied frequently by perifollicular erythema and scale in affected areas [38]. It is quite distinct from any hair loss

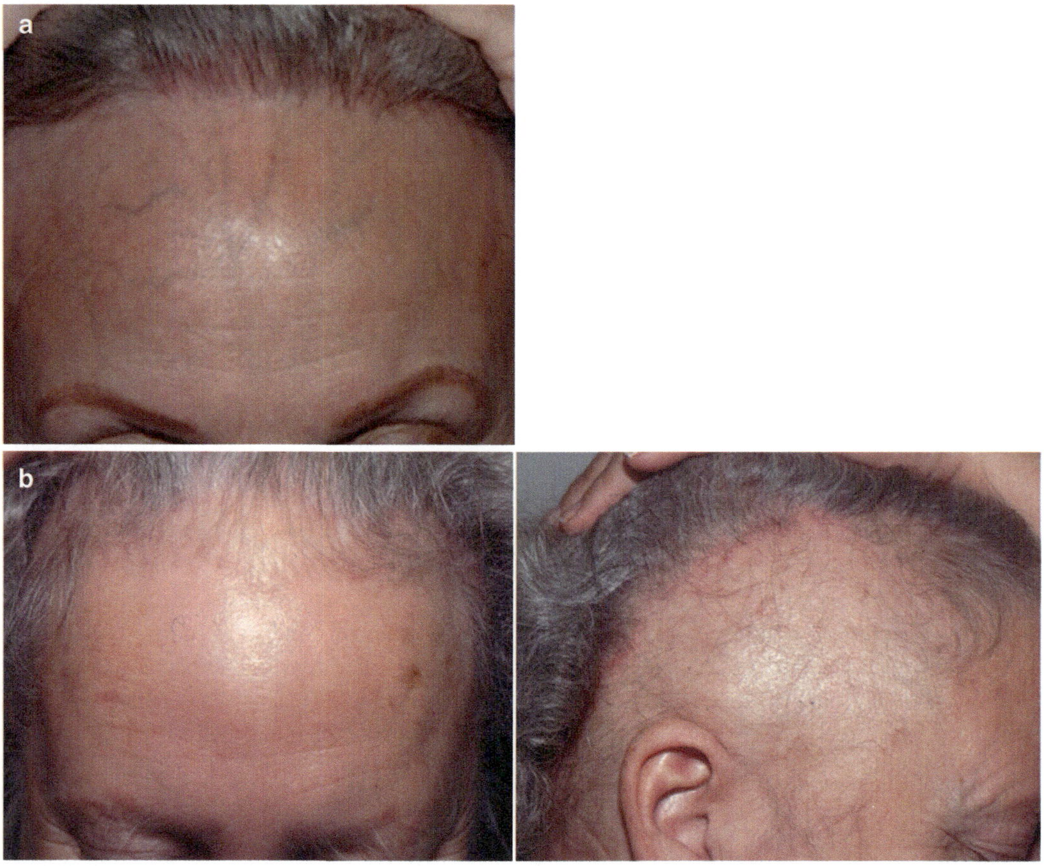

Fig. 18.4 Frontal fibrosing alopecia (FFA). (**a**) Patient with even recession of frontal hairline, perifollicular erythema, and loss of eyebrows. (**b**) Patient with irregular recession of frontal hairline with "lonely hairs" out front, perifollicular erythema, extensive parietal hair loss, and eyebrow loss

condition seen with pCIA, both clinically and pathologically, since this is a type of scarring (destructive) hair loss. However, it may overlap with FPHL.

Central centrifugal cicatricial alopecia (CCCA) occurs in about 5% of African-American women (Fig. 18.5) [39]. It is a slowly expanding process of scarring alopecia in the central scalp. CCCA may occur at any age and may be caused by a compilation of hair care practices, underlying endocrine issues, and/or genetic abnormalities. It is not a pattern seen with pCIA but must be considered as a secondary condition in any African-American woman with pCIA or ET-induced alopecia (EIA).

In addition to scalp hair loss, extremity/axillary/pubic hair, eyelashes, and eyebrows may be persistently decreased in breast cancer survivors post-treatment. Loss of body hair may be related to prior chemotherapy, menopause, or, if present, FFA.

A scalp biopsy in pCIA is important to assess the potential for regrowth and help to confirm the clinical diagnosis. A 4-mm punch biopsy sectioned horizontally is preferred so that the number of follicular units and the anagen/telogen ratio can be determined [34]. In most cases of pCIA, with or without concomitant ET, there are miniaturization and an increase in telogen hairs, analogous to FPHL [30, 40]. Although a few published cases of pCIA showed a perifollicular lymphocytic infiltrate [30, 31], this is also a common pathological finding in biopsies of male- and female-pattern hair loss (PHL). A decrease in follicular density [30, 31, 41] may be seen that aligns histologically with the fea-

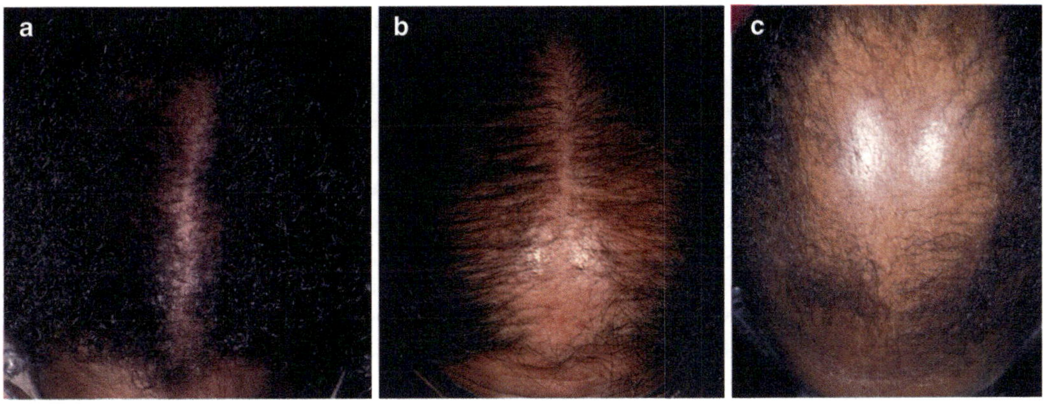

Fig. 18.5 Central Centrifugal Cicatricial Alopecia (CCCA. (**a**) Early central scalp hair loss with widened part width. (**b**) Marked frontal hair loss. (**c**) Extensive central and vertex scalp hair loss

tures of "cicatricial pattern hair loss" [42]. Depending on the degree of loss, patients with pCIA may have little ability to reverse the low hair density. One pathological study of CIA showed dysmorphic telogen germinal units [30], and another showed multiple basaloid aggregates of uncertain significance [41].

Endocrine Therapy-Induced Alopecia

Adjuvant endocrine therapy includes the use of selective estrogen receptor (ER) modulators (SERMs; tamoxifen), aromatase inhibitors (AIs) (anastrozole, letrozole, or exemestane), or gonadotropin-releasing hormone agonists (goserelin or leuprolide). Current recommendations for patients with hormone receptor-positive breast cancer include 5–10 years of ET [43]. In a hospital-based registry of 851 female breast cancer survivors, 22% of those on AIs reported hair loss and 32% reported hair thinning [44]. In a meta-analysis of 13,415 patients treated with various types of ET in 35 different cancer clinical trials, the incidence of alopecia (defined as CTCAE Grade 1 or 2) was reported for the following specific agents [45]: anastrozole 2.5% (15/599), exemestane 2.2% (24/1096), letrozole 2.5% (101/4056), and higher rates for leuprorelin 9.5% (28/294), tamoxifen 9.3% (314/3379), tamoxifen with goserelin 10% (51/511), and tamoxifen followed by anastrozole 14.7% (274/1865).

Text Box

Common Terminology Criteria for Adverse Events (CTCAE) for alopecia:

- Grade 0 = no hair loss
- Grade 1 = hair loss of <50% of normal for that individual that is not obvious from a distance, but only on close inspection; a different hairstyle may be required to cover the hair loss, but it does not require a wig or hairpiece to camouflage.
- Grade 2 = hair loss of ≥50% of normal for that individual that is readily apparent to others; a wig or hairpiece is necessary if the patient desires to completely camouflage the hair loss; associated with psychosocial impact.

The percentage of patients with Grade 2 CTCAE alopecia was seen with the following ETs: 1.3% with exemestane, 0.2% with letrozole, 1.0% with leuprorelin, and highest with tamoxifen (6.4%) [45]. In a study specifically looking at breast cancer patients with ET-induced alopecia (EIA), 67% were taking an AI and 33% tamoxifen [46]. Patients with EIA have the hair loss pattern, trichoscopic findings on dermoscopy (including variation of diameter/miniaturization of hairs, yellow dots) [46], and scalp biopsy findings similar to naturally occurring FPHL. The mechanism of hair loss may be related to the relative increase in tissue androgen [47] and the loss of anagen prolongation normally supported by estradiol [48].

Treatment of pCIA or EIA

Except for alopecia areata, acute telogen effluvium, and infectious causes, patients with hair loss disorders, including those that are designated non-scarring such as FPHL and CTE, may have only partial regrowth despite the use of all potential current treatments. Managing expectations for pCIA and EIA is, therefore, very important. A biopsy of a representative area of hair loss will help determine the density of viable follicles and/or miniaturized hairs (which have the potential to become larger again) and will rule out other causes of hair loss. When trying to discern whether a given treatment of hair loss is helpful, the most valuable aid is standardized photographs taken before chemotherapy, after recovery, and at regular intervals after treatment, something typically not performed in oncology offices.

Text Box

Potential treatments for use by all patients with pCIA or EIA:

- Topical minoxidil
- Oral minoxidil
- Low-level laser treatment
- Topical prostaglandins (for eyelashes and eyebrows)
- Camouflage

Potential additional treatments for patients with EIA:

- For hormone receptor-negative patients:
  - 5-alpha-reductase inhibitors
  - Spironolactone
- For hormone receptor-positive patients:
  - Spironolactone with caution
- Platelet-rich plasma (PRP): with caution

Topical Minoxidil

Minoxidil is the safest and one of the most effective agents for treatment of hair loss in breast cancer survivors. It is a useful treatment for any hair loss condition where a decrease in density is secondary to a miniaturization of hair or a problem in hair cycling, such as FPHL, EIA, pCIA, or CTE. Topical minoxidil has been shown to cause premature entry of telogen follicles into anagen in animal models, which likely explains the rapid onset of effect (6–8 weeks) [49] and the typical shedding that one may see during the first month of treatment as anagen is synchronized and promoted. Minoxidil also prolongs anagen and increases the diameter of miniaturized hairs. Topical minoxidil is highly effective if applied correctly and consistently. Although only 2% topical minoxidil solution twice a day and 5% topical minoxidil foam once a day are FDA approved for use in women, 5% topical minoxidil foam or solution applied twice a day is more effective [21, 22] and is safe for women. To enhance absorption, based on data from radioactive labeling and urinary excretion studies [50, 51], any blow-drying of hair should be done prior to application, no applications of other medications should be applied to the scalp during the 4–6-h absorption time for minoxidil, and application should be directly onto the scalp. Assessment of efficacy should not be made before 6 months of treatment to allow new hair growth to reach a length that contributes to overall density. Topical minoxidil application may also be prescribed to treat thin eyebrows [52].

The most common potential side effects of topical minoxidil, all of which are reversible upon stopping the drug, are skin irritation, allergic contact dermatitis, and facial hair growth, the latter which is usually limited to the sides of the face. Once stopped, any hair growth gained may be lost, but the process of hair loss will not accelerate.

Oral Minoxidil

Oral minoxidil has advantages over topical minoxidil, especially when the hair loss process involves the entire scalp. There is some data that blood levels of 0.5–1 mg per day of oral minoxidil are approximately equivalent to 5% topical minoxidil applied twice a day (personal communication, Rod Sinclair, MD). There are now publications noting the safety and efficacy of very-low-dose oral minoxidil 1–1.25 mg per day in PHL and CTE [53–55]. There is at least one case report of oral minoxidil use in pCIA [56] but no large placebo-controlled studies to date. Cardiovascular side effects can occur with use of oral minoxidil. It acts as vasodilator with rapid onset, leading to augmented cardiac output, salt and water retention, and an increase in plasma renin [57], which can lead to electrocardiographic changes, congestive heart failure, and peripheral edema. Physicians choosing to use this method of delivery for minoxidil for hair loss should be aware of the potential cardiovascular effects and monitor accordingly, especially those patients at highest risk of side effects due to coexisting hypertension and/or renal disease.

Spironolactone

Spironolactone, a steroid analog and aldosterone antagonist, is FDA approved for heart failure, hypertension, edema, and primary hyperaldosteronism. It has also been shown to have antiandrogen properties, probably through its negative effect on cytochrome P450-dependent 17-alpha-hydroxylase (key to testosterone production) in the adrenal gland and testes and through inhibition of dihydrotestosterone (DHT) binding to the androgen receptor [58]. Because of its antiandrogen properties, spironolactone is commonly used to treat FPHL [59, 60]. Spironolactone may clinically cause gynecomastia in men and menstrual irregularities and painful breast enlargement in women. Because of its endocrine effects, there has been reluctance to use this medication in breast cancer survivors with pCIA or EIA. Although a review of the literature found reported increases in estrogen in some men [58] and some women [61] with use of spironolactone, there was no increase in breast cancer in two large studies of (1) 28,032 women over 55 years age who received spironolactone vs 56,961 controls [62] and (2) 19,284 hypertensive women aged 50–67 treated with antihypertensive therapy (including 751 who had received a potassium-sparing diuretic) vs 49,950 controls [63]. In addition, the International Agency for Research on Cancer deemed that there is inadequate evidence for carcinogenicity of spironolactone in humans [64]. Additional recent data on safety comes from a review of the Humana Insurance database of breast cancer patients stratified by spironolactone use: the results showed no association of spironolactone and increased breast cancer recurrence [65]. Spironolactone is a potassium-sparing diuretic, and elevation of potassium levels can occur, so labs, including a metabolic panel, should be checked during the first month of treatment.

Finasteride

Finasteride, a type 2 5-alpha-reductase (5aR) inhibitor that decreases the metabolism of testosterone (T) to DHT [66], is FDA approved for male-pattern hair loss (MPHL) and benign prostatic hypertrophy in 1 mg and 5 mg dose forms, respectively. Use of either dose in male-pattern hair loss (MPHL) leads to a 68% decrease in DHT and a corresponding 9–10% increase in testosterone [67, 68]. Despite some initial negative reports, likely related to study subject selection [69], finasteride has proven to be an effective and commonly used treatment for FPHL [70]. However, because testosterone is a prohormone for both estradiol and DHT production, inhibition of the 5aR pathway that produces higher levels of testosterone could lead to higher aromatase conversion to estradiol, a concern in breast cancer patients. In an evaluation of 284 women in 21 studies with idiopathic hirsutism, presumably many or most premenopausal, who were treated with finasteride, 34% had an increase in serum estrogen and 38% an increase in total testosterone [61]. For postmenopausal women who have very low testosterone levels, the potential for an increase in serum estrogen with finasteride is much lower. In one controlled study of finasteride 1 mg per day in postmenopausal women with a proven 5aR effect (a mean decrease in DHT of 42%), there was no significant effect on total serum testosterone or estradiol [69]. It is only in the presence of supplemental androgens or estrogens in postmenopausal women on 5aR inhibitors that increased estradiol levels are more likely. However, because of the small risk of elevation of estrogen, until further safety data is available, both finasteride and dutasteride, the other FDA-approved 5aR inhibitors, are best avoided in survivors of hormone receptor-positive breast cancer. These agents may be acceptable for use in survivors of hormone receptor-negative breast cancer.

Low-Level Laser Treatment

Low-level laser treatment (LLLT), with primarily red to near-infrared wavelengths (600–1000 nm) and low power densities, has been shown to promote hair growth in animal and human dermal papillae studies and in clinical trials of FPHL and MPHL [71]. There are several LLLT devices on the market including laser combs and laser helmets, all available on the Internet for direct purchase by the consumer. The efficacy of LLLT in FPHL, as determined by target area hair counts, is similar to that of topical minoxidil in the initial months of treatment but lower with long-term use [72]. There are currently no studies that show efficacy of LLLT in pCIA or EIA in breast cancer survivors, but there is a suggestion of efficacy in a CIA rat model [73]. There are no safety concerns for breast cancer survivors with LLLT.

Platelet-Rich Plasma

Injections of platelet-rich plasma (PRP), which contain a high concentration of growth factors, have recently been used to treat a variety of hair loss conditions. The procedure to obtaining the PRP involves collection of the patient's own blood and centrifugation into the component of PRP. The majority of data on efficacy has been in patients with PHL [74], but there remains a lack of standardization of mode of preparation, addition of activators, centrifugation specifics, platelet concentration needed for efficacy, volume injected, and frequency of injections. Whether PRP might be useful and safe in pCIA or EIA remains to be determined.

Topical Prostaglandins

Bimatoprost, a prostaglandin F analog, is FDA approved for both glaucoma and eyelash hypotrichosis. The 0.03% solution applied to the eyelid margin results in an increase in thickness, length, and darkness of eyelashes [75]. In a double-masked, randomized, parallel-group, multicenter study of 130 breast cancer patients who received cytotoxic chemotherapy, treatment at 6 months with topical bimatoprost vs placebo led to the following comparative results with baseline: longer eyelash length (38% vs 16%) and increased eyelash thickness (245% vs 33%) [76, 77]. The most common side effects of bimatoprost applied topically for eyelashes are conjunctival hyperemia, pruritus, skin hyperpigmentation, ocular irritation, dry eye symptoms, and erythema of the eyelids, which occur in less than 4%. Clinically relevant iris hyperpigmentation (seen with the intraocular treatment for glaucoma), periorbital fat atrophy, or changes in intraocular pressure are unlikely.

Bimatoprost 0.03% solution has also been shown to be useful for thinning eyebrows with increased fullness and darkness compared to placebo [78–80]. No skin pigmentation has been noted.

Hair Transplants

Hair transplants rely on moving viable terminal scalp hair follicles from the occiput to areas of hair loss, typically the top of the scalp involved with pattern hair loss. It is usually of limited value in pCIA or EIA since the donor site may now be of low density as well.

Camouflage

For many breast cancer survivors with extensive persistent hair loss, wearing a wig may seem the easiest solution but may not be comfortable, affordable (at least those that are or look like human hair), or psychologically acceptable. Other options include wiglets, which augment the woman's remaining hair; they sit on the top of the scalp, attach by clips to the remaining hair, and cascade down on the sides. Another alternative is extensions or weaves, but these should not be attached by glue, which damages the hair shaft, or with traction that may pull out and permanently damage the remaining hair. Pigmented fibers, powders, or creams that approximate the color of the hair and are applied to the scalp help to lessen the contrast with the scalp skin but can create a physical barrier to the absorption of topical medications also applied to the scalp. Micropigmentation with tattoo stippling of permanent color between the follicular ostia can also lessen the contrast between scalp and scalp hair. Eyebrows can be tattooed, or for a slightly less permanent approach, microblading can be used. Microblading is a specialized tattooing technique that uses a multi-needle tool to add semipermanent pigments to the skin.

Conclusion

Persistent alopecia, whether chemotherapy or ET related, although not life-threatening, potentially has significant psychological effects including a sadness for loss of one's former self-image and a constant reminder of the cancer one has survived. As opposed to loss of a breast, loss of hair is also obvious to others. Mechanisms to prevent CIA without creating a privileged site from chemotherapy exposure would be a huge advance. Lacking this, there are some promising ways of encouraging regrowth of hair in survivors. More needs to be done in the area of preventing, tracking, and treating both pCIA and EIA.

Conflicts of Interest None.

References

1. Am Cancer Society, Surveillance Research, 2017.
2. U.S. Cancer Statistics Working Group. U.S. Cancer Statistics Data Visualizations Tool, based on 2019 submission data (1999-2017): U.S. Department of Health and Human Services, Centers for Disease Control and Prevention and National Cancer Institute; www.cdc.gov/cancer/dataviz, released in June 2020.
3. Howlder N, Noone Am, Krapcho M et al. Seer cancer statistics review, 1975–2014. https://seer.cancer.gov/csr/1975_2014/17 based on November 2016 SEER data submission, posted to the SEER web site, April 2016. Bethesda, MD; NCI, 2017.
4. Surveillance, Epidemiology, and End Results (SEER) Program (www.seer.cancer.gov) SEER*Stat Database: Incidence – SEER 18 Regs Research Data, Nov 2016 Sub (2000–2014) <Katrina/Rita Population Adjustment> – Linked To County Attributes – Total U.S., 1969–2015 Counties, National Cancer Institute, DCCPS, Surveillance Research Program, released April 2017, based on the November 2016 submission.
5. Miller KD, Siegel RL, Lin CC, et al. Cancer treatment and survivorship statistics, 2016. CA Cancer J Clin. 2016;66:271–89.
6. McGarvey EL, Baum LD, Pinkerton R, Rogers LM. Psychological sequelae and alopecia among women with cancer. Cancer Pract. 2001;9:283–9.
7. Carelle N, Em P, Bellanger A, Germanaud J, Thuikllier A, Khayat D. Changing perceptions of the side effects of cancer chemotherapy. Cancer. 2002;95:155–63.
8. Cotsarelis G, Millar SE, Chan EF. Embryology and anatomy of the hair follicle. In: Olsen EA, editor. Disorders of hair growth: diagnosis and treatment. New York: McGraw-Hill; 2004.
9. Olsen EA. Clinical tools for assessing hair loss. In: Olsen EA, editor. Disorders of hair growth: diagnosis and treatment. New York: McGraw Hill; 2004.
10. Hesketh PJ, Batchelor D, Golant M, Lyman GH, Rhodes N, Yardley D. Chemotherapy-induced alopecia: psychosocial impact and therapeutic approaches. Support Care Cancer. 2004;12:543–9.
11. Beisecker AE, Cook MR, Ashworth J, et al. Side effects of adjuvant chemotherapy: perceptions of node-negative breast cancer patients. Psycho-Oncology. 1997;6:85–93.
12. Lemieux J, Maunsell E, Provencher L. Chemotherapy-induced alopecia and effects on quality of life among women with breast cancer: a literature review. Psycho-Oncology. 2008;17:317–28.
13. Yeager C, Olsen EA. Hair disorders associated with anticancer agents. In: Lacouture M, editor. Dermatologic principles and practice in oncology; conditions of the skin, hair and nails in cancer patients and survivors. Wiley; 2013.

14. Botchkarev VA, Komarova EA, Siebenhaar F, et al. p53 is essential for chemotherapy-induced hair loss. Cancer Res. 2000;60:5002–6.
15. Tobin DJ, Hagen E, Botchkarev VA, Paus R. Do hair bulb melanocytes undergo apoptosis during hair follicle regression (catagen)? J Invest Dermatol. 1998;111:941–7.
16. Crounse RC, van Scott EJ. Change in the scalp hair roots as a measure of toxicity from cancer chemotherapeutic drugs. J Invest Dermatol. 1960;35:83–90.
17. Nangia J, Wang T, Osborne C, et al. Effect of a scalp cooling device on alopecia in women undergoing chemotherapy for breast cancer: the SCALP randomized clinical trial. JAMA. 2017;317:596–605.
18. Watanabe T, Yagata H, Saito M, et al. A multicenter survey of temporal changes in chemotherapy-induced hair loss in breast cancer patients. PLoS One. 2019;14(1):e0208118. https://doi.org/10.1371/journal.pone.0208118.
19. Kanti V, Nuwayhid R, Lindner J, et al. Analysis of quantitative changes in hair growth during treatment with chemotherapy or tamoxifen in patients with breast cancer: a cohort study. Br J Dermatol. 2014;170:643–50.
20. Duvic M, Lemak NA, Valero V, et al. A randomized trial of minoxidil in chemotherapy -induced alopecia. J Am Acad Dermatol. 1996;35:74–8.
21. Olsen EA, Dunlap FE, Funicella T, et al. A randomized clinical trial of 5% topical minoxidil versus 2% topical minoxidil and placebo in the treatment of androgenetic alopecia in men. J Am Acad Dermatol. 2012;47:377–85.
22. Blume-Peytavi U, Shapiro J, Messenger AG, Hordinsky MK, Zhang P, Quiza C, Doshi U, Olsen EA. Efficacy and safety of once daily minoxidil foam 5% versus twice -daily minoxidil solution 2% in female pattern hair loss: a phase III, randomized, investigator blinded study. J Drugs Dermatol. 2016;15:883–9.
23. Bourgeois HP, Kerbrat P, Combe M, et al. Long term persistent alopecia and suboptimal hair regrowth after adjuvant chemotherapy for breast cancer: alert for an emerging side effect: French alpers observatory. Ann Oncol. 2010;21:viii83–viii4.
24. Kang D, Kim I-R, Choi E-K, et al. Permanent chemotherapy induced alopecia in patients with breast cancer: a 3-year prospective cohort study. Oncologist. 2019;24:414–20.
25. Kim GM, Kim S, Park HS, et al. Chemotherapy-induced Irreversible alopecia in early breast cancer patients. Breast Cancer Res Treat. 2017;163:527–33.
26. Bertrand M, Mailliez A, Vercambre S, Kotecki N, Mortier L, Bonneterre J. Permanent chemotherapy induced alopecia in early breast cancer patients after (neo)adjuvant chemotherapy: long term follow up. Cancer Res. 2013; https://doi.org/10.1158/0008-5472.SABCS13-P3-09-15.
27. Paus T, Haslam IS, Sharov AA, Botchkarev VA. Pathobiology of chemotherapy-induced hair loss. Lancet Oncol. 2013;14:e50–9.
28. Purba TS, Haslam IS, Poblet E, et al. Human epithelial hair follicle stem cells and their progeny: current state of knowledge, the widening gap in translational research and future challenges. BioEssays. 2014;36:513–25.
29. Masidonski P, Mahon SM. Permanent alopecia in women being treated for breast cancer. Br J Dermatol. 2009;160(4):883–5.
30. Fonia A, Cota C, Setterfield JF, et al. Permanent alopecia in patients with breast cancer after taxane chemotherapy and adjuvant hormonal therapy: clinicopathologic findings in a cohort of 10 patients. J Am Acad Dermatol. 2017;76:948–57.
31. Kluger N, Jacot W, Frouin E, et al. Permanent scalp alopecia related to breast cancer chemotherapy by sequential fluorouracil/epirubicin/cyclophosphamide (FEC) and docetaxel: a prospective study of 20 patients. Ann Oncol. 2012;23:2879–84.
32. Olsen EA. Female pattern hair loss. J Am Acad Dermatol. 2001;45(3 Suppl):S70–80.
33. Messenger AG, Sinclair R. Follicular miniaturization in female pattern hair loss: clinicopathological correlations. Br J Dermatol. 2006;155:926–30.
34. Whiting DA. Chronic telogen effluvium; increased scalp hair shedding in middle-aged women. J Am Acad Dermatol. 1996;35:899–906.
35. Olsen EA. The midline part: an important physical clue to the clinical diagnosis of androgenetic alopecia in women. J Am Acad Dermatol. 1999;40:106–9.
36. Olsen EA, Tosti A, Cotsarelis G, et al. Consensus guidelines for collecting meaningful data on chronic telogen effluvium. Int J Trichol. 2019;11(3):107–12.
37. Velasco MAM, Vazquez-Herrera NE, Maddy AJ, Asz-Sigall D, Tosti A. The hair shedding visual scale: a quick tool to assess hair loss in women. Dermatol Ther. 2017;7:155–65.
38. Vañó-Galván S, Molina-Ruiz AM, Serrano-Falcón C, et al. Frontal fibrosing alopecia: a multicenter review of 355 patients. J Am Acad Dermatol. 2014;70:670–8.
39. Olsen EA, Callender V, McMichael A, Sperling L, Anstrom K, Bergfeld W, et al. Central hair loss in African American women: incidence and potential risk factors. J Am Acad Dermatol. 2011;64(2):245–52.
40. Miteva M, Misciali C, Fanti A, Vincenzi B, Romanelli P, Tosti A. Permanent alopecia after systemic chemotherapy: a clinicopathological study of 10 cases. Am J Dermatopathol. 2011;33:345–50.
41. Tallon B, Blanchard E, Goldberg LJ. Permanent chemotherapy-induced alopecia:case report and review of the literature. J Am Acad Dermatol. 2010;63:333–6.
42. Olsen EA. Female pattern hair loss and its relationship to permanent/cicatricial alopecia: a new perspective. J Investig Dermatol Symp Proc. 2005;10(3):217–21.
43. Burstein HJ, Temin S, Anderson H, et al. Adjuvant endocrine therapy for women with hormone receptor-positive breast cancer: American Society of Clinical Oncology Clinical Practice Guideline Focused Update. J Clin Oncol. 2014;32:2255–69.

44. Gallicchio L, Calhoun C, Helzlsouer KJ. Aromatase inhibitor therapy and hair loss among breast cancer survivors. Breast Cancer Res Treat. 2013;142:435–43.
45. Saggar V, Wu S, Dickler MN, Lacouture ME. Alopecia with endocrine therapies in patients with cancer. Oncologist. 2013;18:1126–34.
46. Freites-Martinez A, Shapiro J, Chan D, et al. Endocrine therapy-induced alopecia in patients with breast cancer. JAMA Dermatol. 2018;154:670–5.
47. Park J, Kim JI, Yun SK, Kim HU, Ihm CW. Pattern alopecia during hormonal anticancer therapy in patients with breast cancer. Ann Dermatol. 2014;26:743–6.
48. Ohnemus U, Uenalan M, Inzunza J, Gustafsson JA, Paus R. The hair follicle as an estrogen target and source. Endo Rev. 2006;27:677–706.
49. Messenger AG, Rundegren J. Minoxidil: mechanisms of action on hair growth. Br J Dermatol. 2004;150:186–94.
50. Ferry JJ, Shepard JH, Szpunar GJ. Relationship between contact time of applied dose and percutaneous absorption of minoxidil from a topical solution. J Pharm Sci. 1990;79:483–6.
51. Franz TJ. Percutaneous absorption of minoxidil in man. Arch Dermatol. 1985;121:203–6.
52. Lee S, Tenglertsampan C, Tanchotikul M, Worapunpong N. Minoxidil 2% lotion for eyebrow enhancement: a randomized, double-blind, placebo-controlled, spilt-face comparative study. J Dermatol. 2014;41(2):149–52. https://doi.org/10.1111/1346-8138.12275.
53. Ramos PM, Sinclair RD, Kasprzak M, Miot HA. Minoxidil 1 mg oral versus minoxidil 5% topical solution for the treatment of female-pattern hair loss: as randomized clinical trial. J Am Acad Dermatol. 2020;82(1):252–3.
54. Beach RA. Case series of oral minoxidil for androgenetic and traction alopecia: tolerability & the five C's of oral therapy. Dermatol Ther. 2018;31(6):e12707. https://doi.org/10.1111/dth.12707.
55. Perera E, Sinclair R. Treatment of chronic telogen effluvium with oral minoxidil: a retrospective study. F1000 Res. 2017;6:1650.
56. Yang X, Thai K-E. Treatment of permanent chemotherapy-induced alopecia with low dose oral minoxidil. Australas J Dermatol. 2016 Nov;57(4):e130–2. https://doi.org/10.1111/ajd.12350.
57. Linas SL, Nies AS. Minoxidil. Ann Int Med. 1981;94:61–5.
58. Loriauz L, Menard R, Taylor A, Pita JC, Santen F. Spironolactone and endocrine dysfunction. Ann Int Med. 1976;85:630–6.
59. Sinclair R, Wewerinke M, Jolley D. Treatment of female pattern hair loss with oral antiandrogens. Br J Dermatol. 2005;152:466–73.
60. Sinclair FD. Female pattern hair loss: a pilot study investigating combination therapy with low dose oral minoxidil and spironolactone. Int Soc Dermatol. 2018;57:104–9.
61. Rozner RN, Freites-Martinesz A, Shapiro J, Geer EB, Goldfarb S, Lacouture M. Safety of 5a-reductase inhibitors and spironolactone in breast cancer patients receiving endocrine therapies. Breast Cancer Res Treat. 2019;174:15–26.
62. Mackenzie IS, Macdonald TM, Thompson A, Morant S, Wei L. Spironolactone and risk of incident breast cancer in women older than 55 years: retrospective, matched cohort study. BMJ. 2012;345:e4447.
63. Fryzek JP, Poulsen AH, Lipworth L, et al. A cohort study of antihypertensive medication use and breast cancer among Danish women. Breast Cancer Res Treat. 2006;97:231–6.
64. Some thyrotropic agents. IARC monogr eval carcinog risks hum. 2001;79:725.
65. Wei C, Bovonratwet P, Gu A, et al. Spironolactone use does not increase the risk of female breast cancer recurrence: a retrospective analysis. J Am Acad Dermatol. 2020;83(4):1021–7. https://doi.org/10.1016/j.jaad2020.05.081.
66. Steiner JF. Clinical pharmacokinetics and pharmacodynamics of finasteride. Clin Pharmacokinet. 1996;30:16–27.
67. Roberts JL, Fiedler V, Imperato-McGinley JI, Whiting D, Olsen E, Shupack J, et al. Clinical dose ranging studies with finasteride, a type 2 5a-reductase inhibitor, in men with male pattern hair loss. J Am Acad Dermatol. 1994;41:555–63.
68. Olsen EA, Hordinsky M, Whiting D, et al. The importance of dual 5a-reductase inhibition in the treatment of male pattern hair loss: results of a randomized placebo-controlled study of dutasteride versus finasteride. J Am Acad Dermatol. 2006;55:1014–23.
69. Price VH, Roberts JL, Hordinsky M, et al. Lack of efficacy of finasteride in postmenopausal women with androgenetic alopecia. J Am Acad Dermatol. 2000;43:768–76.
70. Boersma IH, Oranje AP, Grimalt R, Iorizzo M, Piraccini BM, Verdonschot EH. The effectiveness of finasteride and dutasteride used for 3 years in women with androgenetic alopecia. Indian J Dermatol Venereol Leprol. 2014;80:521–5.
71. Kalia S, Lui H. Utilizing electromagnetic radiation for hair growth. A critical review of phototrichogenesis. Dermatol Clin. 2013;31:193–200.
72. Jimenez JJ, Wikramanayake TC, Bergfeld W, et al. Efficacy and safety of a low-level laser device in the treatment of male and female pattern hair loss: a multicenter, randomized, sham device-controlled, double-blind study. Am J Clin Dermatol. 2014;15:115–27.
73. Wikramanayake TC, Villasante AC, Mauro LM, et al. Low-level laser treatment accelerated hair regrowth in a rat model of chemotherapy -induced alopecia (CIA). Lasers Med Sci. 2013;28:701–6.
74. Cervantes J, Perper M, Wong LL, et al. Effectiveness of platelet-rich plasma for androgenetic alopecia: a review of the literature. Skin Appendage Disord. 2018;4:1–11.

75. Smith S, Fagien S, Whitcup SM, et al. Eyelash growth in subjects treated with bimatoprost: a multicenter, randomized, double-masked, vehicle-controlled, parallel-group study. J Am Acad Dermatol. 2012;66:801–6.
76. Ahluwalia GS. Safety and efficacy of bimatoprost solution 0.03% topical application in patients with chemotherapy induced eyelash loss. J Invest Dermatol Symp Proc. 2013;16:S73–6.
77. Glaser DA, Hossain P, Perkins W, et al. Long-term safety and efficacy of bimatoprost solution 0·03% application to the eyelid margin for the treatment of idiopathic and chemotherapy-induced eyelash hypotrichosis: a randomized controlled trial. Br J Dermatol. 2015;172(5):1384–94. https://doi.org/10.1111/bjd.13443.
78. Carruthers J, Beer K, Carruthers A, et al. Bimatoprost 0.03% for the treatment of eyebrow hypotrichosis. Dermatol Surg. 2016;42:608–17.
79. Beer KR, Julius H, Dunn M, Wilson F. Treatment of eyebrow hypotrichosis using bimatoprost: a randomized, double blind, vehicle controlled pilot study. Dermatol Surg. 2013;38:1079–87.
80. Chanasumon N, Srihojanart T, Suchonwanit P. Therapeutic potential of bimatoprost for the treatment of eyebrow hypotrichosis. Drug Des Devel Ther. 2018;12:365–72.

19 Skin Reactions Associated with Breast Cancer Treatment

Lauren Pontius Floyd

Introduction

Some of the most common side effects that arise from the treatment of breast cancer are adverse skin reactions. These side effects can lead to significant morbidity, with the severity of the adverse skin reactions ranging from benign to life-threatening [1]. These treatment-related toxicities can occur during treatment, as well as persist or evolve in the years following treatment. Our understanding of these adverse skin reactions has evolved significantly, as new therapeutics have been employed for breast cancer treatment. Many of these medications inhibit specific cell cycle phases, which directly impact normal cell turnover in the skin [2]. These new therapies have led to improved survival and treatment outcomes, but despite their benefits, the adverse skin reactions associated with these treatments can be bothersome and, in some cases, life-threatening. Adverse skin reactions associated with breast cancer therapies can be grouped into several broad categories: chemotherapy reactions, targeted therapy reactions, endocrine therapy reactions, and radiation reactions. Overviews of skin and nail changes related to treatments for breast cancer are provided in Tables 19.1, 19.2, and 19.3.

L. P. Floyd (✉)
Duke University Medical Center, Durham, NC, USA
e-mail: Lauren.Floyd@duke.edu

Chemotherapy Reactions

Conventional chemotherapy remains a vital part of breast cancer management. Different chemotherapeutic agents have been used in various regimens for many years, and the skin toxicities are well described. Each class of chemotherapeutic agent affects different parts of the cell cycle, which leads to disproportionate effects on the skin due to its rapid cell turnover [2, 3].

Taxanes

Taxanes act via inhibition of mitosis and are among the most commonly used chemotherapeutic agents in patients with all stages of breast cancer. Adverse skin reactions are often associated with paclitaxel and docetaxel, the two taxanes most frequently used in breast cancer. Of greatest concern are immediate hypersensitivity reactions, which can occur during or shortly after infusion. These hypersensitivity reactions are typically observed during the first or second cycle of treatment and classically present with urticaria, morbilliform eruption, flushing, angioedema, and pruritus. Prophylactic antihistamines and oral steroids are required premedications for paclitaxel and docetaxel infusions [2, 4]. Taxanes have also been linked with drug-induced lupus erythematosus, most commonly drug-induced subacute cutaneous lupus erythematosus (SCLE).

G. G. Kimmick et al. (eds.), *Common Issues in Breast Cancer Survivors*,
https://doi.org/10.1007/978-3-030-75377-1_19

Table 19.1 Cutaneous reactions that occur during breast cancer treatment, onset, and their management

	Cutaneous reactions	Onset	Management
Taxanes	Immediate hypersensitivity reactions	Occurs during or immediately after an infusion	Premedication with antihistamines and oral steroids
	Taxane-induced hand-foot syndrome	Develops during treatment course	Prophylactic cryotherapy; emollients and topical steroids
	Drug-induced lupus erythematosus	Develops during treatment course	Dose reduction or discontinuation of therapy if severe
	Photosensitivity	Develops during treatment course	Strict sunscreen use and sun avoidance
	Radiation recall	Develops during treatment course	See radiation management
	Scleroderma-like skin changes	Develops during and after treatment course completion; changes can persist	Physical therapy
	Morbilliform eruption	Develops during treatment course	Dose reduction or discontinuation of therapy if severe
Antimetabolites	Hand-foot syndrome	Develops during treatment course	Topical steroids, topical keratolytics, NSAIDs (mild-moderate); decrease or discontinue dose (severe)
	Pigmentary changes (pattern dependent on specific drug)	Develops during treatment course	Monitoring
	Photosensitivity	Develops during treatment course	Strict sunscreen use and sun avoidance
	Inflammation of actinic keratoses	Develops during treatment course	Monitoring
	Radiation recall	Develops during treatment course	See radiation management
	Drug-induced lupus (SCLE and DCLE)	Develops during treatment course	Dose reduction or discontinuation of therapy if severe
Alkylating agents	Hyperpigmentation	Develops during treatment course; can persist for a year after the end of therapy	Monitoring
	Type 1 IgE hypersensitivity (platinum agents)	Occurs during or immediately after infusion	Prophylactic antihistamines and oral steroids, reduce infusion rate
	Porphyria cutanea tarda (cyclophosphamide)	Develops during treatment course	Dose reduction or discontinuation of therapy if severe
	Neutrophilic eccrine hidradenitis (cyclophosphamide)	Develops during treatment course	Dose reduction or discontinuation of therapy if severe
	Radiation recall (cyclophosphamide)	Develops during treatment course	See radiation management

Anthracyclines	Hand-foot syndrome	Develops during treatment course	Topical steroids, topical keratolytics, NSAIDs (mild-moderate); decrease or discontinue dose (severe)
	Mucositis	Develops during treatment course	Dose reduction or discontinuation of therapy if severe
	Diffuse follicular rash (liposomal anthracyclines)	Develops during treatment course	Dose reduction or discontinuation of therapy if severe
	Intertrigo-like eruption (liposomal anthracyclines)	Develops during treatment course	Dose reduction or discontinuation of therapy if severe
	Melanotic macules (liposomal anthracyclines)	Develops during treatment course; can persist indefinitely	Monitoring
	Radiation recall (liposomal anthracyclines)	Develops during treatment course	See radiation management
HER2-targeted therapy	Papulopustular eruption	Develops during treatment course	Antihistamines and topical steroids; tetracyclines (severe)
	Acneiform eruption	Develops during treatment course	Antihistamines and topical steroids; tetracyclines (severe)
Endocrine therapy	Flushing (SERM)	Develops during treatment course	Monitoring
	Morbilliform eruption (SERM)	Develops during treatment course	Dose reduction or discontinuation of therapy if severe
	Porphyria cutanea tarda (SERM)	Develops during treatment course	Dose reduction or discontinuation of therapy if severe
	Radiation recall (SERM)	Develops during treatment course	See radiation management
	Cutaneous vasculitis, erythema nodosum, SCLE (AI)	Develops during treatment course	Discontinuation of AI; topical or oral corticosteroids
Radiation	Acute radiation dermatitis	Develops during treatment course	Wash radiation sites daily, topical steroids (prophylaxis and treatment)
	Radiation recall	Can occur during chemotherapy if this follows radiation	Treat like acute radiation dermatitis
	Hypopigmentation, hyperpigmentation, telangiectasias, atrophy, fibrosis, ulceration (late)	Occurs months to years following radiation	PDL (telangiectasias)
	Skin cancer (melanoma and non-melanoma)	Can occur at any time after radiation	Regular skin examinations

Table 19.2 Nail reactions that occur during breast cancer treatment, onset, and their management

	Nail reactions	Onset/duration	Management
Taxanes	Onycholysis, Beau's lines, onychomelanosis, subungual hemorrhage	Develops during treatment course, can persist for many months after course completion	Prophylactic cryotherapy (frozen socks and gloves)
Antimetabolites	Longitudinal melanonychia (capecitabine), diffuse/transverse/half-and-half melanonychia (5-FU), paronychia (5-FU), nail dystrophy, onychomadesis	Develops during treatment course, can persist for many months after course completion	Monitoring
Alkylating agents	Pigmentary changes (longitudinal, transverse, and/or diffuse pigmentation), onychodystrophy, onycholysis, Beau's lines, Muehrcke lines (cyclophosphamide)	Develops during treatment course, can persist for many months after course completion	Monitoring
HER2-targeted therapy	Painful paronychia, subungual hemorrhages, onycholysis	Develops during treatment course, can persist for many months after course completion	Prophylactic cryotherapy (not well studied in these medications)
	Exacerbation of chemotherapy-induced nail toxicity	Develops during treatment course when simultaneous with chemotherapy	Monitoring

Table 19.3 Nail reactions that occur during breast cancer treatment and their definitions

Nail reaction	Definition
Onycholysis	Separation of the nail from the nail bed
Beau's lines	Indentations that run across the nails, caused by temporary arrest of nail growth
Onychomelanosis	Deposition of pigment in the nail unit
Subungual hemorrhage	Bleeding under the nail
Longitudinal melanonychia	Longitudinally oriented brown-black pigment in the nail
Transverse melanonychia	Transversely oriented brown-black pigment in the nail
Diffuse melanonychia	Brown-black pigment that is present in the entire nail
Paronychia	Inflammation of the tissue surrounding the nail (nail folds)
Onychodystrophy	Any alteration in nail morphology (nail dystrophy)
Muehrcke lines	Parallel, white transverse lines across the nail

This can be clinically indistinguishable from idiopathic SCLE, with annular erythematous lesions in sun-exposed areas. These lesions typically regress within several weeks after discontinuation of chemotherapy [4, 5].

Patients can also develop a taxane-induced form of hand-foot syndrome (HFS) that is distinct from HFS caused by other chemotherapeutic agents. Rather than palmar and plantar erythema, patients develop erythematous plaques on the dorsal hands, the Achilles tendon, and the malleoli, in addition to associated pain and burning in these areas. However, it has only been reported in 5% and 10% of patients (docetaxel and paclitaxel, respectively) [2]. The impact on quality of life and functional impairment is variable, but this can be dose-limiting if severe. These limitations can range from mild burning and pain that are easily tolerated to inability to walk or grip objects. Cryotherapy with the use of frozen gloves and socks during drug infusion has been found to be beneficial in preventing HFS in several studies; emollients and topical steroids are used to treat the condition once it develops. After discontinuation of the taxane chemotherapeutic agent, HFS will typically resolve within several weeks [6].

Uncommon taxane-related cutaneous reactions include photosensitivity, radiation recall, scleroderma-like skin changes, and morbilliform eruptions. While most of these skin reactions occur during treatment and typically resolve following cessation of the drug, the scleroderma-like skin changes can persist. These changes may be preceded by edema, and fibrotic changes develop progressively over several months of therapy. The most common sites are on the distal extremities, and induration and fibrosis that occur may not even be noted until chemotherapy is complete. Discontinuing chemotherapy can sometimes lead to regression of these changes, but secondary sclerosis is still a risk in areas of long-standing edema. Initiating physical therapy is a crucial step in prevention [4, 7].

Taxanes are also frequently associated with common acute changes that have the potential to have a long-lasting negative impact. An example is nail toxicity, such as onycholysis (separation of the nail from the nail bed), Beau's lines (indentations that run across the nails, caused by temporary arrest of nail growth), onychomelanosis (deposition of pigment in the nail unit), and subungual hemorrhage. In addition to nail toxicity, patients will often have paronychia of the lateral and proximal nail folds [8, 9]. There are several studies supporting the use of prophylactic cryotherapy, usually via frozen gloves or socks, to limit nail toxicity. Similar to scalp hypothermia therapy, cold treatments to hands and feet during chemotherapy infusion cause cold-induced vasoconstriction of the distal fingers and toes, which limits the amount of drug that reaches the nail unit. The effect of taxanes on the nail is cumulative [10], and cryotherapy helps to reduce the total nail toxicity [11–14]. The long-term effects on the nail unit are less studied, and duration and resolution are often dictated by the structure of the nail and severity of the insult. Typically, resolution occurs over months, though nail changes can persist if the connection between the nail plate and the nail bed is disrupted [15].

Antimetabolites

Antimetabolites are a class of chemotherapeutic agents that function by substituting nucleotide analogues for the building blocks of DNA and RNA, which damage cells in S phase when they interrupt DNA synthesis and replication. Methotrexate, 5-fluorouracil (5-FU), and the oral prodrug of 5-FU, capecitabine, are all breast cancer chemotherapeutic agents that are part of this class. Methotrexate is less commonly implicated in cutaneous reactions, although photosensitivity can occur during treatment.

Classically, in regard to the skin, patients treated with 5-FU and capecitabine present with HFS, also known as palmoplantar erythrodysesthesia. There is a prodrome of pain and tingling in the extremities, followed by development of symmetric, sharply demarcated erythema across the palms and soles. This will typically arise in the first one to two cycles of treatment. HFS can occur in numerous contexts, including after treatment with several other classes of chemotherapy. Functional impairment can be dose-limiting in severe cases due to pain, blistering, and desquamation. HFS occurs less frequently when 5-FU is given as a bolus, compared to the incidence when given as a slow infusion. Capecitabine has a significantly higher incidence of HFS as compared to 5-FU, and this is believed to be related to the oral medication functioning as a continuous infusion. Data regarding prevention with pretreatment of pyridoxine and oral dexamethasone has been mixed [16]. Management of mild to moderate cases includes high-potency topical steroids (such as clobetasol and betamethasone dipropionate) and topical keratolytics (such as ammonium lactate) one to two times per day and non-steroidal anti-inflammatory drugs (NSAIDs) as needed, while management of severe cases is primarily addressed by decreasing the dose or discontinuing the medication altogether until HFS resolves. Resolution typically occurs within several weeks, with complete resolution in 1–2 months after discontinuation of therapy [16, 17].

Both 5-FU and capecitabine can cause hyperpigmentation and other pigmentary changes. However, the appearance differs depending on the chemotherapeutic agent. While capecitabine and 5-FU are the same drug, different methods of delivery (5-FU as a bolus or IV infusion and capecitabine as an oral medication) cause variation in skin and nail reactions. Capecitabine primarily causes acral hyperpigmentation, while 5-FU can have a variety of hyperpigmentation patterns, including photodistributed, serpentine supravenous from the hand to the shoulder, widespread and reticulate, serpentine streaks over the back and buttocks, and diffuse involvement of the palms. Typically, hyperpigmentation will gradually self-resolve over weeks to months. Other reactions to antimetabolites include photosensitivity, inflammation of actinic keratoses (primarily 5-FU and capecitabine), and radiation recall, which all tend to resolve after resolution of therapy. There are also several case reports of drug-induced SCLE and discoid cutaneous lupus erythematosus (DCLE) caused by 5-FU and capecitabine, which resolve within 2 months following discontinuation of chemotherapy [2, 18].

Nail changes are also variable depending on the specific antimetabolite. Capecitabine can cause longitudinal melanonychia (black or brown pigmentation of the nail) across single or multiple nails, as well as nail dystrophy with onycholysis and onychomadesis (proximal separation of the nail from the nail bed due to temporary arrest of nail growth) [19–21]. Melanonychia induced by 5-FU can be diffuse, transverse, or half and half (distal nail is reddish brown; proximal nail is white), but not typically longitudinal. Melanonychia due to antimetabolites does resolve as the nail grows out, but this process can take many months to years. Additionally, paronychia (inflammation of the nail folds) and diffuse nail thickening can occur during treatment [22].

Alkylating Agents

Alkylating agents are divided into two broad categories: classical alkylating agents, such as cyclophosphamide, and platinum agents, such as carboplatin. They function by cross-linking DNA, which affects all phases of the cell cycle, and they are part of many breast cancer treatment regimens [3]. Cyclophosphamide can cause hyperpigmented macules and patches that occur most commonly on the palms, soles, nails, teeth, and, rarely, the gingiva. The hyperpigmentation typically develops after 4 weeks of therapy, and it can persist for 6–12 months following discontinuation of treatment. The nail changes can be prominent, with development of longitudinal, transverse, or even diffuse pigmentation across all nails. Patients can also develop onychodystrophy, onycholysis, Beau's lines, or Muehrcke lines (paired white transverse lines across the nails) [22]. These nail changes do tend to regress slowly over many months once treatment is complete. More rarely with cyclophosphamide, patients can develop porphyria cutanea tarda (PCT), neutrophilic eccrine hidradenitis (NEH), and radiation recall [23, 24]. PCT can develop after multiple cycles of treatment, and it will typically resolve within several weeks after discontinuing the chemotherapeutic agent [23]. NEH presents with tender nodules, particularly on the trunk and extremities. It is considered a reactive, benign condition that resolves when treatment is discontinued [25].

Platinum agents can also cause hyperpigmentation, although the distribution is less distinctive, tending to be patchy and diffuse. The hyperpigmentation occurs around the second or third course of treatment and primarily is seen on the dorsal surfaces of extremities, elbows, knees, and neck, preferentially occurring in sites of trauma or pressure. The hyperpigmentation is thought to be permanent, although the color change may improve with time [26]. The hyperpigmentation can also occasionally be seen in the nails and oral mucosa, but this is less common [2, 22]. The other significant cutaneous reaction is a type I IgE-mediated hypersensitivity to platinum agents, but this only tends to occur after multiple treatments. As with taxanes, the reaction typically occurs during or immediately after infusion. Most commonly, patients will develop palmar pruritus, flushing, urticaria, and, rarely, anaphylaxis [27]. To prevent this hypersensitivity reaction, antihistamines and oral steroids can be administered prior to each infusion, and the infusion rate can be reduced. Once the hypersensitivity reaction occurs, it will typically resolve within several hours of treatment with antihistamines and oral or intravenous corticosteroids [27].

Anthracyclines

The anthracycline chemotherapeutic agents are antitumor antibiotics and are present in some of the most commonly used chemotherapy regimens. These include both the classic forms of doxorubicin and epirubicin, as well as the liposomal encapsulated forms. Anthracyclines function by interfering with topoisomerase II and are administered intravenously. Patients with anthracycline-induced HFS have a presentation very similar to the reaction caused by antimetabolites (see above). HFS typically occurs much more frequently in the liposomal encapsulated form of anthracyclines, although it has also been reported in the classic form [28]. Onset typically occurs within the first two to three cycles of treatment, and the course is usually self-limiting. Most patients have complete resolution within a month after the completion of treatment [29]. Mucositis is also fairly common in all forms of anthracyclines, and it was reported in 37% of patients in one community-based study [30]. A diffuse follicular rash, an intertrigo-like eruption in the skin folds, the onset of melanotic macules, and radiation recall are all due to the liposomal anthracycline formulations [2]. The development of melanotic macules typically occurs on the trunk and extremities, including the palms and soles. There is melanocytic hyperplasia at the basal layer on histopathologic examination; some of these macules can fade over time, while others persist indefinitely [28, 31].

HER2-Targeted Therapy Reactions

The advent of receptor-targeted therapy has significantly altered treatment regimens and improved the survival in breast cancer patients over the past several decades. Tumors demonstrating elevated expression of human epidermal growth factor receptor 2 (HER2), which serves as a marker for more aggressive tumor activity, are treated with therapeutic agents that specifically target the HER2 receptor [3].

Anti-HER2 agents include monoclonal antibodies (trastuzumab and pertuzumab), an antibody-drug conjugate (ado-trastuzumab emtansine), and tyrosine kinase inhibitors (lapatinib, neratinib, and tucatinib). Trastuzumab, pertuzumab, ado-trastuzumab emtansine, and neratinib are approved for use as adjuvant therapy for patients with HER2+ breast cancer. While skin toxicities have been well documented with the use of a related cell-surface protein called EGFR/HER1, cutaneous reactions occur at much lower rates in HER2-targeted therapies [32]. Trastuzumab and pertuzumab, both humanized monoclonal antibodies that target HER2, have become a vital part of breast cancer treatment [3]. When skin reactions occur, papulopustular eruptions and acneiform eruptions, similar to that seen with the use of EGFR/HER1-targeted therapy, are the most common. Regardless of the inducing agent, treatment of the papulopustular and acneiform eruptions is similar and ranges from antihistamines and topical steroids to systemic treatment with tetracyclines if severe. Patients undergoing treatment with HER2 inhibitors need to understand the vital importance of strict sun precautions as prevention against adverse cutaneous reactions. Topical steroids also play an important role in the prevention and treatment of these sequelae [32–34].

Nail toxicity is not as widely reported in HER2-targeted therapy compared to chemotherapy treatments, although there are case reports of HER2-targeted therapy exacerbating chemotherapy-induced nail toxicity [35]. Additionally, trastuzumab can cause taxane-like toxicity, such as painful paronychia, subungual hemorrhages, and onycholysis [15]. Prophylactic cryotherapy has primarily been studied in taxane-induced nail toxicity, but given the low risk associated with cryotherapy, it can be tried with HER2 inhibitors.

Endocrine Therapy Reactions

Endocrine therapy is the frontline systemic treatment used in patients with hormone receptor-positive (HR+) breast cancer. This therapeutic approach specifically targets ER+ breast cancer with hormonal dependency and includes selective estrogen receptor modulators (SERM), aromatase inhibitors, and others. Skin reactions to endocrine therapies are rare.

SERMs, most notably tamoxifen used in the adjuvant setting, can cause flushing. More rarely they cause morbilliform eruptions, radiation recall, and porphyria cutanea tarda (PCT), in addition to case reports of Stevens-Johnson syndrome [36]. It is theorized that the metabolite by-products of these drugs induce PCT [37]. As with cyclophosphamide, PCT tends to resolve after discontinuation of treatment. If the treatment-related toxicity is sufficiently severe, the medication should be discontinued and another endocrine therapy selected. Additionally, data regarding the long-term risk of skin malignancy (both melanoma and non-melanoma skin cancers) following tamoxifen use have been inconclusive. While data from a study in Denmark indicate no significant difference in skin cancer risk when comparing women treated with tamoxifen and control groups, the limitations of this study prevented stratified analyses in these cohorts [38].

The cutaneous toxicities that have been associated with aromatase inhibitors (AI) as a class include cutaneous vasculitis, erythema nodosum, and subacute cutaneous lupus erythematosus. While uncommon, if one of these cutaneous reactions does occur, treatment includes discontinuation of the AI and the use of topical or oral corticosteroids. Patients can eventually be restarted on a different AI with minimal risk of recurrence of the cutaneous toxicity [3, 39, 40].

Radiation Reactions

Radiation therapy plays a critical role in breast cancer management. It helps eradicate subclinical disease after surgical resection of grossly evident tumors, reduce local recurrence rates, and increase breast cancer-specific survival in certain settings [41]. However, radiation also has short- and long-term effects on skin in the targeted field. Cutaneous radiation reactions are classically divided into two broad categories: (1) acute and (2) late skin reactions [42].

Acute Reactions

Morbidity in the acute setting while radiation therapy delivery is ongoing is limited to the parts of the body within the irradiation field. There are typically very few systemic side effects, such as fatigue, nausea, and vomiting, in this setting. Acute radiation dermatitis typically will occur in the first 2–3 weeks of radiation therapy, and it can vary from mild erythema, dry desquamation, moist desquamation, mild bleeding, and ulceration.

Radiation recall can occur within the first several weeks after initiating various systemic therapies (most chemotherapeutic agents such as taxanes, antimetabolites, alkylating agents, and anthracyclines, as well as tamoxifen), and it mimics acute radiation dermatitis with containment to the irradiated zone. The mechanism of radiation recall has not yet been fully elucidated, although several mechanisms have been postulated. While most acute radiation dermatitis will self-resolve after 3–4 weeks, it can adversely affect quality of life as well as cause treatment delays or premature treatment discontinuation [42]. The severity and extent of acute radiation dermatitis are dependent on dose and tumor site, and treatment areas with close proximity to the skin are more adversely affected [43].

While there have been multiple studies for the prevention and management of radiation recall, the variation in clinical practice and the lack of high-quality data that support a single management strategy have led to challenges and debate [44]. In regard to skin care, patients historically were instructed to not wash radiation sites. However, clinical trial results do not support the proscription of cleansing skin fields involved in radiation treatment. It is now the standard clinical practice for patients to wash radiation sites daily with gentle soap and water [45–47]. Topical steroids can be used as both prophylaxis and treatment of acute radiation dermatitis, with overall improvement in pruritus and discomfort. Cutaneous atrophy due to topical steroid use is typically not an issue, given the limited duration of therapy [42, 48]. There is no evidence of worsening radiation dermatitis due to deodorants or antiperspirants, and there is mixed data regarding other nonsteroidal topical agents, such as aloe vera, sucralfate, oil-in-water emulsions, hyaluronic acid, ascorbic acid, and silver dressing [42, 49].

Late Reactions

The late reactions of radiation therapy typically occur months to years after the radiation exposure. Common skin changes include hypopigmentation, hyperpigmentation, telangiectasias, atrophy, fibrosis, and ulceration. While acute reactions tend to self-resolve over a matter of weeks, late reactions can persist for years, adversely affecting quality of life, especially areas of chronic fibrosis or non-healing ulcerations [44].

Telangiectasias can be treated primarily with pulsed dye laser (PDL), which is safe and effective [50]. Additionally, the likelihood of late reactions to radiation therapy increases with ongoing, unprotected sun exposure, and it is critically important for patients to wear sunscreen, especially on the previously irradiated skin, and follow sun protective measures.

While there are multiple other exceedingly rare cutaneous conditions that can be induced by radiation, one of greater concern is a secondary malignancy. In general, breast cancer survivors are at a small increased risk for secondary dermatologic malignancies after radiation, not limited to the radiation field [51]. This includes both melanoma and non-melanoma skin cancers, particularly in patients who received radiation at a young age. They may develop skin cancers many years after radiation therapy. It is therefore important at regular follow-up visits to conduct appropriate age-related cancer screening and regular skin examinations [52–54].

In addition to the various treatment options that have been discussed for acute and late radiation reactions, it is important to note that technical advancements have enabled more precise delivery of radiotherapy to target treatment sites. The development of techniques such as field-in-field 3D technique and breast intensity-modulated radiation therapy, as well as the ongoing research into hypofractionation, will be important for the prevention and treatment of radiation skin reactions in the future [43].

Conclusion

Here, more commonly seen adverse skin reactions that occur during and after treatment of breast cancer were reviewed. These skin reactions vary based on whether they occur in response to chemotherapeutic agents, targeted therapies, or ionizing radiation. Understanding the types of adverse skin reactions that could arise in response to a specific therapy enables doctors and patients to more readily detect and limit these sequelae, as well as differentiate between those that are annoying and those that are life-threatening. As the treatment of breast cancer improves with technological advancements, our understanding of the side effects and their appropriate management will continue to evolve.

References

1. Mockenhaupt M. Epidemiology of cutaneous adverse drug reactions. Allergol Select. 2017;1(1):96–108.
2. Reyes-Habito CM, Roh EK. Cutaneous reactions to chemotherapeutic drugs and targeted therapies for cancer: part I. Conventional chemotherapeutic drugs. J Am Acad Dermatol. 2014;71(2):203.e201–12; quiz 215–206.
3. Waks AG, Winer EP. Breast cancer treatment: a review. JAMA. 2019;321(3):288–300.
4. Sibaud V, Lebœuf NR, Roche H, et al. Dermatological adverse events with taxane chemotherapy. Eur J Dermatol. 2016;26(5):427–43.
5. Marchetti MA, Noland MM, Dillon PM, Greer KE. Taxane associated subacute cutaneous lupus erythematosus. Dermatol Online J. 2013;19(8):19259.
6. Stravodimou A, Voutsadakis IA. Hand and foot syndrome associated with docetaxel treatment. Acta Oncol. 2012;51(4):554–6.
7. Itoh M, Yanaba K, Kobayashi T, Nakagawa H. Taxane-induced scleroderma. Br J Dermatol. 2007;156(2):363–7.
8. Lau CP, Hui P, Chan TC. Docetaxel-induced nail toxicity: a case of severe onycholysis and topic review. Chin Med J. 2011;124(16):2559–60.
9. Minisini AM, Tosti A, Sobrero AF, et al. Taxane-induced nail changes: incidence, clinical presentation and outcome. Ann Oncol. 2003;14(2):333–7.
10. Can G, Aydiner A, Cavdar I. Taxane-induced nail changes: predictors and efficacy of the use of frozen

gloves and socks in the prevention of nail toxicity. Eur J Oncol Nurs. 2012;16(3):270–5.
11. Huang KL, Lin KY, Huang TW, et al. Prophylactic management for taxane-induced nail toxicity: a systematic review and meta-analysis. Eur J Cancer Care (Engl). 2019;28(5):e13118.
12. Scotté F, Tourani JM, Banu E, et al. Multicenter study of a frozen glove to prevent docetaxel-induced onycholysis and cutaneous toxicity of the hand. J Clin Oncol. 2005;23(19):4424–9.
13. Scotté F, Banu E, Medioni J, et al. Matched case-control phase 2 study to evaluate the use of a frozen sock to prevent docetaxel-induced onycholysis and cutaneous toxicity of the foot. Cancer. 2008;112(7):1625–31.
14. Marks DH, Qureshi A, Friedman A. Evaluation of prevention interventions for taxane-induced dermatologic adverse events: a systematic review. JAMA Dermatol. 2018;154(12):1465–72.
15. Zawar V, Bondarde S, Pawar M, Sankalecha S. Nail changes due to chemotherapy: a prospective observational study of 129 patients. J Eur Acad Dermatol Venereol. 2019;33(7):1398–404.
16. Fabian CJ, Molina R, Slavik M, Dahlberg S, Giri S, Stephens R. Pyridoxine therapy for palmar-plantar erythrodysesthesia associated with continuous 5-fluorouracil infusion. Investig New Drugs. 1990;8(1):57–63.
17. Wilkes GM, Doyle D. Palmar-plantar erythrodysesthesia. Clin J Oncol Nurs. 2005;9(1):103–6.
18. Weger W, Kränke B, Gerger A, Salmhofer W, Aberer E. Occurrence of subacute cutaneous lupus erythematosus after treatment with fluorouracil and capecitabine. J Am Acad Dermatol. 2008;59(2 Suppl 1):S4–6.
19. Chen GY, Chen YH, Hsu MM, Tsao CJ, Chen WC. Onychomadesis and onycholysis associated with capecitabine. Br J Dermatol. 2001;145(3):521–2.
20. Paravar T, Hymes SR. Longitudinal melanonychia induced by capecitabine. Dermatol Online J. 2009;15(10):11.
21. Muñoz A, Barceló R, Rubio I, Mañé JM, Ferreiro J, López-Vivanco G. Onycholysis associated with capecitabine in combination with irinotecan in two patients with colorectal cancer. J Natl Cancer Inst. 2003;95(16):1252–3.
22. Susser WS, Whitaker-Worth DL, Grant-Kels JM. Mucocutaneous reactions to chemotherapy. J Am Acad Dermatol. 1999;40(3):367–98; quiz 399–400.
23. Manzione NC, Wolkoff AW, Sassa S. Development of porphyria cutanea tarda after treatment with cyclophosphamide. Gastroenterology. 1988;95(4):1119–22.
24. Borroni G, Vassallo C, Brazzelli V, et al. Radiation recall dermatitis, panniculitis, and myositis following cyclophosphamide therapy: histopathologic findings of a patient affected by multiple myeloma. Am J Dermatopathol. 2004;26(3):213–6.
25. Harrist TJ, Fine JD, Berman RS, Murphy GF, Mihm MC Jr. Neutrophilic eccrine hidradenitis. A distinctive type of neutrophilic dermatosis associated with myelogenous leukemia and chemotherapy. Arch Dermatol. 1982;118(4):263–6.
26. Al-Lamki Z, Pearson P, Jaffe N. Localized cisplatin hyperpigmentation induced by pressure. A case report. Cancer. 1996;77(8):1578–81.
27. Makrilia N, Syrigou E, Kaklamanos I, Manolopoulos L, Saif MW. Hypersensitivity reactions associated with platinum antineoplastic agents: a systematic review. Met Based Drugs. 2010;2010:207084.
28. Lotem M, Hubert A, Lyass O, et al. Skin toxic effects of polyethylene glycol-coated liposomal doxorubicin. Arch Dermatol. 2000;136(12):1475–80.
29. von Moos R, Thuerlimann BJ, Aapro M, et al. Pegylated liposomal doxorubicin-associated hand-foot syndrome: recommendations of an international panel of experts. Eur J Cancer. 2008;44(6):781–90.
30. Salzberg M, Thurlimann B, Hasler U, et al. Pegylated liposomal doxorubicin (caelyx) in metastatic breast cancer: a community-based observation study. Oncology. 2007;72(3–4):147–51.
31. Yuan Y, Orlow SJ, Curtin J, Downey A, Muggia F. Pegylated liposomal doxorubicin (PLD): enhanced skin toxicity in areas of vitiligo. Ecancermedicalscience. 2008;2:111.
32. Sheu J, Hawryluk EB, Litsas G, Thakuria M, LeBoeuf NR. Papulopustular acneiform eruptions resulting from trastuzumab, a HER2 inhibitor. Clin Breast Cancer. 2015;15(1):e77–81.
33. Macdonald JB, Macdonald B, Golitz LE, LoRusso P, Sekulic A. Cutaneous adverse effects of targeted therapies: part I: inhibitors of the cellular membrane. J Am Acad Dermatol. 2015;72(2):203–18; quiz 219–220.
34. Kowalczyk L, Singer CF, Staudigl C, Weber M, Farr A. Adverse mucocutaneous reaction to pertuzumab in a patient with HER2-positive metastatic breast cancer. Breast J. 2017;23(3):352–3.
35. Alexandrescu DT, Vaillant J, Wiernik PH. Trastuzumab/docetaxel-induced nail dystrophy. Int J Dermatol. 2006;45(11):1334–6.
36. Andrew P, Valiani S, MacIsaac J, Mithoowani H, Verma S. Tamoxifen-associated skin reactions in breast cancer patients: from case report to literature review. Breast Cancer Res Treat. 2014;148(1):1–5.
37. Cruz MJ, Alves S, Baudrier T, Azevedo F. Porphyria cutanea tarda induced by tamoxifen. Dermatol Online J. 2010;16(9):2.
38. Praestegaard C, Kjaer SK, Andersson M, Steding-Jensen M, Frederiksen K, Mellemkjaer L. Risk of skin cancer following tamoxifen treatment in more than 16,000 breast cancer patients: a cohort study. Breast Cancer. 2016;23(6):908–16.
39. Kim YJ, Cohen PR. Anastrozole-induced dermatitis: report of a woman with an anastrozole-associated dermatosis and a review of aromatase inhibitor-related cutaneous adverse events. Dermatol Ther (Heidelb). 2020;10(1):221–9.
40. Santoro S, Santini M, Pepe C, et al. Aromatase inhibitor-induced skin adverse reactions: exemestane-

related cutaneous vasculitis. J Eur Acad Dermatol Venereol. 2011;25(5):596–8.
41. Yang TJ, Ho AY. Radiation therapy in the management of breast cancer. Surg Clin North Am. 2013;93(2):455–71.
42. Chan RJ, Larsen E, Chan P. Re-examining the evidence in radiation dermatitis management literature: an overview and a critical appraisal of systematic reviews. Int J Radiat Oncol Biol Phys. 2012;84(3):e357–62.
43. Kole AJ, Kole L, Moran MS. Acute radiation dermatitis in breast cancer patients: challenges and solutions. Breast Cancer (Dove Med Press). 2017;9:313–23.
44. Wong RK, Bensadoun RJ, Boers-Doets CB, et al. Clinical practice guidelines for the prevention and treatment of acute and late radiation reactions from the MASCC skin toxicity study group. Support Care Cancer. 2013;21(10):2933–48.
45. Roy I, Fortin A, Larochelle M. The impact of skin washing with water and soap during breast irradiation: a randomized study. Radiother Oncol. 2001;58(3):333–9.
46. Westbury C, Hines F, Hawkes E, Ashley S, Brada M. Advice on hair and scalp care during cranial radiotherapy: a prospective randomized trial. Radiother Oncol. 2000;54(2):109–16.
47. Campbell IR, Illingworth MH. Can patients wash during radiotherapy to the breast or chest wall? A randomized controlled trial. Clin Oncol (R Coll Radiol). 1992;4(2):78–82.
48. Haruna F, Lipsett A, Marignol L. Topical management of acute radiation dermatitis in breast cancer patients: a systematic review and meta-analysis. Anticancer Res. 2017;37(10):5343–53.
49. Yee C, Wang K, Asthana R, et al. Radiation-induced skin toxicity in breast cancer patients: a systematic review of randomized trials. Clin Breast Cancer. 2018;18(5):e825–40.
50. Lanigan SW, Joannides T. Pulsed dye laser treatment of telangiectasia after radiotherapy for carcinoma of the breast. Br J Dermatol. 2003;148(1):77–9.
51. Goggins W, Gao W, Tsao H. Association between female breast cancer and cutaneous melanoma. Int J Cancer. 2004;111(5):792–4.
52. Burt LM, Ying J, Poppe MM, Suneja G, Gaffney DK. Risk of secondary malignancies after radiation therapy for breast cancer: comprehensive results. Breast. 2017;35:122–9.
53. Roychoudhuri R, Evans H, Robinson D, Møller H. Radiation-induced malignancies following radiotherapy for breast cancer. Br J Cancer. 2004;91(5):868–72.
54. Karagas MR, McDonald JA, Greenberg ER, et al. Risk of basal cell and squamous cell skin cancers after ionizing radiation therapy. For The Skin Cancer Prevention Study Group. J Natl Cancer Inst. 1996;88(24):1848–53.

Hereditary Cancer Counseling and Germline Genetic Testing

20

Carolyn Menendez, P. Kelly Marcom, and Linda M. Sutton

Introduction

The linkage of early onset breast cancer to a specific gene mutation on chromosome 17q21 by investigators in the lab of Mary-Claire King at the University of California, Berkeley, in 1990 was a pivotal moment in the clinical care of breast cancer. The identification of that specific gene, subsequently known as *BRCA1*, was followed by the identification of many more genes linked to an inherited susceptibility to breast cancers [1–5].

Genes known, as of 2021, to be associated with increased risk of breast cancer:

- BRCA1
- BRCA2
- PALB2
- ATM
- BARD1
- BRIP1
- CDH1
- CHEK2
- NBN
- NF1
- PTEN
- RAD51C
- RAD51D
- STK11
- TP53

Over the past 30 years, counseling and testing for germline genetic mutations that predispose individuals to cancer, which we will call cancer predisposing mutations (CPMs), have matured from an area of research interest to an integral part of the evaluation and treatment of patients with breast cancer. Research has expanded the number of known CPM, and next-generation DNA sequencing technology (NGS) now allows for efficient, relatively inexpensive testing. Currently, detection of a CPM may inform immediate treatment options for local-regional management of breast cancer and/or guide systemic therapy choice [6, 7]. This component of comprehensive cancer care is an important and often easily overlooked element of survivorship care, where the opportunity for updating personal and family history may have far-reaching implications for the patient and their family. The goal of germline genetic testing is to identify CPMs and personalize screening and management strategies to reduce morbidity and mortality. The identification of a CPM can lead not only to augmented

C. Menendez (✉)
Duke University, Duke Cancer Institute, Durham, NC, USA
e-mail: carolyn.menendez@duke.edu

P. K. Marcom
Department of Medicine, Duke Cancer Institute, Durham, NC, USA

L. M. Sutton
Duke University School of Medicine, Duke Cancer Network, Durham, NC, USA

G. G. Kimmick et al. (eds.), *Common Issues in Breast Cancer Survivors*,
https://doi.org/10.1007/978-3-030-75377-1_20

breast cancer screening and preventive approaches but also to screening for and prevention of other cancers. Appreciation of the dynamic nature of personal and family history and the necessity of updated genetic risk assessment at every survivorship visit will lead to increased detection of hereditary cancer syndromes.

Standard-of-Care Genetic Assessment at Diagnosis

All patients with a new diagnosis of breast cancer should be assessed for the possibility of a germline, or inherited, CPM, as a contributor to the development of breast cancer. The clinical utility of germline genetic testing results in the perioperative period is continuously being refined for individual CPMs, supporting aggressive screening for the presence of these mutations. A number of national guidelines provide specific recommendations related to effective identification of individuals with CPM.

Guideline Recommendations

Detailed guidelines regarding germline genetic testing are available from many organizations and societies, including the following: the National Comprehensive Cancer Network (NCCN, www.nccn.org) [5]; the US Preventive Services Task Force [8]; the American Society of Clinical Oncology (ASCO, www.asco.org) [9]; and the American Society of Breast Surgeons (ASBrS, www.breastsurgeons.org) [10]. In general, guidelines attempt to maximize identification of individuals with a CPM while minimizing unnecessary testing that has the potential for providing misleading or confusing results (see interpretation of results below). The differences between the thoughtfully presented guidelines from each well-respected organization reflect the controversies in thresholds for pre-test probability. Options for germline genetic testing looking for CPM have also expanded, and there is debate as to which providers should facilitate the test and which genes should be evaluated. Recommendations for testing will continue to evolve. We recommend that providers engaged in survivorship care consult the aforementioned expert guidelines for the most up-to-date policies.

Guidelines Agree that Genetic Testing should be Offered in the Following

- Males with breast cancer
- Patient younger than age 45 years with diagnosis of breast cancer
- Patient younger than age 60 years with diagnosis of hormone-receptor-negative, HER2-negative (triple-negative) breast cancer
- Patient from ethnicities with high carrier rates, such as Ashkenazi Jews

Who to Refer?

There is uniform agreement to recommend testing for CPM in certain scenarios, such as male breast cancer patient, patients under age 45 with any histology, and patients under age 60 with triple-negative breast cancer (TNBC). The national guideline recommendations are currently disparate regarding the patient over age 45 without TNBC and the characterization of risk for the patient with a family history of primarily post-menopausal breast cancer. ASBrS issued a statement for consideration of germline genetic testing for all patients with a personal history of breast cancer, regardless of histology, age at diagnosis, or family history [7]. NCCN maintains an approach based on risk stratification given multiple variables in the individual pedigree [11].

What Genes to Test?

Testing for CPMs, in genes such as BRCA1, BRCA2, tumor protein 53 (TP53), and phosphatase and tensin homolog deleted on chromosome 10 (PTEN), has been available for over two decades. The use of multi-gene panel testing with next-generation sequencing (NGS) to simultaneously screen multiple genes (multi-gene panel testing) has dramatically expanded since 2012 and is now the standard of care [12]. Several studies have demonstrated a near twofold increase in detection of relevant CPMs using panel testing [12, 13]. In fact, some reasonable arguments can be made for broad testing even in individuals without a relevant cancer diagnosis [14]. However, a thoughtfully selected panel of CPMs determined through curated pedigree is the current national guideline recommendation [11]. Family history and tumor phenotype guide customization of a gene panel. The cost for germline testing has decreased significantly and is no longer a major issue in the selection of the panel of genes to test. For the major diagnostic laboratories, the testing cost is independent of the number of genes sequenced. A well-informed patient may consent for multi-gene panel testing. The NCCN has published guidelines for testing and management of several genes, including estimated lifetime risk of breast cancer, breast cancer risk management considerations, other cancers at increased risk, and other considerations. These guidelines undergo substantive updates regularly, reflecting the rapid evolution of the science of germline testing for breast cancer hereditary predisposition. Further details are available by viewing the entire guideline [5].

Genetic Counseling Pre-/Post-test

Consultation with a certified genetic counselor or a provider with expertise in risk assessment and genetic counseling prior to testing for hereditary predisposition syndromes is regarded as best practice [15].

Elements of Genetic Counseling

1. Appropriateness of genetic testing and potential harms and benefits
2. The medical implications of positive and uncertain test results
3. The possibility that the result may not be informative
4. Implications for family

With the advent of multi-gene panel testing, the depth of knowledge required to advise individuals about the impact of specific mutations has expanded significantly. The 2015 American Cancer Society/American Society of Clinical Oncology Breast Cancer Survivorship Care Guideline recommends that clinicians should offer genetic counseling if potential hereditary risk factors are suspected [16]. The ASBS Consensus Guidelines on Genetic Testing specifically recommends that medical professionals knowledgeable in genetic testing provide education and counseling prior to testing [10]. However, the ASBS goes on to advise that strong consideration should be given to consultation with cancer genetics specialists for those individuals found to have less common mutations. NCCN recommends that medical professionals with requisite expertise and experience in medical genetics be involved in pre-test counseling, test selection, and post-test counseling [5]. Regardless of who performs hereditary cancer risk assessment, the assessment should include discussion of [1] appropriateness of genetic testing and potential harms and benefits, [2] the medical implications of positive and uncertain test results, [3] the possibility that the result may not be informative, and [4] implications for family.

One of the pitfalls in cancer genetic testing is the omission of post-test counseling. A survey related to genetic testing of women diagnosed with stage 0–II breast cancer between July 2013 and September 2014 in the Georgia and Los Angeles SEER registries had 2529 women (71%) who responded. Among respondents with a high pre-test probability of a CPM, only 39.6% had a session with a genetic counselor at any point in time. Even among women who had a high risk of having a CPM and underwent genetic testing, only 61.7% had a session with a genetic counselor [17].

Interpretation and Documentation of Test Results

The technical aspects of genetic testing are complex, so some familiarity with the concepts is helpful for interpreting testing results. Commercial laboratories generate reports by comparing sequence data to a reference human sequence genome, as well as proprietary data, using a variety of in-house software packages for base calling, alignment, variant identification, annotation, and generation of quality metrics [18, 19]. A variety of molecular changes can be reported as mutations, such as single base changes resulting in a single amino acid alterations; insertions, deletions, and duplications that can change the reading frame and result in truncated proteins; splice site variants affecting the inclusion/exclusion of sequence in transcripts; and large chromosomal rearrangements.

Molecular Changes Reported as Mutations

1. Single base changes resulting in a single amino acid alterations
2. Insertions, deletions, and duplications that can change the reading frame and result in truncated proteins
3. Splice site variants affecting the inclusion/exclusion of sequence in transcripts
4. Large chromosomal rearrangements

The final test result makes an assertion about the relationship between the sequence variation, the effect on gene/protein function, and the consequent health risks. The terms "mutation" and "polymorphism" are often confused; a mutation is a permanent change in the nucleotide sequence, while a polymorphism is defined as a variant with a frequency above 1%. It is recommended that in test results, both terms be replaced with the term "variant" [20]. Sequence variants are then classified as "pathogenic," "likely pathogenic," "variant of uncertain significance," "likely benign," or "benign."

Classification of sequence variants:

- *Positive/pathogenic*, in which the detected mutation clearly disrupts gene function and is therefore highly likely to cause clinical consequences
- *Likely pathogenic*
- *Uncertain/variant of uncertain significance (VUS) or uncertain variant (UV, UCV)*, in which it is not known whether the variant has any effect on gene function or if it might confer an increased cancer risk
- *Likely benign*
- *Negative/benign*, in which no variation in DNA sequence is detected

While this classification system has been in place for many years, the American College of Medical Genetics and Genomics and the Association for Molecular Pathology (ACMG-AMP) have promulgated a detailed, formalized system for assigning variants to these categories [20]. Most of the major commercial genetic testing laboratories have adopted this system, although some with modifications [21]. The ClinVar database provides the most comprehensive collection of data supporting the assertions for variant classification [22]. While concerns have been raised about concordance of results reported to ClinVar by clinical laboratories, a careful analysis found only a 2.2% discordance rate [23].

Genetic testing results must be interpreted in clinical context. For unaffected individuals, a pathogenic or likely pathogenic result means an increased risk for cancer. The likelihood of developing cancer differs by gene, specific mutation, and genetic/ethnic background [24, 25]. For survivorship considerations, a positive/pathogenic result indicates that individuals have a CPM and that screening and prevention should be customized according to the specific CPM, as discussed further below. The likely benign and benign categories are usually not included in reports since they are of no known clinical utility, represent background genetic variation, and are filtered out in the bioinformatics analysis pipeline.

A result of variant of uncertain significance (VUS) is a result for which [1] it is not known whether or not there is an effect on gene function and [2] it has not been seen in enough affected individuals/families to make a clear pathogenicity determination. The use of large multi-gene panel testing has led to the identification of more VUS results [6]. VUS results are prone to over-interpretation [26] but should only rarely have any impact on clinical management. Family history provides a more useful guide to management for patients with VUS.

A common pitfall is declaring genetic testing results "negative" without considering the family history. Only in the case of a known familial CPM, when the testing does not find the known mutation, can an individual's test results be declared "negative," and even in this scenario, the declaration only applies for that specific CPM. If testing does not identify a CPM, the more accurate statement is that "no CPM was found in the genes tested." Results should be qualified to acknowledge that not all genetic contributions to cancer risk have been identified, particularly polygenic risks that contribute to familial cancer risk. Clinicians should consult a genetics professional for assistance in cases where testing results are unclear.

Documentation is critical in all cases. While maintenance of confidentiality is important, patients should be encouraged to disclose the results in their medical record and to their family so that they can be appropriately managed [27]. Results should include the specific genes sequenced, the results, the laboratory performing the testing, and the date of the testing. For VUS results, the details (nucleotide changes and change in protein sequence) may be helpful for future reclassification of the result.

Impact of Results on Peri-diagnostic Management

Identification of a CPM can guide local-regional and systemic treatment recommendations and decisions. For example, a patient who might otherwise be a candidate for breast-conserving surgery might instead opt for ipsilateral therapeutic and contralateral prophylactic mastectomy; mutation leading to increased ovarian cancer risk can support including oophorectomy as part of the endocrine therapy plan; and clinical trials investigating targeted therapies for genetically related cancers can be considered [15]. These management options are guided by the specific CPM and the preferences of the patient.

Management strategies for BRCA1/2-related cancers are the most thoroughly developed. For local-regional management, studies show that breast conservation is equally effective in BRCA carriers and non-carriers with respect to in-breast recurrence risk. Decisions regarding the type of surgery should factor in contralateral breast cancer risk, and take into consideration age at diagnosis, family history of breast cancer, overall prognosis from the current or other cancers, ability of patient to undergo appropriate breast surveillance, comorbidities, and life expectancy. If patients opt for mastectomy, either unilateral or bilateral, nipple-sparing procedures can be done if clinically appropriate otherwise. Radiation therapy, whether done for breast conservation or post-mastectomy, is not contraindicated in BRCA carriers and should be guided by standard clinical indications [9]. For systemic therapy, initial enthusiasm supporting inclusion of platinum agents as part of adjuvant chemotherapy has not been borne out in later clinical trials [28]. More accurately, these trials support the conclusion that BRCA-related cancers are generally more sensitive to chemotherapy and that platinum-based therapy should not be added to adjuvant systemic therapy [28–30]. Prognosis for BRCA-related breast cancers is likely similar to that of sporadic breast cancers [31]; however, hormone-receptor-positive BRCA-related cancers have been shown to have higher 21-gene recurrence scores, underscoring the relatively greater role for chemotherapy in early-stage BRCA cancers [32]. Poly-adenosine diphosphate ribose polymerase (PARP) inhibitors, a class of targeted agents developed to cause synthetic lethality in BRCA-related cancers, have shown particular promise for improving systemic therapy. While not approved for early-stage breast cancer, a preoperative treatment trial with the PARP inhibitor talazoparib showed a pathologic complete response rate of 53% with single agent therapy [33]. Ongoing studies are assessing the role of these agents for early-stage breast cancer [34].

Establishing the presence of a genetic predisposition, therefore, widens the range of management options. The experience to date supports the conclusion that clarifying the genetic basis of a patient's cancer will improve initial treatment

Implications of Finding a CPM at the Time of Initial Breast Cancer Diagnosis

- It prompts the discussion about [1] future breast cancer risk and [2] weighing of options: augmented breast cancer screening versus prophylactic surgery
- It demonstrates the potential need for monitoring of other cancers (depending on specific gene mutation).
- It prompts discussion of clinical trial options for gene carriers.
- For patients with metastatic disease, it provides a "target" for treatment.

outcomes. Additional research will further improve the management of breast cancers related to genes other than BRCA1/2. Moreover, the genetic information and decisions made will guide management in survivorship.

Genetics Issues in Survivorship

For the geneticist, the survivorship period is a time for reevaluation. During survivorship follow-up visits, the provider can identify factors that may lead to investigation of hereditary cancer syndromes not previously suspected during the acute phase of care. Additional factors warranting consideration of testing may be uncovered, such as previously unreported family history, new medical conditions (benign and cancerous), pathology from new biopsies, and overlooked physical exam findings such as thyroid nodules, macrocephaly, and neurofibromas. Although increased clinician awareness will likely lead to increased genetic testing rates in the peri-diagnostic period, genetic knowledge and technology will continue to evolve, requiring ongoing reevaluation of survivors.

Missed Testing

When it is discovered that a patient did not have genetic testing previously but now meets national guidelines, it is important to discern why the testing was not performed and attend to the underlying reason. In some cases, the answer will be that the patient did not meet guidelines previously or simply that the opportunity was missed. More often, the reason for omission is concern regarding the implications of testing such as financial concerns, misconceptions regarding testing, and discrimination concerns. It is very helpful to identify and address these concerns [35]. Referral to a trained genetic counselor who can help the patient navigate the barrage of media, marketing, and potential misperceptions regarding the current state of genetic testing is often the most effective way to address these concerns.

Despite its importance, not all appropriate patients have genetic counseling or testing during the peri-diagnostic phase. In the peri-diagnostic phase, genetic evaluation may add distress in an already emotional and overwhelming time, and the patient or provider may have omitted it from the workup. In an early review of the psychologic impact of genetic testing on breast cancer patients, Schlich-Bakker et al. found that genetic testing within the context of a recent diagnosis of breast cancer increases patients' cancer-related distress [36]. However, the distress appeared to be ameliorated by genetic counseling. More recent data from 2529 women aged 20–79 years with stage 0–II breast cancer from two large SEER registries revealed that 80% of 773 women defined as high risk for a genetic predisposition wanted genetic testing but only ~53% had testing [37]. The main reason given for not undergoing genetic testing (56.1%) was not related to psychological factors but rather that the test was not recommended by the doctor.

It is important that the provider initiate and complete the process for germline testing if it was not previously done. In the case of a patient who has considered having genetic testing or who had testing in the past, the family history should be updated in light of updated guidelines. Maintaining a vigilant approach to updating the personal and family history for every patient in the survivorship phase can result in identification of a CPM that will have an impact

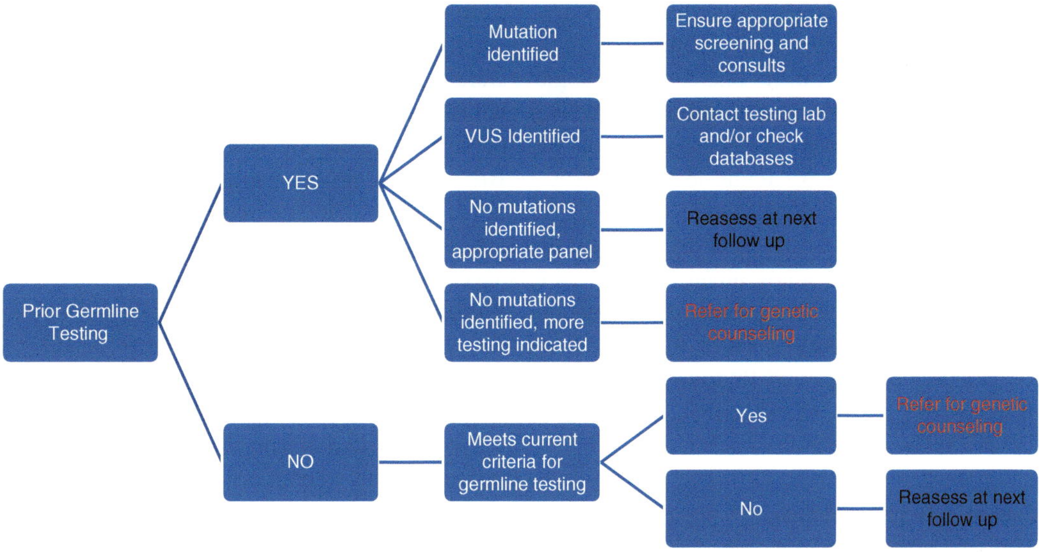

Fig. 20.1 Algorithm for evaluation of genetic testing status during survivorship

on their or their family members' health (Fig. 20.1).

Personalization of Follow-Up Screening/Secondary Prevention

Breast cancer survivors are routinely advised to [1] perform monthly self-breast evaluation with awareness of evolving changes within the breasts, [2] present to a provider for clinical breast exam annually, and [3] undergo mammography annually for female patients with one or two intact breasts. General recommendations regarding health maintenance, including routine dermatology, gynecology, and gastrointestinal cancer screening, are also encouraged. If there is a known CPM, recommendations regarding screening and monitoring for new cancers need to be further personalized. For a CPM that increases the risk of breast cancer, enhanced screening with breast MRI has benefit. The Magnetic Resonance Imaging for Breast Screening (MARIBS) study published in 2005 demonstrated a sensitivity of 77% for MRI, 40% for mammography, and 93% for the combination and established this approach as standard of care for breast screening for patients carrying a breast cancer predisposing CPM [38]. Subsequent studies have refined data for MRI screening [39–42], and this approach is endorsed by the guidelines [5, 43]. Without the knowledge of elevated risks due to a hereditary CPM, opportunities for personalized screening and secondary prevention will likely be missed.

Prophylactic Surgical Interventions

The discovery of hereditary CPM/syndromes may lead a patient to consider risk-reducing surgery. The examples within BRCA1 and BRCA2 are well publicized in the media as celebrities have heightened public awareness and shared their personal stories of prophylactic surgical interventions [44]. Studies done in the years following the identification of BRCA1 and BRCA2 demonstrated the high efficacy of prophylactic mastectomies to reduce the risk of breast cancer in mutation carriers [45]. Rebbeck et al. showed that prophylactic mastectomy reduced risk by 90% at a mean follow-up of 6.4 years in women with intact ovaries; for women undergoing concurrent prophylactic oophorectomy, risk was reduced by 95% [46]. This observation was consistent with the work of Kauff et al. who showed that BRCA carriers who opted for prophylactic salpingo-oophorectomy had a hazard ratio of 0.25 for gynecologic or breast cancer compared to those not having prophylactic surgery [47]. These data can be extrapolated to survivors found to have BRCA1 or BRCA2 mutations.

There are other CPMs that prompt consideration of prophylactic mastectomy, albeit with less data. Like BRCA1/2, these genes also raise the option of prophylactic surgery in other organs such as the stomach (CDH1) and thyroid (PTEN) [48, 49].

Genetic Testing Results, Classification, and Updated Testing

Knowledge about CPM is growing quickly, and new CPMs are identified on a regular basis. Updated genetic testing may, therefore, sometimes be needed. For example, when it was discovered that large gene rearrangements accounted for some portion of BRCA1/2 mutations in breast/ovarian cancer families, testing was expanded to include methodologies to detect these mutations that were missed by traditional Sanger sequencing [50]. Similarly, after the introduction of NGS-based testing in 2012 and the discovery of new breast cancer genes such as PALB2, what was previously adequate testing no longer sufficed [51]. These historical examples illustrate the need to stipulate the incompleteness of genetic testing results; while our knowledge is incomplete, it is also ever-expanding, and updated testing may be needed to address new findings.

VUS results pose a unique challenge during survivorship. As noted, this result category should not guide patient management. However, the result lingers, unresolved until the nature of the variant is clarified. Many laboratories and research groups are actively researching approaches for VUS reclassification. Data regarding this process are most robust for BRCA1/2. Using data from Myriad Laboratories from 2006 to 2016, Mersch et al. examined 59,955 variant reclassification amended reports from testing in 1.45 million individuals [52]. Only 0.7% of pathogenic/likely pathogenic results were reclassified. However, 7.7% of unique VUS results were reclassified: 91.2% to benign/likely benign, but 8.7% to pathogenic or likely pathogenic. Lyra et al. examined VUS missense mutations in BRCA1. Using curated and harmonized functional data for 2701 missense variants, they were able to classify 297 as pathogenic and 2058 variants as non-pathogenic by American College of Medical Genetics and Genomics (ACMG)/ Association for Molecular Pathology (AMP) criteria [53].

While these efforts provide real progress, they raise the question of who is responsible for updating the patient when VUS are reclassified. Most testing laboratories will contact the ordering provider when a VUS is reclassified. However, it is also a good practice to periodically contact the laboratory for individual updates. Updates are also deposited in the ClinVar database (https://www.ncbi.nlm.nih.gov/clinvar/) and can be checked on the database portal. Using these resources, every reported VUS should be reassessed at each follow-up visit until it is reclassified to a definitive category [54] (Fig. 20.1).

Mutations: Somatic vs Germline

A *somatic mutation* occurs in a single cell in the body or in tumor tissue and cannot be inherited.

A *germline mutation* occurs in all cells in the body, including gametes (reproductive cells), and can be passed to offspring.

Somatic Testing on Metastases

Patients with metastatic disease, either following early-stage treatment or with de novo presentation, are in a special survivor category. While treatable, metastatic breast cancer is still ultimately incurable in most patients. For these patients, somatic NGS of tumor tissue is a powerful tool for identifying therapeutic options based on observed mutations.

Inherently, somatic sequencing data has germline sequencing data embedded in the results, and these results of sequencing tumor tissue might indicate the presence of a germline mutation. Detecting germline mutations in genes that lead to homologous recombination deficiency (the inability to repair double-strand breaks), such as BRCA1 and BRCA2, is very important, since these cancers can be treated with PARP inhibitors, including olaparib and talazoparib. As first-line treatment, these agents are superior to chemotherapy [55, 56]. Consequently, the NCCN Breast Cancer guidelines support germline testing for patients with metastatic breast cancer [57]. Whether somatic testing suffices for screening for germline mutations is unknown. Lincoln et al. found that 8.1% of pathogenic germline mutations were missed by somatic tumor testing. It is therefore essential that these somatic NGS results be reviewed critically to confirm that the germline testing is complete. A mutation found on tumor testing does not confirm hereditary predisposition and may be misinterpreted and/or misreported. If a potentially germline mutation is discovered on tumor testing, the provider should facilitate germline testing, and if prior germline testing has been completed, it is imperative to confirm that the specific gene of concern on tumor testing was included in the prior germline testing and remains classified as benign.

Cascade Testing

Once in survivorship, a patient's concern often turns to the cancer risks of family members. Family concern is one of the primary motivators for pursing genetic testing. Sometimes, this motivates proceeding with genetic testing that the patient may have previously declined. Sharing informative testing results with family members is one of the most powerful ways to prevent breast cancer. Cascade testing is the process of extending these results as widely as possible in the family. This process must balance patient confidentiality, the duty to warn, and benefits of cascade testing [58, 59]. Given this, patients should be maximally empowered and assisted with disseminating this knowledge. Consideration of the ramifications for the family should not be overlooked. The role of the genetic counselor is especially relevant in this setting. Frey et al. showed that genetic-counselor-facilitated cascade testing can improve uptake of cascade testing [60]. However, this may not be a practical approach for community practices. The nuances to testing an unaffected relative are quite different from those in the patient who has completed their cancer care and warrant the expertise of a genetic counselor whenever possible. Short of general population screening for CPMs, a currently impractical approach, enhancement of cascade testing is the most effective means for maximizing the population benefits of genetic testing [61].

Future Directions

The inevitable trend for genetic testing is in the direction of broader genome assessment and less stringent patient criteria for testing. This trend will continue as long as providers and patients perceive that ascertainment of these data improves outcomes. Payors too must be convinced, but the experience so far suggests coverage will be provided if outcomes are improved, particularly if costs continue to decline. Genetic insights about low/moderate penetrance mutations, polygenic risk factors, epigenetic factors, and gene-gene modifiers of penetrance will also potentially reshape the field. These possibilities again highlight the importance of ongoing genetic risk assessment in survivors.

References

1. Yang X, Leslie G, Doroszuk A, Schneider S, Allen J, Decker B, Dunning AM, Redman J, Scarth J, Plaskocinska I, Luccarini C, Shah M, Pooley K, Dorling L, Lee A, Adank MA, Adlard J, Aittomaki K, Andrulis IL, Ang P, Barwell J, Bernstein JL, Bobolis K, Borg A, Blomqvist C, Claes KBM, Concannon P, Cuggia A, Culver JO, Damiola F, de Pauw A, Diez O, Dolinsky JS, Domchek SM, Engel C, Evans DG,

Fostira F, Garber J, Golmard L, Goode EL, Gruber SB, Hahnen E, Hake C, Heikkinen T, Hurley JE, Janavicius R, Kleibl Z, Kleiblova P, Konstantopoulou I, Kvist A, Laduca H, Lee ASG, Lesueur F, Maher ER, Mannermaa A, Manoukian S, McFarland R, McKinnon W, Meindl A, Metcalfe K, Mohd Taib NA, Moilanen J, Nathanson KL, Neuhausen S, Ng PS, Nguyen-Dumont T, Nielsen SM, Obermair F, Offit K, Olopade OI, Ottini L, Penkert J, Pylkas K, Radice P, Ramus SJ, Rudaitis V, Side L, Silva-Smith R, Silvestri V, Skytte AB, Slavin T, Soukupova J, Tondini C, Trainer AH, Unzeitig G, Usha L, van Overeem Hansen T, Whitworth J, Wood M, Yip CH, Yoon SY, Yussuf A, Zogopoulos G, Goldgar D, Hopper JL, Chenevix-Trench G, Pharoah P, George SHL, Balmana J, Houdayer C, James P, El-Haffaf Z, Ehrencrona H, Janatova M, Peterlongo P, Nevanlinna H, Schmutzler R, Teo SH, Robson M, Pal T, Couch F, Weitzel JN, Elliott A, Southey M, Winqvist R, Easton DF, Foulkes WD, Antoniou AC, Tischkowitz M. Cancer Risks Associated With Germline PALB2 Pathogenic Variants: An International Study of 524 Families. J Clin Oncol. 2020;38(7):674–85. Epub 2019/12/17. https://doi.org/10.1200/JCO.19.01907. PubMed PMID: 31841383; PMCID: PMC7049229.

2. Schmidt MK, Hogervorst F, van Hien R, Cornelissen S, Broeks A, Adank MA, Meijers H, Waisfisz Q, Hollestelle A, Schutte M, van den Ouweland A, Hooning M, Andrulis IL, Anton-Culver H, Antonenkova NN, Antoniou AC, Arndt V, Bermisheva M, Bogdanova NV, Bolla MK, Brauch H, Brenner H, Bruning T, Burwinkel B, Chang-Claude J, Chenevix-Trench G, Couch FJ, Cox A, Cross SS, Czene K, Dunning AM, Fasching PA, Figueroa J, Fletcher O, Flyger H, Galle E, Garcia-Closas M, Giles GG, Haeberle L, Hall P, Hillemanns P, Hopper JL, Jakubowska A, John EM, Jones M, Khusnutdinova E, Knight JA, Kosma VM, Kristensen V, Lee A, Lindblom A, Lubinski J, Mannermaa A, Margolin S, Meindl A, Milne RL, Muranen TA, Newcomb PA, Offit K, Park-Simon TW, Peto J, Pharoah PD, Robson M, Rudolph A, Sawyer EJ, Schmutzler RK, Seynaeve C, Soens J, Southey MC, Spurdle AB, Surowy H, Swerdlow A, Tollenaar RA, Tomlinson I, Trentham-Dietz A, Vachon C, Wang Q, Whittemore AS, Ziogas A, van der Kolk L, Nevanlinna H, Dork T, Bojesen S, Easton DF. Age- and tumor subtype-specific breast cancer risk estimates for CHEK2*1100delC carriers. J Clin Oncol. 2016;34(23):2750–60. Epub 2016/06/09. https://doi.org/10.1200/JCO.2016.66.5844. PubMed PMID: 27269948; PMCID: PMC5019754 online at www.jco.org. Author contributions are found at the end of this article.

3. Shimelis H, LaDuca H, Hu C, Hart SN, Na J, Thomas A, Akinhanmi M, Moore RM, Brauch H, Cox A, Eccles DM, Ewart-Toland A, Fasching PA, Fostira F, Garber J, Godwin AK, Konstantopoulou I, Nevanlinna H, Sharma P, Yannoukakos D, Yao S, Feng BJ, Tippin Davis B, Lilyquist J, Pesaran T, Goldgar DE, Polley EC, Dolinsky JS, Couch FJ. Triple-negative breast cancer risk genes identified by multigene hereditary cancer panel testing. J Natl Cancer Inst. 2018;110(8):855–62. Epub 2018/08/14. https://doi.org/10.1093/jnci/djy106. PubMed PMID: 30099541; PMCID: PMC6093350.

4. Petridis C, Arora I, Shah V, Moss CL, Mera A, Clifford A, Gillett C, Pinder SE, Tomlinson I, Roylance R, Simpson MA, Sawyer EJ. Frequency of Pathogenic Germline Variants in CDH1, BRCA2, CHEK2, PALB2, BRCA1, and TP53 in Sporadic Lobular Breast Cancer. Cancer Epidemiol Biomarkers Prev. 2019;28(7):1162–8. Epub 2019/07/03. https://doi.org/10.1158/1055-9965.EPI-18-1102.

5. Network NCC. National Comprehensive Cancer Network. Genetic/familial high-risk assessment: breast, ovarian, and pancreatic. Version 1.2021 2020 [cited 2020 Octover 11]. Available from: https://www.nccn.org/.

6. Robson ME, Bradbury AR, Arun B, Domchek SM, Ford JM, Hampel HL, Lipkin SM, Syngal S, Wollins DS, Lindor NM. American society of clinical oncology policy statement update: genetic and genomic testing for cancer susceptibility. J Clin Oncol. 2015;33(31):3660–7. https://doi.org/10.1200/jco.2015.63.0996.

7. Plichta JK, Sebastian ML, Smith LA, Menendez CS, Johnson AT, Bays SM, Euhus DM, Clifford EJ, Jalali M, Kurtzman SH, Taylor WA, Hughes KS. Germline genetic testing: what the breast surgeon needs to Know. Annals of Surgical Oncology. 2019;26(7):2184–90. https://doi.org/10.1245/s10434-019-07341-8.

8. Owens DK, Davidson KW, Krist AH, Barry MJ, Cabana M, Caughey AB, Doubeni CA, Epling JW, Kubik M, Landefeld CS, Mangione CM, Pbert L, Silverstein M, Simon MA, Tseng C-W, Wong JB. Risk assessment, genetic counseling, and genetic testing for BRCA-related cancer. JAMA. 2019;322(7):652. https://doi.org/10.1001/jama.2019.10987.

9. Tung NM, Boughey JC, Pierce LJ, Robson ME, Bedrosian I, Dietz JR, Dragun A, Gelpi JB, Hofstatter EW, Isaacs CJ, Jatoi I, Kennedy E, Litton JK, Mayr NA, Qamar RD, Trombetta MG, Harvey BE, Somerfield MR, Zakalik D. Management of Hereditary Breast Cancer: American Society of Clinical Oncology, American Society for Radiation Oncology, and Society of Surgical Oncology Guideline. J Clin Oncol. 2020;38(18):2080–106. https://doi.org/10.1200/jco.20.00299.

10. Manahan ER, Kuerer HM, Sebastian M, Hughes KS, Boughey JC, Euhus DM, Boolbol SK, Taylor WA. Consensus Guidelines on Genetic` Testing for Hereditary Breast Cancer from the American Society of Breast Surgeons. Annals Surg Oncol. 2019;26(10):3025–31. https://doi.org/10.1245/s10434-019-07549-8.

11. Daly MB, Pilarski R, Yurgelun MB, Berry MP, Buys SS, Dickson P, Domchek SM, Elkhanany A, Friedman S, Garber JE, Goggins M, Hutton ML, Khan S, Klein C, Kohlmann W, Kurian AW, Laronga C, Litton JK, Mak JS, Menendez CS, Merajver SD, Norquist BS, Offit K, Pal T, Pederson HJ, Reiser G, Shannon KM, Visvanathan K, Weitzel JN, Wick MJ, Wisinski KB,

Dwyer MA, Darlow SD. NCCN Guidelines Insights: Genetic/Familial High-Risk Assessment: Breast, Ovarian, and Pancreatic, Version 1.2020. J Nat Comprehen Cancer Network. 2020;18(4):380–91. https://doi.org/10.6004/jnccn.2020.0017.
12. Kurian AW, Ward KC, Hamilton AS, Deapen DM, Abrahamse P, Bondarenko I, Li Y, Hawley ST, Morrow M, Jagsi R, Katz SJ. Uptake, results, and outcomes of germline multiple-gene sequencing after diagnosis of breast cancer. JAMA Oncology. 2018;4(8):1066. https://doi.org/10.1001/jamaoncol.2018.0644.
13. Tung N, Lin NU, Kidd J, Allen BA, Singh N, Wenstrup RJ, Hartman A-R, Winer EP, Garber JE. Frequency of germline mutations in 25 cancer susceptibility genes in a sequential series of patients with breast cancer. J Clin Oncol. 2016;34(13):1460–8. https://doi.org/10.1200/jco.2015.65.0747.
14. Gustafson SL, Raymond VM, Marvin ML, Else T, Koeppe E, Stoffel EM, Everett JN. Outcomes of genetic evaluation for hereditary cancer syndromes in unaffected individuals. Fam Cancer. 2015;14(1):167–74. Epub 2014/09/24. https://doi.org/10.1007/s10689-014-9756-x.
15. Forbes C, Fayter D, De Kock S, Quek RGW. A systematic review of international guidelines and recommendations for the genetic screening, diagnosis, genetic counseling, and treatment of BRCA-mutated breast cancer. Cancer Manage Res. 2019;11:2321–37. https://doi.org/10.2147/cmar.s189627.
16. Runowicz CD, Leach CR, Henry NL, Henry KS, Mackey HT, Cowens-Alvarado RL, Cannady RS, Pratt-Chapman ML, Edge SB, Jacobs LA, Hurria A, Marks LB, Lamonte SJ, Warner E, Lyman GH, Ganz PA. American Cancer Society/American Society of Clinical Oncology Breast Cancer Survivorship Care Guideline. J Clin Oncol. 2016;34(6):611–35. https://doi.org/10.1200/jco.2015.64.3809.
17. Kurian AW, Griffith KA, Hamilton AS, Ward KC, Morrow M, Katz SJ, Jagsi R. Genetic testing and counseling among patients with newly diagnosed breast cancer. JAMA. 2017;317(5):531. https://doi.org/10.1001/jama.2016.16918.
18. O'Leary NA, Wright MW, Brister JR, Ciufo S, Haddad D, McVeigh R, Rajput B, Robbertse B, Smith-White B, Ako-Adjei D, Astashyn A, Badretdin A, Bao Y, Blinkova O, Brover V, Chetvernin V, Choi J, Cox E, Ermolaeva O, Farrell CM, Goldfarb T, Gupta T, Haft D, Hatcher E, Hlavina W, Joardar VS, Kodali VK, Li W, Maglott D, Masterson P, McGarvey KM, Murphy MR, O'Neill K, Pujar S, Rangwala SH, Rausch D, Riddick LD, Schoch C, Shkeda A, Storz SS, Sun H, Thibaud-Nissen F, Tolstoy I, Tully RE, Vatsan AR, Wallin C, Webb D, Wu W, Landrum MJ, Kimchi A, Tatusova T, Dicuccio M, Kitts P, Murphy TD, Pruitt KD. Reference sequence (RefSeq) database at NCBI: current status, taxonomic expansion, and functional annotation. Nucleic Acids Res. 2016;44(D1):D733–D45. https://doi.org/10.1093/nar/gkv1189.
19. Myriad Genetics I. 2020 [updated September 3, 2020; cited 2020 October 26, 2020. Technical sheet for Myriad testing]. Available from: https://s3.amazonaws.com/myriad-library/technical-specifications/BRCA+Tech+Specs_Integrated.pdf.
20. Richards S, Aziz N, Bale S, Bick D, Das S, Gastier-Foster J, Grody WW, Hegde M, Lyon E, Spector E, Voelkerding K, Rehm HL. Standards and guidelines for the interpretation of sequence variants: a joint consensus recommendation of the American College of Medical Genetics and Genomics and the Association for Molecular Pathology. Genetics Med. 2015;17(5):405–23. https://doi.org/10.1038/gim.2015.30.
21. Nykamp K, Anderson M, Powers M, Garcia J, Herrera B, Ho Y-Y, Kobayashi Y, Patil N, Thusberg J, Westbrook M, Topper S. Sherloc: a comprehensive refinement of the ACMG–AMP variant classification criteria. Genetics Med. 2017;19(10):1105–17. https://doi.org/10.1038/gim.2017.37.
22. Landrum MJ, Lee JM, Benson M, Brown GR, Chao C, Chitipiralla S, Gu B, Hart J, Hoffman D, Jang W, Karapetyan K, Katz K, Liu C, Maddipatla Z, Malheiro A, McDaniel K, Ovetsky M, Riley G, Zhou G, Kattman BL, Maglott DR. ClinVar: improving access to variant interpretations and supporting evidence. Nucleic Acids Res. 2018;46(D1):D1062–D7. https://doi.org/10.1093/nar/gkx1153.
23. Nussbaum RL, Yang S, Lincoln SE. Clinical genetics testing laboratories have a remarkably low rate of clinically significant discordance when interpreting variants in hereditary cancer syndrome genes2017. JCO. 2016;70:945. https://doi.org/10.1200/jco.2016.70.9451
24. Mahdavi M, Nassiri M, Kooshyar MM, Vakili-Azghandi M, Avan A, Sandry R, Pillai S, Yin Lam AK, Gopalan V. Hereditary breast cancer; Genetic penetrance and current status with BRCA. J Cell Physiol. 2018; https://doi.org/10.1002/jcp.27464.
25. Taeubner J, Wieczorek D, Yasin L, Brozou T, Borkhardt A, Kuhlen M. Penetrance and expressivity in inherited cancer predisposing syndromes. Trends in Cancer. 2018;4(11):718–28. https://doi.org/10.1016/j.trecan.2018.09.002.
26. Plon SE, Cooper HP, Parks B, Dhar SU, Kelly PA, Weinberg AD, Staggs S, Wang T, Hilsenbeck S. Genetic testing and cancer risk management recommendations by physicians for at-risk relatives. Genetics Med. 2011;13(2):148–54. https://doi.org/10.1097/gim.0b013e318207f564.
27. Witt MM, Witt MP. Privacy and confidentiality measures in genetic testing and counselling: arguing on genetic exceptionalism again? J Appl Genetics. 2016;57(4):483–5. https://doi.org/10.1007/s13353-016-0339-4.
28. Tung N, Arun B, Hacker MR, Hofstatter E, Toppmeyer DL, Isakoff SJ, Borges V, Legare RD, Isaacs C, Wolff AC, Marcom PK, Mayer EL, Lange PB, Goss AJ, Jenkins C, Krop IE, Winer EP, Schnitt SJ, Garber JE. TBCRC 031: Randomized Phase II Study of Neoadjuvant Cisplatin Versus Doxorubicin-Cyclophosphamide in Germline BRCA Carriers With HER2-Negative Breast Cancer (the INFORM trial).

J Clin Oncol. 2020;38(14):1539–48. https://doi.org/10.1200/jco.19.03292.
29. Hahnen E, Lederer B, Hauke J, Loibl S, Kröber S, Schneeweiss A, Denkert C, Fasching PA, Blohmer JU, Jackisch C, Paepke S, Gerber B, Kümmel S, Schem C, Neidhardt G, Huober J, Rhiem K, Costa S, Altmüller J, Hanusch C, Thiele H, Müller V, Nürnberg P, Karn T, Nekljudova V, Untch M, Von Minckwitz G, Schmutzler RK. Germline mutation status, pathological complete response, and disease-free survival in triple-negative breast cancer. JAMA Oncol. 2017;3(10):1378. https://doi.org/10.1001/jamaoncol.2017.1007.
30. Loibl S, O'Shaughnessy J, Untch M, Sikov WM, Rugo HS, McKee MD, Huober J, Golshan M, Von Minckwitz G, Maag D, Sullivan D, Wolmark N, McIntyre K, Ponce Lorenzo JJ, Metzger Filho O, Rastogi P, Symmans WF, Liu X, Geyer CE. Addition of the PARP inhibitor veliparib plus carboplatin or carboplatin alone to standard neoadjuvant chemotherapy in triple-negative breast cancer (BrighTNess): a randomised, phase 3 trial. Lancet Oncol. 2018;19(4):497–509. https://doi.org/10.1016/s1470-2045(18)30111-6.
31. Copson ER, Maishman TC, Tapper WJ, Cutress RI, Greville-Heygate S, Altman DG, Eccles B, Gerty S, Durcan LT, Jones L, Evans DG, Thompson AM, Pharoah P, Easton DF, Dunning AM, Hanby A, Lakhani S, Eeles R, Gilbert FJ, Hamed H, Hodgson S, Simmonds P, Stanton L, Eccles DM. Germline BRCA mutation and outcome in young-onset breast cancer (POSH): a prospective cohort study. Lancet Oncol. 2018;19(2):169–80. https://doi.org/10.1016/s1470-2045(17)30891-4.
32. Shah PD, Patil S, Dickler MN, Offit K, Hudis CA, Robson ME. Twenty-one-gene recurrence score assay inBRCA-associated versus sporadic breast cancers: Differences based on germline mutation status. Cancer. 2016;122(8):1178–84. https://doi.org/10.1002/cncr.29903.
33. Litton JK, Scoggins ME, Hess KR, Adrada BE, Murthy RK, Damodaran S, Desnyder SM, Brewster AM, Barcenas CH, Valero V, Whitman GJ, Schwartz-Gomez J, Mittendorf EA, Thompson AM, Helgason T, Ibrahim N, Piwnica-Worms H, Moulder SL, Arun BK. Neoadjuvant talazoparib for patients with operable breast cancer with a germline BRCA pathogenic variant. J Clin Oncol. 2020;38(5):388–94. https://doi.org/10.1200/jco.19.01304.
34. Tung NM, Garber JE. BRCA1/2 testing: therapeutic implications for breast cancer management. Br J Cancer. 2018;119(2):141–52. https://doi.org/10.1038/s41416-018-0127-5.
35. Jagsi R, Griffith KA, Kurian AW, Morrow M, Hamilton AS, Graff JJ, Katz SJ, Hawley ST. Concerns about cancer risk and experiences with genetic testing in a diverse population of patients with breast cancer. J Clin Oncol. 2015;33(14):1584–91. https://doi.org/10.1200/jco.2014.58.5885.
36. Schlich-Bakker KJ, Warlam-Rodenhuis CC, van Echtelt J, van den Bout J, Ausems MG, ten Kroode HF. Short term psychological distress in patients actively approached for genetic counselling after diagnosis of breast cancer. Eur J Cancer. 2006;42(16):2722–8. Epub 2006/09/05. https://doi.org/10.1016/j.ejca.2006.05.032.
37. Kurian AW, Griffith KA, Hamilton AS, Ward KC, Morrow M, Katz SJ, Jagsi R. Genetic testing and counseling among patients with newly diagnosed breast cancer. JAMA. 2017;317(5):531-4. Epub 2017/02/09. https://doi.org/10.1001/jama.2016.16918. PubMed PMID: 28170472; PMCID: PMC5530866.
38. MARIBS Study Group. Screening with magnetic resonance imaging and mammography of a UK population at high familial risk of breast cancer: a prospective multicentre cohort study (MARIBS). The Lancet. 2005;365(9473):1769–78. https://doi.org/10.1016/s0140-6736(05)66481-1.
39. Le-Petross HT, Whitman GJ, Atchley DP, Yuan Y, Gutierrez-Barrera A, Hortobagyi GN, Litton JK, Arun BK. Effectiveness of alternating mammography and magnetic resonance imaging for screening women with deleterious BRCA mutations at high risk of breast cancer. Cancer. 2011;117(17):3900–7. Epub 2011/03/03. https://doi.org/10.1002/cncr.25971.
40. Kriege M, Brekelmans CT, Boetes C, Besnard PE, Zonderland HM, Obdeijn IM, Manoliu RA, Kok T, Peterse H, Tilanus-Linthorst MM, Muller SH, Meijer S, Oosterwijk JC, Beex LV, Tollenaar RA, de Koning HJ, Rutgers EJ, Klijn JG. Magnetic Resonance Imaging Screening Study G. Efficacy of MRI and mammography for breast-cancer screening in women with a familial or genetic predisposition. N Engl J Med. 2004;351(5):427–37. Epub 2004/07/30. https://doi.org/10.1056/NEJMoa031759.
41. Warner E, Hill K, Causer P, Plewes D, Jong R, Yaffe M, Foulkes WD, Ghadirian P, Lynch H, Couch F, Wong J, Wright F, Sun P, Narod SA. Prospective study of breast cancer incidence in women with a BRCA1 or BRCA2 mutation under surveillance with and without magnetic resonance imaging. J Clin Oncol. 2011;29(13):1664-9. Epub 2011/03/30. https://doi.org/10.1200/JCO.2009.27.0835. PubMed PMID: 21444874; PMCID: PMC4874196.
42. Plevritis SK, Kurian AW, Sigal BM, Daniel BL, Ikeda DM, Stockdale FE, Garber AM. Cost-effectiveness of screening BRCA1/2 mutation carriers with breast magnetic resonance imaging. JAMA. 2006;295(20):2374–84. Epub 2006/05/25. https://doi.org/10.1001/jama.295.20.2374.
43. Saslow D, Boetes C, Burke W, Harms S, Leach MO, Lehman CD, Morris E, Pisano E, Schnall M, Sener S, Smith RA, Warner E, Yaffe M, Andrews KS, Russell CA. American Cancer Society guidelines for breast screening with MRI as an adjunct to mammography. CA Cancer J Clin. 2007;57(2):75–89.
44. Roberts MC, Dusetzina SB. The effect of a celebrity health disclosure on demand for health care: trends

in BRCA testing and subsequent health services use. 2017. https://doi.org/10.1007/s12687-017-0295-7.
45. Meijers-Heijboer H, van Geel B, van Putten WLJ, Henzen-Logmans SC, Seynaeve C, Menke-Pluymers MBE, Bartels CCM, Verhoog LC, van den Ouweland AMW, Niermeijer MF, Brekelmans CTM, Klijn JGM. Breast cancer after prophylactic bilateral mastectomy in women with a BRCA1 or BRCA2 mutation. New England J Med. 2001;345(3):159–64.
46. Rebbeck TR, Friebel T, Lynch HT, Neuhausen SL, Van'T Veer L, Garber JE, Evans GR, Narod SA, Isaacs C, Matloff E, Daly MB, Olopade OI, Weber BL. Bilateral prophylactic mastectomy reduces breast cancer risk in BRCA1 and BRCA2 mutation carriers: the PROSE Study Group. J Clin Oncol. 2004;22(6):1055–62. https://doi.org/10.1200/jco.2004.04.188.
47. Kauff ND, Robson ME, Offit K. Oophorectomy in carriers of BRCA mutations. New England J Med. 2002;347(13):1037–40.
48. Van Der Post RS, Vogelaar IP, Carneiro F, Guilford P, Huntsman D, Hoogerbrugge N, Caldas C, Chelcun Schreiber KE, Hardwick RH, Ausems MGEM, Bardram L, Benusiglio PR, Bisseling TM, Blair V, Bleiker E, Boussioutas A, Cats A, Coit D, Degregorio L, Figueiredo J, Ford JM, Heijkoop E, Hermens R, Humar B, Kaurah P, Keller G, Lai J, Ligtenberg MJL, O'Donovan M, Oliveira C, Pinheiro H, Ragunath K, Rasenberg E, Richardson S, Roviello F, Schackert H, Seruca R, Taylor A, Ter Huurne A, Tischkowitz M, Joe STA, Van Dijck B, Van Grieken NCT, Van Hillegersberg R, Van Sandick JW, Vehof R, Van Krieken JH, Fitzgerald RC. Hereditary diffuse gastric cancer: updated clinical guidelines with an emphasis on germlineCDH1mutation carriers. J Med Genet. 2015;52(6):361–74. https://doi.org/10.1136/jmedgenet-2015-103094.
49. Milas M, Mester J, Metzger R, Shin J, Mitchell J, Berber E, Siperstein AE, Eng C. Should patients with Cowden syndrome undergo prophylactic thyroidectomy? Surgery. 2012;152(6):1201–10. https://doi.org/10.1016/j.surg.2012.08.055.
50. Myriad. Myriad Introduces Enhanced BRACAnalysis® Test for Exceptionally High-Risk Breast Cancer Patients. Myriad Genetics, Inc; 2006.
51. Desmedt C, Voet T, Sotiriou C, Campbell PJ. Next-generation sequencing in breast cancer. 2012;24(6):597–604. https://doi.org/10.1097/cco.0b013e328359554e.
52. Mersch J, Brown N, Pirzadeh-Miller S, Mundt E, Cox HC, Brown K, Aston M, Esterling L, Manley S, Ross T. Prevalence of variant reclassification following hereditary cancer genetic testing. JAMA. 2018;320(12):1266. https://doi.org/10.1001/jama.2018.13152.
53. Lyra PCM, Nepomuceno TC, De Souza MLM, Machado GF, Veloso MF, Henriques TB, Dos Santos DZ, Ribeiro IG, Ribeiro RS, Rangel LBA, Richardson M, Iversen ES, Goldgar D, Couch FJ, Carvalho MA, Monteiro ANA. Integration of functional assay data results provides strong evidence for classification of hundreds of BRCA1 variants of uncertain significance. Genetics Med. 2020; https://doi.org/10.1038/s41436-020-00991-0.
54. Turner SA, Rao SK, Morgan RH, Vnencak-Jones CL, Wiesner GL. The impact of variant classification on the clinical management of hereditary cancer syndromes. Genetics Med. 2019;21(2):426–30. https://doi.org/10.1038/s41436-018-0063-z.
55. Robson M, Im S-A, Senkus E, Xu B, Domchek SM, Masuda N, Delaloge S, Li W, Tung N, Armstrong A, Wu W, Goessl C, Runswick S, Conte P. Olaparib for metastatic breast cancer in patients with a germline BRCA mutation. New England J Med. 2017;377(6):523–33. https://doi.org/10.1056/nejmoa1706450.
56. Litton JK, Rugo HS, Ettl J, Hurvitz SA, Gonçalves A, Lee K-H, Fehrenbacher L, Yerushalmi R, Mina LA, Martin M, Roché H, Im Y-H, Quek RGW, Markova D, Tudor IC, Hannah AL, Eiermann W, Blum JL. Talazoparib in patients with advanced breast cancer and a germline BRCA mutation. New England J Med. 2018;379(8):753–63. https://doi.org/10.1056/nejmoa1802905.
57. Gradishar WJ, Anderson BO, Abraham J, Aft R, Agnese D, Allison KH, Blair SL, Burstein HJ, Dang C, Elias AD, Giordano SH, Goetz MP, Goldstein LJ, Isakoff SJ, Krishnamurthy J, Lyons J, Marcom PK, Matro J, Mayer IA, Moran MS, Mortimer J, O'Regan RM, Patel SA, Pierce LJ, Rugo HS, Sitapati A, Smith KL, Smith ML, Soliman H, Stringer-Reasor EM, Telli ML, Ward JH, Young JS, Burns JL, Kumar R. Breast Cancer, Version 3.2020, NCCN Clinical Practice Guidelines in Oncology. J Nat Comprehen Cancer Network. 2020;18(4):452–78. https://doi.org/10.6004/jnccn.2020.0016.
58. Storm C, Agarwal R, Offit K. Ethical and legal implications of cancer genetic testing: do physicians have a duty to warn patients' relatives about possible genetic risks? J Oncol Pract. 2008;4(5):229–30. https://doi.org/10.1200/jop.0858504.
59. Rothstein MA. Reconsidering the duty to warn genetically at-risk relatives. Genetics Med. 2018;20(3):285–90. https://doi.org/10.1038/gim.2017.257.
60. Frey MK, Kahn RM, Chapman-Davis E, Tubito F, Pires M, Christos P, Anderson S, Mukherjee S, Jordan B, Blank SV, Caputo TA, Sharaf RN, Offit K, Holcomb K, Lipkin S. Prospective feasibility trial of a novel strategy of facilitated cascade genetic testing using telephone counseling. J Clin Oncol. 2020;38(13):1389–97. https://doi.org/10.1200/jco.19.02005.
61. Offit K, Tkachuk KA, Stadler ZK, Walsh MF, Diaz-Zabala H, Levin JD, Steinsnyder Z, Ravichandran V, Sharaf RN, Frey MK, Lipkin SM, Robson ME, Hamilton JG, Vijai J, Mukherjee S. Cascading after peridiagnostic cancer genetic testing: an alternative to population-based screening. J Clin Oncol. 2020;38(13):1398–408. https://doi.org/10.1200/jco.19.02010.

21 Common Considerations in Male Breast Cancer Survivors

Siddhartha Yadav, Karthik V. Giridhar, Kathryn J. Ruddy, and Roberto A. Leon-Ferre

Introduction

Male breast cancer (MaBC) is a rare disease, accounting for approximately 1% of all breast cancer diagnoses. Due to its rarity, recommendations for management are often extrapolated from the female breast cancer literature. However, significant differences in tumor and host biology, drug metabolism and toxicity, and psychosocial issues are known to exist between men and women with breast cancer [1–4]. Clinical trials enrolling breast cancer patients have often excluded men, and those allowing the inclusion of MaBC patients often accrue too few men to provide meaningful information on long-term sex-specific outcomes [5]. Given all this, survivorship guidelines for female breast cancer may not be adequate for MaBC and may not fulfill men's unique needs. In this chapter, we will consider survivorship issues in MaBC and provide guidance on how to address them.

S. Yadav · K. V. Giridhar · K. J. Ruddy
R. A. Leon-Ferre (✉)
Department of Oncology, Mayo Clinic, Rochester, MN, USA
e-mail: Yadav.Siddhartha@mayo.edu; Giridhar.Karthik@mayo.edu; Ruddy.Kathryn@mayo.edu; leonferre.roberto@mayo.edu

Overview of the Differences in the Treatment of MaBC and Female Breast Cancer

Differences in treatment choices for male and female breast cancer have implications for the personalized management of subsequent toxicities and surveillance for recurrence in MaBC survivors. For instance, more than two-thirds of men with localized breast cancer undergo mastectomy rather than lumpectomy [6]. In contrast, the rate of mastectomy in female breast cancer is around 30–40% [7, 8]. Radiation therapy is less frequently administered in the management of MaBC, even for men undergoing lumpectomy compared to women undergoing lumpectomy [6, 9, 10]. The indications for chemotherapy are similar between men and women. Although genomic stratifiers such as Oncotype DX have not specifically been validated in MaBC, they appear to be increasingly used to aid decision-making regarding adjuvant chemotherapy in MaBC [6, 11]. As the recurrence score cutpoints used to guide chemotherapy in women may underappreciate the risk in men, gender-specific thresholds of the recurrence score categorization need further investigation [12]. Approximately 85% of MaBCs are estrogen receptor (ER) positive, compared to around 75% of female breast cancers [10]. As a consequence, the majority of men with breast cancer are recommended to receive endocrine therapy [13]. These differences in the management of MaBC compared to women

G. G. Kimmick et al. (eds.), *Common Issues in Breast Cancer Survivors*,
https://doi.org/10.1007/978-3-030-75377-1_21

with breast cancer should be taken into account when discussing survivorship issues with MaBC patients.

Addressing Psychosocial Issues and Quality of life in MaBC Survivors

Female breast cancer survivors suffer emotional distress, anxiety, depression, and changes in quality of life throughout the course of their disease [14, 15]. In men, there are limited studies evaluating the long-term psychosocial impact of a breast cancer diagnosis. In the few available studies, it was evident that some survivors do experience psychosocial distress and/or poor quality of life [4, 16–18]. Compared to age-matched control men, MaBC survivors have reported significantly poorer physical and mental health, more physical comorbidities and activity limitations, and poorer life satisfaction [17]. However, compared to female breast cancer survivors, male survivors generally do not report more emotional or quality of life impairments. It has been hypothesized that a breast cancer diagnosis could be uniquely distressing to men due to concerns regarding sexuality and masculinity; because breasts are considered female organs, some men have reported that breast cancer is a threat to self-perceived masculinity [19]. MaBC patients have also expressed concerns about mastectomy scars (usually visible when shirtless in hot weather or while swimming) permanently identifying them as MaBC survivors, potentially making them more vulnerable to the stigma associated with an MaBC diagnosis [19, 20]. A lack of awareness of the disease among the general population may be a contributor to social stigmatization. However, differential treatment by health-care providers, as well as the paucity of gender-neutral terminologies or information materials on breast cancer in the health-care systems, may also play a role [21]. Ultimately, this stigma associated with the disease may impact treatment or follow-up compliance among MaBC survivors.

In order to optimally support MaBC patients through their treatment and survivorship, it is important to address their psychosocial concerns. MaBC patients should be asked about anxiety, depression, quality of life, and concerns about masculinity and sexuality during follow-up visits (Fig. 21.1). In addition, using gender-neutral terminologies and information materials specifically designed for MaBC may help decrease the stigma associated with the disease. While support groups are often available to decrease emotional distress related to breast cancer diagnosis in women [22–25], specific support groups for MaBC patients are rare, and support groups comprised predominantly of female survivors may not meet the unique psychosocial needs of MaBC patients [20]. In this context, the creation of institutional pools of MaBC survivors willing to share their stories with other similar patients or referral to online support groups specifically designed for MaBC survivors [26] might be helpful (e.g., American Cancer Society Cancer Survivors Network has an online support group for MaBC patients). Referral to trained professionals adept to addressing psychosocial issues related to MaBC diagnosis may be needed in some cases.

Management of Treatment-Related Toxicities in MaBC Survivors

Sex-specific differences in drug metabolism are known to exist, potentially conferring different toxicity profiles in men and women with breast cancer, even with the same treatment [2, 27]. In addition, a toxicity profile is also dependent on the baseline risk for certain conditions and the hormonal milieu, which are known to be different between men and women. Because men often develop breast cancer at an older age compared to women, the risk of toxicity, drug interactions, and decreased adherence may be increased. Some of the most common short- and long-term toxicities in MaBC survivors with frequently used treatment regimens are highlighted below.

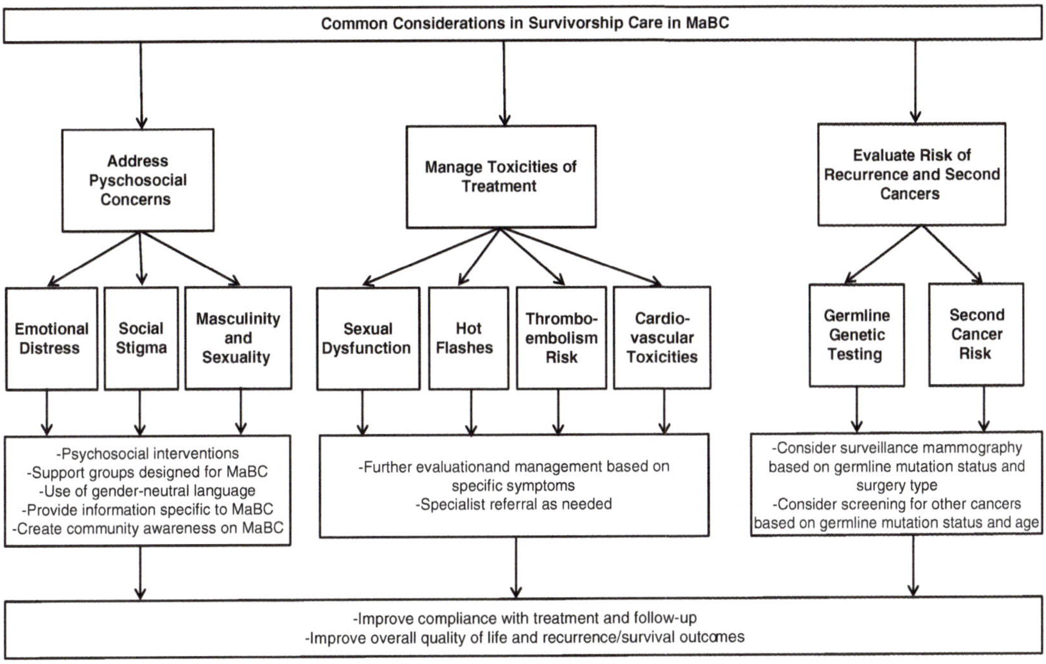

Fig. 21.1 Common considerations in survivorship care in male breast cancer (MaBC)

Endocrine Therapy

Tamoxifen is the preferred drug for the treatment of ER-positive MaBC. The use of aromatase inhibitors in the adjuvant setting is typically restricted to patients who are not able to take tamoxifen and only given in conjunction with gonadotropin-releasing hormone analogues (GnRHa) [28]. Aromatase inhibitor monotherapy is usually not recommended, as it may not adequately reduce estradiol levels in men due to direct production of estrogen from the testis when there is no concomitant use of GnRHa [29]. Tamoxifen is associated with hot flashes, weight gain, sexual dysfunction, and thromboembolic events in MaBC patients [30–32]. More than half of men with breast cancer experience one or more toxicities while taking tamoxifen, and toxicities lead to discontinuation of tamoxifen in approximately 20–25% of patients with MaBC within 1–2 years of treatment [30, 32]. Sexual dysfunction and loss of libido have been reported by a significant proportion (13 to 40%) of patients taking tamoxifen [30–33], though it is unclear how much of this is due to the drug versus due to other comorbidities and aging. Similarly, the cumulative risk of thrombotic events in men treated with tamoxifen for breast cancer is approximately 12%, and the risk is markedly increased in the first 18 months of treatment and in older patients [34]. In contrast, women treated with tamoxifen for breast cancer have a 5-year risk of deep venous thrombosis or pulmonary embolism of around 1.2% [35]. Higher baseline risk for venous thromboembolism (VTE) [36] and the preferred use of tamoxifen in older men (as opposed to aromatase inhibitors in older women) may contribute to some of the differences in the rates of VTE. Although the rate of VTE with tamoxifen appears to be higher in male than female breast cancer survivors, there is no evidence to support prophylaxis with aspirin or other anticoagulants at this time. Evaluation for VTE or other cardiovascular conditions in MaBC survivors should be guided by symptoms, as it is in women with breast cancer.

In men treated with GnRHa plus aromatase inhibitors, the use of prolonged GnRHa may be associated with changes in metabolic states including hyperinsulinemia, hypercholesterolemia, and increase in body fat [37] and may be associated with an increased risk of myocardial infarction and stroke [38–40]. Special efforts should be made to optimize any modifiable cardiac risk factors in MaBC patients treated with these agents.

Health-care professionals should inquire about sexual dysfunction and loss of libido in MaBC patients (Fig. 21.1). While sexual dysfunction may be a result of endocrine therapy, other medical issues (including cardiovascular disease) and psychological factors related to breast cancer diagnosis may contribute, as well. The management of sexual dysfunction in MaBC survivors may require referral to a sex therapist and/or couples counselor. Relationship strain may contribute to or be caused by sexual dysfunction. Pharmacological management of sexual dysfunction with phosphodiesterase 5 inhibitors, e.g., sildenafil, may be helpful, although specific studies evaluating efficacy in MaBC survivors have not been performed. Non-pharmacologic management strategies should also be considered and offered to interested patients, with appropriate referral to urology specialists as needed.

For treatment of hot flashes induced by endocrine therapy, strategies similar to those used in female breast cancer or in men with prostate cancer may be used. Several randomized trials have identified non-hormonal medications that are effective in women, such as selective serotonin reuptake inhibitors (SSRIs), serotonin-norepinephrine reuptake inhibitors [41–54], gabapentinoids [43, 55–60], and oxybutynin [61–63]. However, data specific to men are limited [64]. In terms of specific SSRIs, agents that are not strong inhibitors of CYP2D6 (e.g., venlafaxine) are generally preferred due to the potential concern that inhibition of CYP2D6 will decrease tamoxifen's active metabolite, endoxifen, although the clinical relevance of this interaction remains controversial. Testosterone supplementation for the management of hot flashes or hypogonadism in MaBC patients is typically avoided, especially in those with hormone receptor-positive disease, although it may be considered in select cases after a thoughtful discussion on the risks and benefits [28].

HER2-Directed Therapy

One in ten MaBC patients has HER2-positive tumors [65]. Unique efficacy or toxicity concerns related to anti-HER2-directed therapies have not been reported in MaBC [66], but rates of long-term cardiotoxicity might be important due to a high baseline risk of cardiac diseases in older men [67]. At present, there are no specific recommendations for screening for cardiac diseases in men with HER2-positive breast cancer treated with trastuzumab other than the same echocardiography every 3 months during the year of adjuvant treatment that is recommended for women. Additional evaluation should be guided by symptoms.

Chemotherapy

The most commonly used chemotherapy agents in operable breast cancer therapy are anthracyclines, taxanes, and cyclophosphamide. Animal studies have suggested increased rates of cardiomyopathy and nephropathy and higher mortality from anthracyclines in males compared to females [68, 69]. In studies of patients with lymphoma, male sex has been identified to be associated with adverse cardiac events, cardiac hospitalization, decrease in left ventricular ejection fraction, and cardiomyopathy after doxorubicin therapy [70–72]. Sex-specific differences in the baseline risk of cardiovascular disease may account for some of these findings [67]. Cyclophosphamide is often used in combination with anthracyclines in adjuvant treatment of MaBC. A higher cumulative dose of cyclophosphamide (>6 g) in men is associated with gonadal toxicity and azoospermia [73–75]. In addition, cyclophosphamide is also associated with therapy-related acute myeloid leukemia, which typically occurs 5–7 years after treatment [76]. It is not known if this risk differs by sex. Similarly, studies have not demonstrated different rates of neuropathy with taxanes in males compared to females [77, 78]. At present, there are no specific recommendations in MaBC survivors for any additional screening for cardiac disease, hematological malignancies, or neuropathy except as recommended in the general population. However, further evaluation may be warranted when directed by symptoms or laboratory parameters.

Supporting Compliance with Treatment and Follow-Up

Because >80% of MaBC are ER positive, adjuvant endocrine therapy is recommended for the vast majority of MaBC survivors. However, suboptimal compliance with endocrine therapy and early discontinuation due to multiple factors as discussed above remain significant concerns. Among MaBC patients taking tamoxifen, 20–25% of patients discontinue treatment within the first few years of treatment [30, 32]. In a study of MaBC survivors in China, more than two-thirds of patients had discontinued tamoxifen within 3 years of diagnosis [79]. Similarly, in another study of Medicare patients aged 65 years and older with MaBC in the United States, 61% discontinued tamoxifen before completing 5 years of treatment [80]. Low adherence or early discontinuation of tamoxifen in MaBC is associated with greater risk of recurrence and death [79]. Several factors, including toxicities, lack of social support, and older age, have been associated with tamoxifen discontinuation [79]. Managing toxicities promptly and effectively, addressing psychosocial issues, and frequently reminding patients about the clinical significance of therapies might be particularly helpful in MaBC survivors.

Germline Genetic Testing and Screening for Other Cancers

Among MaBC patients undergoing multigene panel testing, the frequency of germline mutations is noted to be approximately 18% [81]. *BRCA2* is the most common mutation noted in this population, detected in 11% of men, followed by germline *CHEK2* mutations in approximately 4% [81]. Due to the high frequency of germline mutations in *BRCA1/2* and other genes, all MaBC patients are recommended to undergo germline genetic testing (Fig. 21.1) [24]. The results of germline genetic testing may have implications for surveillance of breast cancer recurrence in men (see next section) and screening for other cancers. In particular, current guidelines recommend prostate cancer screening starting at age 40 for germline *BRCA2* mutation carriers, and screening should be considered in *BRCA1* carriers [82]. In addition, *BRCA1*, *BRCA2*, *ATM*, or *PALB2* mutation carriers may also be at a higher risk of pancreatic cancer [82–84]. Although recommendations for pancreatic cancer screening in mutation carriers are not well-defined, screening may be considered, especially in those with a family history of pancreatic cancer, after a careful discussion of the benefits and limitations of screening modalities such as endoscopic ultrasonography, magnetic resonance imaging, and computed tomography [82, 85, 86].

In general, the literature describes higher risk of second cancers (prostate, colon, and pancreatic cancers in particular) in MaBC survivors [87–89]. Some of this risk may be attributed to the presence of a germline mutation. The magnitude of risk of second cancers in MaBC patients without germline mutations is unclear. At present, there are no specific guidelines for screening for other cancers in MaBC survivors without a germline mutation beyond age-appropriate cancer screening.

Surveillance Mammography for MaBC Recurrence

For the majority of MaBC patients—who typically undergo mastectomy—surveillance breast imaging would only have the potential to detect contralateral breast cancers. Even though the risk of contralateral breast cancer is increased by approximately 30-fold in MaBC survivors compared to men in the general population and is highest in men diagnosed with breast cancer under the age of 50 [90], the absolute risk of a second breast cancer in MaBC survivors remains low, less than 2% over a 38-year follow-up according to one study [91]. Hence, the role of surveillance mammography in MaBC survivors is not well-defined but may be of value in specific MaBC survivors at high risk of local recurrence or development of second primary [92]. The American Society of Clinical Oncology guidelines on MaBC management recommend ipsilateral annual mammogram in MaBC patients treated with lumpectomy, whereas contralateral annual mammogram is only recommended for men with a history of breast cancer and a genetic predisposing mutation (Fig. 21.1) [28]. However, the guidelines acknowledge the lack of data on the usefulness or the necessity of surveillance mammography in MaBC survivors. There is no evidence to support the use of magnetic resonance imaging (MRI) for surveillance after treatment for MaBC.

Other Considerations

In postmenopausal women with breast cancer adjuvant bisphosphonate therapy is associated with a small but significant improvement in overall survival [93]. Since the majority of postmenopausal women with breast cancer are treated with aromatase inhibitors, which are associated with bone loss [94], there is an added advantage of reducing the risk of osteoporosis through the use of adjuvant bisphosphonate therapy in these of patients. In addition, due to the concern for bone loss, women treated with aromatase inhibitors typically undergo periodic DEXA scans to evaluate for bone density [83]. However, the role of adjuvant bisphosphonates in MaBC is unclear, and bone loss in MaBC survivors treated with tamoxifen is usually not a major concern. However, bone loss may be an issue in MaBC patients treated with GnRHa in combination with aromatase inhibitors [95–97]. Guidelines for optimal management in this situation are lacking.

In cancer survivors, cardiovascular disease is the leading cause of mortality after cancer-related deaths [98]. Hence, appropriate management of cardiovascular risk factors in MaBC survivors should be considered with age-appropriate screening and primary or secondary prophylaxis as indicated. In addition, management of other comorbidities in MaBC survivors to improve overall health outcomes should be prioritized.

Conclusions

The optimal approach to survivorship care in patients with MaBC is limited by the lack of clinical studies in this field. Differences in tumor biology, treatment modalities, toxicities of treatment, psychosocial issues, and risk of recurrence between men and women with breast cancer suggest that survivorship guidelines designed for women with breast cancer may not be appropriate for MaBC patients. A more nuanced approach to survivorship care in MaBC taking these differences into account is needed to ensure good quality of life and treatment compliance. Ultimately, such personalized approach will hopefully result in improved clinical outcomes for MaBC survivors.

References

1. Ozdemir BC, Csajka C, Dotto GP, Wagner AD. Sex differences in efficacy and toxicity of systemic treatments: an undervalued issue in the era of precision oncology. J Clin Oncol. 2018;36(26):2680–3.
2. Soldin OP, Mattison DR. Sex differences in pharmacokinetics and pharmacodynamics. Clin Pharmacokinet. 2009;48(3):143–57.
3. Ruddy KJ, Winer EP. Male breast cancer: risk factors, biology, diagnosis, treatment, and survivorship. Ann Oncol. 2013;24(6):1434–43.
4. Kipling M, Ralph JE, Callanan K. Psychological impact of male breast disorders: literature review and survey results. Breast Care (Basel). 2014;9(1):29–33.
5. Duma N, Hoversten KP, Ruddy KJ. Exclusion of male patients in breast cancer clinical trials. JNCI Cancer Spectr. 2018;2(2).
6. Yadav S, Karam D, Bin Riaz I, Xie H, Durani U, Duma N, et al. Male breast cancer in the United States: treatment patterns and prognostic factors in the 21st century. Cancer. 2019;
7. Mahmood U, Hanlon AL, Koshy M, Buras R, Chumsri S, Tkaczuk KH, et al. Increasing national mastectomy rates for the treatment of early stage breast cancer. Ann Surg Oncol. 2013;20(5):1436–43.
8. McGuire KP, Santillan AA, Kaur P, Meade T, Parbhoo J, Mathias M, et al. Are mastectomies on the rise? A

13-year trend analysis of the selection of mastectomy versus breast conservation therapy in 5865 patients. Ann Surg Oncol. 2009;16(10):2682–90.
9. Buchholz TA, Theriault RL, Niland JC, Hughes ME, Ottesen R, Edge SB, et al. The use of radiation as a component of breast conservation therapy in national comprehensive cancer network centers. J Clin Oncol. 2006;24(3):361–9.
10. Wang F, Shu X, Meszoely I, Pal T, Mayer IA, Yu Z, et al. Overall mortality after diagnosis of breast cancer in men vs women. JAMA Oncol. 2019;5(11):1589–96.
11. Turashvili G, Gonzalez-Loperena M, Brogi E, Dickler M, Norton L, Morrow M, et al. The 21-gene recurrence score in male breast cancer. Ann Surg Oncol. 2018;25(6):1530–5.
12. Wang F, Reid S, Zheng W, Pal T, Meszoely I, Mayer IA, et al. Sex disparity observed for oncotype DX breast recurrence score in predicting mortality among patients with early stage ER-positive breast cancer. Clin Cancer Res. 2020;26(1):101–9.
13. Leon-Ferre RA, Giridhar KV, Hieken TJ, Mutter RW, Couch FJ, Jimenez RE, et al. A contemporary review of male breast cancer: current evidence and unanswered questions. Cancer Metastasis Rev. 2018;37(4):599–614.
14. Hughes J. Emotional reactions to the diagnosis and treatment of early breast cancer. J Psychosom Res. 1982;26(2):277–83.
15. Andrykowski MA, Cordova MJ. Factors associated with PTSD symptoms following treatment for breast cancer: test of the Andersen model. J Trauma Stress. 1998;11(2):189–203.
16. Robinson JD, Metoyer KP Jr, Bhayani N. Breast cancer in men: a need for psychological intervention. J Clin Psychol Med Settings. 2008;15(2):134–9.
17. Andrykowski MA. Physical and mental health status and health behaviors in male breast cancer survivors: a national, population-based, case-control study. Psycho-Oncology. 2012;21(9):927–34.
18. Kowalski C, Steffen P, Ernstmann N, Wuerstlein R, Harbeck N, Pfaff H. Health-related quality of life in male breast cancer patients. Breast Cancer Res Treat. 2012;133(2):753–7.
19. Donovan T, Flynn M. What makes a man a man? The lived experience of male breast cancer. Cancer Nurs. 2007;30(6):464–70.
20. Williams BG, Iredale R, Brain K, France E, Barrett-Lee P, Gray J. Experiences of men with breast cancer: an exploratory focus group study. Br J Cancer. 2003;89(10):1834–6.
21. Midding E, Halbach SM, Kowalski C, Weber R, Würstlein R, Ernstmann N. Men with a "woman's disease": stigmatization of male breast cancer patients-a mixed methods analysis. Am J Mens Health. 2018;12(6):2194–207.
22. Gray R, Fitch M, Davis C, Phillips C. A qualitative study of breast cancer self-help groups. Psycho-Oncology. 1997;6(4):279–89.
23. Docherty A. Experience, functions and benefits of a cancer support group. Patient Educ Couns. 2004;55(1):87–93.
24. Adamsen L. 'From victim to agent': the clinical and social significance of self-help group participation for people with life-threatening diseases. Scand J Caring Sci. 2002;16(3):224–31.
25. Ussher J, Kirsten L, Butow P, Sandoval M. What do cancer support groups provide which other supportive relationships do not? The experience of peer support groups for people with cancer. Soc Sci Med. 2006;62(10):2565–76.
26. Farrell E, Borstelmann N, Meyer F, Partridge A, Winer E, Ruddy K. Male breast cancer networking and telephone support group: a model for supporting a unique population. Psycho-Oncology. 2014;23(8):956–8.
27. Yadav S, Giridhar KV, Taraba J, Leon-Ferre RA, Ruddy KJ. Safety, efficacy, and tolerability of systemic therapies in male breast cancer: are there sex-specific differences? Expert Opin Drug Saf.In Press.
28. Hassett MJ, Somerfield MR, Baker ER, Cardoso F, Kansal KJ, Kwait DC, et al. Management of male breast cancer: ASCO guideline. J Clin Oncol. 0(0):JCO.19.03120.
29. Doyen J, Italiano A, Largillier R, Ferrero J-M, Fontana X, Thyss A. Aromatase inhibition in male breast cancer patients: biological and clinical implications. Ann Oncol. 2009;21(6):1243–5.
30. Anelli TF, Anelli A, Tran KN, Lebwohl DE, Borgen PI. Tamoxifen administration is associated with a high rate of treatment-limiting symptoms in male breast cancer patients. Cancer. 1994;74(1):74–7.
31. Visram H, Kanji F, Dent SF. Endocrine therapy for male breast cancer: rates of toxicity and adherence. Curr Oncol (Toronto, Ont). 2010;17(5):17–21.
32. Pemmaraju N, Munsell MF, Hortobagyi GN, Giordano SH. Retrospective review of male breast cancer patients: analysis of tamoxifen-related side-effects. Ann Oncol. 2012;23(6):1471–4.
33. Ruddy KJ, Giobbie-Hurder A, Giordano SH, Goldfarb S, Kereakoglow S, Winer EP, et al. Quality of life and symptoms in male breast cancer survivors. Breast. 2013;22(2):197–9.
34. Eggemann H, Bernreiter AL, Reinisch M, Loibl S, Taran FA, Costa SD, et al. Tamoxifen treatment for male breast cancer and risk of thromboembolism: prospective cohort analysis. Br J Cancer. 2019;120(3):301–5.
35. Hernandez RK, Sørensen HT, Pedersen L, Jacobsen J, Lash TL. Tamoxifen treatment and risk of deep venous thrombosis and pulmonary embolism. Cancer. 2009;115(19):4442–9.
36. Cushman M. Epidemiology and risk factors for venous thrombosis. Semin Hematol. 2007;44(2):62–9.
37. Gupta D, Lee Chuy K, Yang JC, Bates M, Lombardo M, Steingart RM. Cardiovascular and metabolic effects of androgen-deprivation therapy for prostate cancer. J Oncol Pract. 2018;14(10):580–7.
38. Levine GN, D'Amico AV, Berger P, Clark PE, Eckel RH, Keating NL, et al. Androgen-deprivation therapy in prostate cancer and cardiovascular risk: a science advisory from the American Heart Association, American Cancer Society, and American Urological Association: endorsed by the American

Society for Radiation Oncology. Circulation. 2010;121(6):833–40.
39. Bosco C, Bosnyak Z, Malmberg A, Adolfsson J, Keating NL, Van Hemelrijck M. Quantifying observational evidence for risk of fatal and nonfatal cardiovascular disease following androgen deprivation therapy for prostate cancer: a meta-analysis. Eur Urol. 2015;68(3):386–96.
40. O'Farrell S, Garmo H, Holmberg L, Adolfsson J, Stattin P, Van Hemelrijck M. Risk and timing of cardiovascular disease after androgen-deprivation therapy in men with prostate cancer. J Clin Oncol. 2015;33(11):1243–51.
41. Loprinzi CL, Kugler JW, Sloan JA, Mailliard JA, LaVasseur BI, Barton DL, et al. Venlafaxine in management of hot flashes in survivors of breast cancer: a randomised controlled trial. Lancet. 2000;356(9247):2059–63.
42. Loprinzi CL, Sloan JA, Perez EA, Quella SK, Stella PJ, Mailliard JA, et al. Phase III evaluation of fluoxetine for treatment of hot flashes. J Clin Oncol. 2002;20(6):1578–83.
43. Loprinzi CL, Sloan J, Stearns V, Slack R, Iyengar M, Diekmann B, et al. Newer antidepressants and gabapentin for hot flashes: an individual patient pooled analysis. J Clin Oncol. 2009;27(17):2831–7.
44. Boekhout AH, Vincent AD, Dalesio OB, van den Bosch J, Foekema-Tons JH, Adriaansz S, et al. Management of hot flashes in patients who have breast cancer with venlafaxine and clonidine: a randomized, double-blind, placebo-controlled trial. J Clin Oncol. 2011;29(29):3862–8.
45. Evans ML, Pritts E, Vittinghoff E, McClish K, Morgan KS, Jaffe RB. Management of postmenopausal hot flushes with venlafaxine hydrochloride: a randomized, controlled trial. Obstet Gynecol. 2005;105(1):161–6.
46. Speroff L, Gass M, Constantine G, Olivier S, Study I. Efficacy and tolerability of desvenlafaxine succinate treatment for menopausal vasomotor symptoms: a randomized controlled trial. Obstet Gynecol 2008;111(1):77–87.
47. Archer DF, Seidman L, Constantine GD, Pickar JH, Olivier S. A double-blind, randomly assigned, placebo-controlled study of desvenlafaxine efficacy and safety for the treatment of vasomotor symptoms associated with menopause. Am J Obstet Gynecol. 2009;200(2):172 e1–10.
48. Stearns V, Beebe KL, Iyengar M, Dube E. Paroxetine controlled release in the treatment of menopausal hot flashes: a randomized controlled trial. JAMA. 2003;289(21):2827–34.
49. Suvanto-Luukkonen E, Koivunen R, Sundstrom H, Bloigu R, Karjalainen E, Haiva-Mallinen L, et al. Citalopram and fluoxetine in the treatment of postmenopausal symptoms: a prospective, randomized, 9-month, placebo-controlled, double-blind study. Menopause. 2005;12(1):18–26.
50. Gordon PR, Kerwin JP, Boesen KG, Senf J. Sertraline to treat hot flashes: a randomized controlled, double-blind, crossover trial in a general population. Menopause. 2006;13(4):568–75.
51. Barton DL, LaVasseur BI, Sloan JA, Stawis AN, Flynn KA, Dyar M, et al. Phase III, placebo-controlled trial of three doses of citalopram for the treatment of hot flashes: NCCTG trial N05C9. J Clin Oncol. 2010;28(20):3278–83.
52. Freeman EW, Guthrie KA, Caan B, Sternfeld B, Cohen LS, Joffe H, et al. Efficacy of escitalopram for hot flashes in healthy menopausal women: a randomized controlled trial. JAMA. 2011;305(3):267–74.
53. Grady D, Cohen B, Tice J, Kristof M, Olyaie A, Sawaya GF. Ineffectiveness of sertraline for treatment of menopausal hot flushes: a randomized controlled trial. Obstet Gynecol. 2007;109(4):823–30.
54. Kimmick GG, Lovato J, McQuellon R, Robinson E, Muss HB. Randomized, double-blind, placebo-controlled, crossover study of sertraline (Zoloft) for the treatment of hot flashes in women with early stage breast cancer taking tamoxifen. Breast J. 2006;12(2):114–22.
55. Guttuso T Jr, Kurlan R, McDermott MP, Kieburtz K. Gabapentin's effects on hot flashes in postmenopausal women: a randomized controlled trial. Obstet Gynecol. 2003;101(2):337–45.
56. Pandya KJ, Morrow GR, Roscoe JA, Zhao H, Hickok JT, Pajon E, et al. Gabapentin for hot flashes in 420 women with breast cancer: a randomised double-blind placebo-controlled trial. Lancet. 2005;366(9488):818–24.
57. Reddy SY, Warner H, Guttuso T Jr, Messing S, DiGrazio W, Thornburg L, et al. Gabapentin, estrogen, and placebo for treating hot flushes: a randomized controlled trial. Obstet Gynecol. 2006;108(1):41–8.
58. Loprinzi CL, Kugler JW, Barton DL, Dueck AC, Tschetter LK, Nelimark RA, et al. Phase III trial of gabapentin alone or in conjunction with an antidepressant in the management of hot flashes in women who have inadequate control with an antidepressant alone: NCCTG N03C5. J Clin Oncol. 2007;25(3):308–12.
59. Bordeleau L, Jugovic O, Ennis M, Pritchard KI, Warr D, Haq R, et al. A randomized crossover trial of venlafaxine (V) versus gabapentin (G) for hot flashes (HF) in breast cancer survivors. ASCO Meeting Abstracts. 2010;28(15_suppl):9023.
60. Loprinzi CL, Qin R, Balcueva EP, Flynn KA, Rowland KM Jr, Graham DL, et al. Phase III, randomized, double-blind, placebo-controlled evaluation of pregabalin for alleviating hot flashes, N07C1. J Clin Oncol. 2010;28(4):641–7.
61. Leon-Ferre RA, Novotny PJ, Wolfe EG, Faubion SS, Ruddy KJ, Flora D, et al. Oxybutynin vs placebo for hot flashes in women with or without breast cancer: a randomized, double-blind clinical trial (ACCRU SC-1603). JNCI Cancer Spectr. 2019;4(1).
62. Smith TJ, Loprinzi CL, Deville C. Oxybutynin for hot flashes due to androgen deprivation in men. N Engl J Med. 2018;378(18):1745–6.
63. Leon-Ferre RA, Majithia N, Loprinzi CL. Management of hot flashes in women with breast cancer receiv-

ing ovarian function suppression. Cancer Treat Rev. 2017;52:82–90.
64. Irani J, Salomon L, Oba R, Bouchard P, Mottet N. Efficacy of venlafaxine, medroxyprogesterone acetate, and cyproterone acetate for the treatment of vasomotor hot flushes in men taking gonadotropin-releasing hormone analogues for prostate cancer: a double-blind, randomised trial. Lancet Oncol. 2010;11(2):147–54.
65. Cardoso F, Bartlett JMS, Slaets L, van Deurzen CHM, van Leeuwen-Stok E, Porter P, et al. Characterization of male breast cancer: results of the EORTC 10085/TBCRC/BIG/NABCG international male breast cancer program. Ann Oncol. 2018;29(2):405–17.
66. Ottini L, Capalbo C, Rizzolo P, Silvestri V, Bronte G, Rizzo S, et al. HER2-positive male breast cancer: an update. Breast Cancer (Dove Medical Press). 2010;2:45–58.
67. Mosca L, Barrett-Connor E, Wenger NK. Sex/gender differences in cardiovascular disease prevention: what a difference a decade makes. Circulation. 2011;124(19):2145–54.
68. van Hoesel QG, Steerenberg PA, Dormans JA, de Jong WH, de Wildt DJ, Vos JG. Time-course study on doxorubicin-induced nephropathy and cardiomyopathy in male and female LOU/M/Wsl rats: lack of evidence for a causal relationship. J Natl Cancer Inst. 1986;76(2):299–307.
69. Moulin M, Piquereau J, Mateo P, Fortin D, Rucker-Martin C, Gressette M, et al. Sexual dimorphism of doxorubicin-mediated cardiotoxicity: potential role of energy metabolism remodeling. Circ Heart Fail. 2015;8(1):98–108.
70. Myrehaug S, Pintilie M, Tsang R, Mackenzie R, Crump M, Chen Z, et al. Cardiac morbidity following modern treatment for Hodgkin lymphoma: supra-additive cardiotoxicity of doxorubicin and radiation therapy. Leuk Lymphoma. 2008;49(8):1486–93.
71. Myrehaug S, Pintilie M, Yun L, Crump M, Tsang RW, Meyer RM, et al. A population-based study of cardiac morbidity among Hodgkin lymphoma patients with preexisting heart disease. Blood. 2010;116(13):2237–40.
72. Clements IP, Davis BJ, Wiseman GA. Systolic and diastolic cardiac dysfunction early after the initiation of doxorubicin therapy: significance of gender and concurrent mediastinal radiation. Nucl Med Commun. 2002;23(6):521–7.
73. Fairley KF, Barrie JU, Johnson W. Sterility and testicular atrophy related to cyclophosphamide therapy. Lancet. 1972;1(7750):568–9.
74. Watson AR, Rance CP, Bain J. Long term effects of cyclophosphamide on testicular function. Br Med J (Clin Res Ed). 1985;291(6507):1457–60.
75. Rivkees SA, Crawford JD. The relationship of gonadal activity and chemotherapy-induced gonadal damage. JAMA. 1988;259(14):2123–5.
76. Smith SM, Le Beau MM, Huo D, Karrison T, Sobecks RM, Anastasi J, et al. Clinical-cytogenetic associations in 306 patients with therapy-related myelodysplasia and myeloid leukemia: the University of Chicago series. Blood. 2003;102(1):43–52.
77. Hwang BY, Kim ES, Kim CH, Kwon JY, Kim HK. Gender differences in paclitaxel-induced neuropathic pain behavior and analgesic response in rats. Korean J Anesthesiol. 2012;62(1):66–72.
78. Yamamoto H, Sekine I, Yamada K, Nokihara H, Yamamoto N, Kunitoh H, et al. Gender differences in treatment outcomes among patients with non-small cell lung cancer given a combination of carboplatin and paclitaxel. Oncology. 2008;75(3–4):169–74.
79. Xu S, Yang Y, Tao W, Song Y, Chen Y, Ren Y, et al. Tamoxifen adherence and its relationship to mortality in 116 men with breast cancer. Breast Cancer Res Treat. 2012;136(2):495–502.
80. Oke O, Niu J, Chavez-MacGregor M, Zhao H, Giordano SH. Adjuvant tamoxifen adherence in men with early stage breast cancer. J Clin Oncol. 2018;36(15_suppl):550.
81. Pritzlaff M, Summerour P, McFarland R, Li S, Reineke P, Dolinsky JS, et al. Male breast cancer in a multi-gene panel testing cohort: insights and unexpected results. Breast Cancer Res Treat. 2017;161(3):575–86.
82. NCCN Clinical Practice Guidelines in Oncology. Genetic/familial high-risk assessment: breast, ovarian and pancreatic version 1.2020. Available at: https://www.nccn.org/professionals/physician_gls/pdf/genetics_bop.pdf. Last accessed: 26 Jan 2020.
83. Hu C, Hart SN, Polley EC, Gnanaolivu R, Shimelis H, Lee KY, et al. Association between inherited germline mutations in cancer predisposition genes and risk of pancreatic cancer. JAMA. 2018;319(23):2401–9.
84. Ibrahim M, Yadav S, Ogunleye F, Zakalik D. Male BRCA mutation carriers: clinical characteristics and cancer spectrum. BMC Cancer. 2018;18(1):179.
85. Canto MI, Almario JA, Schulick RD, Yeo CJ, Klein A, Blackford A, et al. Risk of neoplastic progression in individuals at high risk for pancreatic cancer undergoing long-term surveillance. Gastroenterology. 2018;155(3):740–51.e2.
86. Vasen H, Ibrahim I, Ponce CG, Slater EP, Matthäi E, Carrato A, et al. Benefit of surveillance for pancreatic cancer in high-risk individuals: outcome of long-term prospective follow-up studies from three European expert centers. J Clin Oncol. 2016;34(17):2010–9.
87. Masci G, Caruso M, Caruso F, Salvini P, Carnaghi C, Giordano L, et al. Clinicopathological and immunohistochemical characteristics in male breast cancer: a retrospective case series. Oncologist. 2015;20(6):586–92.
88. Cutuli B, Le-Nir CC-S, Serin D, Kirova Y, Gaci Z, Lemanski C, et al. Male breast cancer. Evolution of treatment and prognostic factors. Analysis of 489 cases. Crit Rev Oncol Hematol. 2010;73(3):246–54.
89. Hemminki K, Scélo G, Boffetta P, Mellemkjaer L, Tracey E, Andersen A, et al. Second primary malignancies in patients with male breast cancer. Br J Cancer. 2005;92(7):1288–92.

90. Auvinen A, Curtis RE, Ron E. Risk of subsequent cancer following breast cancer in men. J Natl Cancer Inst. 2002;94(17):1330–2.
91. Dong C, Hemminki K. Second primary breast cancer in men. Breast Cancer Res Treat. 2001;66(2):171–2.
92. Ferzoco RM, Ruddy KJ. Optimal delivery of male breast cancer follow-up care: improving outcomes. Breast Cancer (Dove Medical Press). 2015;7:371–9.
93. Adjuvant bisphosphonate treatment in early breast cancer: meta-analyses of individual patient data from randomised trials. Lancet. 2015;386(10001):1353–61.
94. Becker T, Lipscombe L, Narod S, Simmons C, Anderson GM, Rochon PA. Systematic review of bone health in older women treated with aromatase inhibitors for early-stage breast cancer. J Am Geriatr Soc. 2012;60(9):1761–7.
95. Hamilton EJ, Ghasem-Zadeh A, Gianatti E, Lim-Joon D, Bolton D, Zebaze R, et al. Structural decay of bone microarchitecture in men with prostate cancer treated with androgen deprivation therapy. J Clin Endocrinol Metab. 2010;95(12):E456–E63.
96. Greenspan SL, Coates P, Sereika SM, Nelson JB, Trump DL, Resnick NM. Bone loss after initiation of androgen deprivation therapy in patients with prostate cancer. J Clin Endocrinol Metab. 2005;90(12):6410–7.
97. Morote J, Orsola A, Abascal JM, Planas J, Trilla E, Raventos CX, et al. Bone mineral density changes in patients with prostate cancer during the first 2 years of androgen suppression. J Urol. 2006;175(5):1679–83.
98. Sturgeon KM, Deng L, Bluethmann SM, Zhou S, Trifiletti DM, Jiang C, et al. A population-based study of cardiovascular disease mortality risk in US cancer patients. Eur Heart J. 2019;40(48):3889–97.

Index

G. G. Kimmick et al. (eds.), *Common Issues in Breast Cancer Survivors*,
https://doi.org/10.1007/978-3-030-75377-1

GPSR Compliance

The European Union's (EU) General Product Safety Regulation (GPSR) is a set of rules that requires consumer products to be safe and our obligations to ensure this.

If you have any concerns about our products, you can contact us on ProductSafety@springernature.com

In case Publisher is established outside the EU, the EU authorized representative is:

Springer Nature Customer Service Center GmbH
Europaplatz 3
69115 Heidelberg, Germany

Batch number: 10731395

Printed by Printforce, the Netherlands